# Neurological Complications of Cancer

# NEUROLOGICAL DISEASE AND THERAPY

*Series Editor*

WILLIAM C. KOLLER

Department of Neurology
University of Kansas Medical Center
Kansas City, Kansas


1. Handbook of Parkinson's Disease, *edited by William C. Koller*
2. Medical Therapy of Acute Stroke, *edited by Mark Fisher*
3. Familial Alzheimer's Disease: Molecular Genetics and Clinical Perspectives, *edited by Gary D. Miner, Ralph W. Richter, John P. Blass, Jimmie L. Valentine, and Linda A. Winters-Miner*
4. Alzheimer's Disease: Treatment and Long-Term Management, *edited by Jeffrey L. Cummings and Bruce L. Miller*
5. Therapy of Parkinson's Disease, *edited by William C. Koller and George Paulson*
6. Handbook of Sleep Disorders, *edited by Michael J. Thorpy*
7. Epilepsy and Sudden Death, *edited by Claire M. Lathers and Paul L. Schraeder*
8. Handbook of Multiple Sclerosis, *edited by Stuart D. Cook*
9. Memory Disorders: Research and Clinical Practice, *edited by Takehiko Yanagihara and Ronald C. Petersen*
10. The Medical Treatment of Epilepsy, *edited by Stanley R. Resor, Jr., and Henn Kutt*
11. Cognitive Disorders: Pathophysiology and Treatment, *edited by Leon J. Thal, Walter H. Moos, and Elkan R. Gamzu*
12. Handbook of Amyotrophic Lateral Sclerosis, *edited by Richard Alan Smith*
13. Handbook of Parkinson's Disease: Second Edition, Revised and Expanded, *edited by William C. Koller*
14. Handbook of Pediatric Epilepsy, *edited by Jerome V. Murphy and Fereydoun Dehkharghani*
15. Handbook of Tourette's Syndrome and Related Tic and Behavioral Disorders, *edited by Roger Kurlan*
16. Handbook of Cerebellar Diseases, *edited by Richard Lechtenberg*
17. Handbook of Cerebrovascular Diseases, *edited by Harold P. Adams, Jr.*
18. Parkinsonian Syndromes, *edited by Matthew B. Stern and William C. Koller*
19. Handbook of Head and Spine Trauma, *edited by Jonathan Greenberg*
20. Brain Tumors: A Comprehensive Text, *edited by Robert A. Morantz and John W. Walsh*

21. Monoamine Oxidase Inhibitors in Neurological Diseases, *edited by Abraham Lieberman, C. Warren Olanow, Moussa B. H. Youdim, and Keith Tipton*
22. Handbook of Dementing Illnesses, *edited by John C. Morris*
23. Handbook of Myasthenia Gravis and Myasthenic Syndromes, *edited by Robert P. Lisak*
24. Handbook of Neurorehabilitation, *edited by David C. Good and James R. Couch, Jr.*
25. Therapy with Botulinum Toxin, *edited by Joseph Jankovic and Mark Hallett*
26. Principles of Neurotoxicology, *edited by Louis W. Chang*
27. Handbook of Neurovirology, *edited by Robert R. McKendall and William G. Stroop*
28. Handbook of Neuro-Urology, *edited by David N. Rushton*
29. Handbook of Neuroepidemiology, *edited by Philip B. Gorelick and Milton Alter*
30. Handbook of Tremor Disorders, *edited by Leslie J. Findley and William C. Koller*
31. Neuro-Ophthalmological Disorders: Diagnostic Work-Up and Management, *edited by Ronald J. Tusa and Steven A. Newman*
32. Handbook of Olfaction and Gustation, *edited by Richard L. Doty*
33. Handbook of Neurological Speech and Language Disorders, *edited by Howard S. Kirshner*
34. Therapy of Parkinson's Disease: Second Edition, Revised and Expanded, *edited by William C. Koller and George Paulson*
35. Evaluation and Management of Gait Disorders, *edited by Barney S. Spivack*
36. Handbook of Neurotoxicology, *edited by Louis W. Chang and Robert S. Dyer*
37. Neurological Complications of Cancer, *edited by Ronald G. Wiley*
38. Handbook of Autonomic Nervous System Dysfunction, *edited by Amos D. Korczyn*

*Additional Volumes in Preparation*

Handbook of Dystonia, *edited by Joseph K. C. Tsui and Donald B. Calne*

Etiology of Parkinson's Disease, *edited by Jonas H. Ellenberg, William C. Koller, and J. William Langston*

# Neurological Complications of Cancer

edited by

Ronald G. Wiley
*Vanderbilt University Medical Center and
Veterans Affairs Medical Center
Nashville, Tennessee*

Marcel Dekker, Inc.　　　New York•Basel•Hong Kong

**Library of Congress Cataloging-in-Publication Data**

Neurological complications of cancer / edited by Ronald G. Wiley.
    p. cm. — (Neurological disease and therapy ; 37)
    Includes bibliographical references and index.
    ISBN 0-8247-8840-0 (hard cover : alk. paper)
    1. Nervous system—Diseases. 2. Cancer—Complications.
3. Cancer—Treatment—Complications. 4. Metastasis. 5. Nervous system—Cancer. I. Wiley, Ronald G. II. Series: Neurological disease and therapy ; v. 37.
    [DNLM: 1. Neoplasms—complications. 2. Neoplasms—therapy.
3. Nervous System Diseases—etiology. 4. Neurological Manifestations.
5. Therapeutics—adverse effects. W1 NE33LD v. 37 1995 / QZ 200
N494 1995]
RC346.N424   1995
616.8'047—dc20
DNLM/DLC
for Library of Congress                                         94-41748
                                                                                                                        CIP

The publisher offers discounts on this book when ordered in bulk quantities. For more information, write to Special Sales/Professional Marketing at the address below.

This book is printed on acid-free paper.

Copyright © 1995 by Marcel Dekker, Inc. All Rights Reserved.

Neither this book nor any part may be reproduced or transmitted in any form or by any means, electronic or mechanical, including photocopying, microfilming, and recording, or by any information storage and retrieval system, without permission in writing from the publisher.

Marcel Dekker, Inc.
270 Madison Avenue, New York, New York 10016

Current printing (last digit):
10  9  8  7  6  5  4  3  2  1

PRINTED IN THE UNITED STATES OF AMERICA

# Series Introduction

*Neurological Complications of Cancer* by Dr. Ronald G. Wiley is the 37th book in the Neurological Disease and Therapy series. This series has covered many neurological topics, including Parkinson's disease, stroke, Alzheimer's disease, sleep disorders, many aspects of epilepsy, multiple sclerosis, tics and Tourette's syndrome, cerebellar diseases, trauma of the head and spine, brain tumors, and myasthenia gravis. The series has also addressed many therapeutic issues— including the use of monoamine oxidase inhibitors and the use of botulinum toxin—and has concentrated on general disease topics, such as neurotoxicology, neurovirology, neuroepidemiology, neurorehabilitation, and tremor disorders. The goal of the series is to provide comprehensive books on topics that are important to the clinical neurologist, covering both the basic neurological aspects as well as practical clinical information for everyday management of patients. It is hoped that these books represent important reference texts in which the clinician can quickly find pertinent information for use in managing patients. Future books in the series will concentrate on emerging knowledge in neurology and how it is being translated into the care of patients in the clinic.

*Neurological Complications of Cancer* addresses many aspects of the relationship between cancer and the nervous system. Neurologists commonly see patients either for the diagnosis of cancer as it affects the nervous system or for the complications of cancer and its treatment. Many clinicians are faced with the challenge of diagnosis and treatment of cancer as it relates to the nervous system on a daily basis. There have been many advances in the area of neuro-oncology, which is now a specific subspecialty in neurology.

The book is divided into three parts. Part I relates to specific management problems of cancer of the nervous system including metastases, direct involvement, and primary tumors of the nervous system. Part II addresses neurological complications of anticancer therapy, including radiotherapy and chemotherapy. Part III addresses neurological complications of specific neoplasms and is composed of 11 chapters that address cancers and neurological complications of specific tumors in anatomical regions.

In keeping with this series, this book provides practical and in-depth clinical information. It is hoped that clinicians will use *Neurological Complications of Cancer* as a frequent reference source as they attempt to solve the challenging issues related to cancer and the nervous system.

*William C. Koller, M.D., Ph.D.*

# Foreword

This book marks the emergence of neuro-oncology as a clinically relevant and important neurological discipline. Although neurosurgeons have been interested in and dealt with metastatic brain and spinal tumors for most of this century, and radiation oncologists began treating metastatic brain tumors in the 1950s, neurologists historically have restricted their interests to the much rarer paraneoplastic syndromes. In recent years that has changed. European neurologists have organized a new interdisciplinary association, "The European Association for Neuro-Oncology," which held its first international meeting in Maastricht, The Netherlands, in October 1994. The organization brings together neurologists, neurosurgeons, radiation oncologists, and medical oncologists to share knowledge and experience. The American Academy of Neurology now has a section on neuro-oncology and special sessions on neuro-oncology are held at the annual meetings of the American Neurological Association and the Academy of Neurology.

It is entirely appropriate that neurologists play a leadership role in the development of this new discipline. Unlike their colleagues in neurosurgery and radiation oncology, they do not offer a specific therapeutic technique and, unlike their colleagues in medical oncology, they better understand nervous system function and how cancer affecting it differs from cancer affecting other organs of the body. Because they have this unique perspective, they can serve as a focal point and coordinator in the diagnosis and management of all neuro-oncological problems.

Among the most important problems that the neuro-oncologist faces are neurological complications of cancer. As many as 15% of the one million people in the United States who each year develop cancer suffer a neurological complication at some time during the course of their illness. Because of the devastating effects of nervous system dysfunction on the quality of an individual's life, and because even with our limited tools we can often ameliorate or even reverse neurological symptoms, early diagnosis and appropriate vigorous management are essential. It is this aspect of neuro-oncology, the effects of cancer on the nervous system, both metastatic and nonmetastatic, that this book addresses. The first part details the current diagnostic approach and management of each of the important neurological complications of cancer. The second part describes the common neurological complications associated with several specific cancers. Thus the book is valuable not only to the general neurologist dealing with a neurological problem in a patient with cancer, but to the oncologist caring for a patient with a specific cancer who develops a neurological problem.

This book can serve both as a clinical guide to neurologists and oncologists caring for patients with neurological complications of cancer and, hopefully, also as an inducement for young physicians to become interested in the discipline. Since this book is written by 30 experts, most of whom are clinical neurologists drawn from 20 different institutions, it gives the reader a broad view of the current practice of neuro-oncology throughout the developed world. It is with particular pride that I note that 23 of the 30 authors did some of their training at Memorial Sloan-Kettering Cancer Center. One role of a specific disease-oriented institution such as Memorial Sloan-Kettering is to train physicians who can then disseminate their knowledge to less specialized institutions. This book indicates that we are fulfilling that role.

*Jerome Posner, M.D.*
*George C. Cotzias Chair in Neuro-Oncology*
*Chairman, Department of Neurology*
*Memorial Sloan-Kettering Cancer Center*
*New York, New York*

# Preface

As diagnosis and treatment of neoplastic diseases have improved, neurological complications of cancer have become increasingly important. Nervous system involvement, either from tumor invasion or from side effects of therapies, can compromise quality and duration of survival. Intelligent, compassionate management of neurological complications can improve quality of life for many, and survival for some cancer patients. The goal of *Neurological Complications of Cancer* is to provide a practically useful reference source for all professionals treating cancer patients and an introduction to clinical trainees.

Understanding of the spectrum of neurological complications of cancer and cancer treatments has advanced rapidly over the past two decades. However, with only one journal specifically dedicated to neuro-oncology, keeping up with these advances requires mastery of a diffuse literature. In this text a wide range of experts have organized and critically presented the current state of knowledge in their fields. Both clinicians taking care of cancer patients and trainees can benefit from the concise presentation of pertinent information in this book. An effort has been made to focus on the key elements of diagnosis and current treatment options. Summary tables organized in parallel with the text have been included to provide rapid access to specific information. References have been chosen with care for key elements of the original data.

Part I, "Specific Management Problems," offers an overview of the most important types of neurological complications. Emphasis in these chapters is on shared clinical manifestations and responses to treatment. Part II, "Neurological Complications of Anticancer Therapy," provides similar information concerning neurological complications of cancer treatments that are common to most patients receiving a particular treatment modality. Part III, "Neurological Complications of Specific Neoplasms," focuses on the neurological complications most often seen with individual neoplasms and any peculiarities of presentation or response to treatment. Emphasis in these chapters is on features unique to a particular primary tissue type. Thus, diagnostic and management information can be found readily on general problems such as brain metastases or complications of chemotherapy, as well as on the particular types of complications most common with a given primary cancer.

Although nihilism often influences management decisions when neurological complications occur in cancer patients, significant palliation is frequently available. In many cases, prompt diagnosis of a neurological complication can shorten the duration of uncontrolled symptoms, improve prognosis, and minimize expense. Patients, relatives, and health care providers benefit from speedy diagnosis, appropriate choice of therapies, and accurate expectations of outcome. This text addresses all of these issues.

Over the past 25 years, the field of neuro-oncology has become a recognized area of clinical specialization. This development owes much to the skill and efforts of Jerome B. Posner, M.D., head of neurology at Memorial Sloan-Kettering Cancer Center. Each chapter of this book is coauthored by a practicing clinician who trained with Dr. Posner, and many of the contributors have made significant contributions of their own to the field of neuro-oncology. We all hope that *Neurological Complications of Cancer* will prove useful to those caring for cancer patients and will be a fitting tribute to Dr. Posner.

*Ronald G. Wiley*

# Contents

Series Introduction (William C. Koller)     *iii*
Foreword (Jerome Posner)     *v*
Preface     *vii*
Contributors     *xiii*

Part I    **Specific Management Problems**

1. Management of Brain Metastases     1
   *Ross S. Goodheart and Roy A. Patchell*

2. Spinal Metastases     23
   *Thomas N. Byrne*

3. Leptomeningeal Metastases     45
   *William R. Wasserstrom*

4. Peripheral Nervous System Complications in Cancer Patients     73
   *Paul L. Moots*

5. Neurological Complications of Malignant Brain Tumors     103
   *Eugenie A.M.T. Obbens and William R. Shapiro*

| | | |
|---|---|---|
| 6 | Cerebrovascular Complications of Cancer<br>*Lisa R. Rogers* | 123 |
| 7 | Nervous System Infections<br>*Neil E. Anderson and Mark G. Thomas* | 145 |
| 8 | Management of Paraneoplastic Neurological Syndromes<br>*Francesc Graus and Josep O. Dalmau* | 167 |
| 9 | Use of Glucocorticoids in Neuro-Oncology<br>*Charles J. Vecht and H.B.C. Verbiest* | 199 |

## Part II  Neurological Complications of Anticancer Therapy

| | | |
|---|---|---|
| 10 | Neurological Complications of Radiotherapy<br>*Mark T. Jennings* | 219 |
| 11 | Neurological Complications of Chemotherapy<br>*Peter A.J. Forsyth and Terrence L. Cascino* | 241 |
| 12 | Neurological Complications of Immunotherapy<br>*Jean-Yves Delattre, Felipe Vega B, and Qiming Chen* | 267 |

## Part III  Neurological Complications of Specific Neoplasms

| | | |
|---|---|---|
| 13 | Neurological Complications of Lung Cancer<br>*Karl E. Misulis and Ronald G. Wiley* | 295 |
| 14 | Neurological Complications of Breast Cancer<br>*Neil E. Anderson* | 311 |
| 15 | Neurological Complications of Malignant Melanoma and Other Cutaneous Malignancies<br>*John W. Henson* | 333 |
| 16 | Neurological Disorders in Head and Neck Cancers<br>*Paul L. Moots and Ronald G. Wiley* | 353 |
| 17 | Neurological Complications of Genitourinary Cancer<br>*Camilo E. Fadul* | 373 |
| 18 | Neurological Complications of Gastrointestinal Cancers<br>*Neil A. Hagen* | 395 |
| 19 | Neurological Complications of Sarcomas<br>*Patricia T. Molloy and Peter C. Phillips* | 417 |

**Contents**

| | | |
|---|---|---|
| 20 | Neurological Complications of Leukemia<br>*Lynne P. Taylor* | 449 |
| 21 | Neurological Complications of Lymphoma<br>*Lawrence D. Recht* | 465 |
| 22 | Neurological Complications of Plasma Cell Dyscrasias<br>*J. Peter Glass* | 489 |
| 23 | Neurological Complications of Childhood Cancer<br>*Mark T. Jennings* | 503 |

*Index*     *535*

# Contributors

**Neil E. Anderson, M.B., Ch.B., F.R.A.C.P.** Department of Neurology, Auckland Hospital, Auckland, New Zealand

**Thomas N. Byrne, M.D.** Clincal Professor, Yale University School of Medicine, New Haven, Connecticut

**Terrence L. Cascino, M.D.** Associate Professor, Department of Neurology, Mayo Clinic, Rochester, Minnesota

**Qiming Chen** Groupe Hospitalier Pitié-Salpêtrière, Paris, France

**Josep O. Dalmau, M.D., Ph.D.** Clinical Assistant, Department of Neurology, Memorial Sloan-Kettering Cancer Center, New York, New York

**Jean-Yves Delattre** Groupe Hospitalier Pitié-Salpêtrière, Paris, France

**Camilo E. Fadul, M.D.** Assistant Professor, Department of Neurology, Dartmouth-Hitchcock Medical Center, Lebanon, New Hampshire

**Peter A.J. Forsyth, M.D., F.R.C.P.C.** Assistant Professor, Department of Clinical Neurosciences, University of Calgary, Tom Baker Cancer Centre, Calgary, Alberta, Canda

**Ross S. Goodheart, M.D., F.R.A.C.P.** Department of Neurology, University of Kentucky Medical Center, Lexington, Kentucky

**J. Peter Glass, M.D.** Associate Professor, Department of Medicine (Neurology), Duke University Medical Center, Durham, North Carolina

**Francesc Graus, M.D.** Assistant Professor, Department of Neurology, University of Barcelona, Barcelona, Spain

**Neil A. Hagen, M.D., F.R.C.P.C.** Assistant Professor, Department of Clinical Neurosciences, University of Calgary, Tom Baker Cancer Centre, Alberta, Canada

**John W. Henson, M.D.** Assistant Professor, Molecular Neuro-Oncology Laboratory, Massachusetts General Hospital and Harvard Medical School, Boston, Massachusetts

**Mark T. Jennings, M.D.** Assistant Professor, Department of Neurology, Vanderbilt University School of Medicine, Nashville, Tennessee

**Karl E. Misulis, M.D.** Vanderbilt University Medical Center, Nashville, and Semmes-Murphey Clinic, Jackson, Tennessee

**Patricia T. Molloy, M.D.** Assistant Professor, Department of Neurology, University of Pennsylvania Medical School, and Children's Hospital of Philadelphia, Philadelphia, Pennsylvania

**Paul L. Moots, M.D.** Assistant Professor, Division of Neuro-Oncology, Department of Neurology, Vanderbilt University Medical Center, Nashville, Tennessee

**Eugenie A.M.T. Obbens, M.D., Ph.D.** Division of Neurology, Barrow Neurological Institute, Phoenix, Arizona

**Roy A. Patchell, M.D.** Chief of Neuro-Oncology, Department of Neurosurgery and Neurology, University of Kentucky Medical Center, Lexington, Kentucky

**Peter C. Phillips, M.D.** Assistant Professor, Divisions of Neurology and Oncology; Director, Pediatric Neuro-Oncology Program, The Children's Hospital of Philadelphia, Philadelphia, Pennsylvania

## Contributors

**Lawrence D. Recht, M.D.** Associate Professor, Department of Neurology, University of Massachusetts Medical Center, Worcester, Massachusetts

**Lisa R. Rogers, D.O.** Associate Professor, Department of Neurology, Wayne State University School of Medicine, Detroit, Michigan

**William R. Shapiro, M.D.** Chairman, Division of Neurology, Barrow Neurological Institute, Phoenix, Arizona

**Lynne P. Taylor, M.D.** Virginia Mason Clinic; Clinical Assistant Professor, Department of Neurology, University of Washington; and Consulting Neurologist, Fred Hutchinson Bone Marrow Transplant Center, Seattle, Washington

**Mark G. Thomas, M.B., Ch.B., F.R.A.C.P.** Department of Infectious Disease, Auckland Hospital, Auckland, New Zealand

**Charles J. Vecht, M.D., Ph.D.** Head, Department of Neuro-Oncology, Daniel den Hoed Cancer Center, Rotterdam, The Netherlands

**Felipe Vega B** Groupe Hospitalier Pitié-Salpêtrière, Paris, France

**H.B.C. Verbiest, M.D.** Department of Neurology, I.C. Hospital the Baronie, Breda, The Netherlands

**William R. Wasserstrom, M.D.** Associate Clinical Professor, Department of Neurology, Robert Wood Johnson Medical School, New Brunswick, New Jersey

**Ronald G. Wiley, M.D., Ph.D.** Professor, Department of Neurology and Pharmacology, Vanderbilt University Medical Center and Veterans Affairs Medical Center, Nashville, Tennessee

# 1
# Management of Brain Metastases

### Ross S. Goodheart and Roy A. Patchell
*University of Kentucky Medical Center, Lexington, Kentucky*

## I. INCIDENCE

Brain metastases are tumors that originate in tissues outside the brain and then secondarily spread to involve the brain. Metastases to the brain are the most common structural neurological complication of systemic cancer and second only to metabolic encephalopathies as a cause of central nervous system dysfunction in cancer patients. The incidence of brain metastases is estimated to be 13,000 cases per year in the United States (1). Parenchymal brain metastases occur most frequently in lung cancer, breast cancer, and melanoma. (See Table 1.)

The exact incidence of brain metastases is difficult to determine. Older estimates, based on historical neurosurgical series, claimed that brain metastases constituted only about 10% of all intracranial tumors (5). With modern neuroimaging techniques and more careful autopsy studies, it is now known that metastases to the brain are actually the most common intracranial tumors and slightly outnumber primary brain tumors (1). The incidence of brain metastases in cancer patients is currently estimated to be 20–40% (3,6,7). Certain subgroups of patients are particularly at risk. For example, a recent study found the cumulative incidence of brain metastases to be 60–80% in patients with squamous cell carcinoma of the lung who survive 2 years or more (8). The percentage of patients with brain metastases may be discovered to be even larger in the future because of the improving ability to detect small tumors with magnetic resonance imaging

**Table 1** Primary Sites of Metastatic Tumors to Brain Parenchyma

| | Takakura et al. (2) | | Delattre et al. (3) | | Zimm et al. (4) | |
|---|---|---|---|---|---|---|
| | Patients (No.) | Relative frequency (%) | Patients (No.) | Relative frequency (%) | Patients (No.) | Relative frequency (%) |
| Primary site | | | | | | |
| Lung | 266 | 48 | 144 | 50 | 122 | 64 |
| Breast | 111 | 20 | 43 | 15 | 26 | 14 |
| Melanoma | 34 | 6 | 30 | 10 | 8 | 4 |
| Pelvis/abdomen | — | — | 27 | 9 | — | — |
|   Gastrointestinal | 43 | 8 | — | — | 6 | 3 |
|   Liver/pancreas | 14 | 3 | — | — | — | — |
|   Urinary tract | 34 | 6 | — | — | 4 | 2 |
|   Prostate | 10 | 2 | — | — | — | — |
| Unknown | — | — | 32 | 11 | 16 | 8 |
| Other sites | 43 | 8 | 12 | 4 | 9 | 5 |
| Total | 555 | 100 | 288 | 100 | 191 | 100 |

(MRI). The prevalence of brain metastases also may be rising due to the longer survival of cancer patients in general.

## II. METHOD OF SPREAD AND DISTRIBUTION

Most tumor cells reach the brain by hematogenous spread, usually through the arterial circulation. Commonly, the metastasis originates in the lung from either a primary lung cancer or from a pulmonary secondary deposit. A small proportion of tumor cells may reach the brain via the vertebral venous system. Batson suggested that this plexus provided a pathway for pelvic and retro-peritoneal cancers to spread to the spine and proximally to the intracranial space (9). He noted a large proportion of posterior fossa metastases with such tumors, often without other evidence of systemic spread.

However, studies have not supported this theory. Delattre et al. (3) did not find an increased incidence of skull and spinal lesions in patients with abdominal or pelvic primary tumors, nor did they find a corresponding decrease in the incidence of pulmonary metastases. The "fertile soil" hypothesis suggests that certain tissues (in this case, brain) have characteristics that support the growth of metastases that are lacking in other organs (3,6). This has been proposed to explain the observed distribution of metastases.

Studies using computed tomography (CT) scan data indicate that metastases to

**Table 2** Metastatic Tumors to Brain Parenchyma (Patients 0–15 Years Old)

| | Vanucci and Batten (10) | | | Graus et al. (11) | | |
|---|---|---|---|---|---|---|
| | Patients with tumor (No.) | Patients with brain metastases (No.) | Percentage with brain metastases | Patients with tumor (No.) | Patients with brain metastases (No.) | Percentage with brain metastases |
| Primary site | | | | | | |
| Neuroblastoma | 37 | 0 | 0 | 75 | 2 | 2.7 |
| Osteogenic sarcoma | 28 | 4 | 14.3 | 12 | 1 | 8.3 |
| Rhabdomyosarcoma | 15 | 2 | 13.3 | 45 | 3 | 6.6 |
| Ewing's sarcoma | 6 | 0 | 0 | 15 | 0 | 0 |
| Wilm's tumor | 5 | 0 | 0 | 31 | 4 | 12.9 |
| Other | 14 | 3[a] | 21.6 | 39 | 3[b] | 7.6 |
| Total | 105 | 9 | 8.5 | 217 | 13 | 6.0 |

[a]Hepatocellular carcinoma, 1; malignant melanoma, 1; ovarian carcinoma, 1
[b]Malignant melanoma, 1; malignant schwannoma, 1; angiosarcoma, 1

the brain are single in slightly less than 50% of cases (3). There are more than five lesions in over 10% of cases (3). Magnetic resonance imaging is more sensitive than CT in the detection of small metastases, and it is likely that when quantitative MRI data become available, the proportion of multiple metastases will be higher.

The phrase *single brain metastasis* refers to those patients with an apparent single cerebral lesion and makes no implication about the extent of cancer elsewhere in the body. *Solitary brain metastasis* is used to describe the uncommon patient who has a single brain metastasis that represents the only known metastasis in the body. Metastases from colon, breast, and renal cell carcinoma are often single, whereas malignant melanoma and lung cancer have a greater tendency to produce multiple cerebral lesions (3).

Cerebral metastatic disease in children, although well recognized, has not been the subject of intensive study. The reported incidence of brain metastases in children with solid tumors is less than the 20–40% reported in adults. Two retrospective pediatric studies estimated the incidence to be 6–10% (10,11). (See Table 2.) The most common childhood solid tumors (other than primary brain tumors) are neuroblastomas and a variety of sarcomas including embryonal rhabdomyosarcoma, Wilm's tumor, Ewing's sarcoma, and osteogenic sarcoma. In patients older than 15 years, germ cell tumors have the highest incidence (11). Neuroblastomas appear to have a very low incidence of cerebral metastases. This is possibly related to the rarity of pulmonary hematogenous spread. Incidence of brain parenchymal involvement in patients with Wilm's tumor decreased between the two reports (1951–72 and 1973–82). The decrement may be the result of more effective systemic chemotherapy for this tumor.

The clinical presentation and neurological manifestations in children with cerebral metastases are similar to those seen in adults. Approach to treatment and response is also comparable: although sarcomas are radioresistant, germ cell tumors respond well to both radiation therapy and chemotherapy.

## III. CLINICAL PRESENTATION

Metastases to the brain are usually symptomatic, and more than two-thirds of patients with brain metastases have some neurological symptoms during the course of their illness (6). The clinical presentation of brain metastases is similar to that of other mass lesions in the brain. (See Tables 3 and 4.) Headache is a common presenting symptom, and this may be followed after an interval of days or weeks by other focal symptoms or signs. The headache may be mild and is rarely of localizing value. Early morning headache (usually thought to be associated with raised intracranial pressure) is a presenting symptom in only 40% of patients with brain metastases who describe headache as a presenting symptom (6).

Headaches are more common with multiple metastases or with single lesions in the posterior fossa. Raised intracranial pressure (and the accompanying headache)

**Table 3** Presenting Symptoms of Brain Metastases

| | Percentage with symptoms[a] | | |
|---|---|---|---|
| Symptom | Posner (12) (162 patients) | Cairncross et al. (6) (201 patients) | Zimm et al. (4) (191 patients) |
| Headache | 53 | 45 | 38 |
| Focal weakness | 40 | 21 | 34 |
| Behavioral or mental change | 31 | 33 | 29 |
| Seizures | 15 | 20 | 21 |
| Gait ataxia | 20 | 22 | 11 |
| Speech disturbance | 10 | 14 | 6 |
| Visual disturbance | — | 11 | 6 |
| Limb ataxia | — | 10 | — |
| Sensory disturbance | — | 10 | 2 |

[a]Some patients with more than one symptom at presentation.

is associated with the clinical sign of papilledema. However, with modern neuroimaging techniques, the reported incidence of papilledema in patients presenting with brain metastases is less than 25%.

Seizures are the presenting event in approximately 10% of patients with brain metastases and are more common in patients with multiple metastases (13). Occasionally the seizure will be focal, and this has hemispheric localizing value. Abnormalities of higher mental functions are very common as presenting symp-

**Table 4** Presenting Signs of Brain Metastases

| | Percentage with signs[a] | | |
|---|---|---|---|
| Sign | Posner (12) (162 patients) | Cairncross et al. (6) (201 patients) | Zimm et al. (4) (191 patients) |
| Altered mental state | 77 | 42 | 29 |
| Hemiparesis | 66 | 54 | 34 |
| Hemisensory loss | 27 | 16 | 2 |
| Papilledema | 26 | 15 | 3 |
| Gait ataxia | 24 | 14 | 11 |
| Aphasia | 19 | 17 | — |
| Visual field alteration | — | 13 | — |
| Limb ataxia | — | 10 | — |
| Coma/stupor | — | — | 10 |

[a]Some patients with more than one sign at presentation.

toms and may take the form of a completely nonfocal encephalopathy (1–2% of patients with metastases) or may relate to localized dysfunction (e.g., aphasia). Focal weakness is second in frequency only to headache as a presenting symptom. Although such weakness accurately reflects contralateral hemispheric involvement, the lesion is often located away from the motor area of the cortex.

Five to ten percent of patients present with acute neurological symptoms caused by hemorrhage into the tumor or cerebral infarction from embolic or compressive occlusion of a blood vessel (6). Hemorrhage into a metastasis is particularly common with choriocarcinoma and melanoma (14). An unusual presentation of brain metastasis is episodic loss of function suggestive of transient ischemic attack. Such symptoms may be manifestations of focal seizures that go unrecognized by the patient (15). However, the signs and symptoms of cerebral metastases are varied and *brain metastases should be suspected in all patients with known systemic cancer in whom new neurological findings develop*.

## IV. DIAGNOSIS

The best diagnostic tests for brain metastases are contrast-enhanced magnetic resonance imaging (MRI) and computed tomography (CT). If the clinical history is typical and lesions are multiple, there is usually little doubt surrounding the diagnosis. However, it is important to distinguish metastases from primary brain tumors (benign or malignant), abscesses, and cerebral infarcts and hemorrhages. Table 5 gives a listing of the most important considerations in the differential diagnosis of brain metastases. It is equally important to identify those patients with single metastases whose management may be different.

Contrast-enhanced MRI has been shown to be more sensitive than enhanced CT scanning (including double-dose delayed contrast) or unenhanced magnetic resonance imaging in detecting lesions in patients suspected of intracranial metastases (16,17). In both scanning methods, multiple lesions often distinguish metastases from glioma or other primary tumors. Other imaging findings that favor metastases include a gray/white junction location, a lesser degree of margin irregularity, and a small tumor nidus with a large amount of associated vasogenic edema (18). (See Fig. 1.)

T2-weighted sequences in MRI are quite sensitive in demonstrating the vasogenic edema as areas of increased signal intensity, but not all metastatic lesions have sufficient edema to be identified (19). Such cryptic lesions are typically less than 5 mm in diameter. However, a recent study has shown that the false-positive rate—even when using contrast MRI for the diagnosis of single brain metastases—is about 11% (20). Other diagnostic tests, such as arteriography or biopsy, may be needed to establish the diagnosis firmly.

Cranial imaging studies also are important in the monitoring of tumor develop-

**Table 5** Differential Diagnosis of Brain Metastases with Some Distinguishing Clinical and Imaging Features[a]

| | Clinical | Imaging |
|---|---|---|
| Brain metastases | Known primary. Systemic metastases present (especially lung). Constitutional symptoms (e.g., weight loss). | May show multiple lesions. Contrast enhancement. Gray/white junction location. Relative margin regularity. |
| Primary neoplasm Glial series | No known primary. | Single lesion. Contrast enhancement. Margin may be irregular. |
| Meningioma | Symptoms over months/years. | May be calcified. Often in relation to dura, falx, or tentorium. |
| Infections (particularly abscess formation) Bacteria | Fever. Unwell. May have history of chronic ear, sinus, or pulmonary infections. | Contrast-enhanced ring. May be multiple. |
| Other organisms (particularly toxoplasmosis) | May be immunosuppressed. | May see response to treatment with subsequent scanning. |
| Cerebrovascular disorders Hemorrhage or infarction | Abrupt or stuttering onset of symptoms. | Changing image over days reflecting change in water content of tissue. Infarction or resolving hematoma may be encapsulated. |
| Radiation necrosis | History of cranial radiotherapy. Subacute/chronic onset. | May contrast enhance. |

[a] Partial listing of differential diagnosis only. The clinical and imaging findings listed may not be present in some cases.

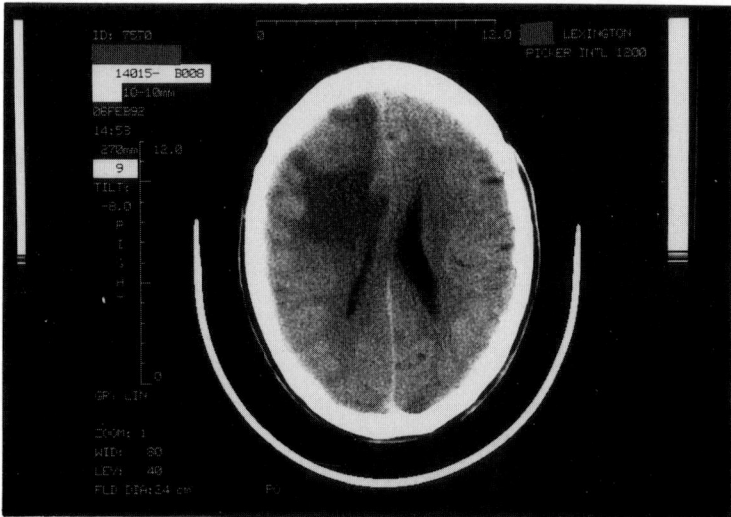

**(A)**

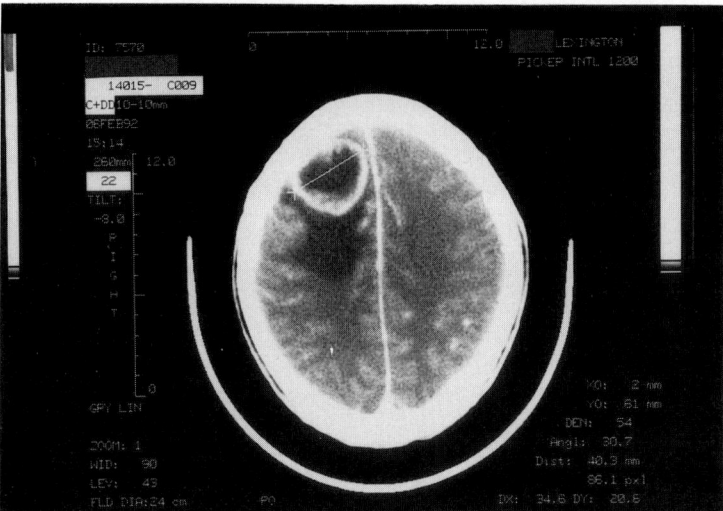

**(B)**

**Figure 1** Four images of a single cortical metastasis from a bronchogenic carcinoma in a 65-year-old man. (Imaging planes differ between CT and MRI.) (A) Noncontrast CT showing surrounding edema, ventricular compression, and midline shift. (B) Administration of contrast results in marked enhancement of the lesion. (C) Postcontrast T1-weighted MR image showing the regularity of the tumor nidus. (D) T2-weighted MR image better illustrated the extent of the surrounding edema.

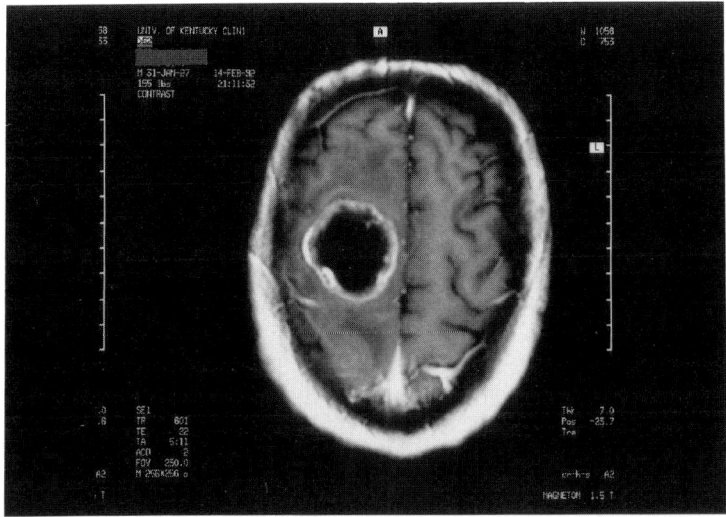

(C)

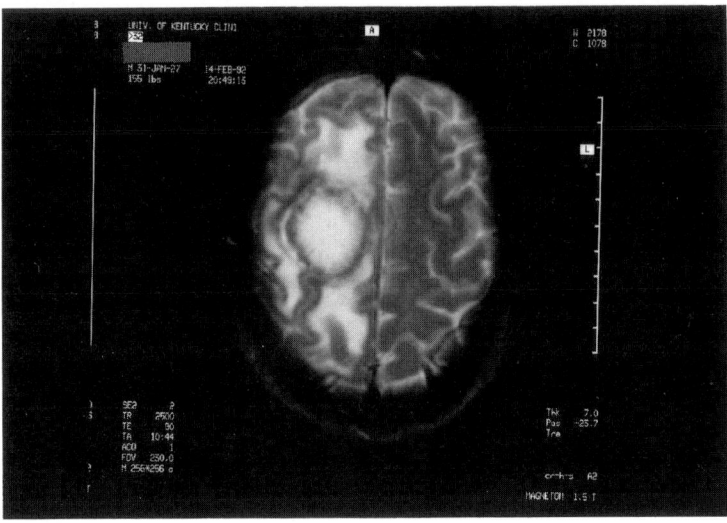

(D)

ment, progression, response to treatment, and the development of associated complications such as bleeding or postradiotherapy changes.

The question often arises as to how far to pursue the search for a primary systemic cancer in a patient with a brain mass demonstrated on a CT or MRI scan and no previous history of cancer. Most metastases reach the brain by hematogenous spread through the arterial circulation. Therefore, the lung is an important source of brain metastases. If the primary tumor is not pulmonary, it has probably spread to the lung before seeding into the arterial circulation and reaching the brain. More than 60% of patients with brain metastases will have a mass demonstrated on chest radiograph that is caused by either a primary lung cancer or a lung metastasis from the primary located elsewhere (21). Therefore, careful radiographic examination of the chest is the most important diagnostic test in patients with suspected brain metastases. When the chest radiograph fails to demonstrate a lesion, CT or MRI of the lung may reveal lesions and suggest the cause of the neurological disorder. Further search for a primary tumor is almost never fruitful, especially if there are no positive findings on physical examination and no features of the history suggesting a specific primary tumor. In the few patients with brain metastases but not identifiable lesions in the lung, the pathogenesis of the brain metastases may be spread through Batson's vertebral venous plexus, tumor embolism through a patent foramen ovale (paradoxical embolus), or tumor filtered through the lungs with only local or microscopic growth.

## V. TREATMENT

### A. Newly Diagnosed Brain Metastases

Brain metastases are associated with a poor prognosis regardless of treatment. Untreated patients have a median survival of only about 4 weeks (22–24), and most die as a direct result of the brain tumor, with increasing intracranial pressure leading to obtundation and terminal cerebral herniation.

Despite more than a half century of clinical experimentation, the optimum treatment of brain metastases (whether single or multiple) remains controversial. Several methods of treatment are available for patients with intracranial metastases. Glucocorticoids, radiotherapy, and surgery all have established places in management. Chemotherapy also is useful in those patients with very chemosensitive tumors.

There are several considerations when selecting the best treatment for a patient, including the extent of systemic disease, neurological status at diagnosis, and the number and site of metastases. An approach to the management of a patient with a suspected brain metastasis is illustrated in Figure 2.

#### 1. Glucocorticoids

All patients with brain metastases should be started on corticosteroid therapy at the time of diagnosis. The mechanism of action of glucocorticoids is not completely

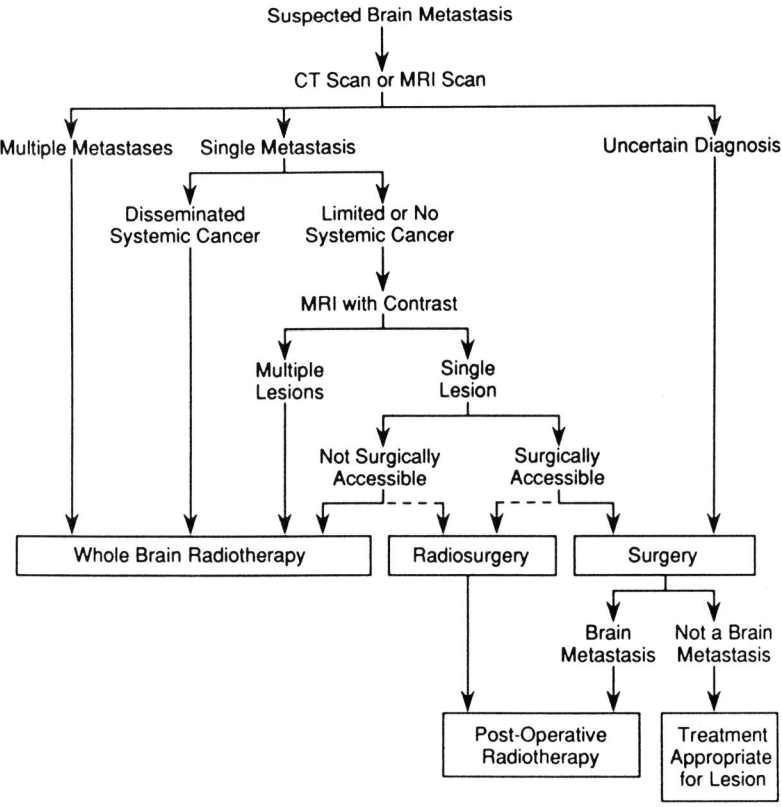

**Figure 2** An approach to the management of a patient with a suspected brain metastasis. No algorithm can apply to all patients; treatment must be individualized to each patient's circumstances. Dashed lines indicate plausible, but unproven, treatments.

understood, although a reduction in the edema surrounding the metastatic tumors is a frequent finding. Dexamethasone is preferred because it has minimal mineralocorticoid activity and a low tendency to induce psychosis (25). More than 70% of patients improve symptomatically following the administration of glucocorticoids (26). Symptoms reflecting generalized neurological dysfunction or brain edema respond more consistently to glucocorticoid treatment than do focal symptoms such as hemiparesis.

The clinical effects of glucocorticoids are noticeable within 6–24 h and maximal within 3 to 7 days (27). Glucocorticoids alone are not tumoricidal (except when used against lymphomas and some leukemias). The main use of glucocorticoids is to induce symptomatic improvement and to buy time for the delivery of more definitive antitumor therapy. The median survival of patients with brain metastases treated with glucocorticoids alone is about 2 months (22,27,28).

The usual starting dose of dexamethasone is 10 mg given intravenously (I.V.) or orally (p.o.), followed by 4 mg four times daily. Occasional patients require higher doses. With stabilization of symptoms and the completion of more definitive treatment, the dose of dexamethasone should be tapered gradually over several weeks and then stopped to minimize long-term toxicity. Some patients may not tolerate reduction in glucocorticoid dosage, redeveloping the signs and symptoms of the tumor and brain edema. In such cases, the lowest effective dose should be continued.

## 2. Radiotherapy

Radiotherapy is the treatment of choice for most patients with brain metastases. Since the initial report of the use of ionizing radiation for palliative benefit in 1954 (29), there have been a number of studies attempting to determine the optimal patient selection criteria and treatment regimens.

There is still no consensus regarding the optimum radiation dose and schedule. Most patients are treated with whole brain radiotherapy (WBRT). This is because over 50% have multiple metastases at the time of diagnosis, preventing success with localized therapy. Data on the effect of dose and schedule for the treatment of brain metastases come from several large-scale multi-institutional trials conducted by the Radiation Therapy Oncology Group (RTOG) (30–32). These studies have shown there is no significant difference in the frequency and duration of response for radiation regimens ranging from 2000 centigrays (cGy) over 1 week to 5000 cGy over 4 weeks. Regimens of 1000 cGy in a single dose, or 1200 cGy in two doses, appear to be less satisfactory and are rarely used.

Whole brain radiotherapy increases the median survival to 2 to 6 months (4,22,23,33–36). However, data from retrospective studies have shown that more than half the patients treated with whole brain radiotherapy die of progressive systemic cancer and not as a direct result of brain metastases (4,33). Further analysis of the RTOG results identified patient subgroups that were more likely to respond to whole brain radiotherapy. Favorable outcome was associated with (1) Karnofsky performance scores over 70 (37); (2) absent or controlled primary tumor; (3) patient age less than 60 years; and (4) metastatic spread limited to the brain (38) (true solitary metastasis).

Increased focal irradiation to the tumor site in the brain is not beneficial. A recent retrospective study has shown that giving a boost dose to the tumor site is no better than whole brain radiotherapy alone in preventing neurologic recurrences or increasing survival (39).

Radiation cell sensitizers have been used in an attempt to increase tumor cell death. The rationale was based on the observation the hypoxic cells (often found centrally in a tumor) are more resistant to the effects of ionizing radiation. The nitroimidazoles can enhance radiation-induced DNA damage in hypoxic cells, potentially increasing tumor cell sensitivity to irradiation. However, none of the radiation cell sensitizers has been shown to provide any additional benefit over conventional palliative radiotherapy courses (40).

Typical treatment schedules for brain metastases consist of short courses (7 to 15 days) of whole brain irradiation with 150 to 400 cGy doses per fraction (per day) to a total dose of 3000 to 5000 cGy. Such schedules minimize the duration of treatment while still delivering adequate amounts of radiation.

Radiotherapy is not without its complications (see Chap. 10). In the short term, patients may have transient worsening of symptoms while receiving therapy. Many physicians believe that maintaining patients on glucocorticoids during radiotherapy will reduce complications of radiotherapy, although there is no conclusive proof of this idea. At the beginning of treatment, symptoms such a nausea, vomiting, headache, and fever are common. This acute reaction may relate to disrupted cerebrovascular autoregulation or increased capillary permeability (41). Radiation-induced parotitis and loss of taste also occur (6).

The long-term ill effects of radiotherapy are not usually a significant issue in the treatment of patients with brain metastases due to their short survival. However, recent reports have suggested that a large percentage of long-term survivors ($>12$ months) will develop symptoms such as dementia, ataxia, and urinary incontinence (42,43). In such patients, imaging studies show cortical atrophy and hyperdense white matter changes. Although the pathogenesis of such alterations is unknown, it is speculated that they relate to high dose and large fractionation schedules. Therefore, in patients expected to survive 12 months or more, a more prolonged course of radiation with smaller doses per fraction should probably be used. A reasonable schedule for patients with a relatively good prognosis is a total dose of 4500 to 5000 cGy given in daily fractions of no more than 200 cGy.

Tumor type does not significantly affect the response of patients treated with brain radiotherapy. However, some rarer causes of brain metastases such as lymphomas and germ cell tumors are more radioresponsive. Complete resolution of abnormal cerebral imaging studies can be obtained following radiotherapy in patients with these tumors (33).

## 3. Radiosurgery

Stereotaxic radiosurgery, a method of delivering intense focal irradiation using a linear accelerator or a gamma knife, has also been used to treat metastatic brain tumors (44,45). These procedures do not replace whole brain radiotherapy but may offer a substitute for surgical therapy. To date, only a few uncontrolled series of highly preselected patients have been published (46,47). The data presented so far are sketchy, and experience with these methods is so limited that no definite conclusion can be drawn about efficacy in the treatment of brain metastases.

Prospective clinical trials are under way that may help determine the role of radiosurgery both in the primary management of patients with single metastases and in the management of recurrent brain metastases (48).

## 4. Interstitial Brachytherapy

Interstitial brachytherapy is a technique involving the placement of radioactive implants within the area of tumor. These implants allow delivery of high-dose focal radiation to the tumor while reducing the risk of significant radiation exposure to the surrounding normal brain tissue because the sources are precalculated to limit radiation exposure to the target area. Both permanent and removable implants have been in use. The sources may be placed stereotaxically or during surgery.

The major complication of brachytherapy is radiation necrosis that may present with the imaging and clinical picture of an expanding mass lesion. The interval may be some months following implantation. Such radiation necrosis may be difficult to distinguish from tumor recurrence and may require surgical resection.

As with radiosurgery, the role of brachytherapy in the primary management of brain metastases and in the management of recurrent brain metastases has yet to be determined.

## 5. Surgery

Surgical therapy is usually not an option for most patients with brain metastases because of multiple lesions or extensive systemic cancer. However, in the subgroup of patients whose only metastatic disease is in the brain, death is more likely to be due to the brain metastases than to progressive systemic disease (4). Therefore, in patients with controlled systemic cancer in whom brain metastases develop, the treatment of the brain disease is the factor that will most likely determine the length of survival. It is in this group that the question of more aggressive therapy, particularly surgery, for the brain metastases is usually raised. There have been several advances over the past 20 years that have decreased the risks associated with the surgical approach. Safer anesthesia, glucocorticoids, the development of cranial imaging technology, and the introduction of stereotaxic approaches have been foremost among these changes.

There are theoretical reasons for believing that the combination of surgical treatment followed by postoperative radiotherapy may be more effective than whole brain radiotherapy alone. Radiotherapy is most successful when used against small tumor volumes. In larger tumors, radiation is usually effective at the periphery of the tumor where cells are small in number and well oxygenated. However, in the center of the tumor, where tumor cells are more numerous and more hypoxic conditions exist, radiation may not destroy the tumor completely. Although there are documented reports of sterilization of brain metastases by radiotherapy alone (49), in most instances, residual tumor probably remains.

While surgical treatment is most successful in removing large volumes of tumor, small numbers of malignant cells may be left behind.

Rational treatment plans combining surgical debulking and radiotherapy have been developed to overcome the deficiencies of both types of treatment (50,51), and combined therapy has shown promise in patients with a variety of tumor types (52). Despite the possible advantages of surgical treatment, the actual role of surgery had been unclear until recently because of an absence of controlled trials showing benefit. Many uncontrolled surgical series had demonstrated longer survivals of surgically treated patients in comparison with historical controls managed with whole brain radiotherapy alone (7,53–55). In addition, retrospective reports of uncontrolled studies of patients treated with whole brain radiotherapy (containing small numbers of patients treated with surgery and postoperative whole brain radiotherapy) generally showed an increased survival in the surgically treated patients (4,6,23,33,55–57).

There have been two prospective randomized trials performed to test the efficacy of surgical treatment for single brain metastases. In the first trial, performed at the University of Kentucky, 48 patients with known systemic cancer were treated with either biopsy of the suspected brain metastasis plus whole brain radiotherapy or complete surgical resection of the metastasis plus whole brain radiotherapy (20). The radiation doses were the same in both groups and consisted of a total dose of 3600 cGy given as 12 daily fractions of 300 cGy each. There was a statistically significant increase in survival in the surgical group (10 months versus 4 months). In addition, the time to recurrence of brain metastases and duration of functional independence were significantly longer in the resection group.

A second randomized trial performed in Holland has produced similar results (58). In the Dutch study, 61 patients with single metastases were treated with either surgical removal plus 4000 cGy of WBRT or with 4000 cGy WBRT alone. The radiation was given as 20 daily fractions of 200 cGy each. Unlike the Kentucky study, patients in the radiation-alone arm did not have biopsies to confirm the presence of metastatic tumor. The Dutch investigators found a statistically significant increase in survival in the surgery arm (11 months versus 6 months). The duration of functional independence was also substantially increased by surgery.

Although these two studies were relatively small, the results clearly show that surgical resection was beneficial. Surgical therapy plus postoperative whole brain radiotherapy is now the treatment of choice for patients with surgically accessible single brain metastases (59).

Despite the demonstration of the efficacy of surgery in the treatment of brain metastases, whole brain radiotherapy alone remains the treatment of choice for most patients who develop brain metastases. Single metastases occur in approximately half of the patients. Unfortunately, nearly half of this group are not surgical candidates due to the inaccessibility of the tumor, extensive systemic disease, and other factors. Therefore, only about 25% of all patients with brain metastases will benefit from surgical resection. The rest should be treated with whole brain radiotherapy.

The best results are seen in those patients with a single surgically accessible lesion and either no remaining systemic disease (true solitary metastasis) or with controlled systemic cancer limited to the primary site only. A study from Memorial Sloan-Kettering Cancer Center (60) has suggested that in patients undergoing resection of brain metastases from non–small cell lung carcinoma, survival is significantly increased in those patients with complete resection of the primary lung disease. There was no correlation of survival with initial cancer stage.

Surgery also is indicated in those patients without known systemic cancer (for tissue diagnosis). Surgery is probably also of benefit in patients with impending herniation due to pressure effects.

## 6. Chemotherapy

The role of chemotherapy in the management of brain metastases has yet to be defined. Although chemotherapy has been used in the treatment of brain metastases from a variety of primary tumors, the results have been unimpressive (61–63). Some reports of responses in patients with certain highly chemosensitive tumors (most noticeably breast, small cell lung cancer, and germ cell tumors) have been published (64,65). However, these are small, uncontrolled studies. Chemotherapy is usually not the primary therapy for most patients, and it is seldom the only therapy.

Since more than half of the patients with brain metastases who are treated with surgery or radiotherapy will die from progression of the systemic disease, a chemotherapeutic agent that is effective against both systemic and brain disease is highly desirable. However, most systemically administered chemotherapeutic agents that are effective against the primary sites of cancer have been ineffective against cerebral metastases from the same cell population (61). Drug delivery appears to be a part of the problem. The transport of material between the bloodstream and cerebral tissue differs from other organs in the body. Tight intercellular junctions allow only the more lipid soluble materials to diffuse across capillaries within the brain. This blood-brain barrier is thought to be one of the major reasons that systemically administered anticancer agents do not reach cerebral metastases in adequate concentrations, or for adequate periods, to achieve efficient tumor cell killing. However, drug delivery cannot be the sole cause of the disappointing results in brain tumors. It is known that the blood-brain barrier is usually broken down at sites of brain cancer and other factors must, therefore, contribute to the relative chemotherapeutic resistance seen with brain metastases (66). It also has been suggested that the blood-brain barrier may increase the incidence of brain metastases following systemic chemotherapy by inducing a relative "pharmacological sanctuary" within the central nervous system (67).

At present a reasonable use for chemotherapy would be in those patients with small asymptomatic tumors that are known to be chemosensitive. If progression occurs with the patient receiving chemotherapy alone, more definitive treatment with surgery or radiation should be given. In the future, brain-specific drug delivery with carrier drugs or multidrug regimens appear to be the most promising options (63). Rigorous controlled trials of such agents will be required before specific recommendations could be made.

## B. Recurrent Brain Metastases

Another difficult and frequently encountered clinical problem is the treatment of recurrent brain metastases. The reappearance of brain metastases is often complicated by extensive systemic disease in many of these patients. In general, the same types of treatment used for newly diagnosed brain metastases are also available for recurrences. However, the type of previous therapy may limit the therapeutic options available at this later time. Commonly, patients with recurrences have already been treated with radiotherapy to the brain, thus limiting the amount of further radiation that can be given safely. The amount of additional radiation that can be offered is usually in the range of 1500–2500 cGy, and this dose range is frequently too low to control tumor growth. Several uncontrolled studies have found no significant increase in survival or control of neurological symptoms in patients who underwent radiotherapy for recurrent brain metastases (68,69). However, these studies consisted of heterogeneous patient groups with extensive disease and a large proportion of radioresistant tumors. Recently it has been suggested that reirradiation may be more beneficial in the subpopulation of patients who showed an initial favorable response to radiotherapy and who remain in good general condition when the cerebral recurrence develops (70). However, even in this favorable subgroup, only 42% of patients showed symptomatic improvement, and the median survival after reirradiation was only 5 months.

Despite such poor results, additional radiotherapy is frequently the only treatment option for patients with recurrent disease. Stereotaxic radiosurgery (gamma knife) has been used to treat recurrent brain metastases. Radiosurgery has the theoretical advantage of being able to deliver large doses of additional radiation to small areas of the brain. A report of 18 patients with recurrent tumors who were treated with stereotaxic radiosurgery via linear accelerator was recently published (71). The treated lesions were apparently controlled, with a decrease in size or stabilization posttreatment. However, quantitative survival data are awaited. Further studies are needed to determine the true value of stereotaxic radiosurgery in the management of recurrent brain metastases.

Conventional surgery for recurrent tumors is an option in patients who have a single recurrence and who are in good general condition. The experience with reoperation is limited. Sundaresan et al. reported a series of 21 patients treated with craniotomy for their initial brain metastases who underwent a second craniotomy for recurrence (72). After the second operation, two-thirds of the patients experienced neurological improvement, and the median survival after operation for the recurrence was 9 months. These patients were a select group with little systemic disease and a single recurrent metastasis.

The results in patients who received radiotherapy alone as the treatment of the initial brain metastases and who were then treated with surgery at recurrence are less favorable. A study from Memorial Sloan-Kettering Cancer Center included patients who were treated with surgery after failing WBRT as initial therapy (54). The median survival after operation for recurrence was 5 months. However, this group fared less well in overall survival than comparable patients undergoing surgery plus WBRT as initial treatment of newly diagnosed brain metastases. Usually, additional radiotherapy is not given after operation for a recurrence. Brachytherapy with implantation of removable radioactive sources has been tried in a few patients with incomplete resections (73). The value of brachytherapy for recurrent metastases is unclear. Chemotherapy has also been used with recurrent tumors, but its benefits, if any, have not been determined.

## REFERENCES

1. Walker AE, Robins M, Weinfeld FD. Epidemiology of brain tumors: the national survey of intracranial neoplasms. Neurology 1985; 35:219–226.
2. Takakura K, Sano K, Hoho S, et al. Metastatic tumors of the central nervous system. Tokyo: Igaku-Shoin, 1982.
3. Delattre JY, Krol G, Thaler HT, et al. Distribution of brain metastases. Arch Neurol 1988; 45:741–744.
4. Zimm S, Wampler GL, Stablein D, et al. Intracranial metastases in solid tumor patients: natural history and results of treatment. Cancer 1981; 48:384–394.
5. Earle KM. Metastatic and primary intracranial tumors of the adult male. J Neuropathol Exp Neurol 1954; 13:448–454.
6. Cairncross JG, Posner JB. The management of brain metastases. In: Walker MD, ed. Oncology of the nervous system. Boston: Martinus Nijhoff, 1983:341–377.
7. Deviri E, Schachner A, Halevy A, et al. Carcinoma of lung with a solitary cerebral metastasis: surgical management and review of the literature. Cancer 1983; 52:1507–1509.
8. Fetall MR. Metastatic tumors and granulomas. In: Rowland, L. P. Merritt's textbook of Neurology, 8th ed. Philadelphia: Lea & Febiger, 1989: 341–349.
9. Batson OV. The role of the vertebral veins in metastatic processes. Ann Intern Med 1942; 16:38–45.
10. Vannucci RC, Baten M. Cerebral metastatic disease in childhood. Neurology 1974; 24:981–985.
11. Graus F, Walker RW, Allen JC. Brain metastases in children. J Pediatr 1983; 103:558–561.
12. Posner JB. Diagnosis and treatment of metastases to the brain. Clin Bull 1974; 4:47–57.

13. Posner JB. Clinical manifestations of brain metastases. In: Weiss L, Gilbert HA, Posner JB, eds. Brain metastases. Boston: G. K. Hall, 1980:189–207.
14. Mandybur TI. Intracranial hemorrhage caused by metastatic tumors. Neurology 1977; 27:650–655.
15. Fisher CM. Transient paralytic attacks of obscure nature: the question of nonconvulsive seizure paralysis. Can J Neurol Sci 1978; 5:267–273.
16. Sze G, Milano E, Johnson C, et al. Detection of brain metastases: comparison of contrast-enhanced MR with unenhanced MR and enhanced CT. AJNR 1990; 11: 785–791.
17. Davis PC, Hudgins PA, Peterman SB, et al. Diagnosis of cerebral metastases: double dose delayed CT vs contrast enhanced MR imaging. AJNR 1991; 12:293–300.
18. Williams AL. Tumors. In: Williams AL, Haughton VM, eds. Cranial computed tomography: a comprehensive text. St. Louis: Mosby, 1985:16.
19. Price AC, Runge VM, Babigian GV Brain: neoplastic disease. In: Runge VM, ed. Clinical magnetic resonance imaging. Philadelphia: Lippincott, 1990.
20. Patchell RA, Tibbs PA, Walsh JW, et al. A randomized trial of surgery in the treatment of single metastases to the brain. N Engl J Med 1990; 322:494–500.
21. Bentson JR, Steckel RJ, Kagan AR. Diagnostic imaging in clinical cancer management: brain metastases. Invest Radiol 1988; 23:335–341.
22. Horton J, Baxter DH, Olson KB. The management of metastases to the brain by irradiation and corticosteroids. Am J Roentgenol Radium Ther Nucl Med 1971; 111:334–335.
23. Markesbery WR, Brooks WH, Gupta GD, et al. Treatment for patients with cerebral metastases. Arch Neurol 1978; 35:754–756.
24. Ruderman NB, Hall TC. Use of glucocorticoids in the palliative treatment of metastatic brain tumors. Cancer 1965; 18:298–306.
25. Fishman RA. Brain edema. N Engl J Med 1975; 293:706–711.
26. Ehrenkranz JR, Posner JB. Adrenocorticosteroid hormones. In: Weiss, L., Gilbert HA, Posner JB, eds. Brain metastases. Boston: G. K. Hall, 1980:340–363.
27. Gutin PH. Corticosteroid therapy in patients with cerebral tumor: benefits, mechanisms, problems, practicalities. Semin Oncol 1975; 2:49–56.
28. Gottlieb JA, Frei E, Luce JK. An evaluation of the management of patients with cerebral metastases from malignant melanoma. Cancer 1972; 29:701–705.
29. Chao JH, Phillips R, Nickson JJ. Roentgen-ray therapy of cerebral metastases. Cancer 1954; 7:682–689.
30. Borgelt B, Gelber R, Kramer S, et al. The palliation of brain metastases: final results of the first two studies by the Radiation Therapy Oncology Group. Int J Radiat Oncol Biol Phys 1980; 6:1–9.
31. Gelber RD, Larson M, Borgelt BB, et al. Equivalent of radiation schedules for the palliative treatment of brain metastases in patients with favorable prognosis. Cancer 1981; 48:1749–1753.
32. Kurtz JM, Gelber RD, Brady LW, et al. The palliation of brain metastases in a favorable patient population: a randomized clinical trial by the Radiation Therapy Oncology Group. Int J Radiat Oncol Biol Phys 1981; 7:891–895.
33. Cairncross JG, Kim JH, Posner JB. Radiation therapy for brain metastases. Ann Neurol 1980; 7:529–541.

34. Order SE, Hellman S, Von Essen CF, et al. Improvement in quality of survival following whole brain irradiation for brain metastases. Radiology 1968; 91:149–153.
35. Berry HC, Parker RG, Gerdes AJ. Irradiation of brain metastases. Acta Radiol [Ther] 1974; 13:535–544.
36. Deeley TJ, Rice Edwards JM. Radiotherapy in the management of cerebral secondaries from bronchial carcinoma. Lancet 1968; 1:1209–1213.
37. Karnofsky DA, Burchenal JH. The clinical evaluation of chemotherapeutic agents in cancer. In: MacLeod CM, ed. Evaluation of chemotherapeutic agents. New York: Columbia University Press, 1949:191–205.
38. Deiner-West M, Dobbins TW, Phillips TL, et al. Identification of an optimal subgroup for treatment evaluation of patients with brain metastases using RTOG study 7916. Int J Radiat Oncol Biol Phys 1989; 16:669–673.
39. Hoskin PJ, Crow J, Ford HT. The influence of extent and local management on the outcome of radiotherapy for brain metastases. Int J Radiat Oncol Biol Phys 1990; 19:111–115.
40. Komarnicky LT, Phillips TL, Martz K, et al. A randomized phase III protocol for the evaluation of misonidazole combined with radiation in the treatment of patients with brain metastases (RTOG-7916). Int J Radiat Oncol Biol Phys 1991; 20:53–58.
41. Olsson Y, Klatzo I, Carsten A. The effect of acute radiation injury on the permeability and ultrastructure of intracerebral capillaries. Neuropathol Appl Neurobiol 1975; 1:59–68.
42. DeAngelis LM, Delattre JY, Posner JB. Radiation induced dementia in patients cured of brain metastases. Neurology 1989; 39:789–796.
43. Paleologos NA, Imperato JP, Vick NA. Brain metastases: effects of radiotherapy on long term survivors. Neurology 1991; 41(suppl 1):129.
44. Leksell L. Stereotactic radiosurgery. J Neurol Neurosurg Psychiatry 1983; 46:797–803.
45. Lutz W, Winston KR, Maleki PV. A system for stereotactic radiosurgery with a linear accelerator. Int J Radiat Oncol Biol Phys 1988; 14:373–381.
46. Lunsford LD, Flickinger J, Coffey RJ. Stereotactic gamma knife radiosurgery: initial North American experience in 207 patients. Arch Neurol 1990; 47:169–175.
47. Sturm V, Kober B, Hover J, et al. Stereotactic percutaneous single dose irradiation of brain metastases with a linear accelerator. Int J Radiat Oncol Biol Phys 1987; 13:279–282.
48. Loeffler JS, Wen Py, Alexander E, et al. Radiosurgery for brain metastases. Principles and practice of oncology. Philadelphia: Lippincott, 1991; 2:1–12.
49. Cairncross JG, Chernik NL, Kim JH, et al. Sterilization of cerebral metastases by radiation therapy. Neurology 1979; 29:1195–1202.
50. Bergonie J, Tribondeau L. Interpretation of some results of radiotherapy and an attempt at determining a logical technique of treatment. Radiat Res 1959; 11:587–588.
51. Suit HD, Todoroki T. Rationale for combining surgery and radiation therapy. Cancer 1985; 55:2246–2249.
52. Hellman S. Improving the therapeutic index in breast cancer treatment. Cancer 1980; 40:4335–4342.

53. Distefano A, Yap HY, Hortobagyi GN, et al. The natural history of breast cancer patients with brain metastases. Cancer 1979; 44:1913–1918.
54. Sundaresan N, Galicich JH, Beattie EJ. Surgical treatment of brain metastases from lung cancer. J Neurosurg 1983; 58:666–671.
55. Winston KR, Walsh JW, Fischer EG. Results of operative treatment of intracranial metastatic tumors. Cancer 1980; 45:2639–2645.
56. Montana GS, Meacham WF, Caldwell WL. Brain irradiation for metastatic disease of lung origin. Cancer 1972; 29:1477–1480.
57. Patchell RA, Cirrincione C, Thaler HT, et al. Single brain metastases: surgery plus radiation or radiation alone. Neurology 1986; 36:447–453.
58. Haaxma-Reiche H, Vecht C, Padberg G, et al. The outcome of single brain metastasis after treatment with irradiation alone or combined with neurosurgery. Ann Neurol 1992; 32:286–287.
59. Posner JB. Surgery for metastases to the brain (editorial). N Engl J Med 1990; 322:544–545.
60. Burt M, Wronski M, Arbit E, et al. Resection of brain metastases from non-small-cell lung carcinoma. J Thorac Cardiovasc Surg 1992; 103:399–411.
61. Greig NH. Chemotherapy of brain metastases: current status. Cancer Treat Rev 1984; 11:157–186.
62. Hildebrand J. Chemotherapy of brain metastases. Eur J Cancer Clin Oncol 1988; 24:1097–1098.
63. Seigers HP. Chemotherapy for brain metastases: recent developments and clinical considerations. Cancer Treat Rev 1990; 17:63–76.
64. Kristjansen PE, Hansen HH. Brain metastases from small cell lung cancer treated with combination chemotherapy. Eur J Radiat Oncol Biol Phys 1990; 19:111–115.
65. Rosner D, Nemoto T, Lane WW. Chemotherapy induces regression of brain metastases in breast carcinoma. Cancer 1986; 58:832–839.
66. Greig N, Jones H, Cavanagh J. Blood brain barrier integrity and host responses in experimental metastatic brain tumors. Clin Exp Metastasis 1983; 1:229–246.
67. Tsukada Y, Fouad A, Pickren JW, et al. Central nervous system metastases from breast carcinoma: autopsy study. Cancer 1983; 52:2349–2354.
68. Hazuka MB, Kinzie JJ. Brain metastases: results and effects of reirradiation. Int J Radiat Oncol Biol Phys 1988; 15:433–437.
69. Kurup P, Reddy S, Hendrickson FR. Results of re-irradiation for cerebral metastases. Cancer 1980; 46:2587–2589.
70. Cooper JS, Steinfeld AD, Lerch IA. Cerebral metastases: value of reirradiation in selected patients. Radiology 1990; 174:883–885.
71. Loeffler JS, Kooy HM, Wen PY, et al. The treatment of recurrent brain metastases with stereotactic radiosurgery. J Clin Oncol 1990; 8:576–582.
72. Sundaresan N, Sachdev VP, DiGiancinto GV, et al. Reoperation for brain metastases. J Clin Oncol 1988; 6:1625–1629.
73. Prados M, Leibel S, Barnett CM, et al. Interstitial brachytherapy for metastatic brain tumors. Cancer 1989; 63:657–660.

# 2
# Spinal Metastases

**Thomas N. Byrne**

*Yale University School of Medicine, New Haven, Connecticut*

Spinal neoplasms are classified according to location, i.e., epidural, intradural-extramedullary (leptomeningeal), and intramedullary. While the histology of primary spinal tumors that occur in these locations reflect the tissues found in each of these sites, metastases from any primary elsewhere may grow in the epidural, leptomeningeal, or intramedullary locations. The present chapter emphasizes the clinical management of epidural metastases and briefly discusses intramedullary metastases. The latter were once considered a rare event but now are recognized more frequently with the advent of gadolinium-enhanced magnetic resonance imaging (MRI). The management of leptomeningeal metastases is discussed elsewhere in this volume (Chap. 3).

## I. METASTATIC EPIDURAL SPINAL CORD COMPRESSION

### A. Magnitude of the Clinical Problem

Metastatic epidural spinal cord compression (MESCC) occurs in about 5% of patients dying from cancer (1). If untreated, it ultimately causes unrelenting pain, paraplegia, sensory loss, and sphincter paralysis. Alternatively, if MESCC is recognized and treated before neural injury occurs, most patients maintain neurological function.

In about 85% of cases of MESCC (2), the metastasis begins in the vertebral column and extends into the epidural space to cause neural compression. Vertebral metastases have been reported to occur in 15–41% of patients dying from cancer (3). All patients with vertebral metastases are at risk for developing MESCC, and vertebral metastases can be clinically indistinguishable from early MESCC. Among the 400,000 patients dying annually from cancer in the United States, between 60,000 and 160,000 harbor vertebral metastases and 20,000 suffer from MESCC. The two challenges confronting the clinician are (1) determining which patients will benefit from extensive spinal canal imaging; and (2) selecting therapy for MESCC.

## B. Pathogenesis of Spine Metastasis

The pathogenesis of cancer metastasis has been debated for decades. Paget described the "seed and soil" hypothesis in which metastases develop where the metabolic environment is propitious for growth of these cells. Alternatively, Ewing maintained that hemodynamic and anatomic factors were the most important determinants in defining the sites of metastases. In the hemodynamic model the sequence of metastases is determined by the anatomy of the draining veins. Thus lung metastases precede spread to bone. Clinical experience reveals, however, many exceptions to the cascade (3).

In an attempt to explain the discrepancy that spine metastases occur so frequently in the absence of lung and other visceral metastases, Batson studied the epidural venous plexus which now bears his name (4). In human cadavers, he showed that this valveless system acts as a source of collateral circulation for veins draining the chest, abdomen, pelvis, and breast. In living primates, he demonstrated that the epidural plexus did not fill following injection of the dorsal vein of the penis unless the abdomen was compressed, mimicking a Valsalva maneuver (see Fig. 1). Batson hypothesized that in the human this vertebral venous plexus of low intraluminal pressure could be filled from venous effluent draining breast, intrathoracic, and intra-abdominal organs during coughing, sneezing, and straining. Furthermore, because the vertebral system is valveless, blood could flow in a rostral or caudal direction unimpeded.

Batson's hypothesis was confirmed by Coman and DeLong (5), who injected cancer cells into the femoral veins of animals either with or without external abdominal pressure. In the control group, only lung metastases were seen in the majority of animals. Spine metastases occurred in the majority of the experimental group. The significance of these findings has been challenged recently by Arguello and coworkers (6), who found that intracardiac injection of tumor cells resulted in metastases to the subchondral regions of vertebral bodies. They attributed this localization to the fact that bone marrow contains hematopoietic growth factors that have been shown to stimulate cancer cells to grow in vitro. Thus both Paget's

# Spinal Metastases

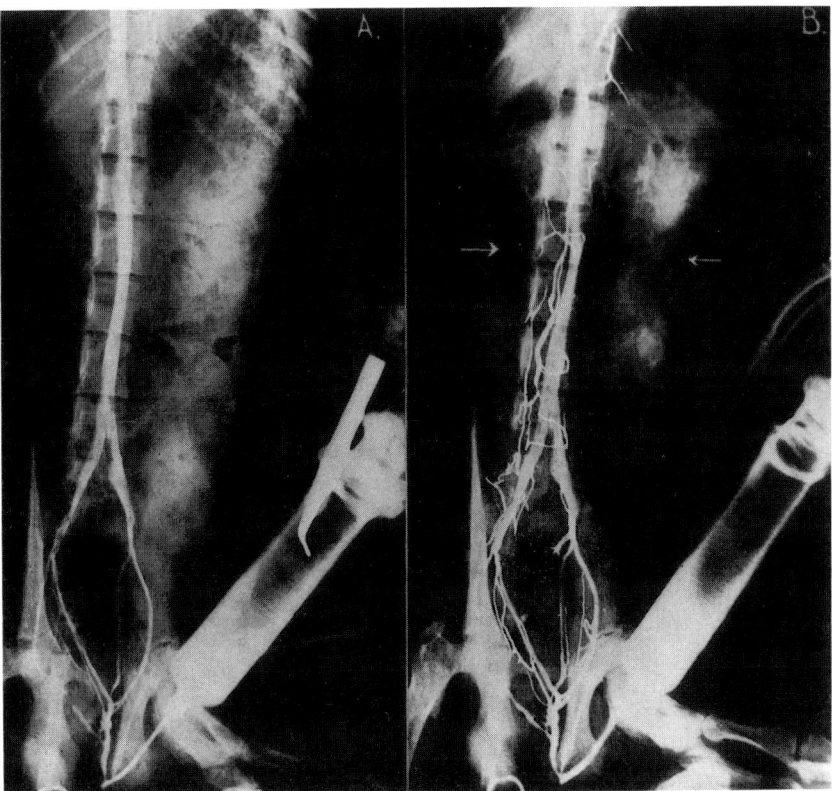

**Figure 1** The plain x-ray of a living primate during the injection of radiopaque material into the deep dorsal vein of the penis. (A) The injected material flows into the inferior vena cava without entering the vertebral veins. (B) With the primate's abdomen compressed, mimicking a Valsalva maneuver, the dye is diverted into the vertebral venous plexus. (From Ref. 4.)

"seed and soil" hypothesis and Ewing's hemodynamic mechanism may help explain the high incidence of spine metastases.

## C. Location of Tumor in Relation to Spinal Cord

Malignant epidural spinal cord compression arises from metastases to one of three locations: the vertebrae in 85% of cases, the paravertebral tissues in 10–15%, or, rarely, the epidural space itself.

The vertebral body is the most common site of metastases. Less frequently the pedicle or posterior arch is involved. Compression of the spinal cord by tumor or, less frequently, bone fragments occurs as tumor expands and destroys the vertebra. Thus, tumor is usually anterior or anterolateral to neural structures, a fact that has implications for surgical therapy. Plain x-rays and radionuclide bone scans are typically positive in these cases.

Paravertebral tumors may extend into the vertebral canal through the intervertebral foramina. Two-thirds of cases of MESCC due to lymphoma and pediatric neoplasms occur via this mechanism. Plain x-rays of the spine and radionuclide bone scans are usually negative. However, computed tomography (CT) and magnetic resonance imaging (MRI) can image paravertebral tumors well.

## D. Pathology

Spinal cord pathology in cases of MESCC includes edema, demyelination, hemorrhage, and cystic necrosis. McAlhany and Netsky (7) reported a clinicopathological study among 19 patients with extramedullary spinal cord compression. There was no correlation between the axial location of the neoplasm and the presenting symptoms. Pathological findings were present both ipsilateral and contralateral to the mass. In some cases, the contralateral damage was more marked than the ipsilateral injury. White matter was more severely affected than the gray matter but the distribution of demyelination and infarction did not conform to the arterial supply.

More recent autopsy studies (8) have found "pencil-shaped softenings" of the spinal cord at the level of epidural tumors. These softenings extended over several segments of the spinal cord in a cephalad or, less frequently, caudad direction. The necrotic cavity is usually located in the ventral portion of the posterior column or dorsal horn. This corresponds to the region involved in cases of venous infarction but is also considered a watershed zone for arterial circulation (9,10). Mechanical factors also may be responsible for pathogenesis (8) of these cystic lesions, that can be imaged using delayed CT myelography and magnetic resonance imaging (11).

## E. Pathophysiology of Neurological Signs and Symptoms

Both circulatory disturbance and direct neural compression have been proposed as causes of neurologic injury in MESCC. Elsberg (12) observed venous engorgement and diminished arterial pulsation at operation. Ushio et al. (13) injected Walker 256 carcinoma into the epidural space of the rat and demonstrated that vasogenic edema of the spinal cord was an early pathological finding. The marker horseradish peroxidase, which is normally excluded from the spinal cord, entered the cord at the site of compression suggesting a breakdown of the blood–spinal cord barrier as a cause of edema. Diminution of vasogenic edema derived from the administration of glucocorticoids to the animals correlated with improvement in neurological function.

In another animal model of MESCC, Siegal and colleagues (14) examined somatosensory-evoked responses and the role of prostaglandins in the evolution of pathological changes and myelopathy. These authors found abnormalities in spinal somatosensory-evoked responses precede neurological signs of myelopathy. Furthermore, electron microscopic studies showed that both mechanical compression and ischemia caused demyelination. Increased prostaglandin $E_2$ ($PGE_2$) synthesis that accompanies vasogenic cord edema was inhibited by steroidal and nonsteroidal anti-inflammatory agents (15). These investigators also found that cyproheptadine, a serotonin antagonist, reduces $PGE_2$ synthesis, vascular permeability, and cord edema and delays the development of paraplegia in rats (15). These experimental results suggest new therapeutic approaches.

## F. Primary Tumors

There are several reports that address the relative frequency of the various primary tumors that cause MESCC. Many of these studies report surgical series and therefore reflect a select group of patients. Among studies that include all patients, breast, lung, and prostate cancer make up nearly 50% of all primaries (16). Other frequent primary neoplasms include lymphoma, renal tumors, melanoma, multiple myeloma, and sarcoma (1,2,17,18). Among children with MESCC, the most common tumors are sarcoma, neuroblastoma, and lymphoma (19,20).

Metastatic epidural spinal cord compression usually occurs in the setting of disseminated disease, although it can be the presenting manifestation of malignancy or the sole site of recurrence. The interval between the diagnosis of cancer and spinal cord compression was 0 to 19 years in the series from Memorial Sloan-Kettering Cancer Center (MSKCC) (2). Lung cancer is more likely to present initially as a spine metastasis than breast cancer. Breast cancer usually causes MESCC late in the course of the disease (17).

## G. Level of Spinal Cord Compression

Several studies have confirmed that the thoracic spine is the most common level of spinal metastasis. The spinal level of MESCC is thoracic in approximately 70% of cases, cervical in 10%, and lumbar in 20% (2,17). MESCC occurs at multiple noncontiguous levels in 10–38% of cases (2,17,21–23).

## H. Clinical Presentation of MESCC

The major presenting clinical signs and symptoms of MESCC are pain, weakness, sensory loss, and autonomic disturbance. Progressive pain, either axial or referred or radicular, is the most common initial complaint of both vertebral metastases and

MESCC. Pain is reported by 95% of adults (2) and 80% of children (20) with MESCC. In a study of patients with suspected MESCC, Bernat and colleagues (24) found that the character of pain did not distinguish vertebral metastasis alone from MESCC. Thus each patient with pain due to spine metastasis must be considered at risk for MESCC.

In the Memorial Sloan-Kettering series of MESCC (2), pain was the first symptom in 96% of 130 cases. The pain was radicular in 79% of cervical lesions, 55% of thoracic lesions, and 90% of lumbosacral lesions. Radicular pain was typically bilateral when it occurred in the thoracic region. Although frequently sought, vertebral tenderness was reported in only 42 of 130 patients (2).

The pain of MESCC is frequently misdiagnosed as degenerative joint disease (DJD). Both types of pain may be aggravated by movement, Valsalva maneuver, straight-leg raising, and neck flexion. Alternatively, DJD rarely occurs outside of the low cervical or lumbar spine and the pain of DJD is usually familiar to the patient. Another characteristic that serves to distinguish the two sources of pain is the response to recumbency. The pain of DJD is usually lessened by bedrest, whereas that of MESCC is commonly made worse by recumbency, such that patients may sleep in a chair (2,3). Furthermore, the pain of MESCC is progressive, in contrast to degenerative joint disease, that tends to cause episodic pain. Finally, since plain films or bone scan will usually confirm incidental DJD in patients over 50 years of age, caution must be exercised in attributing their complaints to DJD (3).

The duration of pain prior to diagnosis of spinal cord compression may vary with different primary tumors (17). Among all patients with tumors in the London Hospital series, pain was present on average for 5 months (range 3 days to 3.8 years) before diagnosis. This duration was significantly shorter for spine metastases from lung cancer (mean, 4 months) than for breast cancer (mean, 7 months). In the MSKCC series (2), the median duration of pain was 2 months for all patients irrespective of their primary tumor.

Weakness nearly always is accompanied by pain in MESCC and is rarely the sole manifestation. As shown in Table 1, only 2 of 130 patients in the MSKCC series (2) had weakness as the initial manifestation of cord compression. Alternatively, at the time of diagnosis subjective weakness was found in over 76% and objective signs of weakness in 87% of patients, which reflects the typical delay in making the diagnosis of MESCC.

As with weakness, sensory loss is rare as a sole presenting manifestation of MESCC. Although sensory disturbance was not the presenting complaint in any of the 130 patients from MSKCC (2), numbness and paresthesias were reported at the time of diagnosis by 51% of patients (see Table 1). On examination, sensory loss was found in 78% of patients. As the somatotopically arranged spinothalamic tracts are progressively compressed, an ascending sensory level may occur. Thus the sensory level may be several segments below the level of compression. This

**Table 1** Signs and Symptoms of Epidural Spinal Cord Compression in 130 Patients

| Sign/symptom | First symptom | | Symptoms at diagnosis | |
|---|---|---|---|---|
| | (No.) | (%) | (No.) | (%) |
| Pain | 125 | 96 | 125 | 96 |
| Weakness | 2 | 2 | 99 | 76 |
| Autonomic dysfunction | 0 | 0 | 74 | 57 |
| Sensory complaints | 0 | 0 | 66 | 51 |
| Ataxia | 2 | 2 | 4 | 3 |
| Herpes zoster | 0 | 0 | 3 | 2 |
| Flexor spasms | 0 | 0 | 2 | 1 |

Source: Ref. 2.

has clinical implications because a sensory level may mislead the examiner, underscoring the need for imaging the entire spinal canal in patients with symptoms or signs of MESCC.

Sphincter disturbances are rare presenting manifestation of MESCC unless the lesion is located at the conus medullaris or cauda equina (2). Among the series of 600 patients reported by Constans and coworkers (18), sphincter disturbances were the sole presenting complaint in only 2%. In the MSKCC series (2), no patients presented with sphincter dysfunction alone. At the time of diagnosis, however, sphincter disturbances were present in 57% (see Table 1). Sphincter dysfunction was a poor prognostic indicator for ambulation after therapy. However, patients with caudal tumors may present with bladder difficulties and impotence (25,26). In such cases large volumes of urine may be retained with secondary overflow incontinence.

Rare clinical presentations of MESCC include Brown-Séquard's syndrome, herpes zoster (shingles), and truncal ataxia (1–3). In the MSKCC series, three of 130 patients had a zoster eruption at the site of cord compression (2). Gait ataxia was the sole presenting symptom in 2% of cases in the MSKCC series and was present in an additional seven patients on examination. The mechanism of gait ataxia did not involve position sense loss. Gait ataxia may be secondary to compression of the spinocerebellar tracts and, initially, may suggest cerebellar or cerebral disease if back or neck pain is not prominent. Once a neurological deficit appears it can evolve rapidly to paraplegia over a period of hours or days. Such rapid evolution is unpredictable and the main argument for rapid diagnosis and treatment of patients with MESCC.

## I. Laboratory Studies

### 1. Cerebrospinal Fluid Analysis and Lumbar Puncture

Cerebrospinal fluid (CSF) abnormalities in cases of MESCC are nonspecific. The protein content is typically elevated, as expected in cases of partial or complete spinal block, and the cell count usually is normal (1,2,17). Occasionally, a mild CSF pleocytosis occurs, reflecting inflammation from a parameningeal tumor or concomitant metastases involving the leptomeninges (27). The CSF glucose is typically normal in cases of MESCC.

Since Cushing reported on the phenomenon of cerebral and cerebellar herniation following lumbar puncture in the presence of increased intracranial pressure, there has been concern over a similar risk of spinal herniation in patients harboring spinal tumors. Although not all investigators have had similar experiences (1), some reports suggest that lumbar puncture may result in neurological deterioration in patients with extramedullary neoplasms (28,29). For instance, Elsberg (12) commented that radicular pain and neurological disturbances worsened after the removal of spinal fluid in some patients with spinal tumors. Hollis and coworkers (28) reviewed their experience with neurological deterioration after lumbar puncture for myelography below the level of a complete spinal subarachnoid block. In this retrospective series, 14% of 50 patients had "significant neurological deterioration" after lumbar puncture. No deterioration was seen in patients undergoing myelography via a cervical (C1-2) puncture. The mechanism for neurological deterioration in such patients is uncertain but has been thought to be secondary to impaction of the spinal cord tumor, also known as "spinal coning" (30). Elsberg (12) believed it is due to removal of CSF, which acted as a "buffer" between the tumor and the spinal cord.

Despite these occasional reports, the quantitative risk is difficult to establish. For example, among several hundred patients, no postmyelography neurological deterioration was reported in several other series (1,31). Since there is little information to be gained from CSF analysis alone that would assist in making the diagnosis of MESCC, a lumbar puncture should not be performed to "rule in" or "rule out" this diagnosis. However, if CSF analysis is indicated to diagnose infectious or neoplastic meningitis, close neurological observation following lumbar puncture is indicated along with neurosurgical consultation. Furthermore, although MRI may obviate the need for myelography in most patients, it often is not available in a timely fashion in many centers and patients with pacemakers or claustrophobia are not candidates for MRI. In this setting, myelography should not be delayed or avoided if needed to establish promptly the diagnosis of MESCC and plan therapy (see below).

### 2. Diagnostic Imaging

Plain x-ray findings that predict the presence or absence of MESCC are important. About 85% of adult patients with MESCC have spinal abnormalities upon x-ray.

The most characteristic appearances include a lytic or blastic metastasis, erosion of a pedicle, or vertebral body collapse (1–3,32).

Tumor type determines the frequency of bony abnormality. Spinal metastases arising from carcinoma of the breast are much more likely to demonstrate abnormalities on plain x-ray (94%) than those arising from carcinoma of the lung (74%). Alternatively, plain films reveal abnormality only in approximately one-third of cases due to lymphoma or pediatric neoplasms (20,33,34).

Rodichok et al. (31,35) reported the frequency of MESCC to be greater than 60% in cancer patients with back pain, no neurological deficit, *and spinal metastasis on radiograph*. In a study of 41 cancer patients with back pain, weakness, and/or sensory loss undergoing myelography, Portenoy et al. retrospectively determined the frequency of epidural tumor based on clinical and plain x-ray findings. The three segments of spine—cervical, thoracic, and lumbar—were each identified as symptomatic or asymptomatic. The plain films of each segment were identified as showing the presence or absence of vertebral metastases. When plain films were positive at symptomatic segments, myelography showed epidural disease 86% of the time. On the other hand, epidural tumor was present in only 8% of symptomatic segments with normal radiographs. In asymptomatic segments with abnormal plain films, myelography showed epidural tumor in 43% compared to 3% of asymptomatic segments with normal radiographs.

Graus et al. (37) found that the appearance of the vertebral metastasis correlated with the risk of MESCC. They found epidural lesions adjacent to 7% of vertebrae with tumor limited to the vertebral body without collapse; at 31% with pedicle erosion; and at 87% of vertebrae with more than 50% collapse.

Generally, radionuclide bone scans are more sensitive than plain films in detecting bone metastases (except in multiple myeloma). The development of a new spinal abnormality on bone scan in cancer patients is due to metastases in 72% of cases based on findings from plain films and CT scans (23,38). On the other hand, among 18 patients with abnormal bone scans and normal plain films, CT showed metastases in 12 (67%), and three had epidural extension. This has led to the recommendation that new spinal abnormalities on bone scans in cancer patients should be evaluated with plain films and CT scanning to differentiate benign from metastatic disease (38). Portenoy et al. (15) found that a high frequency of false positives limited the usefulness of a positive bone scan. They also reported that the combination of a negative study in an asymptomatic region with negative plain films reduced the risk of MESCC from 0.02 to 0.001 using decision analysis. However, Rodichok et al. (31) found that 54% of cancer patients with back pain and a positive myelogram had a normal bone scan, underscoring the fact that a normal bone scan in a symptomatic patient does not exclude MESCC.

Spinal CT is more sensitive and specific than plain films or radionuclide scanning for identifying and distinguishing benign from malignant disease and visualizing paravertebral masses (21,23,38). Spinal CT can be used to investigate unexplained pain or abnormalities on plain films and radionuclide studies in the cancer patient with a normal neurologic examination (23). Alternatively, in patients with clinical manifestations of MESCC the entire spinal axis must be visualized, making spinal CT impractical. Also, without myelography, the sensitivity of CT for detecting MESCC has not been adequately validated.

Carmody et al. (39), Smoker et al. (40), and others (3,39,41,42) have found unenhanced MRI equivalent to myelography in detecting MESCC and superior in detecting vertebral metastases and paravertebral masses. This has led to MRI becoming the preferred imaging method in centers where MRI is readily available. Alternatively, myelography should be performed if there is delay in obtaining MRI in a timely fashion, in patients unable to undergo MRI (e.g., those with pacemakers and pain precluding recumbency), or when a technically adequate MRI cannot be obtained. Since recumbency can be painful for patients with MESCC, adequate analgesics should be given as needed to ensure patient comfort and cooperation.

Contrast-enhanced MRI is superior to unenhanced studies for detecting leptomeningeal metastases (43,44) and intramedullary tumors (45), and may provide additional information regarding epidural disease. Sze et al. (46) have found that contrast enhancement may provide additional information in cases of MESCC. These authors found that regions of vertebral enhancement may correspond to areas of active tumor proliferation and may be useful for directing biopsies. (See Fig. 2.)

## J. Clinical Approach to the Patient with Symptoms and Signs Suggestive of Spinal Metastasis

Cancer patients with clinical evidence of spinal metastases can be divided into four groups and approached accordingly: (1) patients with back or neck pain, normal neurological examination, and abnormal plain radiographs; (2) those with back or neck pain, normal neurological examination, and normal radiographs; (3) patients with radiculopathy; and (4) those with the clinical picture of MESCC (47).

### 1. Neck/Back Pain, Normal Neurological Examination, and Positive Plain Films

The appropriate management of the cancer patient with neck or back pain, normal neurological examination, and metastatic disease demonstrated by conventional radiographs is controversial. Although myelography or MRI is recommended by many authors (38,48,49) to define radiotherapy ports, many physicians (31,50) irradiate such symptomatic vertebral metastases without further imaging. Advocates of definitive canal imaging argue that unexpected epidural disease outside the planned radiotherapy port can be identified and treated and that this is worth the attendant inconvenience, delay, and expense of further imaging (36). If all

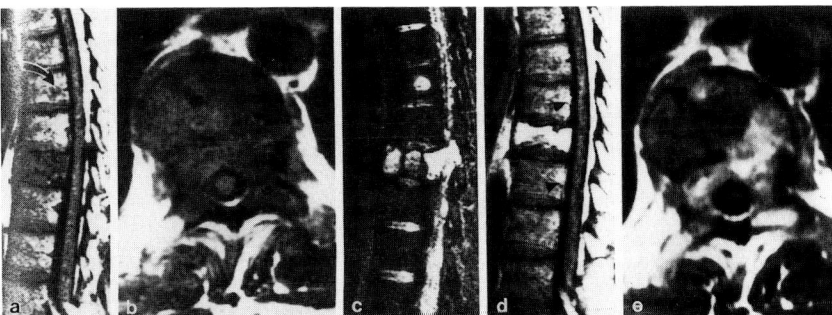

**Figure 2** Gadolinium-enhanced MRI of the spine of a 36-year-old patient with cancer is shown. (a,b) Sagittal (a) and axial (b) images show partial collapse of the T-10 vertebral body and replacement of normal high signal of bone marrow with low-intensity tumor. Moreover, a poorly defined hypointense focus is present in the T-8 vertebral body (arrow, a). (c) Both lesions are seen on T2-weighted images. (d,e) Following the administration of gadolinium-DTPA, the T1-weighted sagittal (*D*) and axial (*E*) images demonstrate enhancement of the T-10 vertebral body. The previously seen hypointense region of tumor in T-8 is not visualized because it is isointense with the remainder of the vertebral body on this enhanced study. The axial scan (e) demonstrates greater enhancement on the left than the right side of the vertebral body. Although neoplasm may extend through the entire vertebral body, results from multiple biopsies on the right side were negative, whereas results of biopsy on the left revealed tumor. (From Ref. 46.)

epidural disease is not identified at the time of initial radiotherapy, future radiotherapy may be compromised because of the risk of overlapping treatment fields. There is no prospective data to identify which patients can bypass definitive canal imaging. The retrospective data cited above (23,31,36–38) suggest that the risk of missing adjacent or distant epidural disease is low only in patients with well-documented solitary metastases or limited adjacent metastases. Rodichok and coworkers (31) recommended that all patients with multiple vertebral metastases undergo myelography (the study was performed before the availability of MRI). They also concluded that when metastatic disease was limited to two or three adjacent vertebrae in the region of symptoms and demonstrated by plain films, then a radiation port extending two segments above and below these lesions is likely to include all epidural tumor. More recent studies (23,36,38) would argue that if radiotherapy is to be performed without the advantage of MRI or myelography, then conventional radiographs of the entire spine and radionuclide bone scan should be performed to establish that disease is restricted to a limited region of the spine (one to three vertebrae). If definitive canal imaging is not performed, a greater responsibility is placed upon the physician, not only to be confident of a normal neurological examination initially, but to remain vigilant for early symptoms of MESCC.

Definitive spinal canal imaging is indicated in order to confirm that MESCC is not present in patients with back pain, a normal neurological examination, and plain radiographs or bone scan showing metastases who are not scheduled for radiotherapy (51).

### 2. Pain, Normal Neurological Examination, and Normal Plain Films

In cancer patients who develop unexplained back, neck, or radicular pain, have a normal neurological examination, and have negative plain films, MRI of the involved region is indicated to distinguish benign from malignant disease. If MRI is unavailable, CT and myelography should be considered (23,31).

### 3. Radiculopathy

The manifestations of radiculopathy include pain, weakness, sensory loss and/or reflex loss in a single nerve root distribution unilaterally or bilaterally. MESCC is present in up to 88% of such cancer patients with positive plain films and up to 25% of those with normal x-rays (35). MRI is indicated for these patients in order to identify adjacent levels of vertebral metastases that could cause confounding referred or radicular pain (3) and to define the extent of epidural tumor. If MRI is unavailable, myelography with CT is an alternative.

### 4. Clinical Manifestations of MESCC

Cancer patients with mild, stable, or equivocal clinical manifestations of MESCC should undergo total spine MRI or myelography by the next day (48). It is essential to image the entire spine since unsuspected MESCC at other levels may go unrecognized. Patients with significant neurological signs should be given intravenous glucocorticoids (see below) and undergo an emergent total spine MRI or myelography, if MRI is unavailable or not feasible.

Since spinal MRI and myelography occasionally may yield false-negative results in cases of spinal cord compression, the physician often must consider other diagnostic studies following a "negative" MRI or myelogram in the cancer patient with a myelopathy. For example, if the noncontrast spinal MRI is negative, a contrast-enhanced spinal MRI and CSF analysis may identify leptomeningeal metastases or an intramedullary metastasis not seen on unenhanced MRI or myelography. Myelography should still be considered in cancer patients with myelopathy in whom the clinical suspicion for a compressive lesion remains but is not identified on the spinal MRI.

## K. Therapy

The mainstays of treatment of MESCC have been glucocorticoids and radiation therapy in most patients, but recent excellent results with anterior decompression in selected patients have renewed interest in surgery. Chemotherapy has occasionally been reported to be effective in exceedingly chemosensitive tumors (52,53).

Although the value of glucocorticoids in improving neurological outcome has not been demonstrated, clinical and laboratory studies have demonstrated that these compounds improve neurological function and alleviate pain acutely (54). Glucocorticoids are indicated for MESCC at the time of confirmation by diagnostic imaging or when the clinical circumstances strongly suggest the diagnosis pending diagnostic imaging confirmation. The dosage and form of corticosteroid varies (see Chap. 21). Some investigators recommend dexamethasone, 4 milligrams (mg) four times daily (q.i.d.) (33,54,55). Laboratory studies have shown a dose-related benefit with dexamethasone (13,56) that prompted study of a loading dose of 100 mg followed by 24 mg q.i.d. (48). We usually give 10–100 mg of dexamethasone intravenously stat followed by 4 to 24 mg q.i.d. The lower doses are used in patients with mild or no signs of myelopathy. The highest doses are reserved for patients with prominent, or rapidly progressive, myelopathy. Occasional patients report pain in the perineal region when high-dose glucocorticoids are rapidly administered intravenously. Glucocorticoids are usually continued through the course of radiotherapy. Tapering can usually begin within 2 to 3 days of initiating glucocorticoids. As the steroids are tapered, patients must be observed for neurological deterioration. The dose is increased if deterioration occurs. In many patients, steroids can be tapered off within 2 to 3 weeks (54). Patients must be followed closely to identify steroid-induced complications such as glucose intolerance (54).

Radiation therapy has become the primary definitive treatment of MESCC because most patients often harbor widespread metastatic disease and are poor surgical candidates. When radiotherapy is selected, it should begin promptly once the diagnosis of MESCC is established. Radiotherapy ports should include adjacent asymptomatic epidural deposits as well as the symptomatic MESCC. If these sites are untreated and the adjacent asymptomatic deposits become symptomatic, future radiotherapy may be compromised because of the radiotherapeutic problem of overlapping treatment field margins.

While the neurological prognosis depends in some measure on the primary tumor, the more important prognostic criterion is the level of neurological function at the beginning of radiotherapy. The proportion of patients who ambulate following radiotherapy declines from greater than 80% for patients who are ambulatory at the start of treatment to less than 50% for patients who are paraparetic at the initiation of treatment. Less than 10% of patients who are paraplegic eventually walk (2,57,58).

The role of surgery in the management of MESCC is evolving. Many retrospective (2,48,58,59) and one small prospective study (60) found no difference in neurological outcome between radiotherapy versus laminectomy followed by radiotherapy. Alternatively, laminectomy has been associated with a significant increase in morbidity, including spinal instability (58). However, the concept of decompressing the spinal cord from the effects of MESCC by removing tumor or bone rather than just enlarging the spinal canal by laminectomy is attractive. Since most cases of MESCC begin as metastases to the vertebral body, these principles and observations have led to the procedure of anterior decompression and stabilization, in carefully selected patients (61–63). Harrington (62) reported the results of this operation in 40 patients who had major neurological deficits preoperatively; 21 had complete neurological recovery postoperatively. Furthermore, of 13 plegic patients, seven had normal neurological examinations postoperatively. This surgical technique is difficult and carries a risk of major complications and thus should be performed only by experienced surgeons (32). Moreover, many patients are too debilitated from their underlying disease to permit major surgery even in the presence of vertebral collapse or instability with neurological compromise. Further studies are needed to determine the clinical and diagnostic imaging criteria that might be indications for surgery as initial therapy.

At present, the indications for surgical decompression of MESCC are controversial. Among patients whose general medical condition permits surgery, surgical decompression should be considered in (1) patients in whom the diagnosis of the spinal lesion is in doubt; (2) cases of symptomatic spinal instability or bone compression of neural structures; (3) patients with progressive neurological deterioration during radiation therapy; or (4) those who develop neurological deterioration due to MESCC at a previously irradiated level. Surgery also can be considered in patients with radioresistant tumors and intractable pain.

## II. INTRAMEDULLARY METASTASIS

Metastases to the substance of the spinal cord are rare and present difficult diagnostic and management problems. Grem and associates (64) found approximately 100 reported cases as of 1985. The risk of intramedullary metastases varies with the primary tumor. In a review of 55 cases culled from the literature (64), 49% were due to lung cancer. Breast cancer was next in frequency, accounting for 15%, followed by lymphoma (9%), colorectal (7%), head and neck (6%), renal cell (6%), and miscellaneous other neoplasms.

The spinal level of intramedullary spinal cord metastasis roughly corresponds to the length of spinal cord. Grem et al. (64) found the cervical region involved in 31%; the thoracic cord was the site in 42%; and the lumbar region accounted for 15%. The cervicothoracic and thoracolumbar areas accounted for the remaining cases.

The spinal cord at the level of the tumor may or may not be enlarged (65), which accounts for the lack of myelographic abnormalities often found in many cases. A metastasis may extend from one to several segments along the rostro-caudal axis.

The pathogenesis of metastasis to the spinal cord may be either by direct hematogenous spread to the cord or from leptomeningeal metastases with secondary extension into the spinal parenchyma. One pathological study reported nine of 13 cases were due to direct metastasis to the spinal cord and four cases resulting from extension from the subarachnoid space to the spinal parenchyma.

## A.  Clinical Features

As in the case of epidural metastases or leptomeningeal metastases from systemic cancer, intramedullary spinal cord metastases may herald the diagnosis of malignancy or develop years after the original diagnosis. The clinical manifestations of 55 cases reviewed by Grem and colleagues (64) are shown in Table 2. The most

**Table 2**  Neurological Manifestations at the Time of Initial Evaluation of 55 Patients with Intramedullary Spinal Cord Metastases

| Symptoms | Number of patients (%) |
|---|---|
| Pain | 34 (62) |
|    Nonradicular | 16 (29) |
|    Radicular | 18 (33) |
| Motor deficit | 35 (64) |
| Paresthesias | 15 (27) |
| Bowel/bladder dysfunction | 5 (9) |

| Signs | Number of patients (%) |
|---|---|
| Motor deficit | 55 (100) |
| Sensory level to pain, etc. | 27 (49) |
| Dermatomal sensory loss | 7 (13) |
| Paresthesias | 15 (27) |
| Atrophy of musculature | 3 (5) |
| Bowel/bladder dysfunction | 39 (71) |
| Upgoing toes | 17 (31) |
| Tenderness over spine | 4 (7) |
| Pain on straight-leg raising or neck flexion | 6 (12) |
| Horner's syndrome | 2 (4) |
| Completed neurological deficit | |
|    Flaccid paralysis | 25 (45) |
|    Spastic paresis/plegia | 5 (9) |
|    Brown/Séquard's syndrome | 6 (11) |

Source: Ref. 64.

frequent presenting complaints are pain and weakness. Paresthesias and sphincter dysfunction occurred in 27% and 9%, respectively, as presenting manifestations.

All 55 patients had weakness or paralysis on the initial examination. The motor weakness—which may be paraparesis, quadriparesis, monoparesis or hemiparesis—was asymmetric in half the patients. Sensory deficits were found in 64%, with a sensory level being present in 49%. Despite a low incidence of bowel and bladder symptoms, signs of sphincter disturbance were present in the majority (71%) by the time of diagnosis.

The temporal profile between the onset of symptoms and the development of the full neurological deficit was under 1 week in 22%, between 1 week and 1 month in 49%, and 5 weeks to 6 months in 24%. In 5% of cases the neurological syndrome developed over more than 6 months (64). Vertebral tenderness appears to be less common with intramedullary metastases than with MESCC. Intramedullary metastases usually develop in the setting of widespread metastatic visceral and CNS disease.

## B. Laboratory and Diagnostic Imaging Studies

Cerebrospinal fluid abnormalities are usually nonspecific, with the protein often elevated and a pleocytosis. In cases of leptomeningeal metastases with secondary invasion of the spinal cord, the CSF may contain malignant cells.

Diagnostic imaging studies are usually necessary to confirm the clinical impression. Myelography was the most important diagnostic study prior to development of MRI (45,66). Enhancement with gadolinium has been reported with MRI in cases of intramedullary metastases (44,67).

## C. Differential Diagnosis

When the cancer patient develops symptoms and signs of myelopathy and the diagnostic imaging workup fails to reveal an epidural metastasis, the physician is confronted with a difficult diagnostic problem. The differential diagnosis in such cases includes metastatic disease (e.g., leptomeningeal metastases, intramedullary spinal cord metastasis); complications of antineoplastic therapy (e.g., radiation myelopathy and myelopathy caused by intrathecal chemotherapy); paraneoplastic necrotizing myelopathy; and a cause unrelated to the cancer or its treatment, such as spondylosis or demyelinating disease. The clinical differentiation of intramedullary metastasis from radiation myelopathy, paraneoplastic necrotizing myelopathy, and leptomeningeal metastases can be a daunting task (see Table 3).

The various clinical syndromes of radiation myelopathy are more fully discussed in Chapter 10. Chronic progressive radiation myelopathy may be difficult to distinguish from intramedullary spinal cord metastasis. However, the tempo of

**Table 3** Clinical Neurological Manifestations of Differential Value in the Diagnosis of a Noncompressive Myelopathy in the Cancer Patient

| Myelopathy | Pain | Tempo progression of spinal disease | | Ascending or descending | Size of affected spinal segments as seen on myelogram | | | Tumor cells in CSF |
| --- | --- | --- | --- | --- | --- | --- | --- | --- |
| | | Subacute | Chronic | | Normal | Enlarged | Small | |
| Intramedullary spinal cord metastasis | + | + | – | + | + | + | – | – |
| Leptomeningeal metastases | + | + | – | NA | + | – | – | + |
| Radiation myelopathy | – | – | + | – | – | + | + | – |
| Necrotizing myelopathy | – | + | – | +/– | + | + | – | – |

CSF indicates cerebrospinal fluid; NA, not applicable; plus sign, present; minus sign, absent; and plus-minus sign, may be present or absent.

Source: Ref. 70.

evolution of intramedullary spinal cord metastasis is usually abrupt with a rapid progression (68). Radiation myelopathy may worsen abruptly but usually evolves over several months or years and may arrest at a stage of incomplete myelopathy.

The total dose, fractionation schedule, and specific radiation treatment field location are important in the diagnosis of radiation myelopathy. Consideration of the primary tumor also may help distinguish the risk (69). Head and neck cancer is the most frequent primary tumor in cases of radiation myelopathy—82% of cases according to one report (70)—whereas the most common tumors associated with intramedullary spinal cord metastasis are lung and breast cancer (70). In the irradiation of these latter primary malignancies, the spine does not usually receive radiation at doses sufficient to cause chronic progressive radiation myelopathy.

Intramedullary metastasis may be difficult to differentiate clinically from leptomeningeal metastases (see Table 3). While leptomeningeal metastases usually cause symptoms and signs at multiple levels throughout the neuraxis, the cauda equina syndrome caused by metastases to this site alone may be identical to the clinical presentation of an intramedullary metastasis to the conus medullaris. In leptomeningeal metastases, the CSF cytology is usually positive (27,71). Although enhanced MRI is insensitive in the evaluation of intramedullary tumors or leptomeningeal invasion of the cord (72), contrast-enhanced MRI is more sensitive (43,45). Because some patients develop intramedullary tumors secondary to leptomeningeal spread, the two may coexist (65).

Paraneoplastic necrotizing myelopathy is a very rare remote effect of cancer that is in the differential diagnosis of myelopathy in the cancer patient and must be differentiated from intramedullary spinal cord metastasis (73). Unlike intramedullary metastasis, paraneoplastic myelopathy does not cause local or radicular pain (74,75). Patients usually report vague, intermittent paresthesias in the lower extremities for weeks or months before an ascending transverse myelopathy develops. The thoracic spine is the most common initial site; the myelopathy then ascends and descends through the cord. Thus patients may initially have spastic paraplegia which is followed by flaccid, areflexic paraplegia (70). Radiological and CSF studies are nondiagnostic in paraneoplastic necrotizing myelopathy.

## D. Therapy

Since there are no large prospective studies of intramedullary metastases, management recommendations are based on anecdotal reports. Intramedullary metastases are often multiple or associated with intracerebral and/or leptomeningeal metastases and treatment should consider the full extent of central nervous system dissemination. Radiation therapy has been the primary treatment in most cases. The location and size of the radiation treatment field is determined by imaging studies, clinical involvement, and consideration of bone marrow tolerance. When leptomeningeal metastases are present, intrathecal chemotherapy also may be used. The prognosis for patients with intramedullary spinal cord metastasis is poor, with over 80% of patients dying within 3 months, usually due to uncontrolled systemic disease (64).

## REFERENCES

1. Barron KD, Hirano A, Araki S, et al. Experiences with metastatic neoplasms involving the spinal cord. Neurology 1959; 9:91–106.
2. Gilbert RW, Kim JH, Posner JB. Epidural spinal cord compression from metastatic tumor: diagnosis and treatment. Ann Neurol 1978; 3:40–51.
3. Byrne TN, Waxman SG. Spinal cord compression: diagnosis and principles of treatment. Contemporary Neurology Series. Philadelphia: F. A. Davis Co., 1990.
4. Batson OV. The function of the vertebral veins and their role in the spread of metastases. Ann Surg 1940; 112:138–148.
5. Coman DR, DeLong RP. The role of the vertebral venous system in the metastasis of cancer to the spinal column. Cancer 1951; 4:610–618.
6. Arguello F, Baggs RB, Duerst RE, et al. Pathogenesis of vertebral metastasis and epidural spinal cord compression. Cancer 1990; 65:98–106.
7. McAlhany HJ, Netsky MG. Compression of the spinal cord by extramedullary neoplasms: a clinical and pathological study. J Neuropathol Exp Neurol 1955; 14:276–287.
8. Hashizume Y, Iljima S, Kishimoto H, Hirano A. Pencil-shaped softening of the spinal cord: pathologic study in 12 cases. Acta Neuropathol (Berl) 1983; 61:219–224.
9. Hughes JT. Venous infarction of the spinal cord. Neurology 1971; 21:794–800.
10. Henson RA, Parsons M. Ischaemic lesions of the spinal cord: an illustrated review. Q J Med 1967; 36:205–222.
11. Al-Mefty O, Harkey LH, Middleton TH, Smith RR, Fox JL. Myelopathic cervical spondylotic lesions demonstrated by magnetic resonance imaging. J Neurosurg 1988; 68:217–222.
12. Elsberg CA. Surgical diseases of the spinal cord, membranes and nerve root. New York: Hoeber, 1941.
13. Ushio Y, Posner R, Posner JB, et al. Experimental spinal cord compression by epidural neoplasms. Neurology 1977; 27:422–429.
14. Siegal T, Siegal TZ, Sandbank U, et al. Experimental neoplastic spinal cord compression: evoked potentials, edema, prostaglandins, and light and electron microscopy. Spine 1987; 12:440–448.
15. Siegal T, Siegal TZ. Participation of serotonergic mechanisms in the pathophysiology of experimental neoplastic spinal cord compression. Neurology 1991; 41:574–580.
16. Grant R, Papadopoulos SM, Greenberg HS. Metastatic epidural spinal cord compression. Neurol Clin 1991; 9:825–841.
17. Stark RJ, Henson RA, Evans SJW. Spinal metastases: a retrospective survey from a general hospital. Brain 1982; 105:189–213.
18. Constans JP, De Divitiis E, Donzelli R, et al. Spinal metastases with neurological manifestations: review of 600 cases. J Neurosurg 1983; 59:111–118.

19. Klein SL, Sanford RA, Muhlbauer MS. Pediatric spinal epidural metastases. J Neurosurg 1991; 74:70–75.
20. Lewis DW, Packer RJ, Raney B, et al. Incidence, presentation, and outcome of spinal cord disease in children with systemic cancer. Pediatrics 1986; 78:438–442.
21. Weissman DE, Gilbert M, Wang H, et al. The use of computed tomography of the spine to identify patients at high risk for epidural metastases. J Clin Oncol 1985; 3:1541–1544.
22. Ruff RL, Lanska DJ. Epidural metastases in prospectively evaluated veterans with cancer and back pain. Cancer 1989; 63:2234–2241.
23. O'Rourke T, George CB, Redmond J, et al. Spinal computed tomography and computed tomographic metrizamide myelography in the early diagnosis of metastatic disease. J Clin Oncol 1986; 4:576–583.
24. Bernat JL, Greenberg ER, Barrett J. Suspected epidural compression of the spinal cord and cauda equina by metastatic carcinoma. Cancer 1983; 51:1951–1957.
25. Levitt P, Ransohoff J, Spielholz N. The differential diagnosis of tumors of the conus medullaris and cauda equina. In: Vinken PJ, Bruyn GW, eds. Handbook of clinical neurology. Vol. 19. Amsterdam: North-Holland Publishing Co., 1975:77–90.
26. Norstrom CW, Kernohan JW, Love JG. One hundred primary caudal tumors. JAMA 1961; 178:1071–1077.
27. Bleyer WA, Byrne TN. Leptomeningeal cancer in leukemia and solid tumors. Curr Probl Cancer 1988; 12:185–238.
28. Hollis PH, Malis LI, Zappulla RA. Neurological deterioration after lumbar puncture below complete spinal subarachnoid block. J Neurosurg 1986; 64:253–256.
29. Eaton LM, Craig WM. Tumor of the spinal cord: sudden paralysis following lumbar puncture. Proc Staff Meet Mayo Clin 1940; 15:170–172.
30. Jooma R, Hayward RD. Upward spinal coning: impaction of occult spinal tumors following relief of hydrocephalus. J Neurol Neurosurg Psychiatry 1984; 47:386–390.
31. Rodichok LD, Ruckdeschel JC, Harper GR, et al. Early detection and treatment of spinal epidural metastases: the role of myelography. Ann Neurol 1986; 20:696–702.
32. Harrington KD. Anterior decompression and stabilization of the spine as a treatment for vertebral body collapse and spinal cord compression from metastatic malignancy. Clin Orthop 1988; 233:177–197.
33. Rodriguez M, Dinapoli RP. Spinal cord compression: with special reference to metastatic epidural tumors. Mayo Clin Proc 1980; 55:442–448.
34. Haddad P, Thaell JF, Kiely JM, et al. Lymphoma of the spinal extradural space. Cancer 1976; 38:1862–1866.
35. Rodichok LD, Harper GR, Ruckdeschel JC, et al. Early diagnosis of spinal epidural metastases. Am J Med 1981; 70:1181–1188.
36. Portenoy RK, Galer BS, Salamon O, et al. Identification of epidural neoplasm: radiography and bone scintigraphy in the symptomatic and asymptomatic spine. Cancer 1989; 64:2207–2213.
37. Graus F, Krol G, Foley KM. Early diagnosis of spinal epidural metastases (SEM): correlation with clinical and radiological findings. Proc Am Soc Clin Oncol 1985; 4:269.
38. Redmond J, Freidl KE, Cornett P, Stone M, O'Rourke T, George CB. Clinical

usefulness of an algorithm for the early diagnosis of spinal metastatic disease. J Clin Oncol 1988; 6:154–157.
39. Carmody RF, Yang PJ, Seeley GW, et al. Spinal cord compression due to metastatic disease: diagnosis with MR imaging versus myelography. Radiology 1989; 173: 225–229.
40. Smoker WRK, Godersky JC, Knutzon RK, Keyes WD, Norman D, Bergman W. The role of MR imaging in evaluating metastatic spinal disease. AJR Am J Roentgenol 1987; 149:1241–1248.
41. Li KC, Poon PY. Sensitivity and specificity of MRI in detecting malignant spinal cord compression and in distinguishing malignant from benign compression fractures of vertebrae. Magn Reson Imaging 1988; 6:547–556.
42. Zimmerman RA, Bilaniuk LT. Imaging of tumors of the spinal canal and cord. Radiol Clin North Am 1988; 26:965–1007.
43. Sze G, Abramson A, Krol G, et al. Gadolinium-DTPA in the evaluation of intradural extramedullary spinal disease. AJNR 1988; 9:153–163.
44. Sze G. Gadolinium-DTPA in spinal disease. Radiol Clin North Am 1988; 26:1009–1024.
45. Sze G, Krol G, Zimmerman RD, Deck MDF. Intramedullary disease of the spine: diagnosis using gadolinium-DTPA-enhanced MR imaging. AJNR 1988; 9:847–858.
46. Sze G, Krol G, Zimmerman RD, Deck MDF. Gadolinium-DTPA: malignant extradural spinal tumors. Radiology 1988; 167:217–223.
47. Byrne TN. Spinal cord compression from epidural metastases. N Engl J Med 1992; 327:614–619.
48. Posner JB. Back pain and epidural spinal cord compression. Med Clin North Am 1987; 71:185–204.
49. Portenoy R, Lipton RB, Foley KM. Back pain in the cancer patient: an algorithm for the evaluation and management. Neurology 1987; 37:134–137.
50. Calkins AR, Olson MA, Ellis JH. Impact of myelography on the radiotherapeutic management of malignant spinal cord compression. Neurosurgery 1986; 19:614–616.
51. Kim RY, Spencer SA, Meredith RF, et al. Extradural spinal cord compression: analysis of factors determining functional prognosis—prospective study. Radiology 1990; 176:279–282.
52. Manabe S, Tanaka H, Higo Y, et al. Experimental analysis of the spinal cord compressed by spinal metastases. Spine 1989; 14:1308–1315.
53. Posner JB, Howieson J, Cvitkovic E. "Disappearing" spinal cord compression: oncolytic effect of glucocorticoids (and other chemotherapeutic agents) on epidural metastases. Ann Neurol 1977; 2:409–413.
54. Weissman DE. Glucocorticoid treatment for brain metastases and epidural spinal cord compression: a review. J Clin Oncol 1988; 6:543–551.
55. Vecht CHJ, Haaxma-Reiche H, van Putten WLJ, et al. Initial bolus of conventional versus high-dose dexamethasone in metastatic spinal cord compression. Neurology 1989; 39:1255–1257.
56. Delattre JY, Arbit E, Thaler HT, et al. A dose-response study of dexamethasone in a model of spinal cord compression caused by epidural tumor. J Neurosurg 1989; 70: 920–925.

57. Greenberg HS, Kim J-H, Posner JB. Epidural spinal cord compression from metastatic tumor: results with a new treatment protocol. Ann Neurol 1980; 8:361–366.
58. Findlay GFG. Adverse effects of the management of malignant spinal cord compression. J Neurol Neurosurg Psychiatry 1984; 47:761–768.
59. Siegal T, Siegal TZ. Current considerations in the management of neoplastic spinal cord compression. Spine 1989; 14:223–228.
60. Young RF, Post EM, King GA. Treatment of spinal epidural metastases: randomized prospective comparison of laminectomy and radiotherapy. J Neurosurg 1980; 53:741–748.
61. Sundarasen N, DiGiacinto GV, Krol G, Hughes JEO. Spondylectomy for malignant tumors of the spine. J Clin Oncol 1989; 7:1485–1491.
62. Harrington KD. Anterior cord decompression and spinal stabilization for patients with metastatic lesions of the spine. J Neurosurg 1984; 61:107–117.
63. Siegal T, Siegal T. Surgical decompression of anterior and posterior malignant epidural tumors compressing the spinal cord: a prospective study. Neurosurgery 1985; 17:424–432.
64. Grem JL, Burgess J, Trump DL. Clinical features and natural history of intramedullary spinal cord metastasis. Cancer 1985; 56:2305–2314.
65. Costigan DA, Winkelman MD. Intramedullary spinal cord metastasis: a clinicopathological study of 13 cases. J Neurosurg 1985; 62:227–233.
66. Scientific Affair Council. Magnetic resonance imaging of the central nervous system. JAMA 1988; 259:1211–1222.
67. Fredericks RK, Elster A, Walker FO. Gadolinium-enhanced MRI: a superior technique for the diagnosis of intraspinal metastases. Neurology 1989; 39:734–736.
68. Edelson RN, Deck MDF, Posner JB. Intramedullary spinal cord metastases: clinical and radiological findings in 9 cases. Neurology 1972; 22:1222–1231.
69. Kagan AR, Wollin M, Gilbert HA, et al. Comparison of the tolerance of the brain and spinal cord to injury by radiations. In: Gilbert HA, Kagan AR, eds. Radiation damage to the nervous system. New York: Raven Press, 1980:183–190.
70. Winkelman MD, Adelstein DJ, Karlins NL. Intramedullary spinal cord metastasis: diagnostic and therapeutic considerations. Arch Neurol 1987; 44:526–531.
71. Grogan, JP, Daniels DL, Williams AL, et al. The normal conus medullaris: CT criteria for recognition. Radiology 1984; 151:661–664.
72. Barloon TJ, Yuh WTC, Yang CJC, Schultz DH. Spinal subarachnoid tumor seeding from intracranial metastasis: MR findings. J Comput Assist Tomogr 1987; 11:242–244.
73. Mancall EL, Remedios KR. Necrotizing myelopathy associated with visceral carcinoma. Brain 1964; 87:639–655.
74. Handforth A, Nag S, Sharp D, et al. Paraneoplastic subacute necrotic myelopathy. Can J Neurol Sci 1983; 10:204–207.
75. Ojeda VJ. Necrotising myelopathy associated with malignancy: a clinicopathological study of two cases and literature review. Cancer 1984; 53:1115–1123.

# 3

# Leptomeningeal Metastases

## William R. Wasserstrom

*Robert Wood Johnson Medical School, New Brunswick, New Jersey*

## I. BACKGROUND

Leptomeningeal metastases are an important form of diffuse or multifocal tumor infiltration of pial and arachnoidal membranes enveloping brain, spinal cord, and spinal roots. The primary neoplasm may be a carcinoma, sarcoma, melanoma, leukemia, or lymphoma. Probably first described by Eberth in the late nineteenth century, meningeal infiltration was not initially recognized as a form of metastatic complication of cancer; rather, it was thought to be a coexistent primary "endothelioma" of the leptomeninges in a patient with a known lung carcinoma (1). Later cases reported in German and English in the early 20th century began to recognize metastatic spread to the leptomeninges from distant extraneural primaries, particularly stomach but also breast, lung, and other gastrointestinal primaries (2,3). First termed "meningeal carcinomatosis" by Beerman in 1912 (4), numerous case reports appeared over the next half century, most of which emphasized the rarity of this type of cancer metastasis, the singularly poor prognosis, and the infrequency of antemortem discovery (5,6). By 1974, with almost 250 cases reported, Olson et al. (7) suggested that the disease may not be as rare as previously thought and might in fact be diagnosed in life by careful history, physical examination, and appropriate diagnostic studies. Leptomeningeal metastases now are recognized as an important form of metastatic dissemination to the central nervous system. Although precise epidemiological studies are lacking, the incidence of leptomeningeal metastases appears to be increasing, at least in certain tumor types, as systemic treatment of neoplasms improves. Treatment protocols designed to treat leptomeningeal disease per se have been established, but effective treatment remains an elusive and ongoing challenge for medical and neurological oncologists.

## II. PATHOLOGY

The gross inspection of brain, spinal cord, and spinal roots in leptomeningeal metastases is variable. In milder cases, the nervous system may appear grossly normal. In some cases, the leptomeninges has a thickened, fibrotic, opacified appearance, which may be seen adjacent to blood vessels. In some cases, disease may be confined to brain leptomeninges or only the spinal cord or roots may be involved. Most often, the entire central nervous system (CNS) is involved in a diffuse or multifocal fashion. If spinal roots are involved, they may be thickened with beaded nodules separated by intervening tumor-free areas. A predilection for certain areas of the nervous system seems clear in many cases. Tumor frequently concentrates in basal cisterns enveloping the base of the brain (Fig. 1). Tumor may extend rostrally to the optic chiasm and infundibular areas through the cisterns to the Sylvian fissures and over the cerebral convexities (Fig. 2). Hydrocephalus may appear by virtue of obstruction of the cerebrospinal fluid (CSF) pathways at the level of the basal cisterns. Leptomeningeal tumor around the brainstem may infiltrate cranial nerves. Tumor often extends caudally over the surface of the spinal cord with a proclivity for the posterior surface. Exiting spinal roots may be encased. Tumor cells accumulate in areas where there is relative stasis of CSF flow, where subarachnoid channels are lined by culs-de-sac and weblike membranes (such as the basal cisterns, hippocampal sulci, and cauda equina). Tumor cell growth is less frequent on smooth membranes and in areas of rapid CSF flow (such as the aqueduct or ventricles).

The essential histological finding is diffuse or multifocal infiltration of pia mater and arachnoid membranes by neoplasm filling the subarachnoid space with cancer cells (Fig. 3). Extension of tumor infiltration into the perivascular spaces of Virchow and Robin and the periradicular sleeves of cranial nerves and spinal nerve roots is common. The latter may be seen as diffuse nodular infiltrates of intradural nerve roots. Cancer cells may grow in layers or glandular formations along the pial and arachnoid surfaces with a tendency to concentrate around penetrating blood vessels and nerve roots. Tumor appears bound to the underlying meningeal membranes, which provide a medium for growth and spread of tumor. Tumor cells concentrate microscopically in the same areas seen grossly, mainly the basilar cisterns, chiasmal-infundibular area, parahippocampal sulci, cerebellar pontine angle cisterns, ambient cisterns, and quadrigeminal cisterns. Tumor may ensheathe penetrating meningeal arteries and veins, forming perivascular cuffs that

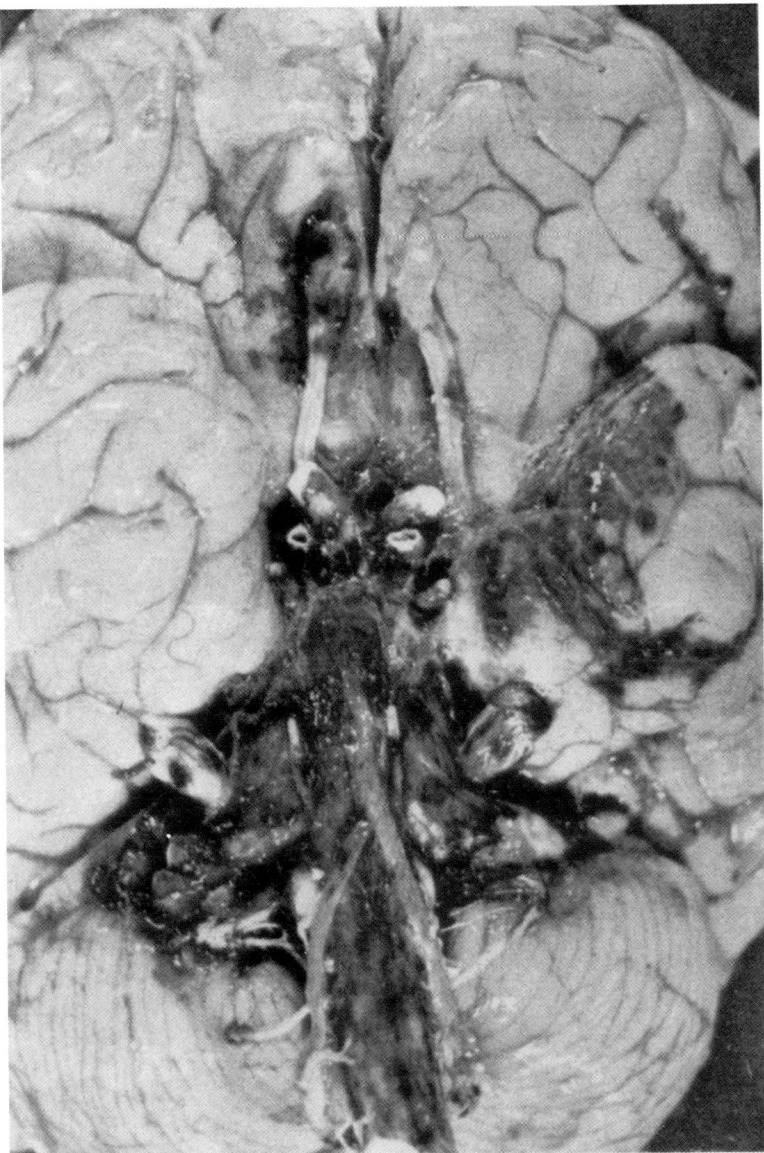

**Figure 1** Anterior surface of the brain showing tumor concentrated in the basal cisterns extending to the optic chiasm and cistern of the Sylvian fissure in a patient with metastatic malignant melanoma. (Reprinted from Arch Neurol 1974; 30:122–137.)

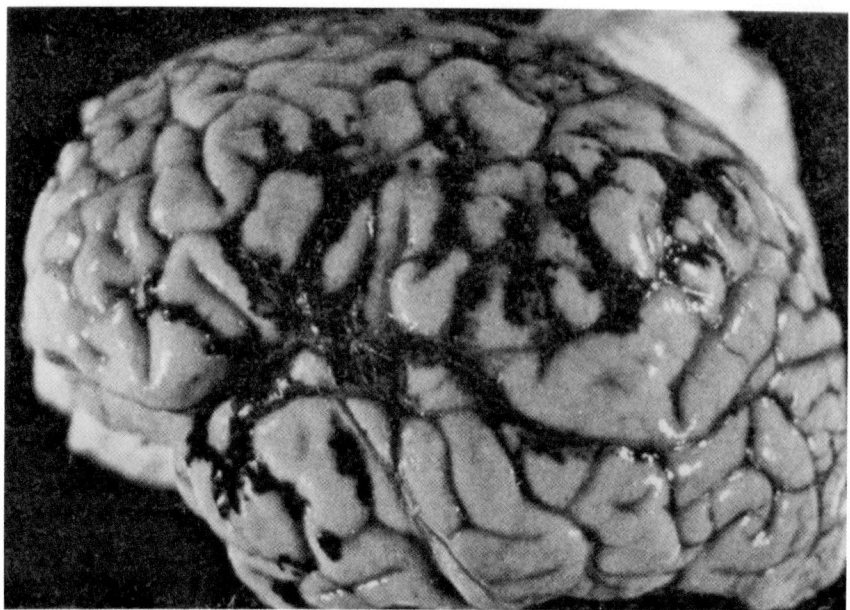

**Figure 2** Lateral view of cerebral hemisphere with tumor concentrated in Sylvian fissure and communicating sulci over the brain surface in a patient with malignant melanoma. (Reprinted from Arch Neurol 1974; 30:122–137.)

extend into the brain and spinal cord parenchyma through the pial membrane. Tumor may grow along brain and spinal cord surfaces encasing perineurium of spinal and cranial nerves. Affected nerves may undergo demyelination and eventually axonal degeneration. Meningeal fibrosis with a mild round cell inflammatory reaction is sometimes present. If the leptomeninges are seeded focally, this fibrotic reaction may wall off the tumor preventing further propagation. If this fibrotic reaction does not occur, tumor cells can spread throughout the subarachnoid space, usually coming to rest and growing along the membranes forming the walls of subarachnoid channels in a linear or multifocal nodular pattern. If the tumor is more than a few cells thick, neovascularization occurs. The new vessels are fenestrated capillaries, which have no blood-brain barrier, a finding of potential therapeutic importance.

## III. PATHOGENESIS

The mechanism by which cancer metastases reach the pia-arachnoid surfaces is still speculative. Knierim in 1908 found direct infiltration of tumor cells from a

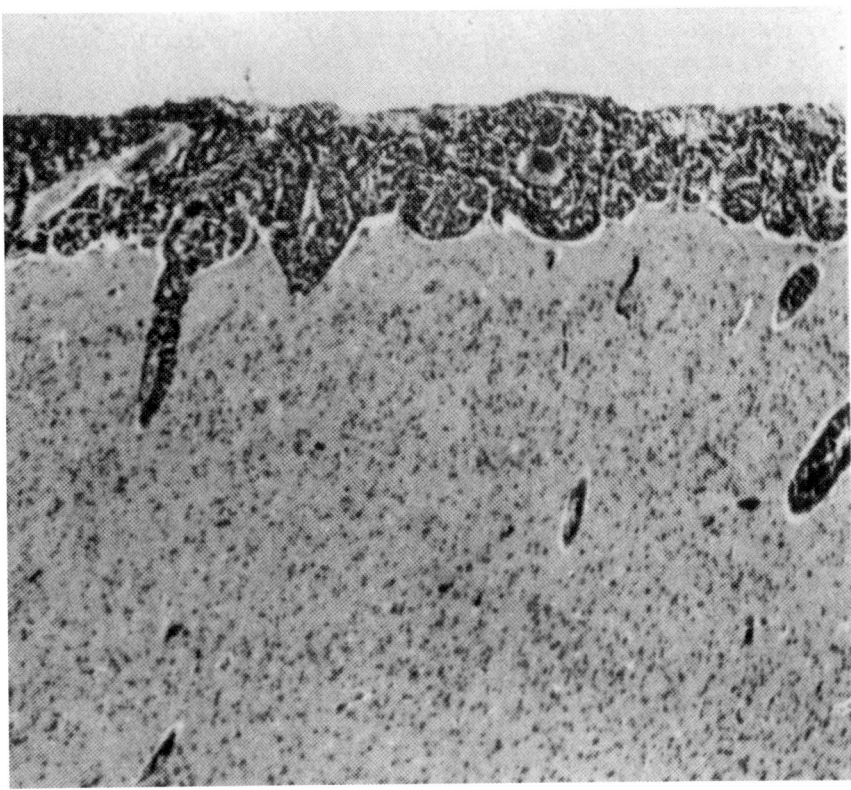

**Figure 3** Microscopic infiltration of pia and arachnoid membranes obliterating underlying architecture of the meninges. Tumor encases meningeal vessels and continues within the perivascular space of the penetrating vessels (hematoxylin-eosin, original magnification ×25). (Reprinted from Arch Neurol 1974; 30:122–137.)

gastric carcinoma along perineural and endoneural lymphatics of spinal nerves and ganglia. He concluded that this was the route taken by tumor to invade the spinal leptomeninges (8). Since that time, others have speculated on different mechanisms. Cancers likely reach the leptomeninges in several ways, perhaps depending on tumor type. In acute leukemias, leukemic cells may enter the leptomeninges via thin-walled microscopic veins in the arachnoid membrane. The studies of Price and Johnson (9) have demonstrated that CNS leukemia is primarily a perivascular arachnoidal disease. The earliest evidence of leukemia is detected in the walls of superficial arachnoid veins. Then, leukemic infiltrates extend to the deep perivascular spaces confined by the pia-glial membrane. Depending on the severity of arachnoidal involvement, transgression of the pia-glial membrane then occurs with varying degrees of parenchymal infiltration by collections of leukemic cells.

In at least some cases of breast and lung cancer metastases, tumor cells may reach the leptomeningeal surfaces by extension from vertebral and paravertebral metastases (10). Tumor in vertebral bone marrow or other tissue near the spinal canal may spread along perivascular spaces of intravertebral veins or paravertebral venous plexuses. Tumor growth may then extend through the dural and arachnoidal sleeves of nerve roots joined to the subarachnoid space. In some cases of cancers from gastrointestinal primaries, infiltration of perineural spaces of spinal nerves is the path for eventual dissemination into the subarachnoid space (10). The study of Gonzales-Vitale and Garcia-Bunuel (11) infers that most cases of tumor reach the leptomeninges from axial lymph nodes and blood vessels through intervertebral and possibly cranial foramina via perineural and perivascular pathways to the leptomeninges.

Rupture of brain metastases into the cerebral ventricles and subarachnoid space has been proposed as an alternative mechanism but is likely infrequent and may only apply to those few cases in which deep parenchymal metastases coexist with leptomeningeal metastases. Hematogenous metastases to the choroid plexus with escape into the cerebrospinal fluid and metastatic spread via Batson's venous plexus also are likely to be rare. Tumors believed to spread in this fashion (prostatic adenocarcinoma) rarely invade the leptomeninges. Hematogenous spread of tumor to the arachnoid itself, although important in acute leukemia, may not be as common in solid tumors. Kokkoris (10) found no tumor within leptomeningeal vessels of patients with solid tumor primaries and Gonzales-Vitale (11) found only a rare such example.

## IV. CLINICAL FINDINGS

Clinical signs and symptoms parallel the pathological findings (7). Because the disease is manifested by diffuse and multifocal seeding of the leptomeninges, a multiplicity of signs and symptoms are usually present. Signs may initially predominate over symptoms. Therefore, a careful and thorough neurological examination is mandatory. Virtually any system malignancy has the potential to metastasize to the leptomeninges. Leukemias (particularly acute lymphoblastic leukemia and to a lesser extent acute myelogenous leukemia), lymphomas (particularly intermediate and high-grade non-Hodgkin's lymphomas), and certain solid tumors (breast carcinoma, lung carcinoma, and malignant melanoma) are the most common causes of neoplastic meningitis. Gastric carcinoma, the most common primary tumor described in the early literature, is now relatively rare, likely a reflection of reduced incidence of this tumor in western civilizations. Adenocarcinomas predominate over other types of carcinomas. Age and gender appear to reflect the primary tumor type. In a large autopsy series, leptomeningeal metastases accounted for 4% of metastatic disease to the central nervous system (12). The incidence of leptomeningeal metastases is increasing, particularly with the enhanced longevity associated with improved systemic therapies for some tumors. This observation was initially made in the early 1970s in children with acute lymphoblastic leukemia (ALL) (13–15). As chemotherapy for the systemic illness became more effective, leukemic meningitis, once considered a rare complication, appeared with increasing frequency, such that 50% of the children treated for ALL developed leptomeningeal metastases. A similar phenomenon has occurred with myelogenous leukemias, as well as certain histological subtypes of lymphomas (16–19). Other solid tumors, such as breast carcinoma (20), small cell lung carcinoma (21), ovarian carcinoma (22), sarcomas (23), and genitourinary tract carcinomas (24) seem to be following the same pattern.

Leptomeningeal metastases usually are a late complication of systemic cancers. The metastases tend to occur 6 months to 3 years after the primary tumor is discovered. However, in approximately 5–8% of cases (25) and perhaps as high as 11% (26), meningeal involvement is the presenting manifestation of malignancy. Only after the leptomeningeal tumor is discovered does the primary cancer become evident. In some cases, there is a long interval between the discovery of the primary tumor and the leptomeningeal relapse (up to 10 years or more with breast carcinoma and malignant melanoma). Leptomeningeal metastases usually occur in association with active disease outside the central nervous system. However, tumor occasionally appears confined to the leptomeninges. Leptomeningeal metastases may occur with or without other sites or types of CNS metastases.

The clinical diagnosis of leptomeningeal metastases rests on finding focal neurological signs and symptoms involving more than one level of the neuraxis (25). Although signs and symptoms may be confined initially to one anatomical area, multiple levels of the neuraxis become involved as the disease progresses. In the cerebrum, headache and change in mental status are the most common symptoms. Headache is often bifrontal and bioccipital, with nuchal radiation, and may have characteristics associated with increased intracranial pressure such as nausea, vomiting, and lightheadedness. Lethargy, confusion, and memory loss are common. Focal cerebral signs and symptoms, including focal seizures, aphasia, hemiparesis, papilledema and wide-based ataxic gait can occur but are less common (25). Table 1 shows cerebral findings in 90 patients with leptomeningeal metastases from solid tumor primaries.

Cranial nerve signs and symptoms are the result of infiltration of cranial nerves by leptomeningeal tumor. Diplopia, the result of involvement of sixth, third, or fourth cranial nerves, is the most common finding. A sixth nerve palsy in a cancer patient should arouse suspicion of leptomeningeal neoplasm. Facial weakness and facial numbness due to involvement of seventh and fifth cranial nerves occur next most frequently. Subacute blindness and diminished hearing are less common. Diminished visual acuity may occur as a result of infiltration of optic nerves and

**Table 1** Cerebral Symptoms and Signs in 90-Patient Series of Leptomeningeal Metastases from Solid Tumors

| Symptoms | | Signs | |
|---|---|---|---|
| Headache | 30 | Mental change | 28 |
| Mental change | 15 | Seizures | 5 |
| Difficulty walking | 12 |    Generalized | 3 |
| Nausea/vomiting | 10 |    Focal | 2 |
| Unconsciousness | 2 | Papilledema | 5 |
| Dysphasia | 2 | Diabetes insipidus | 2 |
| Dizziness | 2 | Hemiparesis | 1 |
| | | Total: 45 Patients | |

Reprinted from Cancer 1982; 49:759–772.

optic chiasm by leptomeningeal tumor. Table 2 shows cranial nerve findings and solid tumor metastases in the 90-patient series.

Spinal cord and spinal root signs and symptoms are common and predicted by the pathological findings. Segmental weakness, paresthesia, or radicular pain affecting the legs usually conform to one or multiple lumbosacral nerve roots. A partial or complete cauda equina syndrome is seen in at least one-third of patients initially. Bowel and bladder dysfunction occur when sacral roots are involved. Neck and back pain are often present (27). Careful clinical examination reveals asymmetrical reflex changes, segmental weakness and sensory changes, often

**Table 2** Cranial Nerve Symptoms and Signs in 90-Patient Series of Leptomeningeal Metastases from Solid Tumors

| Symptoms | | Signs | |
|---|---|---|---|
| Diplopia | 18 | Ocular muscle paresis (III, IV, VI) | 18 |
| Hearing loss | 7 | Facial weakness (VII) | 15 |
| Visual loss | 5 | Diminished hearing (VIII) | 9 |
| Facial numbness | 5 | Optic neuropathy (II) | 5 |
| Decreased taste | 3 | Trigeminal neuropathy (V) | 5 |
| Tinnitus | 2 | Hypoglossal neuropathy (XII) | 5 |
| Hoarseness | 2 | Blindness | 3 |
| Dysphagia | 1 | Diminished gag (IX, X) | 3 |
| Vertigo | 1 | | |
| | | Total: 50 Patients | |

Reprinted from Cancer 1982; 49:759–772.

**Table 3** Spinal Symptoms and Signs in 90-Patient Series of Patients with Leptomeningeal Metastases from Solid Tumors

| Symptoms | | Signs | |
|---|---|---|---|
| Lower motor neuron weakness | 34 | Reflex asymmetry | 64 |
| Paresthesias | 31 | Weakness | 54 |
| Radicular pain | 19 | Sensory loss | 24 |
| Back/neck pain | 23 | Straight-leg raising | 11 |
| Bowel/bladder dysfunction | 12 | Decreased rectal tone | 10 |
| | | Nuchal rigidity | 7 |
| Total: 74 Patients | | | |

Reprinted from Cancer 1982; 49:759–772.

with laxity of the rectal sphincter. Signs of meningeal irritation, including nuchal rigidity and positive straight-leg raising tests, are present in a minority of patients. Table 3 shows spinal findings in solid tumor metastases.

The multiplicity of signs and symptoms affecting more than one level of the neuraxis suggests the diagnosis (7,25,27). Although similar findings may occur with multiple parenchymal metastases or epidural spinal cord or cauda equina metastases, this pattern should evoke a high index of suspicion. In some patients, signs and symptoms may be confined to one level of the neuraxis on initial presentation but eventually other areas become involved as the disease progresses. In some patients, focal findings are absent initially only to emerge with time.

The natural history of the disease is inexorably progressive. As the tumor grows within the subarachnoid space and within penetrating vessels of the brain and spinal cord parenchyma, patients experience increasing signs and symptoms. The literature suggests that untreated patients survive 1 to 3 months (28,29). Spontaneous stabilization is rare, although an occasional patient has been reported to survive 6 to 12 months with indolent tumor.

## V. DIAGNOSTIC STUDIES

### A. Cerebrospinal Fluid Examination

Examination of cerebrospinal fluid by lumbar puncture is the most important diagnostic study. The cerebrospinal fluid profile varies from patient to patient depending on the degree of leptomeningeal infiltration. Most patients have some CSF abnormality. Approximately 50% of patients have elevated cerebrospinal fluid pressure (over 180 mm) with pressures often as high as 400–500 mm. A significant number of patients have a CSF pleocytosis with predominantly mononuclear cells, most of which are lymphocytes presumably reactive to tumor in the leptomeninges. Occasional polymorphonuclear leukocytes are seen. In some patients, normal numbers of cells are seen (less than 6 white blood cells per cubic millimeter [WBC/mm$^3$]) while some may have a pleocytosis as high as 1800–2000 white blood cells. Protein may be normal but generally is elevated in more than 80% of cases (7,25) and may be as high as 2500 mg/dl. Cerebrospinal fluid glucose is depressed in approximately 30% of patients with glucose concentrations as low as 2 mg/dl. Hypoglycorrhachia may result from decreased transport of glucose into the CSF or increased utilization of glucose by malignant cells in the leptomeninges. Cerebrospinal fluid lactate levels are inversely related to CSF glucose levels, suggesting increased glycolysis by tumor in the leptomeninges with accumulation of lactate (the end product) in the CSF (25).

Malignant cells in the cerebrospinal fluid occur in approximately 90% of patients, although multiple samples of CSF are often needed. First described by Stadelmann in 1908 (30), malignant cells are found in cerebrospinal fluid specimens in 55–60% of patients on initial lumbar puncture. With repeated sampling, 90% of patients have at least one positive cytology. In 8–10% of patients, cytological examination remains normal despite multiple taps suggesting that cells remain adherent to the pia-arachnoid surfaces without desquamating into the CSF. The study of Glass et al. (31) infers that malignant cells in the cerebrospinal fluid indicate widespread leptomeningeal metastases. The more extensive the disease, the more likely cells will be recovered in the CSF. The study of Bigner and Johnston (32) confirms this impression. Spinal subarachnoid hemorrhage in a cancer patient also may indicate widespread leptomeningeal metastases (33).

Variations in cerebrospinal fluid composition at different levels of the CSF pathways has been observed with leptomeningeal metastases (34). This finding is likely the result of focal disruption of the blood-CSF barrier by the meningeal neoplasm. Evaluation of cisternal or ventricular CSF may occasionally yield positive cytology when lumbar CSF is negative in patients with primarily cerebral or cranial nerve manifestations. The use of monoclonal antibody immunocytology may improve the diagnostic sensitivity of CSF cytology in some laboratories (35) and may have advantages over conventional cytological techniques (36). The contribution of such techniques, however, has been disputed (37). The site and nature of the primary tumor may be inferred in some cases in which immunocytology is utilized (35).

Cerebrospinal fluid tumor markers (such as carcinoembryonic antigen, beta glucuronidase, beta 2 microglobulin, lactic dehydrogenase isoenzymes, and HMFG1 antigen, among others) have also been widely studied (38–44). These markers appear sensitive for certain tumors infiltrating the leptomeninges. Elevated concentrations in nonmalignant leptomeningeal inflammations, however, limit the diagnostic usefulness of these markers (45). The exact clinical role of these markers remains to be proven; a likely use will be as prognosticators or indicators of disease activity in patients aggressively treated (46). A suggestion that such markers may be early predictors of leptomeningeal metastases is speculative (41).

## B. Radiographic Studies

Gadolinium-enhanced magnetic resonance imaging (MRI) of the brain shows abnormal enhancement of leptomeningeal surfaces adjacent to the inner table of the skull in approximately two-thirds of patients studied with leptomeningeal metastases (47). This technique appears superior to contrast-enhanced computed tomography (CT) of the brain, which also reveals abnormalities in a smaller percentage of patients. Unenhanced MRI does not show advantage over CT (48). Similar meningeal enhancement appears on MR imaging in other nonmalignant inflammatory diseases of the leptomeninges (49). Nodular enhancement of tumor along cerebral sulci or basal cisterns may be seen by enhanced MRI scans as well as contrast-enhanced CT scans (Figs. 4 and 5). Communicating hydrocephalus is present in some patients and suggests occlusion of the subarachnoid absorptive pathways by leptomeningeal tumor. Enhancement in the basal cisterns or along cerebral sulci in the absence of clearly established infectious meningitis suggests tumor in the leptomeninges in patients with known neoplastic disease. In some patients, MRI or CT scan may be normal or may show other findings, such as parenchymal metastases, subdural effusions, or other nonmetastatic complications.

Myelography is of benefit in some patients who have spinal root or spinal cord signs and symptoms. Irregular filling defects in the subarachnoid space due to thickening and nodularity of cauda equina nerve roots is seen in 25% of patients studied (25,50,51) (Fig. 6). Contrasted MR imaging of the spine may uniquely visualize subarachnoid disease in some patients (51), but unenhanced spinal MRI is less sensitive (48,51).

In an occasional patient with symptoms suggesting cerebral vascular disease, cerebral angiography may show irregular narrowing of arteries at the base of the brain, due to either spasm of pial vessels or infiltration of their walls by leptomeningeal neoplasm. In other patients without symptoms of vascular events, cerebral angiograms are normal and of limited value.

## VI. DIFFERENTIAL DIAGNOSIS

The differential diagnosis includes other subacute and chronic meningitides, including tuberculous, fungal, sarcoid, syphilitic, and perhaps Lyme meningitis. These infectious meningitides are generally distinguished by appropriate smear and culture studies. Systemic clinical signs and symptoms and serological tests for syphilis, cryptococcus, and Lyme disease generally distinguish these entities from leptomeningeal metastases. Chest radiograph and serum angiotensin-converting

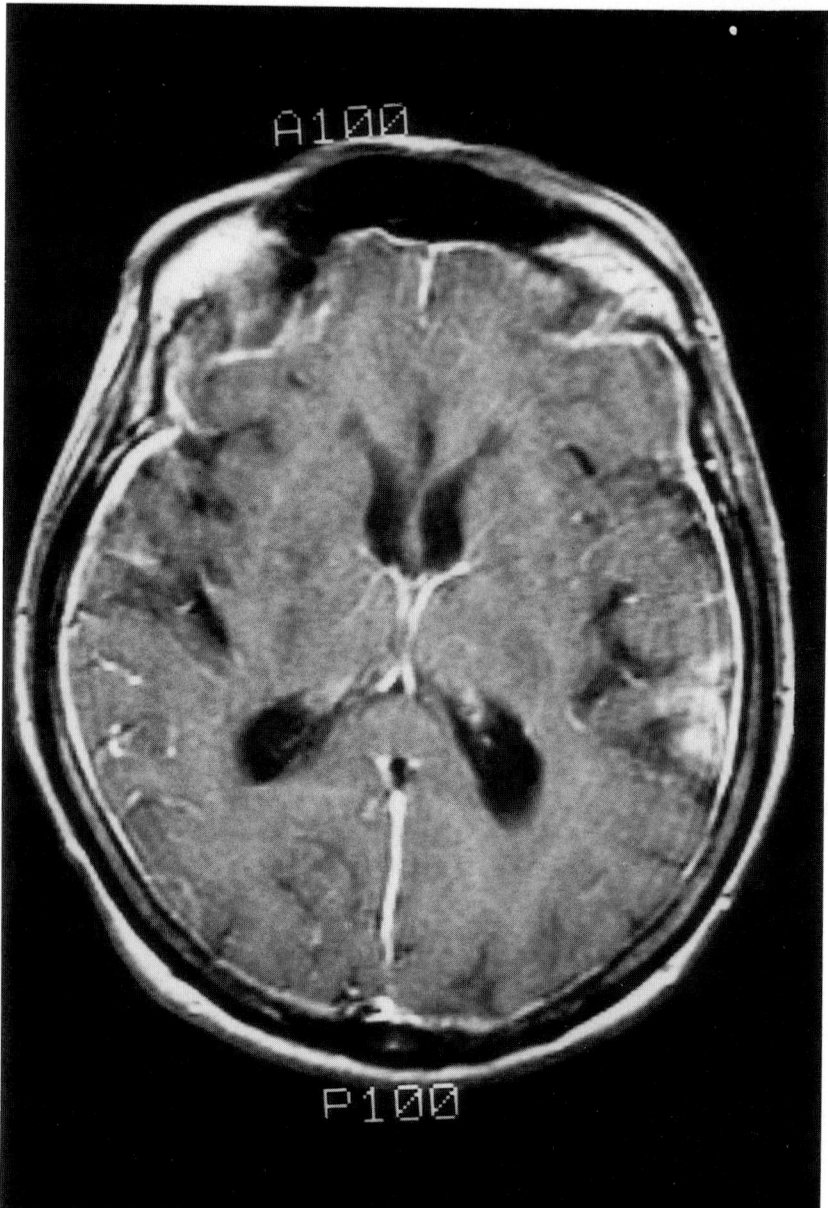

**Figure 4** Magnetic resonance image in a patient with breast cancer showing intense meningeal enhancement in a para-Sylvian location. (Radiograph courtesy of Dr. Howard Lee.)

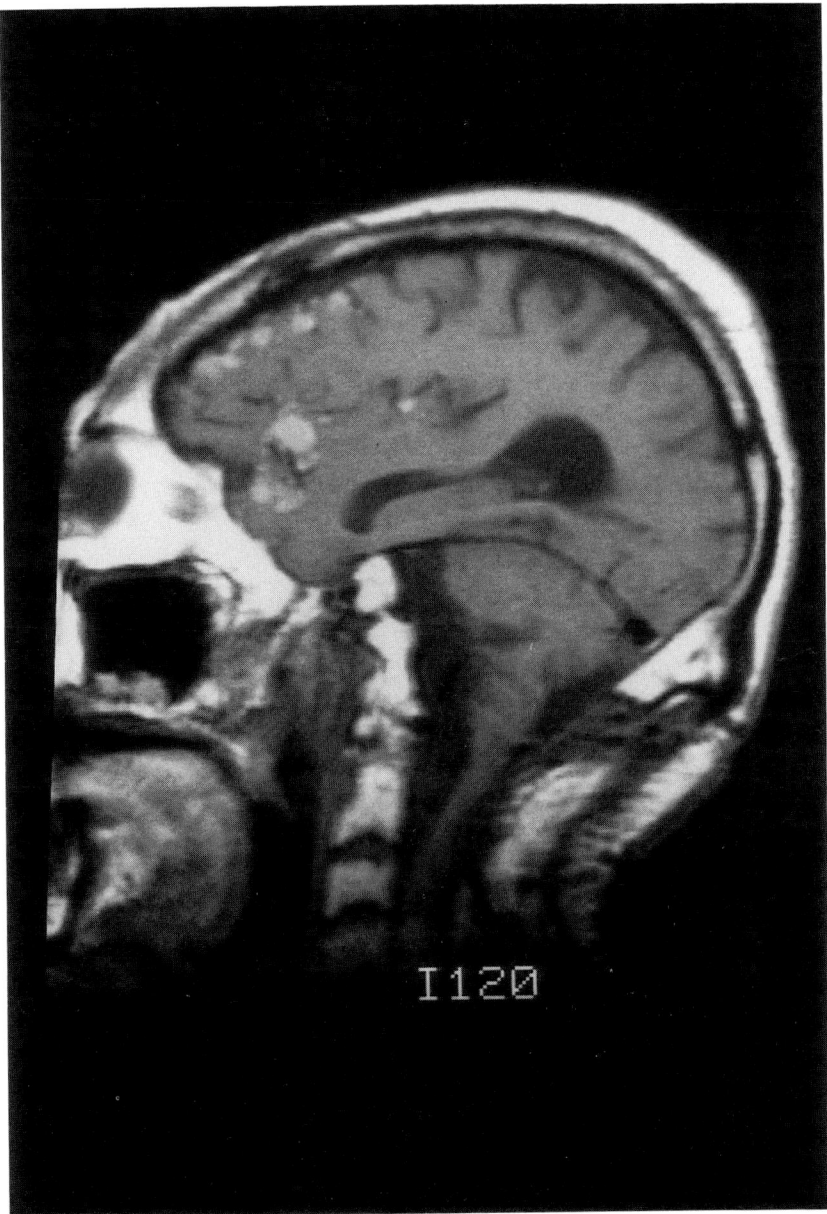

**Figure 5** MRI scan of the head showing intense nodular meningeal enhancement in the frontal region of a patient with metastatic malignant melanoma. (Radiograph courtesy of Dr. Howard Lee.)

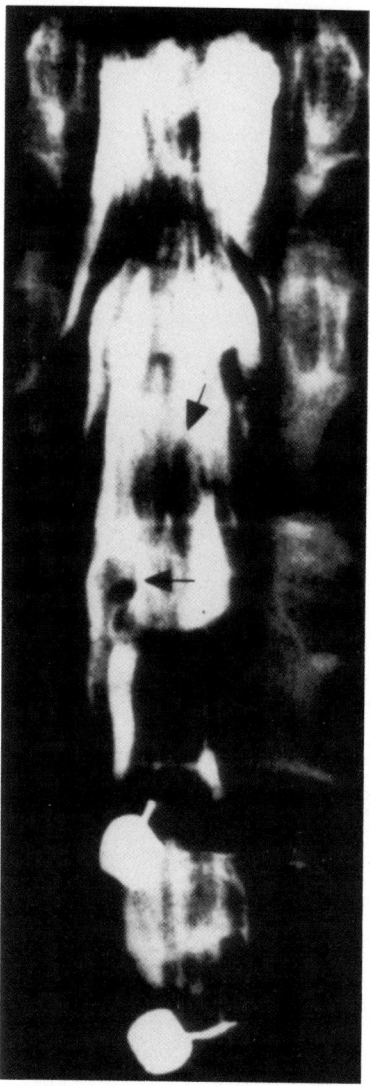

**Figure 6** Lumbar myelogram from a patient with carcinoma of the lung showing irregular nodular thickenings and beadlike filling defects (*arrows*) in the cauda equina representing nodular tumor growth. (Reprinted from Ref. 25.)

enzyme can suggest sarcoidosis, but meningeal or other biopsy may be necessary to establish this diagnosis.

In patients with known primary cancers, the diagnosis is usually not in doubt. In those patients without a known tumor primary, the diagnosis of neoplastic meningitis may be more difficult. In some circumstances, a meningeal biopsy of a portion of the meninges which enhances on MRI or CT scan may be considered. Computed tomography or MRI scanning can distinguish parenchymal metastases from leptomeningeal metastases. Myelography or gadolinium (Gd)-enhanced spinal MRI can detect epidural spinal cord or cauda equina compression with or without leptomeningeal infiltration.

## VII. TREATMENT

Leptomeningeal disease is probably the most difficult form of CNS metastasis to treat. Because of proximity to neural tissue and the large anatomical breadth of disease disseminated diffusely and multifocally throughout brain and spinal subarachnoid spaces, treatment has remained a challenge. In spite of over two decades' experience treating meningeal leukemia and lymphoma and more than one decade of experience with solid tumor metastases, safe and effective treatment remains elusive. This topic has been recently reviewed (52).

### A. Radiotherapy

Most treatment protocols have used a combination of radiation therapy and chemotherapy. Radiation therapy delivered to the entire brain and spinal subarachnoid space may be effective in some cases. This approach would reach tumor layered in the pia and arachnoid and also penetrate into deep perivascular extensions of disease within the brain and spinal cord. However, because of the attendant suppression of bone marrow in the skull and vertebral column related to craniospinal radiation therapy, this approach has limited usefulness. The majority of patients with leptomeningeal metastases have active disease outside the central nervous system. Therefore, other systemic therapies are needed and would be compromised by the bone marrow suppression caused by total craniospinal radiation. Accordingly, most treatment protocols have used focal radiation to the site or sites of symptomatic involvement only. In many patients, this involves radiation therapy to the brain and perhaps to the cauda equina. In the large series of patients reported by the Memorial Sloan-Kettering Cancer Center group, 2400 cGy were delivered in 10 doses over approximately 2 weeks (25).

### B. Chemotherapy

Since tumor will be present in locations not focally irradiated, and these areas will be likely to propagate and disseminate, eventually reseeding the irradiated areas, chemotherapy remains a necessary part of effective treatment. Systemic chemotherapy remains largely ineffective. The traditional rationale offered for the failure of this treatment relates to the inability of water-soluble agents to cross the blood-brain barrier to reach leptomeningeal tumor. Experimental evidence, however, has shown in animals that leptomeningeal tumor has fenestrated capillaries which allow for leakage of water-soluble tracers (53). Nevertheless, systemically administered drugs, either water or lipid soluble, appear not to achieve or maintain tumoricidal concentrations in the CSF. Therefore, introduction of chemotherapy directly into the CSF has been a part of most treatment protocols over the past two decades.

The placement of an Ommaya device (54) into the lateral ventricle with a subcutaneous reservoir for instillation of drugs has been found superior to repeated lumbar punctures (55). The use of the Ommaya device allows for drugs to consistently enter cerebrospinal fluid and to permeate throughout the entire subarachnoid channels with CSF flow. The studies of Shapiro et al. (56) and Bleyer et al. (57) indicate that drug given by the intraventricular route is superior in producing prolonged remissions. Nevertheless, in some patients with extensive leptomeningeal disease partly obliterating and compartmentalizing subarachnoid channels, the delivery of chemotherapy directly into the ventricle may still fail to reach areas of persistent leptomeningeal tumor (34). Indium 111-DTPA CSF flow studies have documented this compartmentalization of the CSF system in some patients (58).

Many effective chemotherapeutic agents are excessively neurotoxic when administered intrathecally. Drugs that have received human trials for intraventricular use include triethylenethiophosphoramide (thio-TEPA), arabinosylcytosine, methotrexate, nimustine hydrochloride (ACNU) (59), interleukin-2 (60), and diaziquone (AZQ). Potentially useful agents recently studied in animals include ACNU (61) and 1-β-D-arabinofuranosylcytosine packaged in liposomes (62). *Thio-TEPA*, an alkylating agent, has been used in the treatment of malignant meningeal disease since 1976. In a dose of 2–10 mg/m$^2$, it is safe and somewhat effective in leukemias and perhaps breast carcinoma, but has limited usefulness because of its rapid transport out of the subarachnoid space resulting in significant systemic absorption and toxicity (51,63,64). *Arabinosylcytosine* (Ara-C), a synthetic pyrimidine nucleoside given in a dose of 30 mg/m$^2$, has activity against leukemias and some lymphomas but appears to be largely ineffective in solid tumor primaries (65). Intrathecal therapy with Ara-C produces high CSF concentrations but elimination times are short (66,67).

*Methotrexate* (MTX), effective in leukemias, lymphomas and breast carcinoma, but marginally effective in other solid tumors, has been the most widely used drug injected directly into the cerebrospinal fluid. Methotrexate is an antimetabolite which competitively interferes with the folic acid cycle, thereby inhibiting DNA synthesis. It typically is given at a dose of 7 mg/m$^2$ or 12 mg/dose.

## Leptomeningeal Metastases

In the large treatment series reported by the Memorial Group in 1982 (25), 90 patients with solid tumor primaries were treated with radiation therapy to the site or sites of clinical involvement. An Ommaya device was placed. Methotrexate was instilled intraventricularly twice weekly at the beginning of treatment and then less frequently as the clinical condition dictated (Fig. 7). Citrovorum factor (9 mg, p.o. twice daily for 4 days after chemotherapy) was given to reduce systemic effects of methotrexate diffusing from the CSF. Arabinosylcytosine was used infrequently and only when methotrexate presented a problem. Patients were followed closely with serial examinations and CSF samples. Patients with breast carcinoma showed the greatest response, with approximately 60% showing improvement or stabilization of neurological signs and symptoms within a range of 2 to 20 months. Median survival for this group was approximately 7 months. Other solid tumor primaries (lung carcinoma, malignant melanoma, and others) fared less well. Only 30% showed evidence of stabilization or improvement. The median survival of 3½ to 4 months only marginally exceeded the upper limits of the natural history of survival in untreated patients. Ten to fifteen percent of patients with breast cancer and

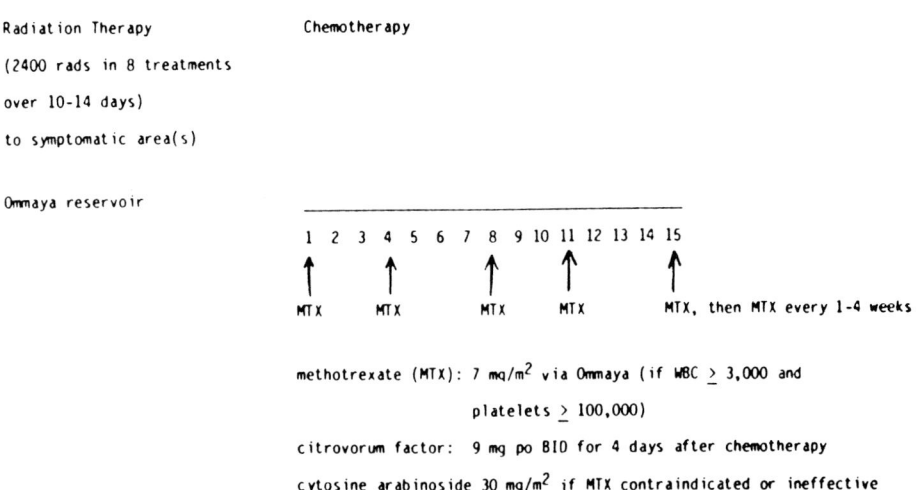

**Figure 7** Treatment protocol for leptomeningeal metastases from solid tumors. Radiation therapy is directed at the area or areas of clinical involvement, and an Ommaya device is placed in the right lateral ventricle. Intraventricular chemotherapy (methotrexate 7 mg/mm$^2$) or arabinosylcytosine 30 mg/mm$^2$ is instilled into the Ommaya device at intervals indicated on the graph, initially twice per week and then once per week to once per month, depending on clinical response. (Reprinted from Ref. 25.)

leptomeningeal metastases survived 1 year or longer. Only an infrequent patient with other solid tumor primaries survived 1 year. It appeared that among patients who did respond, most died of disease outside the nervous system with stable central nervous system disease. Objective evidence of improvement in CSF parameters such as cell counts, protein, glucose, and CSF markers can substantiate the efficacy of treatment in some patients when clinical signs and symptoms are equivocal.

Other studies (68–74) have reported similar results in treating leptomeningeal metastases with radiation therapy and intraventricular methotrexate. Recent smaller studies using combinations of intraventricular chemotherapeutic agents have shown no significant benefits afforded by multiple agents over the use of methotrexate alone (75–78). Multiple agents may produce undesirable side effects, particularly neurotoxicity (79,80) and bone marrow suppression. Pharmacokinetics of methotrexate in the CSF have shown highly variable results in patients with meningeal neoplasms (81–83). Drug distribution may be unpredictable in such patients (34). An attempt to improve the risk/benefit ratio for intrathecal MTX has included repeated small doses (5 mg) with frequent testing CSF drug levels (69). This protocol attempted to keep the CSF MTX concentration in the range between $10^{-6}$ M and $10^{-5}$ M in order to maximize efficacy and minimize toxicity. In spite of these efforts, a number of patients treated in this fashion have developed the serious delayed complication of leukoencephalopathy (84).

A report using intrathecal diaziquone, an alkylating agent that penetrates the blood-brain barrier, has recently been shown safe and active in refractory meningeal malignancies, particularly childhood leukemia (85). Pharmacokinetic data indicate significant CNS tissue penetration with negligible systemic levels (86). Additional trials are needed to judge the effectiveness of this promising agent.

## C. Antibody-Mediated Therapies

Recent clinical trials using radioimmunotherapy with $^{131}$I coupled to monoclonal antibodies directly injected into the CSF have had promising though preliminary results (87–89). These monoclonal antibodies serve as vectors to deliver radiation to tumors enclosed in the limited subarachnoid cavity, minimizing radiation dose to underlying brain and spinal cord. In the study of Lashford et al. (87), two patients with widespread leptomeningeal metastases from lymphoma and malignant melanoma, who had failed conventional therapy, were treated with intrathecal radiolabeled antibody. Therapy was well tolerated and both patients showed objective clinical responses for 8 to 12 months. In the study of Moseley and coworkers (88), intrathecal $^{131}$I–labeled monoclonal antibody HMFG1 (to a tumor-associated antigen) was administered to seven patients with widely disseminated leptomeningeal metastases. Aseptic meningitis, seizures, and myelosuppression were seen in some. Two patients improved clinically (ovarian and breast primaries) with survival of 7 and 26 months, respectively.

Moseley et al. (89) studied six patients with leptomeningeal metastases from solid tumor primaries after treatment with $^{131}$I–radiolabeled monoclonal antitumor antibody doses between 11 and 60 millicuries (mCi). Of those evaluable, three improved (two with malignant melanoma and one with breast carcinoma) with survival of 12, 32, and 26 months, respectively. One patient with lung carcinoma progressed to death in 4 months.

In laboratory experiments, Zovickian and Youle (90) examined the therapeutic effect of a monoclonal anti–ferritin receptor antibody–ricin A chain immunotoxin delivered directly into the subarachnoid space in a guinea pig model of leptomeningeal neoplasia. Immunotoxin therapy extended survival and yielded significant tumor kill without detectable toxicity. Johnson et al. (91) used a similar genetically engineered immunotoxin which showed significant tumor kill in laboratory studies of cell cultures of CSF–borne tumors. Antitumor immunotoxins composed of monoclonal antibodies armed with cytotoxins are in early clinical trials for carcinomatous meningitis (92).

## D. Toxicities and Complications

Treatment of leptomeningeal disease is not without its side effects. Radiation therapy administered in usual doses has minimal side effects (see also Chap. 10). Most patients are treated concurrently with corticosteroids when receiving brain radiation therapy to reduce headache, nausea, or vomiting. Likewise, the placement of an Ommaya device (54) by the method described by Galicich and Guido has few side effects (93). In the Memorial Hospital series of patients with solid tumors described by Wasserstrom et al. in 1982, there were few complications and no patient worsened neurologically as a result of the placement of an Ommaya device (25). However, other authors (94,95) have reported complication rates up 15% in the first year. A major difference between these two series is the incidence of bleeding complications in the later series, primarily among patients with leukemia or lymphoma. In a large series (404 placements) of Ommaya placements in cancer patients (96), 70% had breast cancer, leukemia, or lymphoma, and the perioperative mortality rate for reservoir placement was 0.5%. Perioperative morbidity was 2.5%, late infections occurred in 6%, and chemotherapy complications occurred in 3%.

In patients with increased intracranial pressure, cerebrospinal fluid can track along the catheter, resulting in subgaleal collections of CSF, which may become infected. In such patients, the device may require revision or replacement with a ventriculoperitoneal shunt. If a shunt is placed, an on-off valve is attached to the Ommaya device to allow instillation of chemotherapeutic agents. Occasionally, the Ommaya catheter may be misplaced, requiring repositioning. Infections of the

Ommaya device with ventriculitis and meningitis most often are due to coagulase-negative Staphylococcus (*epidermidis*) (97–100) and can be successfully treated with intravenous antibiotics and removal of the device, at least temporarily.

Methotrexate or any of the other intraventricular drugs, including monoclonal antibodies, may occasionally cause an aseptic meningitis syndrome or acute meningoencephalopathy (84). This syndrome occurs several hours after the instillation of drug and is manifested by headache, fever, and sometimes stiff neck, confusion, and disorientation. Cerebrospinal fluid is usually unchanged but occasionally may be associated with a mild pleocytosis and protein elevation above preinstillation levels. Cultures are sterile and the symptoms resolve within 1 to 3 days. Patients may continue to receive methotrexate after the acute meningoencephalopathy and experience no side effects, suggesting that the syndrome is idiosyncratic. Systemic glucocorticoids (dexamethasone) may provide symptomatic relief.

Methotrexate leukoencephalopathy is encountered in some patients who have been treated for greater than 6 months and received total doses of methotrexate averaging 140 mg. The leukoencephalopathy is manifested by the insidious evolution of dementia associated with pseudobulbar signs, ataxia, focal cerebral deficits, or paraplegia in some patients (25,84,101,102). This syndrome appears more common with concurrent brain radiation or if intravenous methotrexate has also been used. Periventricular white matter hypodensities seen on CT scan or hyperintense signals on T2-weighted MRI scans correlate with the pathological findings. Throughout the cerebral white matter and to a lesser extent in the brain stem, there are foci of coagulation necrosis of varying size and severity. In smaller lesions, a perivascular location is evident. The pathogenesis of this disorder is uncertain. Radiation injury may be an important factor, altering the blood-brain barrier such that methotrexate is more prone to injure myelin. The condition is more likely to occur if there is obstruction to normal bulk CSF flow (101). Similar lesions have been reported around Ommaya catheters in patients with hydrocephalus who received methotrexate for neoplastic meningitis (103).

Thio-TEPA has been associated with an acute paraparesis with pathological findings showing demyelination of lumbosacral nerve roots and posterior columns of the spinal cord (64). Arabinosylcytosine has been associated with a transient meningitis and rarely with paraplegia (65) or ascending myelopathy (104–106). Headache and nausea were observed in some patients receiving AZQ (85).

## VIII. FUTURE CONSIDERATIONS

The past century has shown an increased recognition of leptomeningeal metastases as an important and not uncommon neurological complication of systemic cancers. Improved diagnostic methods, including cytological and biochemical analyses of cerebrospinal fluid and technological imaging procedures, have been developed. Refinements of these diagnostic methods offer promise that diagnosis may be made in earlier stages of the disease, perhaps before devastating and permanent neurological signs and symptoms occur.

Effective treatment has lagged behind diagnostic advances. Although some patients with responsive tumors improve clinically and manifest objective laboratory improvements, the treatment of leptomeningeal metastases remains unsatisfactory. The prognosis for patients with leptomeningeal disease remains poor.

The advent of monoclonal antibody technology has offered hope for new treatment possibilities. While this technology is in its infancy, preliminary animal and human clinical studies are promising. Animal models of the disease (53,90,107–109) offer means of study that may enhance understanding of fundamental issues such as the role of the CSF-brain and blood-brain barriers in human disease, the activity of immunotoxins in regional CSF disease, and the pharmacokinetics of newer, more effective chemotherapeutic agents.

## REFERENCES

1. Eberth CJ. Zur entwickelung des epitheliomas (cholesteatomas) der pia und der lung. Virchows Arch 1870; 49:51–63.
2. Siebert E. Uber die Multiple Karzinomastose des Zentralnerven-Systems. Munch med Wochen Schr 1902; 49:826–828.
3. Lilienfeld BC. Fall von Metasticher Karcinose der Neivenund Hirnhaute. Berl Klin Wochenschr 1901; 38:729–730.
4. Beerman WF. Meningeal carcinomatosis. JAMA 1912; 58:1437–1439.
5. Fischer-Williams M, Bosanquet FD, Daniel PM. Carcinomatosis of the meninges: a report of three cases. Brain 1955; 78:42–58.
6. Grain GO, Karr JP. Diffuse leptomeningeal carcinomatosis: clinical and pathological characteristics. Neurology 1955; 5:706–722.
7. Olson ME, Chernik NL, Posner JB. Infiltration of the leptomeninges by systemic cancer: a clinical and pathologic study. Arch Neurol 1974; 30:122–137.
8. Knierim G. Uber diffuse meningeal karcinose mit Amaurose and Tauhheit bie Magenkrebs. Beitr Pathol Anat 1908; 44:409–427.
9. Price RA, Johnson WW. The central nervous system in childhood leukemia: I. The arachnoid. Cancer 1973; 31:520–533.
10. Kokkoris CP. Leptomeningeal carcinomatosis—How does cancer reach the pia-arachnoid? Cancer 1983; 51:154–160.
11. Gonzales-Vitale J, Garcia-Bunuel R. Meningeal carcinomatosis. Cancer 1976; 37: 2906–2911.
12. Posner JB, Chernik NL. Intracranial metastases from systemic cancer. Adv Neurol 1978; 19:579–592.
13. Evans AE, Gilbert ES, Landstra R. The increasing incidence of central nervous system leukemia in children. Cancer 1970; 26:404–409.
14. Nies BA, Thomas LB, Freireich EJ. Meningeal leukemia: a follow-up study. Cancer 1965; 18:546–553.

15. Simone J. Acute lymphocytic leukemia in childhood. Semin Hematol 1974; 11: 25–39.
16. Griffith J, Thompson N, Mitchinson M, deKiewiet J, Welland F. Lymphomatous leptomeningitis. Am J Med 1971; 51:200–208.
17. Levitt L, Dawson D, Rosenthal D, Maloney W. CNS involvement in the non-Hodgkin's lymphomas. Cancer 1980; 45:545–552.
18. Bunn PA, Schein PS. Meningeal involvement in lymphoma. N Engl J Med 1974; 290–517.
19. Bunn PA, Schein PS, Banks PM, De Vita VT. Central nervous system complications in patients with diffuse histiocytic and undifferentiated lymphoma: leukemia revisited. Blood 1976; 47:3–9.
20. Yap HY, Yap BS, Tashima CK, DiStefano A, Blumenschein GR. Meningeal carcinomatosis in breast cancer. Cancer 1978; 42:283–286.
21. Rosen S, Aisner J, Makuch R, Mathews M, Ihde D, Whitacre M, Glatstein E, Wiernik P, Lichter A, Bunn P. Carcinomatous leptomeningitis in small cell lung cancer: a clinico-pathologic review of The National Center Institute experience. Medicine (Baltimore) 1982; 61:45–53.
22. Mayer RJ, Berkowitz RS, Griffiths CT. Central nervous system involvement by ovarian carcinoma: a complication of prolonged survival with metastatic disease. Proc AACR/ASCO 1978; 19:318 (abstract).
23. Marsa GW, Johnson RE. Altered patterns of metastases following treatment of Ewings sarcoma with radiotherapy and adjuvant chemotherapy. Cancer 1971; 27:1051–1054.
24. Hussein AM, Savaraj N, Feun LG, Ganjei P, Donnelly E. Carcinomatous meningitis from transitional cell carcinoma of the bladder: case report. J Neurooncol 1989; 7:255–260.
25. Wasserstrom WR, Glass JP, Posner JB. Diagnosis and treatment of leptomeningeal metastases from solid tumors: experience with 90 patients. Cancer 1982; 49: 759–772.
26. Bigner S, Johnston W. The diagnostic challenge of tumors manifested initially by the shedding of cells into cerebrospinal fluid. Acta Cytol 1984; 28:29–36.
27. Kaplan JG, DeSouza TG, Farkash A, Shafran B, Pack D, Rehman F, Fuks J, Portenoy R. Leptomeningeal metastases: comparison of clinical features and laboratory data of solid tumors, lymphomas and leukemias. J Neurooncol 1990; 9:225–229.
28. Little J, Dale A, Okazak H. Meningeal carcinomatosis—clinical manifestations. Arch Neurol 1974; 30:138–143.
29. Sorenson S, Eagen R, Scott M. Meningeal carcinomatosis in patients with primary breast or lung cancer. Mayo Clin Proc 1984; 59:91–94.
30. Stadelmann E. Zur diagnose der meningitis carcinomatosis. Berl Klin Wochenschr 1908; 45:2262.
31. Glass JP, Melamed M, Chernik NL, Posner JB. Malignant cells in the cerebrospinal fluid: the meaning of a positive CSF cytology. Neurology 1979; 29:1369–1375.
32. Bigner S, Johnston W. The cytopathology of cerebrospinal fluid. II. Metastatic cancer meningeal carcinomatosis and primary central nervous system neoplasma. Acta Cytol 1981; 25:461–479.

33. Losses A, Siegal T. Spinal subarachnoid hemorrhage associated with leptomeningeal metastases. J Neurooncol 1992; 12:167–171.
34. Murray J, Greco A, Wolff S, Hainsworth J. Neoplastic meningitis: marked variations of cerebrospinal fluid composition in the absence of extradural block. Am J Med 1983; 75:289–294.
35. Moseley DA, Davies A, Bourne S, Popham C, Carrell S, Monro P, Coakham H. Neoplastic meningitis in malignant melanoma: diagnosis with monoclonal antibodies. J Neurol Neurosurg Psychiatry 1989; 52:881–886.
36. Bigner SH. Cerebrospinal fluid (CSF) cytology: current status and diagnostic applications. J Neuropathol Exp Neurol 1992; 51:235–245.
37. Boogerd W, Vroom TM, VanHeerde P, Brutel de la Riviere G, Pederse J, Vander Sande J. CSF cytology versus immunocytology in meningeal carcinomatosis. J Neurol Neurosurg Psychiatry 1988; 51:142–145.
38. Suttleworth E, Allen N. CSF B-glucoronidase assay in the diagnosis of neoplastic meningitis. Arch Neurol 1980; 37:634–687.
39. Fleisher M, Wasserstrom WR, Schold S, Schwartz M. Posner JB. Lactic dehydrogenase isoenzymes in the cerebrospinal fluid of patients with systemic cancer. Cancer 1981; 47:2654–2659.
40. Schold S, Wasserstrom WR, Fleisher M, Schwartz M, Posner JB. Cerebrospinal fluid biochemical markers of central nervous system metastases. Ann Neurol 1980; 8:597–604.
41. Wasserstrom WR, Schwartz M, Fleisher M, Posner JB. Cerebrospinal fluid biochemical markers in central nervous system tumors: a review. Ann Clin Lab Sci 1981; 11:239–251.
42. Mavligit A, Stuckey S, Cahanillas F, Keating M, Tourtellotte W, Schold S, Freireich E. Diagnosis of leukemia or lymphoma in the central nervous system by B-microglobulin determination. N Engl J Med 1980; 303:718–722.
43. Twijins A, Ongerhoer de Visser B, VanZanten A, Hart A, Nobyen W. Serial lumbar and ventricular CSF biochemical marker measurements in patients with leptomeningeal metastases from solid and hematologic tumors. J Neurooncol 1989; 7:57–63.
44. Moseley R, Oge K, Shafqat S, Moseley, C., Sullivan, N., Badley, R., Burcheli J, Taylor-Papadimitriou J, Coakham H. HMFG1 Antigen: A new marker for carcinomatous meningitis. Int J Cancer 1989; 44:440–444.
45. Adachi N. Beta-2-microglobulin levels in the cerebrospinal fluid: their value as a disease marker. Eur Neurol 1991; 31:181–185.
46. Twijnstra A, Ongerboer de Visser BW, van Zanten AP, Hart AAM, Nooyen WJ. Serial lumbar and ventricular cerebrospinal fluid biochemical marker measurements in patients with leptomeningeal metastases from solid and hematological tumors. J Neurooncol 1989; 7:57–63.
47. Sze G, Soletsky S, Bronen R, Krol G. MR imaging of the cranial meninges with emphasis on contrast enhancement and meningeal carcinomatosis. AJNR 1989; 10:965–975.
48. Krol G, Sze G, Malkin M, Walker R. MR of cranial and spinal meningeal carcinomatosis. AJNR 1988; 9:709–714.
49. Lee H. Personal communication.

50. Pedersen AG, Paulson OB, Gyldensted C. Metrizamide myelography in patients with small cell carcinoma of the lung suspected of meningeal carcinomatosis. J Neurooncol 1985; 3:85–89.
51. Schuknecht B, Huber P, Buller B, Nadjm M. Spinal leptomeningeal neoplastic disease: evaluation by MR, myelography and CT myelography. Eur Neurol 1992; 32(1):11–16.
52. Blaney SM, Balis FM, Poplack DG. Current pharmacological treatment approaches to central nervous system leukaemia. Drugs 1991; 41:702–716.
53. Siegal T, Sandhank U, Gahizon A, Siegal T, Mizrachi R, Ben-David E, Catano R. Alteration of blood-brain-CSF barrier in experimental carcinomatosis: a morphologic and adriamycin penetration study. J Neurooncol 1987; 4:233–242.
54. Ommaya AK. Subcutaneous reservoir and pump for sterile access to ventricular cerebrospinal fluid. Lancet 1963; i:983–984.
55. Shapiro W, Young D, Mehta B. Methotrexate: distribution in cerebrospinal fluid after intravenous, ventricular, and lumbar injections. N Engl J Med 1975; 293: 161–166.
56. Shapiro W, Posner J, Ushio Y, Chernik N, Young D. Treatment of meningeal neoplasms. Cancer 1977; 61:733–743.
57. Bleyer W, Poplak D. Intraventricular versus intralumbar methotrexate for central nervous system leukemia: prolonged remission with the Ommaya reservoir. Med Pediatr Oncol 1979; 6:207–213.
58. Chamberlain M, Corey-Bloom J. Leptomeningeal metastases: indium-DTPA CSF flow studies. Neurology 1991; 41:1765–1769.
59. Levin VA, Chamberlain M, Silver P, Rodriguez L, Prados M. Phase I/II study of intraventricular and intrathecal ACNU for leptomeningeal neoplasia. Cancer Chemother Pharmacol 1989; 23:301–307.
60. List J, Moser RP, Steuer M, Loudon WG, Blacklock JB, Grimm EA. Cytokine responses to intraventricular injection of interleukin 2 into patients with leptomeningeal carcinomatosis: rapid induction of tumor necrosis factor alpha, interleukin 1 beta, interleukin 6, gamma-interferon, and soluble interleukin 2 receptor (Mr 55,000 protein). Cancer Res 1992; 52:1123–1128.
61. Arita N, Ushio Y, Hayakawa T, Nagatani M, Huang T-Y, Izumoto S, Mogami H. Intrathecal ACNU—a new therapeutic approach against malignant leptomeningeal tumors. J Neurooncol 1988; 6:221–226.
62. Kim S, Kim DJ, Geyer MA, Howell SB. Multivesicular liposomes containing 1-B-D-arabinofuranosylcytosine for slow-release intrathecal therapy. Cancer Res 1987; 47:3935–3937.
63. Gutin P, Levi J, Wiernik P, Walker, M. Treatment of malignant disease with intrathecal thio-TEPA: a phase II study. Cancer Treat Rev 1977; 61:885–887.
64. Strong J, Collins J, Lester C, Poplak D. Pharmacokinetics of intraventricular and intravenous N,N1,N11-triethyl enethiophosphoramide (Thiotepa) in Rhesus monkeys and humans. Cancer Res 1986; 46:6101–6104.
65. Band P, Holland J, Bernard J, Weil M, Walker M, Rall D. Treatment of central nervous system leukemia with intrathecal cytosine arabinoside. Cancer 1973; 32: 744–748.

66. Zimm S, Collins JM, Miser J, Chatterji D, Poplack DG. Cytosine arabinoside cerebrospinal fluid kinetics. Clin Pharmacol Ther 1984; 35:826–830.
67. Bekassy AN, Liliemark J, Garwicz S, Wiebe T, Gulliksson H, Peterson C. Pharmacokinetics of cytosine arabinoside in cerebrospinal fluid and of its metabolite in leukemic cells. Med Pediatr Oncol 1990; 18:136–142.
68. Yap H, Yap B, Rasmussen S, Levens M, Hortobagyi G, Blumenschein G. Treatment for meningeal carcinomatosis in breast cancer. Cancer 1982; 49:219–222.
69. Ongerhoer de Visser B, Somers R, Nooyen W, VanHeede P, Hart A, McVie G. Intraventricular methotrexate therapy of leptomeningeal metastasis from breast cancer. Neurology 1983; 33:1565–1572.
70. Sause W, Crowley J, Fyre H, Riukin S, Pugh R, Quagliana J, Taylor S, Molnar B. Whole brain irradiation and intrathecal methotrexate in the treatment of solid tumor leptomeningeal metastases. J Neurooncol 1988; 6:107–112.
71. Boogerd W, Hart A, Vander Sande J, Engelsman E. Meningeal carcinomatosis in breast cancer: prognostic factors and influence of treatment. Cancer 1991; 67:1685–1695.
72. Schabet M, Kloeter I, Adam T, Heidemann E, Wietholter H. Diagnosis and treatment of meningeal carcinomatosis in ten patients with breast cancer. Eur Neurol 1986; 25:403–411.
73. Pfeffer MR, Wygoda M, Siegal T. Leptomeningeal metastases—treatment results in 98 consecutive patients. Isr J Med Sci 1988; 24:611–618.
74. Nakagawa H, Murasawa A, Kubo S, Nakajima S, Nakajima Y, Izumoto S, Hayakawa T. Diagnosis and treatment of patients with meningeal carcinomatosis. J Neurooncol 1992; 13:81–89.
75. Trump D, Grossman S, Thompson G, Mullay K, Wharam M Treatment of neoplastic meningitis with intraventricular Thiotepa and methotrexate. Cancer Treat Rev 1982; 66:1549–1551.
76. Giannone L, Greco A, Hainsworth J. Combination intraventricular chemotherapy for meningeal neoplasia. J Clin Oncol 1986; 4:68–73.
77. Hutchins R, Bell D, Woods R, Levi J. A prospective randomized trial of single-agent versus combination chemotherapy in meningeal carcinomatosis. J Clin Oncol 1987; 5:1655–1662.
78. Stewart D, Maroun J, Hugenholtz H, Benoit B, Girard A, Richard M, Rusell N, Huebsch L, Drouin J. Combined Intraommya methotrexate, cytosine arabinoside hydrocortisone and thio-TEPA for meningeal involvement by malignancies. J Neurooncol 1987; 5:315–322.
79. Colamaria V, Caraballo R, Borgana-Pignatti C, Marradi P, Balter R, Mazza C, Procacci C, Della Bernardine B. Transient focal leukoencephalopathy following intraventricular methotrexate and cytarabine. A complication of Ommaya reservoir: case report and review of the literature. Childs Nerv Syst 1990; 6:231–235.
80. Boogerd W, Moffie D, Smets LA. Early blindness and coma during intrathecal chemotherapy for meningeal carcinomatosis. Cancer 1990; 65:452–457.
81. Ettinger LJ, Chervinsky DS, Freeman AI, Creaven PJ. Pharmacokinetics of methotrexate following intravenous and intraventricular administration in acute lymphocytic leukemia and non-Hodgkin's lymphoma. Cancer 1982; 50:1676–1682.

82. Collins JM. Pharmacokinetics of intraventricular administration. J Neurooncol 1983; 1:283–291.
83. Miller KT, Wilkinson DS. Pharmacokinetics of methotrexate in the cerebrospinal fluid after intracerebroventricular administration in patients with meningeal carcinomatosis and altered cerebrospinal fluid flow dynamics. Ther Drug Monit 1989; 11:231–237.
84. Boogerd W, vd Sande JJ, Moffie D. Acute fever and delayed leukoencephalopathy following low dose intraventricular methotrexate. J Neurol Neurosurg Psychiatry 1988; 51:1277–1283.
85. Berg S, Balis F, Zimm S, Murphy R, Holcenberg J, Sato J, Reaman G, Steinherz P, Gillespie A, Doherty K, Poplack D. Phase I/II trial and pharmacokinetics of intrathecal diaziquone in refractory meningeal malignancies. J Clin Oncol 1992; 10(1):143–148.
86. Zimm S, Collins JM, Curt GA, O'Neill D, Poplack DG. Cerebrospinal fluid pharmacokinetics of intraventricular and intravenous aziridinylbenzoquinone. Cancer Res 1984; 44:1698–1701.
87. Lashford L, Davies G, Richardson R, Bourne S, Bullimore J, Eckert H, Kemshead J, Coakham H. A pilot study of I$^{131}$ monoclonal antibodies in the therapy of leptomeningeal tumors. Cancer 1988; 61:857–868.
88. Moseley R, Benjamin J, Ashpole R, Sullivan N, Bullimore J, Coakham H, Kemshead J. Carcinomatous meningitis: antibody guided therapy with I-131 HMFG1. J Neurol Neurosurg Psychiatry 1991; 54:260–265.
89. Moseley R, Davies A, Richardson R, Zalutsky M, Carrell S, Fahre J, Slack N, Bullimore J, Pizer B, Papanastassiou V, Kemshead J, Coakham H, Lashford L. Intrathecal administration of I$^{131}$ radiolabelled monoclonal antibody as a treatment of neoplastic meningitis. Br J Cancer 1990; 62:637–642.
90. Zovickian J, Youle R. Efficacy of intrathecal immunotoxin therapy in an animal model of leptomeningeal neoplasia. J Neurosurg 1988; 68:767–774.
91. Johnson V, Wrohel C, Wilson D, Zovickion J, Greenfield L, Oldfield E, Youle R. Improved tumor-specific immunotoxins in the treatment of CNS and leptomeningeal neoplasia. J Neurosurg 1989; 70:240–248.
92. Hall W, Fodstad O. Immunotoxins and central nervous system neoplasia. J Neurosurg 1992; 76:1–12.
93. Galicich J, Guido L. Ommaya device in carcinomatous and leukemic meningitis: surgical experience in 45 cases. Surg Clin N Am 1974; 54:915–922.
94. Lishner M, Perrin R G, Feld R, Messner HA, Tuffnell PG, Elhakim T, Matlow A, Curtis JE. Complications associated with Ommaya reservoirs in patients with cancer. The Princess Margaret Hospital experience and a review of the literature. Arch Intern Med 1990; 150:173–176.
95. Perrin RG, Lishner M, Guha A, Curtis J, Feld R, Messner H. Experience with Ommaya reservoir in 120 consecutive patients with meningeal malignancy. Can J Neurol Sci 1990; 17:190–192.
96. Obbens EAMT, Leavens ME, Beal JW, Lee Y-Y. Ommaya reservoirs in 387 cancer patients: a 15-year experience. Neurology 1985; 35:1274–1278.
97. Sutherland GE, Palitang EG, Marr JJ, Luedke SL. Sterilization of Ommaya reservoir by instillation of vancomycin. Am J Med 1981; 71:1068–1070.

98. Connors JM. Cure of Ommaya reservoir associated Staphylococcus epidermidis ventriculitis with a simple regimen of vancomycin and rifampin without reservoir removal. Med Pediatr Oncol 1982; 10:549–552.
99. Trump DL, Grossman SA, Thompson G, Murray K. CSF infections complicating the management of neoplastic meningitis: clinical features and results of therapy. Arch Intern Med 1982; 142:583–586.
100. Siegal T, Pfeffer MR, Steiner I. Antibiotic therapy for infected Ommaya reservoir systems. Neurosurgery 1988; 22:97–100.
101. Shapiro W, Chernik N, Posner JB. Necrotizing encephalopathy following intraventricular instillation of methotrexate. Arch Neurol 1973; 28:96–102.
102. Ojeda VJ, Necrotizing leukoencephalopathy associated with intrathecal/intraventricular methotrexate therapy. Med J Aust 1982; 2:289–293.
103. Lemmon W, Wiley R, Posner J. Leukoencephalopathy complicating intraventricular catheters: clinical, radiographic and pathologic study of 10 cases. J Neurooncol 1988; 6:67–74.
104. Breuer AC, Pitman SW, Dawson DM, Schoene WC. Paraparesis following intrathecal cytosine arabinoside: a case report with neuropathological findings. Cancer 1977; 40:2817–2822.
105. Mena H, Garcia JH, Velandia F. Central and peripheral myelinopathy with systemic neoplasia and chemotherapy. Cancer 1981; 48:1724–1737.
106. Dunton SF, Nitschke R, Spruce WE, Bodensteiner J, Krouse HF, Progressive ascending paralysis following administration of intrathecal and intravenous cytosine arabinoside: a Pediatric Oncology Group study. Cancer 1986; 57:1083–1088.
107. Fuchs H, Archer G, Colvin M, Bisner S, Shuster J, Fuller G, Muhlbaier L, Schold S, Friedman H, Bigner D. Activity of intrathecal 4-Hydro-peroxycyclophosphamide in a nude rat model of human neoplastic meningitis. Cancer Res 1990; 50:1954–1959.
108. Ushio Y, Chernik N, Posner JB, Shapiro W. Meningeal carcinomatosis: development of an experimental model. J Neuropathol Exp Neurol 1977; 36:228–244.
109. Ushio Y, Posner JB, Shapiro W. Chemotherapy of experimental meningeal carcinomatosis. Cancer Res 1977; 37:1232–1237.

# 4

# Peripheral Nervous System Complications in Cancer Patients

**Paul L. Moots**

*Vanderbilt University Medical Center, Nashville, Tennessee*

## I. INTRODUCTION

Peripheral nervous system (PNS) disorders are a common source of morbidity in the general population. Neuropathies, both inherited and acquired, motor neuron syndromes, disorders of the neuromuscular junction, and myopathies are all common problems seen in the general practice of neurology. Both in diversity and frequency, the problem of peripheral nervous system disorders is magnified in the cancer population. In addition to direct involvement by cancer, treatment-related peripheral nerve toxicities and paraneoplastic disorders stand out as peculiar to this group of patients. A variety of other problems, including herpes zoster, nerve compression syndromes, and weakness due to corticosteroids, are also encountered in cancer patients. Some of these problems are reviewed elsewhere in this volume in relation to specific neoplasms. The purpose of this chapter is to provide a framework for classifying and diagnosing the peripheral nervous system disorders encountered in cancer patients. For a comprehensive review of disorders of peripheral nerve and muscle, a number of excellent texts are available (1,2).

## II. POLYNEUROPATHY

### A. Clinical Features

The clinical classification of peripheral neuropathies considers the rate of onset, the course, the severity, and the nature of the symptoms and the degree to which sensory, motor, and autonomic functions are variously affected. Neuropathies that evolve acutely (hours to days) are uncommon in cancer patients. Subacute neuropathies, evolving over many days or weeks, include several important entities, i.e., some common chemotherapy-related toxic neuropathies and paraneoplastic neuropathies. Few chronic neuropathies, those evolving over many months or years, have a specifically defined relationship to cancer. Many of the cancer-related neuropathies are progressive or progress to a certain level of involvement and then stabilize. Relapsing neuropathies are uncommon. Many patients experience moderate to severe neurological impairment. There is a prominent dose effect in the common chemotherapy-related toxic neuropathies. Most peripheral neuropathies include a mixture of motor and sensory impairment. Certain paraneoplastic neuropathies and cisplatin-related neuropathy are remarkable for the predominance of sensory symptoms. Pure motor and autonomic neuropathies are rare but intriguing disorders often seen with paraproteinemias.

In the most typical cases, peripheral neuropathies present with symmetric, distal greater than proximal sensory and motor symptoms. The feet are often affected earlier than the hands. Tingling *paresthesias*, which are often intermittent initially, evolve into persistent numbness. In the predominantly sensory neuropathies, painful *dysesthesias* are common. Repeated testing with painful stimuli (e.g., pin prick) may result in an increased appreciation of the stimulus, termed *hyperpathia*. Dysfunction of the larger myelinated sensory fibers is associated with diminished proprioception and vibration. This is often accompanied by difficulty walking—so-called sensory ataxia, which can be a major disabling feature of platinum-related and some paraneoplastic neuropathies. Fine movements of the fingers, such as buttoning, may be impaired by this mechanism also. Weakness is initially most prominent in the toes and ankles. Difficulty dorsiflexing the ankle is common, and tripping or spraining the ankle is often described as an early symptom. Moderate or severe weakness of ankle dorsiflexion produces footdrop. Whether predominantly sensory, predominantly motor, or mixed sensorimotor, the tendon reflexes are symmetrically reduced and often absent. This is an important sign strongly indicating that the disorder involves the peripheral rather than central nervous system. Additionally, the absence of reflexes is unusual in disorders of muscle or the neuromuscular junction and thus helps to identify the peripheral nerve as the site of involvement.

In addition to the clinical classification, neuropathies may be classified based on electrophysiological characteristics. The main diagnostic value of nerve conduction studies and electromyography is distinguishing between processes that affect myelin, leading to slowed conduction velocity, and those that produce axonal loss, resulting in muscle denervation. The latter are often accompanied by other changes in the motor unit. With chronicity, most neuropathies show electrophysiological features of both demyelination and axonal loss with denervation. Conduction block along the course of a nerve and marked asymmetries indicating mononeuropathies superimposed on a diffuse polyneuropathy are additional features useful in characterizing peripheral neuropathies which can be shown by electrophysiological testing, but that may not be apparent on bedside examination.

## B. Iatrogenic Polyneuropathies

*Vincristine* is the agent most commonly associated with polyneuropathy (see Table 1). All patients acquire diminished tendon reflexes after four to six courses. Areflexia is common. While paresthesias are very common, detectable sensory disturbance on examination is not. Weakness of the dorsiflexors of the toes and ankles is common, obvious foot-drop less so. In the upper extremities the finger and wrist extensors are notably affected early in the course. The rate of onset and severity of the neuropathy are a function of the dose and frequency of administration (3). Except for bowel hypomotility, autonomic symptoms are rarely of major significance (4). Symptoms appear earlier and are more severe in adults than in children. In the absence of a preexisting neuropathy, discontinuation of the drug due to neurological toxicity is usually unnecessary. Patients with hereditary sensorimotor neuropathies, i.e., subtypes of Charcot-Marie-Tooth, have experienced severe peripheral neurotoxicity with vincristine (5). Patients with acquired neuropathies (e.g., diabetes) also may be unusually sensitive to the neuropathic effects of vincristine. The neuropathy associated with vincristine is reversible, although recovery may be slow. A number of agents have been studied as prophylaxis, but as yet none has documented efficacy.

*Cisplatin* (CDDP) is also frequently associated with a diffuse symmetric polyneuropathy. This is dose related, frequently occurring after a cumulative dose of 400 mg/m$^2$, and is seen in over half of the patients who receive more than 600 mg/m$^2$ (6,7). However, it also may occur with lower doses (8). Sensory symptoms predominate, and on clinical examination vibration and proprioception are often impaired, indicating involvement of large myelinated nerve fibers. This feature helps to distinguish CDDP neuropathy from the paraneoplastic subacute sensory neuropathy in which all sensory modalities are equally affected. Deep tendon reflexes are diminished or absent. Strength is minimally affected, if at all. Recovery is often slow and incomplete (6,7). Some progress has been made in preventing this complication with the administration of synthetic derivatives of corticotropin (ACTH), with sulfhydryl compounds, and with nerve growth factor (6,9,10).

Neuropathies have also been reported with procarbazine, etoposide (VP-16),

**Table 1** Characteristics of Chemotherapy-Related Neuropathies

| | Dose relationship | Symptoms and signs | | | | | Prophylaxis | Prognosis |
| --- | --- | --- | --- | --- | --- | --- | --- | --- |
| | | Sensory | Motor | Autonomic | Reflexes | Gait | | |
| Vincristine | Cumulative; >50% after 4–8 mg over 2–4 weeks | Distal paresthesias with mild sensory deficits | Wrist/finger extensors and ankle dorsiflexors affected early | Constipation or ileus common; not cumulative | Absent | "Foot-drop" | None | Usually full recovery |
| Cisplatin | Cumulative; >50% after 400–600 mg/m² | Vibration and proprioception severely affected | None or very mild weakness | Minor | Absent | "Ataxic" | Corticotropin (ACTH) derivatives Sulfhydryl compounds Nerve growth factor (NGF) | Poor |

and arabinosylcytosine (Ara-C) (11–13). A number of agents that are relatively new to clinical trials have been reported to produce neuropathy, including suramin and taxol (14,15).

Patients with multi-organ failure and sepsis requiring intensive care therapy have been reported to develop a severe neuropathy characterized by axonal degeneration with muscle denervation that has been labeled *critical illness polyneuropathy* (16). This neuropathy occurs in about 5% of patients requiring extended intensive care unit treatment. The presenting feature of the neuropathy is usually failure to wean from assisted ventilation. The cause of this neuropathy is uncertain. Specific toxic, nutritional, and metabolic factors have not been identified. Critical illness polyneuropathy may represent a component of the multiorgan failure syndrome. Patients receiving intensive chemotherapy, particularly in the setting of autologous and allogeneic bone marrow transplantation when complicated by sepsis and multi-organ failure, are at risk for developing this neuropathy.

## C. Paraneoplastic

*Paraneoplastic disorder* is a term used to represent a group of disorders seen in association with cancer, but not due to metastatic disease, and not the result of nutritional, infectious, metabolic, or treatment-related toxic abnormalities. Recent work, most notably by Posner and colleagues, has provided strong support for the concept that some of these neurological disorders result from an immunological process initiated against tumor antigens that are also present on normal neural tissue (17). These syndromes often appear before the development of any symptoms due to the tumor itself. Thus, despite the rarity with which they occur, identification of patients with these particular clinical syndromes, more recently with the aid of specific serological tests, provides the clinician an opportunity to diagnose certain cancers at an early stage.

Paraneoplastic disorders affecting peripheral nerve, nerve roots, and ganglia, presynaptic and postsynaptic elements of the neuromuscular junction, and muscle have all been described. Mostly, these are rare disorders. For example, in large series of patients with small-cell carcinoma of the lung, paraneoplastic neurological disorders (peripheral and central), are observed in less than 1% of patients. Many of these disorders present with a short history (weeks) of progressive, disabling weakness and/or sensory disturbance (Table 2).

Peripheral neuropathies occurring as a paraneoplastic phenomenon may involve predominantly the sensory fibers, or motor fibers, or may be mixed sensorimotor disorders. *Subacute sensory neuropathy* is a prototypic paraneoplastic neurological disorder (18–20) (see Table 2). The syndrome presents as paresthesias, which are often painful, involving the hands and feet, then progressing over a few weeks to involve the entire body and sometimes the face. All

Table 2  Noniatrogenic Polyneuropathies in Cancer Patients

| Neuropathy | Associated malignancy | Distinctive features |
|---|---|---|
| Subacute sensory neuropathy | Small-cell cancer of lung<br>Breast carcinoma<br>Ovarian carcinoma | *All* sensory modalities affected<br>Painful paresthesias common<br>Other syndromes (e.g., cerebellar degeneration) coexist<br>Anti-Hu antibody |
| Chronic sensorimotor neuropathy | Lung cancer | Poor temporal relation to diagnosis of cancer<br>Diagnosis of exclusion |
| Neuropathy associated with paraproteinemia | Multiple myeloma<br>Lymphoma<br>Hodgkin's disease | POEMS syndrome (sclerotic myeloma)<br>Subacute mixed sensorimotor or predominantly sensory<br>Anti-MAG antibodies with IgM monoclonal proteins |
| Motor neuronopathy | Hodgkin's disease<br>Lymphoma | Atrophy and fasciculations indicating anterior horn cell disease<br>Resemble multifocal motor neuropathy with conduction block |
| Acute inflammatory polyradiculopathy (Landry-Guillain-Barré syndrome) | Hodgkin's disease | Axonal variant with greater severity and poorer recovery rate than typical LGB |
| Diffuse metastatic involvement of peripheral nerves | Lymphoma<br>Leukemia | Rare<br>Coexistent meningeal disease common |

sensory modalities are affected to an equal degree. Although strength is less affected, these patients often are unable to walk because of sensory ataxia. In addition, half of these patients have coexistent involvement of other portions of the nervous system by the same paraneoplastic/degenerative process (21). Other areas frequently involved are the cerebral cortex (e.g., limbic encephalitis), the cerebellum (e.g., subacute cerebellar degeneration) and the brainstem (e.g., brainstem encephalitis). This combination of different areas involved by the same process has led to the use of the more general, inclusive term, paraneoplastic encephalomyeloradiculoneuritis. The syndrome is most often seen in patients with small-cell carcinoma of the lung, but also may be seen with Hodgkin's disease and other neoplasms. Some of these patients harbor antibodies to specific tumor antigens that are also expressed in certain nerve cells, such as the anti-Hu antibody defined by Posner and colleagues (21). This antibody recognizes a 35 to 40 kd neuronal nuclear protein. The identification of this antigen has led to the development of a diagnostic test for patients presenting with this neurological syndrome. The demonstration of the anti-Hu antibody in serum or CSF necessitates a detailed investigation aimed at detecting an occult small-cell carcinoma of the lung.

Chronic, slowly progressive sensorimotor polyneuropathy of mild to moderate severity is the most common form of neuropathy encountered in the general population. A defined systemic illness (e.g., diabetes or vasculitis), toxin, nutritional disorder, or other specific etiology is often not identifiable. Some of these neuropathies are familial and a careful analysis of the family history is critical in their evaluation (22). A chronic sensorimotor polyneuropathy is also the most common form of neuropathy encountered in cancer patients. While cancer and neuropathy may be coincidental illnesses, most authors consider chronic neuropathies without other underlying illness in the setting of cancer as paraneoplastic disorders (23). The mechanism responsible for this paraneoplastic phenomenon is not understood.

*Chronic sensorimotor polyneuropathy* is most often seen in association with lung cancer (23,24) (see Table 2). Based on electrophysiological criteria, up to 50% of lung cancer patients have evidence of peripheral nerve dysfunction (25). Most of these patients are asymptomatic. About 5% of cancer patients have clinically significant neuropathies, most of which fall into this category (24). The neuropathy may antedate the diagnosis of cancer by years, and the course of the neuropathy does not appear to reflect the evolution of the cancer or its response to treatment. A prospective study of neuropathy in small-cell lung cancer patients suggests that progression of the neurological disorder may relate to the degree of weight loss (25). Electrodiagnostic studies of these patients usually show evidence of axonal loss. However, as with most chronic neuropathies, electrical features of both axonal degeneration and demyelination are often observed together (23).

Even more commonly in the cancer population, one observes patients with mild, predominantly proximal weakness and hyporeflexia or areflexia. Characteristically the Achilles reflexes are lost. Sensory symptoms and signs are slight if present at all. These findings are often but not invariably seen in the setting of advanced cancer. In early clinical series describing peripheral nerve complications of cancer, these disorders were grouped under the heading of carcinomatous neuromyopathy, an ill-defined category that also included some of the more well-characterized peripheral nerve and muscle syndromes (26). While intending to designate the complex of proximal weakness and hyporeflexia as paraneoplastic, this term at the same time indicated that a clear distinction between peripheral nerve and muscle as the source of the process could not be established clinically. With increasing diagnostic sophistication, many of these patients can now be given a more specific diagnosis, and thus the term has largely been abandoned. However, cachexia, disuse, and steroid myopathy often serve as modern substitutes for this vaguely defined category of "neuromyopathy," and like their predecessor, these diagnoses also suffer from considerable diagnostic imprecision.

## D. Neuropathy Associated with Paraproteinemia (see also Chap. 22)

Monoclonal gammopathies are not uncommon in the general population, occurring with a frequency of 0.5% at age 40 years and increasing to 3% at age 70. In 85% of these, the excessive immunoglobulin is IgG, and the remainder are IgA or IgM. Approximately 20–25% of patients discovered to have a monoclonal gammopathy will eventually develop multiple myeloma, lymphoma, macroglobulinemia, amyloidosis, or other disorder. Conversely, 6–8% of patients with lymphomas of diffuse histology have a coexistent monoclonal gammopathy. Paraproteinemias are much less common in patients with nodular lymphomas or Hodgkin's disease, and rare in the acute leukemias, but occur in 5% of patients with chronic lymphocytic leukemia. Paraproteinemias are, of course, a hallmark feature of the plasma cell neoplasms.

Peripheral neuropathy is seen in about 20% of patients with monoclonal gammopathies, apparently irrespective of the presence or absence of a coexisting malignancy (27) (see Table 2). The type of neuropathy varies among these patients. A predominantly sensory neuropathy, and a mixed sensorimotor neuropathy are the most common. These often show evidence of demyelination on electrophysiological testing and on pathological examination. Less common is a motor neuropathy or neuronopathy with features that simulate anterior horn cell diseases, including amyotrophic lateral sclerosis (ALS). Preserved nerve conduction velocities with evidence of denervation and axonal loss are seen on EMG and pathological investigation. The course of these neuropathies is subacute or chronic and progressive in most cases. Acute deterioration or a relapsing-remitting course occurs in about 20%.

The pathogenesis of neuropathies associated with paraproteinemias is a subject of intensive research. Over 50% of patients with monoclonal IgM proteins and neuropathy have antibodies to myelin-associated glycoprotein (MAG) and a demyelinating neuropathy (28). Other antibodies to peripheral nerve components have been identified, and also may be related to particular types of neuropathies; these include antichondroitin sulfate antibodies with axonal neuropathies, anti-sulfatide antibodies with sensory neuropathies, and antiganglioside antibodies associated with motor neuropathies (29–31). Identical antibodies sometimes are found in patients with neuropathy unassociated with gammopathy, and in this context the neuropathy may be considered an autoimmune phenomenon. However, the role of antibodies in the pathogenesis of these neuropathies remains uncertain. While a specific antibody-mediated attack on myelin is likely the cause of the neuropathy associated with anti-MAG antibodies, amyloid deposition, hyperviscosity, and vasculitis are other mechanisms that might apply in patients with gammopathies.

While neuropathy is not common in multiple myeloma, a subgroup of patients with osteosclerotic myeloma, approximately 2% of myeloma patients, develop sensorimotor demyelinating polyneuropathy. Coexisting features may include endocrinopathies, acromegaly, and dermatologic abnormalities. Progression of the neoplasm tends to be slow, but the neuropathy is often disabling (32,33).

The association between cancer and *motor neuron disease* is an issue of debate, yet to be resolved. Epidemiological studies of patients with ALS have generally not demonstrated an increase in the incidence of cancer in patients with this relatively common neurological disorder (annual incidence 1 per 100,000 persons) (34). There are, however, some case reports documenting improvement of neurological syndromes that are indistinguishable from ALS after treatment of a coexistent neoplasm (35). Lower motor neuron involvement has been observed in a small percent of patients with cancer harboring the anti-Hu antibody, but it is rarely a prominent feature of that disorder. A subacute motor neuronopathy or atypical polio has been observed in patients with Hodgkin's disease and in non-Hodgkin's lymphoma (36,37). These patients present with moderately severe weakness accompanied by atrophy, fasciculations, and absent tendon reflexes without appreciable sensory disturbance. Some of these patients manifest upper as well as lower motor neuron findings making the clinical picture at times indistinguishable from classical ALS. The temporal relationship between the neurological syndrome and the course of the neoplasm is variable, but it most often arises after treatment of the neoplasm. Some of these patients have paraproteinemias, and thus may form a subgroup of patients with peripheral neuropathy associated with circulating antibodies to peripheral nerve. Some patients may be distinguished from classical ALS by the demonstration of multifocal conduction block on electrophysiological testing.

## E. Infectious and Postinfectious Neuropathies

In the gray area that excludes a sharp distinction between infectious and postinfectious neurological disorders lies the syndrome of *acute inflammatory polyradiculopathy*, historically the Landry-Guillain-Barré (LGB) syndrome (38) (see Table 2). This syndrome classically presents with progressive, symmetric weakness starting in the legs and spreading to the arms, trunk, and face. The weakness may progress rapidly (e.g., over hours) to the point of requiring respiratory assistance. More often the nadir is reached about the eighth day. Deep tendon reflexes are absent. Mild, symmetric paresthesias and sensory findings are typical. Autonomic dysfunction may occur, and occasionally severe cardiac arrhythmias and labile blood pressure produce life-threatening management problems. Nerve conduction velocities are decreased after the first week of illness. The CSF characteristically contains an elevated protein concentration with normal or minimally increased white blood cell count. There are a number of variants based on different clinical presentations and different electrophysiological results. Plasma exchange has been shown to reduce the time to recovery and decrease the length of time ventilatory assistance is needed. High-dose intravenous gamma globulin may be as effective (39). Without treatment, 75% of patients eventually will recover well.

The relationship between the LGB syndrome and cancer is not clear. Epidemiological studies indicate that 65% of patients have an antecedent "viral syndrome" within 4 weeks before the neuropathy. Many viruses have been implicated, as has *Campylobacter* infection. While studies have failed to identify an association between cancer and LGB syndrome, they have tended to focus on antecedent rather than subsequent illnesses. A number of case reports suggest a relationship between the LGB syndrome and Hodgkin's disease. These reports describe a severe form of acute/subacute polyneuropathy often with prominent axonal abnormalities and a recovery rate that appears lower than seen in most series of LGB syndrome. For these reasons some authors consider LGB syndrome in this setting a paraneoplastic disorder (40,41). LGB syndrome has also been observed in patients with non-Hodgkin's lymphomas and leukemias (41). It is reported as a complication of high-dose Ara-C therapy prior to bone marrow transplantation (12), and as a complication of ricin-conjugated immunotoxins (42).

## F. Neoplastic

Diffuse involvement of peripheral nerves by metastatic cancer in a manner that produces the clinical picture of a diffuse symmetric, predominantly distal sensorimotor deficit characteristic of many polyneuropathies is exceptional. Diffuse infiltration of peripheral nerves has been reported in leukemia, usually in the setting of meningeal involvement (43,44) and in both B and T cell lymphomas (45). The clinical picture may evolve rapidly, simulating the Landry-Guillain-

Barré syndrome, but in most cases the evolution is slower, and in all cases the course is progressive. Cranial nerve involvement is noted in half of these patients. Electrodiagnostic studies usually demonstrate evidence of axonal damage, but mixed axonal/demyelinating changes also may be seen. Elevated CSF protein and mild pleocytosis are found in most patients. Evidence of coexisting meningeal lymphoma is found in about 33% by cytological examination of CSF, and in 50% at autopsy (45). While destruction of nerve fibers and fascicles may result directly from tumor infiltration, some patients also have paraproteinemias that may be involved in the genesis of the neuropathy.

Meningeal carcinomatosis with widespread nerve root involvement may simulate a symmetric sensorimotor polyneuropathy, although this is uncommon (46,47). More commonly, meningeal metastases produce patchy, asymmetric sensory and motor dysfunction (see Chap. 3). Frequently, cranial nerve deficits and mental status abnormalities also are present. The high frequency of radicular signs and symptoms makes it an important diagnostic consideration in patients who on clinical grounds appear to have plexus lesions, isolated cranial neuropathies, or single or multiple peripheral nerve lesions. Magnetic resonance imaging scans with contrast enhancement can show neoplastic involvement of the meninges. However, a variety of inflammatory conditions produce an identical MRI appearance. Cerebrospinal fluid pleocytosis and elevated protein are characteristic findings. Cerebrospinal fluid cytology remains the most valuable diagnostic test.

## III. MONONEUROPATHIES AND MULTIPLE MONONEUROPATHIES

### A. Clinical Features

The involvement of isolated portions of the peripheral nervous system in cancer patients raises a group of diagnostic considerations that overlap to some extent with those diffuse polyneuropathies. However, infections, particularly herpes zoster, and direct invasion by tumor are much more frequently responsible, while iatrogenic and paraneoplastic processes are less common (Table 3).

### B. Infectious Mononeuropathies

Herpes zoster is the single most common peripheral nerve disorder in cancer patients. This disorder presents as tingling or burning paresthesias in a dermatomal distribution followed in 1 to 3 days by a vesicular eruption. Occasionally the antecedent pain is severe. The vesicles evolve to a crusted dry appearance over 5 to 10 days. The pain and paresthesias usually resolve over 1 to 4 weeks. In 10% of patients the pain will persist for many months in the form of recurrent, severe lancinating pain (postherpetic neuralgia). Postherpetic neuralgia is more common in older patients ($>50$ years) than in young patients (48).

**Table 3** Common Causes of Isolated Peripheral Nervous System Lesions in Cancer Patients

| A. *Cranial neuropathies* | *Etiology* | *Comment* |
|---|---|---|
| Trigeminal | Varicella zoster | Ophthalmic division ($V_1$) |
| | Tic douloureux | Mimicked by endoneural metastasis (e.g., basal cell carcinoma) |
| | Mental neuropathy | Mandibular metastases, especially with breast and prostatic cancer |
| | Meningeal/skull base metastases | |
| Facial | Idiopathic Bell's palsy | "Idiopathic" Bell's palsy should be diagnosed by exclusion |
| | Endoneural invasion from parotid tumors | |
| | Meningeal/skull base metastases | |
| Auditory | Cisplatin | Dose-related |
| | Aminoglycosides | |
| Other | Rarely idiopathic | Meningeal and base of skull metastases must be excluded |
| | Vincristine | Ptosis, diplopia, VII and IX-X palsies described |

| B. *Radiculopathies* | *Etiology* | *Comment* |
|---|---|---|
| Solitary | Varicella zoster | Rash; positive Tzank test |
| | Meningeal metastases | Coexistent cognitive and cranial nerve symptoms |
| | Degenerative disk disease | Frequently affected levels include C-6, C-7, L-4, L-5, and S-1 |
| Multiple | Meningeal metastases | |
| | Paraspinal metastases | Often involves contiguous levels; high incidence of epidural spread (see plexopathy) |

| C. *Plexopathies* | *Etiology* | *Comment* |
|---|---|---|
| Brachial | Metastatic | Breast, lung, lymphoma |
| | | Painful |
| | | Lower roots (i.e., C-7–T-1) most severely affected and epidural involvement common |
| | Radiation | Breast, lung, lymphoma |
| | | Not painful |
| | | Entire plexus involved |
| | Other | Traction (e.g., surgical) |
| | | Postinfectious |
| | | Familial |

**Table 3** Continued

| Plexopathies | Etiology | Comment |
|---|---|---|
| Lumbosacral | Metastatic | Colon, cervical, sarcoma |
| | | Painful |
| | Radiation | Not painful |
| | Other | Hematoma, abscess |
| D. *Mononeuropathies* | *Etiology* | *Comment* |
| Median | Compression at carpal tunnel | Weakness and atrophy of thenar muscles |
| | | Must be distinguished from C-6 radiculopathy and upper brachial plexus lesion |
| Ulnar | Compression at the elbow | Weakness of intrinsic hand muscles |
| | | May be superimposed on neuropathy (e.g., vincristine) |
| | | May mimic C8 or T1 root lesions or lower brachial plexus lesions |
| Peroneal | Compression at the fibula | Associated with foot-drop |
| | | May mimic L5 roots or sacral plexus lesion |
| Lateral femoral cutaneous | Compression at inguinal ligament | Paresthesias without motor symptoms or reflex changes |
| | | May mimic L3 root lesion |

Epidemiological studies show the incidence of zoster in the general population is extremely low in children and increases steadily with age. By 80 years of age over 25% of individuals will have had one episode of zoster. Studies of cancer patients reveal an increased incidence of zoster in patients with Hodgkin's disease (22%), acute lymphocytic leukemia (10%), and non-Hodgkin's lymphomas (49). In bone marrow transplant patients who have received high-dose chemotherapy and radiation, the frequency is higher still, approaching 50%. Although the course of the infection in most cancer patients is similar to that of noncancer patients, patients with deficiencies of cellular immunity have a higher risk of involvement of multiple dermatomes and of disseminated skin and visceral lesions (49). Pneumonia, hepatitis, and encephalitis are associated with the highest morbidity and mortality. Zoster is rarely the presenting manifestation of meningeal carcinomatosis. Zoster remains uncommon in such patients even in the presence of advanced root disease from cancer.

Early treatment of acute herpes zoster in immunocompromised patients with Acyclovir (500 mg/m$^2$ every 8 h) decreases the duration of pain, hastens healing of the lesions, and limits dissemination of the infection (50). This is the primary mode of therapy for such patients. Nonopioid and opioid analgesics should be aggressively titrated to achieve pain relief. Occasionally, sympathetic blockade may be helpful in patients with a persistent burning discomfort. Glucocorticoids reduce the pain associated with acute herpes zoster and may reduce the incidence of postherpetic neuralgia, but are not recommended for immunocompromised patients because of the preexisting risk of dissemination (48).

Postherpetic neuralgia is similar in character to the pain of the acute attack. It is often itching or burning in quality, and may be triggered by gentle stimulation of the affected skin. Severe lancinating attacks may occur along with a more continuous burning discomfort. Pharmacological treatment of postherpetic neuralgia is similar to that used in a variety of neuropathic pain syndromes, i.e., tricyclic antidepressants, particularly amitriptyline. Anticonvulsants, especially carbamazepine, have been found useful in the management of lancinating pains (48). Topical capsaicin (0.025–1.0%) provides relief in one-third of patients, but in as many patients produces burning pain on application that requires discontinuation of treatment (51). Again, patients with a prominent burning, dysesthetic quality to their pain may benefit from sympathetic blockade. Surgical treatments (i.e., rhizotomy) generally fail to provide long-term pain control.

## C. "Benign" Mononeuropathies

### 1. Cranial Nerve Syndromes

In addition to zoster—which most often affects the trigeminal nerve—other cranial neuropathies, some of which are considered "post-infectious" and others "idiopathic," are relatively common in general neurology practice. When encountered in a patient with cancer, the possibility of metastatic disease must be strongly considered, even in the most typical-appearing case.

The single most common cranial neuropathy observed in general neurological practice is unilateral facial paralysis or Bell's palsy (incidence 23 per 100,000 yearly) (52). The onset of weakness is often preceded by pain, particularly behind the ear, for a few days. The onset of weakness is acute and in most cases reaches a maximum by 48 to 72 h. Impairment of taste and hyperacusis are common. Few patients report hypesthesia in small areas on the affected side of the face. The CSF analysis often will show a mild pleocytosis. Magnetic resonance imaging may show an abnormal signal often with enhancement along the proximal segment of the nerve contained within the temporal bone. Most patients recover nearly full facial movement within a few months.

Epidemiological studies do not suggest an association between idiopathic Bell's palsy and cancer (52). However, the facial nerve is commonly involved by meningeal neoplasia and by bone metastases to the skull base (46,53). The facial nerve may also be involved by intraparotid neoplasms that show a propensity for endoneurial spread and represents an important part of anatomical staging (54).

Thus, the diagnosis of idiopathic Bell's palsy in a patient with cancer should be made with caution. Magnetic resonance imaging and CSF for cytology are appropriate for patients with active metastatic disease elsewhere and for patients whose cancers commonly involve the meninges or bone (i.e., lung, breast). Detailed investigation is also appropriate for those with pain persisting beyond the onset of the weakness and if auditory, vestibular, or prominent sensory disturbance on the face is present. Weekly follow-up examinations may obviate the need for imaging studies and lumbar puncture in selected solid tumor patients without evidence of active cancer.

Excluding disorders of the optic nerves, which are CNS tracts, the other common idiopathic cranial neuropathy is trigeminal neuralgia or tic douloureux (annual incidence 15 per 100,000) (55). This disorder is characterized by severe, unilateral lancinating facial pain in the distribution of the second or third divisions of the fifth nerve. A trigger point is often present, but otherwise there are no motor or sensory deficits, and the corneal reflex is intact in idiopathic cases. The mean age of onset of idiopathic trigeminal neuralgia is between 50 and 60 years, and there is a female-to-male predominance of 3:2.

The ophthalmic, maxillary, and mandibular branches of the trigeminal nerve exit the skull through the superior orbital fissure, the foramen rotundum, and the foramen ovale respectively. The mandibular branch then traverses a long canal through the mandible to exit the mental foramen. Thus in its course the nerve is subject to involvement by bone metastases at multiple locations. The most notable is involvement of the mandibular branch which produces mental neuropathy, e.g., the numb chin syndrome (56). This may be accompanied by bone pain, but rarely has the lancinating quality characteristic of tic douloureux.

A syndrome of progressive facial pain that may mimic tic douloureux has been observed in patients with endoneurial spread of squamous cell or basal cell carcinomas along the distal ramifications of the trigeminal nerve (57,58). Progression of the neoplasm to more proximal segments of the nerve may lead to involvement of the trigeminal ganglion and intracranial extension.

Idiopathic palsies of the other cranial nerves are uncommon in the general population. When these occur in cancer patients a detailed investigation for evidence of metastatic disease or treatment-related toxicity is warranted. Vincristine is notable for its association with isolated cranial neuropathies, particularly ptosis, jaw pain, and abducens and facial palsies (11,59). Cisplatin often causes sensorineural hearing loss (60).

## 2. Peripheral Nerve Syndromes

Injury to peripheral nerves due to entrapment or compression are common problems in general neurology and in cancer patients. There are few instances in which entrapment (in the absence of metastasis) is associated with particular neoplasms, as, for example, the increased incidence of carpal tunnel syndrome in patients with acromegaly. However cachexia, confinement to bed or chair, and peripheral nerve toxicity, for example from vincristine, are factors that increase the likelihood of compression palsies in the cancer population.

The compression syndromes encountered most frequently involve the median nerve (carpal tunnel), the peroneal nerve, the ulnar nerve, and the lateral femoral cutaneous nerve. These lesions usually present with intermittent paresthesias that progress over weeks to become persistent. Pain may be an important presenting feature. Lesions involving mixed sensorimotor branches tend to manifest weakness well after the onset of sensory symptoms. Obvious weakness and muscle atrophy are late findings.

Carpal tunnel syndrome often occurs in patients with a history of work or hobbies requiring repetitive hand and wrist movements. Pain and paresthesias are often most apparent at night. These symptoms are classically localized to the thumb, index, and middle fingers, but often the pain also involves the forearm, and occasionally the shoulder and neck. Weakness and atrophy are most apparent in the thenar muscles. Not infrequently, the process is bilateral. Tinel's sign, electrical or shocklike sensations in the distribution of a peripheral nerve on tapping over the nerve, may be elicited at the wrist. While the diagnosis of carpal tunnel syndrome is often straightforward, the clinical features may be very difficult to differentiate from radiculopathies involving the C6 or C7 nerve roots and the forms of brachial plexopathy involving the upper portion of the plexus (e.g., postinfectious plexopathy, brachial neuritis). Meningeal carcinomatosis, bone or paraspinal metastases with root compression, and uncommonly metastatic plexopathy can produce similar symptoms. Cervical degenerative disk disease and other forms of brachial plexopathy (postirradiation) must also be considered.

Ulnar and common peroneal neuropathies probably are more common in the setting of cancer than in the general population. Cachexia, poor nutrition, immobility, and treatment with agents that cause peripheral nerve toxicity (e.g., vincristine) are important predisposing factors. Ulnar neuropathies produce weakness of the intrinsic hand muscles and numbness over the ulnar edge of the palm which may closely resemble lesions of the lower portion of the brachial plexus. In cancer patients, lower plexopathies commonly are due to metastatic disease.

Peroneal neuropathies produce numbness over the lateral aspect of the lower leg and foot, and weakness of dorsiflexion of the ankle that often is described as foot-drop when severe. This lesion may resemble a sciatic neuropathy, sacral plexopathy, or L5 radiculopathy. Degenerative disease of the spine commonly affects the L5 root. Vertebral, epidural, paraspinal and meningeal metastases may also produce root lesions that are difficult to distinguish from a peroneal neuropathy.

Compression of the lateral femoral cutaneous nerve (meralgia paresthetica) produces numbness and, in a minority of cases, pain over the anterolateral aspect of the thigh. Obesity, heavy or tight-fitting garments (e.g., tool belt), pregnancy, and diabetes mellitus are common predisposing factors. There is no weakness or reflex loss associated with this nerve palsy. The nerve arises from the L2 and L3 roots, passes through the psoas muscle, and maintains a retroperitoneal course until it passes through the inguinal ligament where most benign compressions of the nerve are presumed to arise. The clinical picture of meralgia paresthetica may be difficult to distinguish from dermatomal sensory loss in the L3 distribution. However, the L2 and L3 roots are uncommon sites of root irritation due to disk herniation. Thus, the presence of paresthesias over the anterolateral aspect of the thigh in a cancer patient, particularly if painful, should raise the suspicion of meningeal, epidural, paraspinal, or retroperitoneal metastasis.

The femoral nerve, derived from the L2, L3, and L4 nerve roots, is rarely the site of a benign compression neuropathy. However, isolated femoral palsies most frequently are seen in diabetes mellitus. Hematomas in the iliac muscle and pelvic tumors are the next most common etiologies. Anterior thigh pain with hip extension, sensory loss, quadriceps weakness, and loss of the patellar reflex are associated findings. Proximal injury also produces weakness of hip flexion due to psoas and iliacus weakness.

Compression of the sciatic nerve that derives from the L4, L5, S1, and S2 nerve roots is uncommon, but not rare. Prolonged immobility, particularly in the sitting or lotus position, may produce a compression injury. Paresthesias extending down the posterior aspect of the leg to the sole of the foot are observed along with weakness of the hamstrings and all muscles below the knee. Proximal injury to the nerve also produces gluteal weakness. A common scenario is the cachectic patient with respiratory compromise due to lung cancer who sleeps sitting up and awakens with bilateral sciatic compression neuropathies.

## D. Metastatic Peripheral Nerve Disorders

Involvement of peripheral nerves by tumors most often is due to compression and invasion by metastases in adjacent structures. Most of the proximal nerve segments include sensory, motor, and autonomic fibers. Tumors usually produce well-delineated sensory deficits and characteristic patterns of weakness. Slight weakness and disability early in the evolution of the lesion often is much more apparent to the patient than to the examiner. Muscle atrophy generally is apparent after 3 to 6 weeks, but may be masked by local processes such as lymphedema. Tumor invasion of the nerve usually is painful. Pain in this situation may conform to a characteristic distribution, but often is superimposed on pain arising from adjacent structures, pain related to autonomic involvement, and not infrequently referred pain. For these reasons the distribution of pain is not as helpful in localizing the site of nerve involvement as are sensory and motor deficits. Absence of a deep tendon reflex can be a valuable indicator of lesion location in the peripheral nervous system. Although important exceptions exist, most peripheral nervous system lesions due to metastases produce asymmetric neurological findings with characteristic anatomical distributions.

Metastatic involvement of the brachial plexus is documented in 1–5% of cancer patients referred for neurological consultation, but the exact incidence is not clearly defined (61). Seventy percent of these patients have breast or lung cancers. Pain is the typical presenting symptom, antedating other signs by weeks or sometimes months. The pain, which is often severe, may involve the shoulder diffusely, but more characteristically extends along the inner aspect of the arm and ulnar side of the forearm and hand. Weakness and paresthesias are found in more than 70% of patients in a distribution corresponding to the lower portion of the plexus (e.g., C8-T1 root levels). In the remainder, the entire plexus is involved (61). Idiopathic, postinfectious, and familial brachial plexopathies usually involve the upper portions of the plexus (e.g., C5-C7 root levels) predominantly. Radiation injury often involves the entire plexus.

Tumor involvement in close proximity to the cervical spinal canal is common. Epidural extension, often through the neural (intervertebral) foramen, is seen in at least one-third of patients with neoplastic brachial plexopathy. The presence of a Horner's syndrome or involvement of the entire plexus (e.g., C5-T1 root levels) by tumor is associated with a higher incidence of epidural extension. Computed tomography and MRI scanning are very helpful in demonstrating abnormalities in the brachial plexus, but will not always distinguish neoplastic involvement from postradiation fibrosis. Surgical exploration is required for diagnosis in a small number of patients (62). Antineoplastic therapy, commonly focal radiation, may be beneficial for pain control, but recovery of neurological function is uncommon. For this reason and the high frequency of coexisting spinal epidural involvement, early diagnosis is essential for limiting neurological morbidity from brachial plexus metastases.

Lumbosacral plexopathy due to neoplasia is most commonly related to colorectal cancer, but sarcoma, breast cancer, lymphoma, cervical carcinoma, and a variety of less common pelvic and retroperitoneal tumors may involve the plexus (63). Direct extension of tumor from adjacent soft tissue or bone is the mechanism of involvement in 75% of cases. Like brachial plexus invasion, pain is by far the most common initial symptom, occurring in 70%. Patients often describe a combination of local pelvic/sacral discomfort and pain radiating into the leg. Pain is often present for weeks or months before other neurological signs and symptoms are apparent. The sensory disturbance, weakness, and reflex loss involve the lower (L4-S2/3 root levels) and upper (L1-L4 root levels) portions of the plexus with approximately equal frequency. Involvement of the entire plexus occurs in about 20% of cases. In less than 10% the involvement is bilateral. In bilateral cases, the lowest sacral roots from each side are involved as they exit the sacral foramen in close proximity. Low sacral metastases may cause incontinence and impotence without epidural extension. Myelography demonstrates epidural extension in almost 50% of patients with lumbosacral plexopathy. Both CT and MRI scanning may be useful in demonstrating tumor involvement of the lumbosacral plexus. CT is helpful for detecting bone abnormalities in the sacrum and for imaging the paravertebral spaces. Magnetic resonance imaging provides a better demonstration of the epidural space. As with brachial plexopathy, the treatment of lumbosacral plexopathy when initiated after the onset of sensory and motor deficits rarely produces neurological recovery. Most often, radiotherapy arrests progression of deficits and provides some pain relief.

Metastatic involvement of the more distal peripheral nerve ramifications is relatively uncommon, although again accurate figures regarding incidence are not available. Extension of the neoplasm from adjacent structures is the most common mechanism. Pathologically, the nerve is often encased by tumor without true invasion of the nerve fascicles. When the tumor does invade the endoneurium, it may extend considerable distances along the nerve. Lesions of the phrenic and recurrent laryngeal nerves often are associated with carcinoma of the lung involving the mediastinum. Breast cancer, lymphoma, and germinoma also may involve nerves in the mediastinum (43). Of the nerves emanating from the lumbosacral plexus, the sciatic and obturator nerves most often are involved by pelvic tumors, particularly rectal and cervical carcinomas. Although rare, chloromas (granulocytic sarcomas) have been observed to cause isolated neuropathies (personal observation). Computed tomography scanning may be needed to distinguish these more peripheral lesions from involvement in the plexus that often is accompanied by epidural extension. Bone metastases in the vertebral bodies extending into the epidural space and impinging on nerve roots, or nerve root involvement by meningeal spread of tumor, also must be considered.

Single or multiple cranial neuropathies due to metastases are well-documented complications of tumors that frequently metastasize to bone. Although calvarial metastases are about three times more common than base of skull metastases, the latter frequently are associated with cranial nerve dysfunction because they exit the skull through the bony foramen (53). Headache often precedes the development of neurological deficits. The nerves most frequently involved are the third and seventh. Involvement at sites peripheral to the neural foramen are less common. As mentioned above, involvement of the mental nerve, a branch of the trigeminal that traverses a long bony canal through the mandible, often reflects bone involvement (56), and involvement of branches of the facial nerve is an important feature of parotid gland neoplasms (54).

Endoneurial spread, the contiguous spread of tumor within the confines of nerve fascicles, is a rare form of metastasis. While this may occur at any site, involvement of a cranial nerve is notable because of a relationship to seemingly cured basal cell carcinomas. Such patients often present with pain and paresthesias in a portion of the trigeminal nerve distribution. At times, the symptoms mimic trigeminal neuralgia. The process may be complicated by mass-like expansion of the trigeminal ganglion and occasionally meningeal dissemination of tumor. Biopsy of the nerve will show tumor cell infiltration. Melanoma may advance in a similar fashion, e.g., so-called neurotropic melanoma. Pathological demonstration of endoneural spread is of prognostic value in the assessment of parotid, pancreatic, and prostatic carcinomas. Radiotherapy may offer some benefit in treating cranial or major nerve infiltration. Surgical resections produce permanent neurological deficits, a result that is often inappropriate in the overall clinical context.

## E. Iatrogenic Mononeuropathies

In addition to a diffuse polyneuropathy, vincristine has been associated with other PNS complications. Pain in the jaw and less frequently localized to the limbs or trunk occasionally is seen in the days after treatment. The origin of this pain is unclear. Ileus and other symptoms of autonomic dysfunction are relatively common in the first few days following treatment. Occasionally isolated cranial neuropathies are observed without any other identifiable cause (11,59).

Radiation damage to peripheral nerve is an uncommon problem. Demyelination of the optic and other cranial nerves has been reported, but well-documented cases are rare. Radiation injury to the brachial plexus is an important diagnostic concern in women who have received local radiation for breast cancer and occasionally in patients similarly treated for lung cancer (61). The distinction from neoplastic involvement of the brachial plexus may be difficult. Radiation plexopathy is rare during the first 6 months after the treatment. The onset of symptoms usually is gradual. Often, the entire plexus is involved, compared with tumor-related plexopathies that more commonly are limited in distribution, usually to the lower plexus. Most distinctive is the lack of pain as a presenting feature of radiation neuropathy (64–66). Radiation-induced neoplasms of the peripheral nerves, malignant nerve sheath tumors, are a rare complication of therapeutic irradiation. These tumors typically present with pain and well-localized sensorimotor dysfunction. There is a considerable delay from the time of treatment to appearance of the tumor, the median interval being 16 years. Many patients with this complication have neurofibromatosis. Resection is the only therapy (67).

## F. Mononeuritis Multiplex

The term mononeuritis multiplex applies to the simultaneous or sequential involvement of multiple peripheral nerves. This form of peripheral nerve disorder is classically seen with vasculitides that produce multiple nerve infarctions. When advanced, the clinical picture may be difficult to distinguish from diffuse polyneuropathy. However, patients will often describe the onset and evolution as patchy and asymmetric rather than as a symmetric distal-to-proximal progression. In some patients, mononeuritis multiplex will occur along with a distal, symmetric polyneuropathy.

In cancer patients, vasculitic mononeuritis multiplex may be associated with the paraproteinemias as mentioned above (see also Chap. 3). More commonly, however, this clinical picture is seen in patients with solid tumors, and usually represents multiple root involvement due to carcinomatous meningitis rather than multiple peripheral nerve lesions. Thus, any cancer patient presenting with a clinical picture suggesting multiple mononeuropathies should be carefully evaluated for carcinomatous meningitis.

Multiple mononeuropathies due to vincristine or cisplatin toxicity are rare, although minor asymmetries in these diffuse neuropathies are not. The superimposition of pressure palsies, particularly of the peroneal or ulnar nerve, on a chemotherapy-related polyneuropathy may simulate very closely the picture of vasculitic mononeuritis multiplex. Multiple mononeuropathies have also been reported in patients with graft-versus-host disease.

## IV. NEUROMUSCULAR JUNCTION DISORDERS AND MYOPATHIES

### A. Clinical Features

The cardinal feature of disorders affecting the neuromuscular junction and muscle is weakness. Typically the weakness is symmetric and most apparent in proximal muscle groups, i.e., the shoulders and pelvic girdle. Difficulty working with the arms above the head, such as combing the hair, and difficulty rising from a seated position or climbing stairs are frequent symptoms. In addition to the distribution of weakness, features that serve to distinguish these disorders from peripheral neuropathies and other causes of weakness are the preservation of reflexes and the absence of sensory symptoms or signs.

The other major symptom of neuromuscular junction and muscle disease is fatigue. Excessive fatigue and exertional intolerance are extremely common complaints in patients undergoing treatment for cancer. For most patients, this complaint can be attributed to cardiopulmonary, hematological, toxic, or metabolic derangements, central nervous system or psychological complications of disseminated cancer, or its treatment. In the absence of such an explanation, the complaint of excessive fatigue should direct attention to the possibility of a muscle or neuromuscular junction disorder. Fatigue is a property of normal muscles. Weak muscles fatigue more readily than normal muscles. Dramatic fatigability on repetitive strength testing is characteristic of myasthenia gravis, whereas enhancement with repeat contraction is sometimes seen in Lambert-Eaton syndrome (Table 4).

**Table 4** Paraneoplastic Disorders of Neuromuscular Junction and Muscle

| Disorder | Associated malignancy | Clinical features |
| --- | --- | --- |
| Lambert-Eaton syndrome | Small-cell lung cancer | Proximal weakness without extraocular weakness |
| | | Autonomic symptoms (i.e., dry mouth, constipation) |
| | | Facilitation of DTRs after brief voluntary contraction |
| | | EMG: Repetitive stimulation (20 to 50 Hz) leads to increased amplitude of motor response |
| | | Tensilon test ($-$) |
| | | Autoantibodies to presynaptic $Ca^{2+}$ channels |
| Myasthenia gravis | Thymoma | Proximal weakness with excessive fatigue |
| | Post-allogeneic BMT | Extraocular, pharyngeal, and respiratory involvement common |
| | | EMG: Repetitive stimulation at low frequencies ($<10$ Hz) leads to a decrease in the amplitude of the motor response |
| | | Tensilon test ($+$) |
| | | Autoantibodies to postsynaptic acetylcholine receptor |
| Inflammatory myopathy | Ovarian cancer | Proximal weakness without extraocular muscle involvement |
| | Breast cancer | Elevated CK |
| | Lung cancer | EMG: Myopathic features including polyphasic motor units |
| | | Tensilon test ($-$) |

# B. Neuromuscular Junction Disorders

## 1. Lambert-Eaton [Myasthenic] Syndrome (LEMS)

Lambert-Eaton syndrome is a disorder of neuromuscular transmission that is clinically manifest as weakness, particularly involving the proximal muscles (68). Initial complaints usually relate to weakness of the pelvic girdle, with difficulty climbing stairs or rising from a seated position. Some patients will notice a transient improvement in strength after initial attempts at exertion. Unlike myasthenia gravis, ocular involvement is rare. Bulbar and respiratory impairment are uncommon. Many patients complain of diffuse muscle aches and of symptoms related to cholinergic autonomic dysfunction, particularly dry mouth, constipation, and difficulty with urination. The exam shows diminished tendon reflexes; however, the demonstration of an increase in a reflex after brief voluntary contraction of the muscle is a particularly valuable sign. Electromyography is a valuable addition to the clinical exam in the diagnosis of LEMS. The compound muscle action potential is reduced, but low-frequency repetitive stimulation or brief voluntary contraction will result in a transient increase in the size of the potential. This finding is highly characteristic, and, prior to the development of diagnostic tests demonstrating antibodies to the presynaptic calcium channel, electromyography was the best diagnostic test available.

Lambert-Eaton syndrome is strongly associated with small-cell carcinoma of the lung that is found in about 50% of patients. The neoplasm is often found at an early stage, and in fact the neurological manifestations may precede the demonstration of the neoplasm by months or rarely years. The longest observed interval between the onset of neurological symptoms and diagnosis of the associated neoplasm is 4 years (68).

Lambert-Eaton syndrome is due to the presence of autoantibodies that interfere with calcium entry into the presynaptic terminal that is necessary for the release of acetylcholine. Diagnosis can be supported by detecting the autoantibodies in the blood. Treatment of the underlying neoplasm may result in improvement of the neurological symptoms (69). Symptomatic treatment with agents that promote the release of acetylcholine are beneficial for both cancer-related and non–cancer-related LEMS. The agent of choice is 3,4-diaminopyridine (70). Plasmapheresis and immunosuppressive therapies are also effective.

## 2. Myasthenia Gravis

The prevalence of myasthenia gravis is 5 per 100,000. In 95% of patients, autoantibodies directed against the postsynaptic acetylcholine receptors are present in the serum. These antibodies diminish the availability of muscle acetylcholine receptors and thus decrease the depolarization of the postsynaptic membrane that is necessary to produce muscle contraction. The disease is characterized by fluctuating weakness and excessive fatigue. Ptosis and diplopia due to extraocular muscle weakness are the most common presenting symptoms. In 15% of patients the process is limited to the extraocular muscles. More commonly, proximal arm and leg weakness of variable degree are also found. Bulbar symptoms including dysphagia, dysphonia, and aspiration, along with respiratory muscle weakness, represent the most morbid aspects of the illness (2).

Myasthenia gravis is associated with thymoma in about 10% of cases. These tumors are usually benign lymphoepithelial T-cell neoplasms that on occasion are locally invasive, but very rarely metastasize. In another 70% of patients, thymic hyperplasia is found. All patients with myasthenia should undergo a CT scan of the chest, and in a large percentage of patients thymectomy is recommended as a therapeutic procedure regardless of the presence of a thymoma. Immunosuppressive treatments such as corticosteroids or azathioprine, plasma exchange, and anticholinesterase medications are the major therapeutic options along with thymectomy.

Autoimmune myasthenia gravis has been reported in a small number of patients following allogeneic bone marrow transplants in the setting of chronic graft-versus-host disease (71,72). Symptoms generally present 2 years or more after transplantation, often at a time when immunosuppressants used for graft-versus-host disease are being discontinued. Thymomas are not found. Most of the described cases have acetylcholine receptor autoantibodies, with evidence indicating that engrafted donor cells are responsible for antibody production.

### 3. Iatrogenic Neuromuscular Transmission Disorders

Aside from anesthesiology, iatrogenic impairment of neuromuscular transmission is rare. Patients with preexisting neuromuscular transmission disorders may have unusually prolonged recovery from anesthesia using competitive acetylcholine receptor blocking agents. Several antibiotics are known to interfere with neuromuscular transmission. None of the antitumor antibiotics are reported to affect neuromuscular transmission.

## C. Myopathies

### 1. Iatrogenic

Toxic and metabolic myopathies probably are underrecognized in patients receiving treatment for cancer. The agents most often incriminated are glucocorticoids. Mild to moderate symmetric shoulder and pelvic girdle weakness with preserved reflexes are considered typical. Sensory deficits and pain are not found. The disorder may be related to dose and duration of treatment, but neither of these parameters are well defined. Synthetic fluoro-corticosteroids (e.g., dexamethasone) are more often incriminated than nonfluorinated drugs such as prednisone (73,74). Laboratory investigations are of limited value in diagnosing this condition. Muscle enzymes (e.i., creatine kinase [CK] and aldolase) are normal. Electromyography and muscle biopsy are either normal or show nonspecific abnormalities. Thus, the diagnosis of steroid myopathy is clinical, based on the exclusion of other causes of weakness. The observation of improvement following discontinuation of the corticosteroid is probably the best evidence in support of the diagnosis. However, since discontinuation often is not possible, dose reduction may be the best option.

Didemnin B, a cyclic peptide currently in phase II clinical trials, causes a severe myopathy characterized by elevated CK with myotonic discharges on electromyogram (EMG). Myopathy is the dose-limiting toxicity for didemnin B (75).

## 2. Paraneoplastic

Dermatomyositis and polymyositis in adults are associated with an increased incidence of cancer (76). The incidence of cancer in these patients is 10–15%. The relative risk of cancer is increased by 1.7 to 3.4 as determined in a population-based cohort study. The highest risk was found in females with dermatomyositis. In this subgroup the risk of ovarian cancer was increased 17-fold. However, unlike many other paraneoplastic neurological syndromes, myopathies may be associated with a variety of malignancies. The most common associations are with breast, lung, ovarian, colorectal, gastric, and pancreatic neoplasms. The myopathy precedes the cancer about half of the time. Cancer and dermatomyositis tend to occur in close temporal proximity, i.e., within 1 to 2 years. The temporal relationship is less pronounced in polymyositis. The risk of cancer does not appear to be increased in children with inflammatory myopathies.

The inflammatory myopathies present as proximal muscle weakness, accompanied by elevated serum creatine kinase, characteristic "myopathic" abnormalities on EMG studies, and inflammatory changes on muscle biopsy. Muscle pain is present in less than half of these patients. The weakness typically progresses over weeks or, rarely, days. The course of the illness and its response to therapy with glucocorticoids are indistinguishable from that of inflammatory myopathies not associated with cancer.

## 3. Disuse Atrophy

A variety of factors, including cachexia, immobilization, intercurrent illnesses such as infections, and poorly controlled pain, can lead to disuse and muscle atrophy. Although some of these factors are strongly associated with advanced cancer, bone marrow transplantation, postoperative and hospitalized chemotherapy patients, and patients with chronic or difficult-to-control pain, also may be at increased risk. Disuse atrophy is most readily appreciated in the anterior thigh muscles where obvious wasting may evolve over the course of 1 to 2 weeks. The symptoms of pelvic girdle weakness, commonly described as difficulty rising from lying to sitting, from sitting to standing, or difficulty getting up from the toilet or bath, usually are mild in these patients. Occasionally the weakness is sufficient to interfere with ambulation. The examination usually shows symmetric, mild pelvic girdle weakness proportionate to the degree of atrophy. Fasciculations are not found, and tendon reflexes are preserved. The presence of pain, sensory deficits, or bladder and bowel dysfunction should raise serious doubts about the diagnosis of disuse atrophy. The condition is important to recognize for two reasons. First, treatment including mobilization, physical therapy, and attention to nutritional status may significantly benefit these patients. Second, a variety of more serious neurological syndromes, including myopathies, acute and subacute polyneuropathies, and central disorders, particularly spinal cord compression, may have similar initial presentations.

## REFERENCES

1. Dyck PJ, Thomas PK, eds. *Peripheral neuropathy*, 3rd ed., vol 1 & 2. Philadelphia: W. B. Saunders Co., 1993.
2. Brooke MH. *A clinician's view of neuromuscular diseases*, 2nd ed. Baltimore: Wilkins & Wilkins, 1986.
3. Casey EB, Jellife AM, LeQuesne PM, Millett YL. Vincristine neuropathy: clinical and electrophysiological observations. Brain 1973; 96:69–86.
4. Hirvonen HE, Salmi TT, Heinonen E, Antila KJ, Valimake AT. Vincristine treatment of acute lymphoblastic leukemia induces transient autonomic cardioneuropathy. Cancer 1989; 64:801–805.
5. McGuire SA, Gospe SM, Dahl G. Acute vincristine neurotoxicity in the presence of hereditary motor and sensory neuropathy type I. Med Pediatr Oncol 1989; 17: 520–523.
6. Mollman JE, Glover DJ, Hogan WM, et al. Cisplatin neuropathy: risk factors, prognosis, and protection by WR-2721. Cancer 1988; 61:2192–2195.
7. Hamers FPT, Gispen WH, Neijt JP. Neurotoxic side-effects of cisplatin. Eur J Cancer Clin Oncol 1991; 27(3):372–376.
8. Greenspan A, Treat J. Peripheral neuropathy and low dose cisplatin. Am J Clin Oncol 1988; 11(6):660–662.
9. Van der Hoop RJ, Vecht CJ, van der Burg ME, et al. Prevention of cisplatin neurotoxicity with an ACTH(4-9) analogue in patients with ovarian cancer. N Engl J Med 1990; 322:89–94.
10. Apfel SC, Arezzo JC, Lipson LA, Kessler JA. Nerve growth factor prevents experimental cisplatin neuropathy. Ann Neurol 1992; 31:76–80.
11. Weiss HD, Walker MD, Wiernik PH. Neurotoxicity of commonly used antineoplastic agents (second of two parts). N Engl J Med 1974; 291:127–133.
12. Johnson NT, Crawford SW, Sargur M. Acute acquired demyelinating polyneuropathy with respiratory failure following high-dose systemic cytosine arabinoside and marrow transplantation. Bone Marrow Transplant 1987; 2:203–207.
13. Borgeat A, DeMuralt B, Stalder M. Peripheral neuropathy associated with high-dose Ara-C therapy. Cancer 1986; 58:852–854.
14. LaRocca RV, Meer J, Gilliatt RW, Stein CA, Cassidy J, Myers CE, Dalakas MC. Suramin-induced polyneuropathy. Neurology 1990; 40:954–960.
15. Lipton RB, Apfel SC, Dutcher JP, et al. Taxol produces a predominantly sensory neuropathy. Neurology 1989; 39:368–373.
16. Zochodne DW, Bolton CF, Wells GA, Gilbert JJ, Hahn AF, Brown JD, Sibbald WA. Critical illness polyneuropathy: a complication of sepsis and multiple organ failure. Brain 1987; 110:819–842.
17. Anderson NE, Cunningham JM, Posner JB. Autoimmune pathogenesis of paraneoplastic neurological syndromes. Crit Rev Neurobiol 1987; 3(3):245–299.
18. Graus F, Elkon KB, Cordon-Cardo C, Posner JB. Sensory neuropathy and small cell lung cancer: antineuronal antibody that also reacts with the tumor. Am J Med 1986; 80:45–52.
19. Graus F, Cordon-Cardo C, Posner JB. Neuronal antinuclear antibody in sensory neuronopathy from lung cancer. Neurology 1985; 35:538–543.

20. Budde-Steffen C, Anderson NE, Rosenblum MK, Posner JB. Expression of an antigen in small cell lung carcinoma lines detected by antibodies from patients with paraneoplastic dorsal root ganglionopathy. Cancer Res 1988; 48:430–434.
21. Anderson NE, Roseblum MK, Graus F, Wiley RG, Posner JB. Autoantibodies in paraneoplastic syndromes associated with small-cell lung cancer. Neurology 1988; 38:1391–1398.
22. Dyck PJ, Oviatt KF, Lambert EH. Intensive evaluation of referred unclassified neuropathies yields improved diagnosis. Ann Neurol 1981; 10:222–226.
23. McLeod JG. Carcinomatous neuropathy. In: Dyck PJ, Thomas RK, Lambert EH, et al., eds. Peripheral neuropathy, 2nd ed, vol II. Philadelphia: W. B. Saunders, 1984:2180–2191.
24. Croft PB, Urich H, Wildinson M. Peripheral neuropathy of sensorimotor type associated with malignant disease. Brain 1967; 90:31–66.
25. Hawley RJ, Cohen MH, Saini N, et al. The carcinomatous neuropathy of oat cell lung cancer. Ann Neurol 1980; 7:65–72.
26. Croft PB, Wilkinson M. The incidence of carcinomatous neuromyopathy in patients with various types of carcinoma. Brain 1965; 88:427–434.
27. Gosselin S, Kyle RA, Dyck PJ. Neuropathy associated with monoclonal gammopathies of undetermined significance. Ann Neurol 1991; 30:54–61.
28. Yee WC, Hahn AF, Hearn SA, Rupar AR. Neuropathy in $IgM_\lambda$ paraproteinemia: immunoreactivity to neural proteins and chondroitin sulfate. Acta Neuropathol (Berl) 1989; 78:57–64.
29. Pestronk A, Li F, Griffin J, Feldman EL, Cornblath D, Trotter J, Zhu S, Yee WC, Phillips D, Peeples DM, Winslow B. Polyneuropathy syndromes associated with serum antibodies to sulfatide and myelin-associated glycoprotein. Neurology 1991; 41:357–362.
30. Vital A, Vital C, Julien J, Baquey A, Steck AJ. Polyneuropathy associated with IgM monoclonal gammopathy: immunological and pathological study in 31 patients. Acta Neuropathol (Berl) 1989; 79:160–167.
31. Nobile-Orazio E, Legname G, Daverio R, Carpo M, Giuliani A, Sonnino S, Scarlato G. Motor neuron disease in a patient with a monoclonal IgMκ directed against GM1, GD1b, and high-molecular-weight neural-specific glycoproteins. Ann Neurol 1990; 28:190–194.
32. Bardwick PA, Zvaifler NJ, Gill GN, et al. Plasma cell dyscrasia and polyneuropathy, organomegaly, endocrinopathy, M protein, and skin changes: the POEMS syndrome: report of two cases and a review of the literature. Medicine (Baltimore) 1980; 59:311.
33. Kelly JJ Jr, Kyle RA, Miles JM, Dyck PJ. Osteosclerotic myeloma and peripheral neuropathy. Neurology 1973; 33:202.
34. Rosenfeld MR, Posner JB. Paraneoplastic motor neuron disease. Adv Neurol 1991; 56:445–459.
35. Evans BK, Fagan C, Arnold T, et al. Paraneoplastic motor neuron disease and renal cell carcinoma: improvement after nephrectomy. Neurology 1990; 40:960–962.
36. Schold SC, Cho ES, Somasandaram, et al. Subacute motor neuronopathy: a remote effect of lymphoma. Ann Neurol 1979; 5:271–287.
37. Younger DS, Rowland LP, Latov N, Hays AP, Lange, DJ, Sherman W, Inghirami G,

Pesce MA, Knowles DM, Powers J, Miller JR, Fetell MR, Lovlace RE. Lymphoma, motor neuron diseases, and amyotrophic lateral sclerosis. Ann Neurol 1991; 29: 78–86.
38. Asbury AK, Cornblath DR. Assessment of current diagnostic criteria for Guillain-Barré syndrome. Ann Neurol 1990; 27:S21–S24.
39. Van der Meche FGA, Schmitz PIM, and the Dutch Guillain-Barré Study Group. A randomized trial comparing intravenous immune globulin and plasma exchange in Guillain-Barré syndrome. N Engl J Med 1992; 326:1123–1129.
40. Lisak RP, Mitchell M, Sweiman B, et al. Guillain-Barré syndrome and Hodgkin's disease: 3 cases with immunological studies. Ann Neurol 1977; 1:72–78.
41. Case Records of the Massachusetts General Hospital (Case 39-1990). N Engl J Med 1990; 323:895–908.
42. Peterson K, Verma R, Kernan NA, Moots PL. Reversible demyelinating polyneuropathy possibly associated with the use of an anti-T cell ricin A chain immunotoxin in the treatment of acute graft versus host disease. Ann Neurol 1991; 30:274.
43. Henson RA, Urich H. Diffuse infiltration by lymphoma and leukemia. In: Cancer and the nervous system. Boston: Blackwell Scientific Publications, 1982:227–268.
44. Kuroda Y, Nakata H, Kakigi R, Oda K, Shibasaki H, Nakashiro H. Human neurolymphomatosis by adult T-cell leukemia. Neurology 1989; 39:144–146.
45. Diaz-Arrastia R, Younger DS, Hair L, et al. Neurolymphomatosis: a clinicopathologic syndrome re-emerges. Neurology 1992; 42:1136–1141.
46. Olson ME, Chernik NL, Posner JB. Infiltration of the leptomeninges by systemic cancer: a clinical and pathologic study. Arch Neurol 1974; 30:122–137.
47. Wasserstrom WR, Glass P, Posner JB. Diagnosis and treatment of leptomeningeal metastases from solid tumors: experience with 90 patients. Cancer 1982; 49: 759–772.
48. Portenoy RK, Duma C, Foley KM. Acute herpetic and postherpetic neuralgia: clinical review and current management. Ann Neurol 1986; 20:651–664.
49. Feldman S, Hughes WT, Kim HY. Herpes zoster in children with cancer. Am J Dis Child 1973; 126:178–184.
50. Shepp DH, Dandliker PS, Meyers JD. Treatment of varicella-zoster virus infection in severely immunocompromised patients: A randomized comparison of acyclovir and vidarabine. N Engl J Med 1986; 314:208–212.
51. Watson CP, Evans RJ, Watt VR. Post-herpetic neuralgia and topical capsaicin. Pain 1988; 33:333–340.
52. Hauser WA, Karnes WE, Annis J, Kurland LT. Incidence and prognosis of Bell's palsy in the population of Rochester, Minnesota. Mayo Clinic Proc 1971; 46: 258–264.
53. Greenberg HS, Deck MDF, Vikram B, Chu FCH, Posner JB. Metastasis to the base of the skull: clinical findings in 43 patients. Neurology 1981; 31:530–537.
54. Theriault C, Fitzpatrick PJ. Malignant parotid tumors: prognostic factors and optimum treatment. Am J Clin Oncol 1986; 9:510–516.
55. Sweet WH. The treatment of trigeminal neuralgia (tic douloureux). N Engl J Med 1986; 315:174–177.

56. Massey EW, Moore J, Schold SC. Mental neuropathy from systemic cancer. Neurology 1981; 31:1277–1281.
57. Carter RL, Pittam MR, Tanner NSB. Pain and dysphagia in patients with squamous carcinomas of the head and neck: the role of perineural spread. J R Soc Med 1982; 75:598–604.
58. Vrielinck LJG, Ostyn F, van Damme B, van den Bogaert, Fossion E. The significance of perineural spread in adenoid cystic carcinoma of the major and minor salivary glands. Int J Oral Maxillofac Surg 1988; 17:190–193.
59. Sandler SG, Tobin W, Henderson ES. Vincristine-induced neuropathy: a clinical study of fifty leukemic patients. Neurology 1969; 19:367–374.
60. Walker RW, Allen JC. Cisplatin in the treatment of recurrent childhood primary brain tumors. J Clin Oncol 1988; 6:62–66.
61. Kori S, Foley KM, Posner JB. Brachial plexus lesions in patients with cancer: 100 cases. Neurology 1981; 31:45–50.
62. Payne R, Foley K. Exploration of the brachial plexus in patients with cancer. Neurology 1986; 36:329.
63. Jaeckle KA, Young DF, Foley KM. The natural history of lumbosacral plexopathy in cancer. Neurology 1985; 35:8–15.
64. Bagley FH, Walsh JW, Cady B, Salzman FA, Oberfield RA, Pazianos A. Carcinomatous versus radiation-induced brachial plexus neuropathy in breast cancer. Cancer 1978; 41:2154–2157.
65. Lederman RJ, Wilbourn AJ. Brachial plexopathy: recurrent cancer or radiation? Neurology 1984; 34:1331–1335.
66. Thomas JE, Cascino TL, Earle JD. Differential diagnosis between radiation and tumor plexopathy of the pelvis. Neurology 1985; 35:1–7.
67. Folley KM, Woodruff JM, Ellis FT, Posner JB. Radiation-induced malignant and atypical nerve sheath tumors. Ann Neurol 1980; 7:311–318.
68. O'Neill JH, Murray NMF, Newson-Davis J. The Lambert-Eaton myasthenic syndrome: a review of 50 cases. Brain 1988; 111:577–596.
69. Chalk CH, Murray NMF, Newson-Davis J, et al. Response of the Lambert-Eaton myasthenic syndrome to treatment of associated small-cell lung carcinoma. Neurology 1990; 40:1552–1556.
70. McEvoy KM, Windebank AJ, Daube JR, et al. 3,4-Diaminopyridine in the treatment of Lambert-Eaton myasthenic syndrome. N Engl J Med 1989; 321:1567–1571.
71. Grau JM, Casademont J, Monforte R, Marín P, Grañena A, Rozman C, Urbano-Márquez A. Myasthenia gravis after allogeneic bone marrow transplantation: report of a new case and pathogenetic considerations. Bone Marrow Transplant 1990; 5: 435–437.
72. Bolger GB, Sullivan KM, Spence AM, Appelbaum FR, Johnston R, Sanders JE, Deeg HJ, Witherspoon RP, Doney KC, Nims J, Thomas ED, Storb R. Myasthenia gravis after allogeneic bone marrow transplantation: relationship to chronic graft-versus-host disease. Neurology 1986; 36:1087–1091.
73. Bowyer L, LaMothe MP, Hollister JR. Steroid myopathy: incidence and detection in a population with asthma. J Allergy Clin Immunol 1985; 76:234–242.

74. Ellis EF. Steroid myopathy. J Allergy Clin Immunol 1985; 76:431–432.
75. Shin DM, Holoye PY, Murphy WK, Forman A, Papasozomenos SC, Hong WK, Raber M. Phase I/II clinical trial of didemnin B in non-small-cell lung cancer: neuromuscular toxicity is dose-limiting. Cancer Chemother Pharmacol 1991; 29:145–149.
76. Sigurgeirsson B, Lindelof B, Edhag O, Allander E. Risk of cancer in patients with dermatomyositis or polymyositis: a population-based study. N Engl J Med 1992; 326:363–367.

# 5
# Neurological Complications of Malignant Brain Tumors

**Eugenie A. M. T. Obbens and William R. Shapiro**

*Barrow Neurological Institute, Phoenix, Arizona*

## I. INTRODUCTION

Primary brain tumors form a significant part of any neuro-oncology practice. Incidence has been defined in several large-scale studies, the two largest coming from the State of Connecticut Registry (1,2) and from the Rochester, Minnesota, Registry (3). The median age-adjusted incidence is between four and five cases per 100,000 per year. These estimates may be below the true rates because tumor registries typically record information on nervous system tumors inconsistently, making comparison difficult.

Brain tumors are more common in men than in women, except for meningiomas. Analysis of age-specific incidence shows a small peak in childhood and a higher peak later, reaching a maximum in adults between 60 and 80 years of age. In adults, the most common tumor is glioblastoma multiforme, followed by meningioma and astrocytoma. Glioblastomas represent more than half of the total of intracranial primary brain tumors. In children, medulloblastoma is the most common tumor, accounting for about a quarter of all intracranial primary tumors in childhood (2). Other tumors in childhood occurring about equally are astrocytomas, often in the cerebellum and usually fairly benign, and the more malignant glioblastoma. Brainstem tumors are usually astrocytomas or glioblastomas multiforme (4).

Histological diagnosis of brain tumors is essential, not only for appropriate treatment decisions but also for prognosis. Tumors such as meningioma or juvenile pilocytic astrocytoma have the best prognosis, whereas survival is shortest in the malignant gliomas. Malignant gliomas are defined as tumors arising from glial elements (astrocytes, oligodendrocytes, ependymal cells) that have an anaplastic histologic appearance and an aggressive biological behavior. This includes glioblastoma multiforme, anaplastic astrocytomas, ependymomas, and oligodendrogliomas, or combinations of any of these. The aggressiveness of a malignant glioma correlates with the presence of necrosis and the proliferation of small anaplastic cells. Other prognostic factors for survival are signs and symptoms at time of diagnosis and the patient's age. Surgical morbidity and mortality are higher in patients presenting with increased intracranial pressure, hemiplegia, or severe personality or mental changes. These patients are also less likely to remain independent and often suffer from a rapid downhill course despite treatment. Adults under age 40 at the time of diagnosis have a significantly longer survival in general than older patients with the same tumor histology.

## II. CLINICAL MANIFESTATIONS

The symptoms and signs of primary brain tumors depend on the size of the tumor, its location, and its rate of growth. The *characteristic clinical feature is a progression of symptoms*. The rate of progression ranges from an acute apoplectic onset following a hemorrhage or seizure to a slowly progressive mental deterioration. Clinical signs and symptoms may be divided into general and focal manifestations. Examples of the former are headache, mental changes, generalized seizures, nausea, and vomiting. Focal signs include focal seizures, weakness, sensory abnormalities, speech disturbances, and visual defects. Brain tumors produce generalized symptoms because tumor growth increases intracranial pressure by expansion of tumor volume, by associated cerebral edema, or by obstruction of cerebrospinal fluid pathways. Focal symptoms occur by direct compression of, or infiltration into, the surrounding brain tissue. In addition to its size, the location of the tumor in the brain strongly influences signs and symptoms. Thus, a small tumor in the speech or visual association cortex may produce more signs than a large frontal tumor. In addition, the clinical presentation will differ according to whether a generalized increase in intracranial pressure accompanies a specific focal dysfunction. Mental changes associated with increased intracranial pressure consist primarily of psychomotor retardation, lethargy, and eventually obtundation or coma. Division of signs and symptoms into general and focal may be useful in understanding the presenting picture of a brain tumor patient.

## A. General Symptoms and Signs

### 1. Mental Changes

Mental changes are often subtle, progressing gradually, and often not recognized until someone notices the patient's behavior changes. They are characterized as psychomotor retardation and include impersistence in routine tasks, emotional lability, inertia, faulty insight and forgetfulness, reduction in the range of mental activity, indifference to social practices, reduced initiative and spontaneity, and blunted affect. The patient rarely recognizes the change but instead may complain of fatigue, tiredness, dizziness, lethargy, and hypersomnia. There may be temporal retardation and delay in responsiveness in thinking and motor function. Changes in personality may be described in psychological terms (5). Thus, a patient may appear to be depressed, in that he is apathetic and indifferent to his surroundings, or he may appear euphoric, with reduced inhibitions, disheveled in his appearance, and unconcerned about inappropriate social behavior. The sudden occurrence of flamboyance, loss of inhibition, or impulsive behavior with impaired cognition should immediately raise the suspicion of a progressive intracranial space-occupying lesion. Many of these symptoms appear related to increased intracranial pressure and not to the site and nature of the lesion.

Apathy and indifference (pseudodepression) or euphoria are personality changes most often seen with frontal lobe lesions (6,7). Lesions in this area also may cause early impairment of intellectual function. When the tumor crosses the corpus callosum to involve both frontal lobes (butterfly glioma), mental changes are often accompanied by gait ataxia.

While mental dullness often accompanies large masses, mental changes may accompany small focal tumors in the temporal lobe or may be part of the speech abnormalities associated with small lesions in speech areas of the brain. The mental changes seen in temporal lobe lesions often include bizarre thinking and immature emotional behavior.

### 2. Headache

Headache as an initial symptom occurs in 20–25% of patients with brain tumor and in as many as 90% at some time during the illness (8). The head pain from brain tumor is often intermittent and may be described as deep, aching, or pressure-like rather than the more characteristic throbbing pain of migraine. It is often aggravated by the Valsalva maneuver, as in coughing or straining, and frequently is worse with change of posture. The patient with a slow-growing neoplasm may complain of headache for months or years. The headache that occurs in the early morning hours appears to be related to the recumbent posture and may be associated with increased intracranial pressure that is exacerbated by lying down. Such patients may actually sleep in a semirecumbent position to relieve the pain and may often trivialize the pain because it subsides once they awaken and begin the day's activities. Later, the headache becomes more persistent and severe.

Headache is more prominent and may occur earlier when the tumor is located below the tentorium rather than above, because an infratentorial tumor can obstruct cerebrospinal fluid (CSF) flow at an earlier stage. Headache more frequently occurs with rapidly growing tumors than slow-growing neoplasms. A patient with a glioblastoma multiforme is more likely to have headache than a patient with a meningioma. Of special importance are headaches that (1) have recently changed in character; (2) are worse in the morning or awaken the patient at night; (3) are of a recurrent nature; and (4) are increased by reduced atmospheric pressure.

The location of the tumor may influence the location and character of the headache, although usually not diagnostically. Cerebral hemispheral tumors initially produce headache in about one-third of patients. When it begins, the headache is often located over the tumor, but the pain spreads bilaterally as the tumor grows. Third ventricular tumors produce headache in as many as 85% of the patients. Tumors in the posterior fossa, especially the fourth ventricle (for example, medulloblastomas in children), may produce vomiting rather than headache because of pressure on the medulla. Cerebellar hemisphere tumors similarly produce pain in the occipital region but usually only after causing neurological symptoms related to the cerebellum.

Some tumors obstruct intracerebral cerebrospinal fluid pathways. If the ventricular system is obstructed there will be hydrocephalic ventricular dilatation. If the tumor obstructs the aqueduct or distal fourth ventricle, symmetric enlargement of the lateral ventricles occurs. Intracranial pressure rises, usually exceeding 200 mm water, producing brain shifts, cerebral dysfunction, and headache.

Headache that occurs with change in posture and lasts for 20–30 min may be associated with both an abrupt worsening in mental state and vomiting. This symptom complex may be due to the occurrence of plateau pressure waves. Originally defined by Lundberg (9), plateau waves have been reported in many neurological conditions, including brain tumor, head injury, benign intracranial hypertension, hydrocephalus, and subarachnoid hemorrhage. They are observed most often in cases with a marked degree of intracranial hypertension. The patients are usually alert during the plateau waves despite the severity of their intracranial condition. Occasionally, however, they may lose consciousness. Studies performed in patients with plateau waves demonstrate alterations in vasomotor tone associated with marked increase in intracranial pressure that may remain elevated for 5–30 min. The mechanism of plateau waves is thought to be related to the presence of a space-occupying mass that interferes with the compensatory changes in vasomotor tone that normally accompany postural changes and serve to stabilize intracranial pressure. Despite deficient autoregulation, such patients retain the ability to vasodilate the cerebral vessels and the increase in pressure appears to be associated with vasodilatation (10).

## 3. Seizures

Seizures, both generalized and focal, are a common manifestation of intracranial tumor. *Generalized* convulsions, along with focal seizures, occur in 35% of patients with cerebral tumors (11). They are more likely to accompany slower-growing tumors than they are the more rapid-growing malignant neoplasms (12). The location of the tumor and its infiltrative or expansive properties probably determine the risk of epilepsy. Generalized seizures may occur with a large mass producing increased intracranial pressure. Neoplasms of the white matter and those below the tentorium are less likely to produce seizures than are tumors situated in the cortical or subcortical regions of the cerebral hemispheres. Most tumors that produce seizures are located in the centroparietal regions. Generalized seizures may occur with tumors in a variety of locations, while focal seizures are more common with tumors in the motor or sensory cortical regions. Psychomotor seizures are much more frequent with tumors of the temporal lobe than with tumors located anywhere else in the brain; however, sphenoidal meningiomas also may produce temporal lobe seizures. While there is no consistent relationship between the type of seizure and the histological type of tumor, oligodendrogliomas produce seizures more frequently than other tumors and are more likely to induce generalized rather than focal seizures (11). Compared with other types of tumors, low-grade astrocytomas and oligodendrogliomas are more likely to present with seizures. Seizures infrequently accompany childhood brain tumors because most such tumors are infratentorial. Metastatic brain tumors are less likely to induce seizures than are primary brain tumors, with the possible exceptions of malignant melanoma and choriocarcinoma. The incidence of seizures in metastatic disease is approximately 20% (13).

*Focal* seizures may be produced by a specific cortical tumor. Seizures occurring for the first time in adults usually are due to focal cerebral disease, especially neoplasms. Seizures may be precipitated by alcohol or withdrawal of barbiturates or other sedative drugs.

Jacksonian seizures that progress from one body part to another usually imply a lesion of the motor or sensory cortex. Gliomas of the temporal lobe characteristically give rise to psychomotor seizures that may be associated with olfactory hallucinations (uncinate fits), disorders of visual or auditory perception, or episodes of déjà vu or automatic behavior. Petit mal epilepsy is never due to a neoplasm, but minor temporal lobe seizures that resemble petit mal attacks may accompany temporal lobe tumors. Parietal lobe tumors may provoke either generalized convulsions or sensory focal seizures. Seizures caused by occipital lobe lesions may be preceded by an aura of flashing lights but not formed images.

Seizures developing late after primary therapy for intracranial neoplasms imply recurrence of tumor and indicate a need to reevaluate the patient. Seizures recurring after primary therapy may reflect tumor recurrence/progression but electrolyte concentrations and anticonvulsant blood level measurements also are indicated. Hyponatremia, drug interactions, or noncompliance are well-recognized reasons for seizures in a patient treated for brain tumor.

## 4. Increased Intracranial Pressure

Hydrocephalus and increased intracranial pressure may cause significant signs and symptoms in glioma patients and lead to herniation syndromes. As a tumor enlarges, with any associated cerebral edema adding to the mass effect, brain tissue may be displaced through the fixed intracranial openings, producing various herniation syndromes. For example, the medial surface of the brain may be forced beneath the falx cerebri or transtentorial and tonsillar herniation may occur because of displacement of brain tissue through, respectively, the tentorial notch and foramen magnum. The clinical manifestations of transtentorial herniation depend in part on the site of the mass lesion. If the mass is unilateral, especially temporal, the medial temporal lobe is displaced inferiorly (caudally) and medially through the tentorial notch, producing uncal herniation. When the mass effect is near the midline, bilateral, or symmetrical, there is downward displacement of the diencephalon and the upper brainstem producing central herniation. The clinical manifestations of the two overlap, although there are differences in the specific nature and temporal sequence of individual symptoms (14).

Raised intracranial pressure may cause papilledema characterized by swelling of the optic nerve head with engorgement of the retinal veins and hemorrhages into the nerve and adjacent retina. Papilledema most often results from raised intracranial pressure (15). In 1971, Huber reported that of his 1166 patients with brain tumor, 59% had papilledema (16). Almost all of these patients had bilateral papilledema. Unilateral papilledema most commonly means intraorbital disease. In recent years, however, the overall incidence of papilledema in patients with brain tumor has decreased; now, only about 25% of such patients have papilledema. The reduced incidence appears to be related to earlier diagnosis, the use of corticosteroid hormones to control raised intracranial pressure, and earlier specific therapy. The likelihood of papilledema relates more to the location of the tumor than to its histological type. According to Huber, papilledema is more common in patients with infratentorial tumors (70%) than in those with supratentorial tumor (60%). Papilledema is more common when tumors interfere with CSF circulation and produce internal hydrocephalus. It is possible to have markedly increased intracranial pressure associated with brain tumor and not have papilledema. Local factors and variability from patient to patient appear to be important in determining if papilledema will occur in any given patient. Generally, tumor-associated papilledema occurs without visual change, differentiating it from papillitis. However, patients with choked disks occasionally complain of a graying-out phenomenon or other visual obscurations probably associated with plateau waves. On examination, such patients frequently have enlarged blind spots (16).

Vomiting, with or without nausea, often accompanies increased intracranial pressure and occurs most frequently with brainstem displacement secondary to herniation, bleeding into the CSF, or tumors of the posterior fossa. Patients with lower brainstem gliomas, medulloblastomas, and metastatic tumors in the cerebellar peduncles frequently experience nausea and vomiting. The symptom may be accompanied by a nonspecific, nonrotational sense of giddiness or dizziness. Vasomotor and autonomic changes, such as bradycardia, hypertension, and respiratory abnormalities, accompany expanding intracranial tumors when the pressure becomes high enough to compress the medulla.

## B. Focal Manifestations

Focal clinical manifestations of intracranial tumor depend on localized impairment of nervous system function and, by definition, vary with the location of the process (Table 1).

### 1. Motor Symptoms

Motor abnormalities caused by frontal lobe tumors include postural disturbances, incoordination, weakness, and tremor. Subcortical tumors commonly involve the internal capsule and produce contralateral weakness. Invasion of the basal ganglia may result in athetosis, bizarre tremors, or dystonic posturing. Posterior fossa tumors frequently produce long-tract signs accompanied by weakness and incoordination, along with associated cranial nerve signs and symptoms.

### 2. Sensory Loss

Sensory disturbances include unusual pains, paresthesias, or numbness, and imply lesions in the cerebral hemispheres or posterior fossa. With parietal lobe tumors, thresholds for cutaneous tactile, pain, and temperature senses are intact, but contralateral stereognosis and the cortical sensory modalities (position sense, two-point discrimination) are impaired. Contralateral homonymous hemianopsia (or inferior quadrantanopsia), apraxia, and anosognosia (nonrecognition of bodily defects) may also be present. Thalamic invasion often produces contralateral cutaneous sensory impairment that includes an elevated threshold for pain and temperature perception.

### 3. Speech Disturbance

Tumors of the dominant hemisphere are frequently associated with disturbances in language. Generally, tumors involving the dominant posterior inferior frontal lobe produce an expressive aphasia. Those involving the posterior parietal or posterior temporal lobe produce a mixed receptive-expressive aphasia. With parietal lobe

**Table 1** Focal Symptoms and Signs

Motor symptoms:
  Contralateral weakness, postural disturbances, incoordination, tremor
Sensory loss:
  Loss of cortical sensory modalities in parietal lobe tumors;
  Cutaneous sensory impairment due to thalamic invasion
Speech disturbance:
  Expressive and/or receptive aphasia, anomia, dysarthria
Visual abnormalities:
  Reduced visual acuity, diplopia, visual field defects
Cerebellar and brainstem dysfunction:
  Ataxia, intention tremor, nystagmus
  Unilateral facial palsy, hearing loss, palatal weakness
False localizing signs:
  Lateral rectus palsy due to sixth nerve compression
  Homolateral hemiplegia
  Homolateral visual field defects caused by compression of the opposite posterior cerebral artery
Other symptoms:
  Anosmia due to infrafrontal tumor
  Precipitate urination
  Neuroendocrine disturbances caused by hypothalamic and pituitary tumors

tumors, agraphia and finger agnosia may occur in addition to a receptive aphasia or mixed expressive-receptive aphasia. Tumors involving the surface of the dominant temporal lobe also produce a mixed expressive and receptive aphasia or dysphasia, chiefly anomia. The latter is especially common in brain tumor patients.

Dysarthria can accompany tumors of the posterior fossa, cerebral hemisphere, or meningeal gliomatosis. Occasionally a frontal lobe tumor produces a "cortical" dysarthria.

## 4. Visual Abnormalities

Visual loss—either reduced visual acuity, field defects, or diplopia—implies involvement of the visual apparatus anywhere from the eye to the occipital cortex or to the oculomotor nerves. Occipital lobe tumors usually cause a contralateral quadrantic visual field defect or a homonymous hemianopsia with sparing of the macula. Parietal lesions and temporal lobe lesions produce corresponding, variably congruent homonymous quandrantanopsias. Sellar tumors may produce compression of the optic chiasm with a corresponding bitemporal hemianopsia, or a combination of partial bitemporal hemianopsia and unilateral optic atrophy with blindness. Pupillary abnormalities and oculomotor abnormalities may occur with tumors along the base of the brain involving the third, fourth, or sixth cranial nerve. A sixth nerve paresis may accompany mass lesions as a false localizing sign of increased intracranial pressure, brain shift, or meningeal spread.

## 5. Focal Seizures

Focal seizures may occur alone or as part of a generalized seizure. They are therefore discussed under the heading of General Symptoms and Signs (see Table 2).

## 6. Cerebellar and Brainstem Dysfunction

Gliomas of the brainstem may destroy brainstem nuclei or cause paralysis of the lower cranial nerves (V–XII), resulting in a variety of associated symptoms. Damage to the motor or sensory pathways in the brainstem causes hemiplegia, hemianesthesia, or cerebellar disturbance. Increased intracranial pressure appears late in intrinsic brainstem tumors such as gliomas.

On the other hand, tumors of the fourth ventricle and cerebellum, such as medulloblastomas, typically interfere with CSF fluid circulation, causing symptoms of increased pressure early. Occasionally, headache, nausea, vomiting, and papilledema may develop acutely. Ataxic gait, intention tremor, nystagmus, and other signs of cerebellar dysfunction may appear before or after onset of increased intracranial pressure.

**Table 2** Generalized Symptoms and Signs of Primary Brain Tumor

Mental changes:
  Psychomotor retardation
  Cognitive impairment
  Mood changes
Headaches:
  Intermittent, deep, pressure-like pain worsened by recumbent posture
Seizures:
  Generalized tonic-clonic seizures, with or without focal onset
  Partial-complex seizures
  Focal motor or sensory seizures
Increased intracranial pressure:
  Herniation syndromes—subfalcine, transtentorial, tonsillar
  Papilledema—more common in infratentorial tumors and often accompanied by hydrocephalus
  Vomiting—most common in lower brainstem and posterior fossa tumors
  Vasomotor and autonomic changes—bradycardia, syncope, hypertension, altered respiration

Cerebellopontine angle tumors, particularly acoustic schwannomas, are characterized by tinnitus, unilateral hearing impairment, and sometimes vertigo. Pressure on the adjacent cranial nerves, brainstem, and cerebellum produces loss of corneal reflex, facial weakness and anesthesia, palatal weakness, signs of cerebellar dysfunction, and, rarely, contralateral hemiplegia or hypesthesia.

### 7. False Localizing Signs

These include unilateral or bilateral lateral rectus palsy from sixth nerve compression, hemiplegia on the same side as the tumor from compression of the opposite cerebral peduncle against the tentorium, and visual field defects on the same side as the tumor from compression of the contralateral posterior cerebral artery.

False localizing signs may accompany prolonged elevation of intracranial pressure with midline shift and are more common in slowly growing neoplasms like meningiomas (17).

### 8. Other Symptoms

Anosmia may be associated with infrafrontal meningiomas. Precipitate urination (urgency incontinence) may be caused by bifrontal gliomas. Neuroendocrine disturbances such as diabetes insipidus, hypopituitarism, or precocious puberty frequently occur in hypothalamic or pituitary tumors.

## III. DIAGNOSIS

The diagnostic study of choice is magnetic resonance imaging (MRI). This technique demonstrates the normal anatomy of the brain better than any other imaging modality. The addition of gadolinium enhancement has made MRI the procedure of choice in diagnosing brain tumors. Malignant tumors appear as altered signal with associated edema and displacement of adjacent structures. $T_2$-weighted sequences are very effective in showing tumor-associated edema. In general, malignant tumors enhance after administration of gadolinium, while low-grade gliomas do not enhance after gadolinium administration. The MRI is invaluable in the diagnosis of low-grade astrocytoma or oligodendroglioma in which computed tomography (CT) may show only low density without contrast enhancement that is indistinguishable from infarction. The MRI is also more accurate in diagnosing posterior fossa tumors.

## IV. DIFFERENTIAL DIAGNOSIS

Intracranial neoplasms are characterized by *progressive neurological dysfunction*. The onset may be abrupt, e.g., following a hemorrhage or seizure, or may be gradual, as the brain tumor grows. A large number of brain disorders can produce similar symptoms and, therefore, can be confused with intracranial neoplasm. However, tumor should be sought early while considering other diagnoses. The advent of MRI and CT has made diagnosis easier than in former years, when invasive procedures were required and were approached with reluctance. Patients with stroke characteristically present with acute onset of neurological dysfunction, although occasionally a "stuttering" onset may be confused with the tumor. Patients with subdural hematoma may have headache, drowsiness, papilledema, and hemiparesis; the diagnosis is usually made by CT or MRI scan. Patients with dementia from Alzheimer's disease usually have nonfocal cognitive deficits with minimal motor abnormalities. Differential diagnosis between tumor and abscess may require surgery to obtain tissue.

## V. THERAPY

The goal of brain tumor therapy is cytoreduction, i.e., to decrease the total tumor mass to a size that the body's immune system might suppress and eventually kill—approximately 0.0001 g or $1 \times 10^5$ cells (18). Brain tumors can produce symptoms when they are quite small (e.g., seizures), but most patients presenting with neurological symptoms usually have tumors 30 to 60 g in size ($3-6 \times 10^{10}$ cells). Depending on location of the tumor, the neurosurgeon may be able to remove between 20 and 90 percent of it. More commonly less than 50 percent can be resected, thus leaving a residual tumor burden of $1-5 \times 10^9$ cells. Radiation therapy (RT) may kill two additional logs of cells, reducing the tumor to $1 \times 10^7$ cells. Chemotherapy must then kill two additional logs to reduce the cell burden to the desired $1 \times 10^5$ cells. However, available chemotherapeutic agents produce a net cell kill of only about 1 log, with the result that the tumor grows despite the drug. The above considerations imply that present multi-modality therapy can palliate infiltrative brain tumors but can rarely cure them. Nevertheless, vigorous therapy permits many patients to live longer with a better quality of life than is possible without such intervention.

### A. Surgery

There are five surgical goals in managing neuroectodermal tumors (Table 3). The first is to establish a diagnosis. While modern radiographic techniques frequently give a presumptive diagnosis with considerable accuracy, both the number of instances where the tissue diagnosis is different and the need to tailor treatment to specific histological tumor type require that a pathological diagnosis be established. A second role for surgery is cytoreduction. It is the only form of cytoreductive therapy in which the tumor cells are not only killed but actually removed. Because the body's capacity to remove debris from the brain may be less than that for other organs of the body, removal of dead tumor tissue is valuable for relief of symptoms due to mass effect. A third goal of surgery is prompt relief of symptoms. As a tumor mass grows it compresses surrounding brain, producing

**Table 3** Goals of Brain Tumor Surgery

1. To establish a diagnosis
2. To decrease the total tumor mass (cytoreduction)
3. To improve symptoms
4. To prolong life
5. To increase the potential benefits of other forms of treatment

increased intracranial pressure and general and focal signs and symptoms. A surgical resection can often reduce signs and symptoms, returning the patient to near-normal functioning. A fourth goal for surgery is to prolong life to permit further anticancer therapy. While a neuroectodermal tumor cannot be cured surgically, partial removal frequently prolongs the patient's life enough to permit adjunctive radiation treatment and chemotherapy. A fifth surgical goal derives from studies of the kinetics of cancer growth. If tumor bulk is reduced, quiescent cells enter an active phase of growth, making them more susceptible to radiation and chemotherapy. Thus, tumor resection potentially increases the sensitivity of the tumor to antineoplastic treatment.

The beneficial effects of surgery are related less to the amount of tumor removed than to leaving the least residual tumor possible. Results of recent studies strongly support the surgical removal of the greatest possible volume of tumor that safe operation allows (19). There is little justification in performing only a biopsy or limited resection of accessible tumors. If the surgeon confines his resection to the tumor itself, he rarely induces a major new neurological defect. On the contrary, patients are frequently able to return to a full, active life without the need for large doses of glucocorticoids. In our view, surgical resection should be considered a key part of the therapy for this disease.

In recent series, the risks of surgical resection or biopsy have been quite acceptable, with a 30-day mortality rate of less than 1% and morbidity rates around 8% (20). Morbidity rates are higher after reoperation because of a higher risk of serious infection of bone flap and scalp. Local scalp, bone, and meningeal blood flow typically is already compromised by previous surgeries and radiation therapy.

## B. Radiation Therapy

Radiation therapy represents the single most important cytocidal therapeutic modality for malignant gliomas. Initial controlled trials of the Brain Tumor Study Group (BTSG) demonstrated that whole-brain radiation therapy increased the survival of patients over resection alone (21,22). Patients receiving 5500–6000 cGy live significantly longer than those receiving 5000 cGy or less (23). In the Brain Tumor Cooperative Group (BTCG) CT scan study, patients with no tumor enhancement after radiation therapy had better survival than those with residual tumor. Patients whose tumors shrank by more than 50% survived longer than those whose tumors shrank less than 50% or those whose tumors increased in size (19).

Because radiation damages normal brain tissue, the BTCG restricted the volume of tissue irradiated as much as possible. In a recently reported study, they compared entirely whole-brain radiation therapy for malignant glioma with partial whole-brain, partial coned-down radiation (24). Patients receiving limited-volume radiation survived as long as those receiving whole-brain radiotherapy.

For malignant gliomas, radiation therapy is now delivered through tumor-focused portals for total tumor doses up to 6000 cGy in 6–7 weeks. Radiation therapy has also been recommended as a form of treatment in low-grade astrocytomas and oligodendrogliomas. For such tumors, radiation is usually limited to the region of the tumor at total doses of 5000–5500 cGy.

Brachytherapy is a more local form of irradiation delivered by interstitial implantation of radioactive seeds. Improved survival has been reported in patients with glioblastoma multiforme treated with temporarily implanted $^{125}$I sources after completion of external beam irradiation or when treated for tumor recurrence (25). The high doses of intratumoral irradiation achieved with this method often results in focal radiation necrosis with edema, requiring reoperation for removal of necrotic tissue. The incidence of steroid dependency is high in these patients, with resulting complications.

In addition to local radiation necrosis, external beam whole-brain irradiation, with or without a coned-down boost, has also been associated with a gradual decline in cognitive function or, rarely, a subacute brain atrophy with progressive neurological deterioration (26,27). In a retrospective review of 160 consecutive patients with malignant glioma treated with radiotherapy, Imperato and coworkers found nine patients who had lived more than twice as long as the median survival for their disease entity (26). All but one patient had cognitive impairment, varying from a mild intellectual decline to profound dementia.

## C. Chemotherapy

Chemotherapy of malignant primary brain tumors has many of the problems of chemotherapy of systemic cancer: lack of therapeutic specificity, development of cellular resistance, and excessive toxicity to normal tissue. In addition, brain tumor chemotherapy must contend with problems related to drug delivery, i.e., low tumor blood flow and the blood-brain, or more precisely, the blood-tumor barrier (BTB). The slower blood flow in tumors reduces delivery of lipid-soluble drugs, while the variable permeability of the BTB restricts entry of water-soluble drugs (28). The problem of cerebral edema adds to the difficulties of the chemotherapist, both because edema affects drug entry and because the effect of the chemotherapeutic agents on the tumor must be distinguished from that of corticosteroid hormone treatment of the edema, especially since steroids are so effective initially. The heterogeneity of brain tumor cells plays a role in response to chemotherapy, with chemosensitivity highest in rapidly growing cells and in the more abnormal, often hyperdiploid cells (29).

Chemotherapeutic agents are cellular poisons whose actions are not specific to tumors but also affect normal cells. They may be cell cycle specific, i.e., effective only during certain phases of the cell's life cycle, usually when DNA is synthesized, or cell cycle nonspecific. However, some drugs such as BCNU that are cell-cycle nonspecific are known to be more effective during DNA synthesis (30). Modifying the growth fraction of a tumor with cell-cycle–nonspecific agents, radiation, or surgery may improve the efficacy of cell-cycle–specific agents because the number of cells in active division may be increased. This may be especially valuable in combination chemotherapy where cell-cycle–specific agents can be combined with cell-cycle–nonspecific agents. Such combinations of sequenced therapies are under investigation.

Two methods to increase tumor concentrations of the drugs in brain tumor chemotherapy are intra-arterial drug delivery and blood-brain barrier modification. The former relies on the "first pass" advantage of high drug concentrations due to local intra-arterial injection and should be especially valuable for drugs with high extraction fractions and rapid systemic elimination. A controlled trial by the BTCG used intra-arterial BCNU chemotherapy (31). The drug proved to be too toxic to both the eye and the half of the brain on the infused side. Current studies are testing the more water-soluble drug cisplatin. Attempting to increase drug concentration by opening the BBB using intracarotid (IC) hyperosmolar mannitol has been described by Neuwelt et al. who administered methotrexate (MTX) (32). In a recent report they indicate that the method is safe and effective (33). Animal studies demonstrate that opening the barrier markedly increased concentrations of MTX in the brain, but much less in the tumor (34). Also, there is concern that patients treated in this manner may ultimately develop brain damage from the high brain MTX concentrations.

Chemotherapy for brain tumors carries the same risks as chemotherapy for systemic malignancies. The almost universal side effect is myelosuppression. This is mostly reversible, but with a tendency to incomplete recovery over time. Chemotherapy with BCNU has the added potential of pulmonary fibrosis which, once developed, is often fatal. The vinca alkaloids and cisplatin may cause a sensorimotor polyneuropathy after repeated administration, with slow improvement of symptoms after discontinuation.

## D. Glucocorticoid Therapy

For intracranial neoplasms, glucocorticoids are the treatment of choice for cerebral edema. Steroids appear to work by reducing edema. On CT scan a decrease in tumor enhancement, mass effect, and edema can be seen within 1 week of starting glucocorticoid treatment. Glucocorticoids improve "global" symptoms (headache, lethargy, etc.) and often reduce the frequency and severity of seizures but are less effective against focal clinical signs and symptoms. Dexamethasone in initial doses of 16–32 mg/day is recommended, although attempts should be made to reduce the dosage gradually to the lowest level of drug that controls symptoms adequately. The myriad complications of glucocorticoids are described in Chapter 9.

## E. Treatment of Cerebral Herniation

Herniation requires immediate attention if the condition is to be reversed before the patient dies or further permanent neurological deficits develop (35). Stuporous or comatose patients need to be intubated to maintain the airway, and hyperventilated to lower the $Pa_{CO_2}$ to 25–30 mm Hg in order to reduce cerebral blood flow and thus reduce cerebral blood volume.

Osmotic diuretics such as mannitol or urea may acutely reduce increased intracranial pressure, but their use must be limited to 4 days or less because of the increased osmolality within the CNS. Mannitol initially should be administered rapidly at doses up to 1 g/kg and repeated as needed with careful monitoring of fluid, electrolyte, and volume status. In addition, 100 mg of dexamethasone may be given intravenously. Once herniation is reversed, patients usually are maintained on glucocorticoids.

## F. Anticonvulsant Medication

Thirty-five percent of patients with a primary brain tumor will eventually have one or more seizures. Anticonvulsants are required for patients who have seizures and usually need to be continued indefinitely (36). Patients with gliomas who do not have seizures initially usually do not require long-term anticonvulsant therapy. While the likelihood of a seizure following clean neurosurgical intervention is low, many neurosurgeons routinely administer anticonvulsants. Phenytoin is the drug used most often. Brain tumor patients treated with radiotherapy and phenytoin have an unusually high incidence of side effects such as skin rashes. Often higher dosages, up to 600 or 800 mg per day, are necessary due to an interaction of phenytoin with glucocorticoids that many patients take concurrently.

## G. Management of Metastatic Glioma

Diffuse gliomatous infiltration of the leptomeninges and subarachnoid space produces a syndrome of chronic meningitis similar to meningitis caused by fungi, tuberculosis, sarcoidosis, and meningovascular syphilis. Subarachnoid seeding is most common in patients with ependymoma and medulloblastoma. For malignant gliomas the incidence of meningeal dissemination has increased over the years with improvement in primary treatment and now may be as high as 20% (37). Leptomeningeal gliomatosis is more common in younger patients. Characteristically, there is involvement of more than one CNS location, i.e., cerebral, cranial nerve, spinal cord, and/or nerve root involvement. Common manifestations include headache, mental changes, cranial nerve palsies, paraparesis and signs of meningeal irritation. Areflexia is common, as is urinary retention and other autonomic signs (38). In two-thirds of patients the diagnosis is made antemortem, on clinical and radiographic grounds, and by cerebrospinal fluid (CSF) analysis. Cerebrospinal fluid pressure may be normal or elevated, sugar content is often below 45 mg/dl, protein content is elevated, and cell counts may reveal an increased number of mononuclear cells and, less often, cytological evidence of malignant cells. Computed tomography and MRI scan may show hydrocephalus, contrast-enhanced subarachnoid or cortical nodules, and meningeal enhancement (39). Treatment consists of radiation therapy to the symptomatic area, such as brain or cauda equina, and systemic or intraventricular chemotherapy. In cases of hydrocephalus, symptomatic improvement may be achieved with a ventriculoperitoneal shunt.

Extracranial metastases are quite rare in malignant brain tumors but are more common in medulloblastoma. The most common distant sites of medulloblastoma metastases are lymph nodes and bone (40). Malignant gliomas metastasize most often to lungs and lymph nodes. Oligodendrogliomas have a higher propensity than astrocytomas or meningiomas for extracranial metastases (41). The treatment of choice for extracranial metastases is systemic chemotherapy. The presence of metastases does not appear to affect survival time, as few patients die as a result of systemic glioma metastases.

## H. Management of Vascular Complications

Patients with malignant glioma are at higher risk for venous thromboembolism, especially in the postoperative period, with an incidence as high as 36% (42). This increased incidence is thought to be related to activation of coagulation by the brain tumor itself through the production of plasmin inhibitors (43). The most common presentation is that of a deep vein thrombosis in the lower extremities, followed in frequency by pulmonary embolus. Lower extremity thrombophlebitis is more common in the hemiparetic patient and is most often found in the hemiparetic leg. Anticoagulant therapy is the treatment of choice, although the complication rate and overall survival are similar when patients are treated with an inferior vena cava Greenfield filter only (44). The incidence of intratumoral bleeding in patients on anticoagulants is low and is similar to patients who have not received anticoagulant therapy.

Cerebral hemorrhage into a primary tumor, usually glioblastomas, may occasionally be associated with subarachnoid hemorrhage. This is usually treated conservatively. However, a patient presenting with an atypical hemorrhage may present a diagnostic challenge. Continued vigilance may be necessary to detect the underlying tumor.

## REFERENCES

1. Schoenberg BS. Epidemiology of primary nervous system neoplasms. In: Schoenberg BS, ed. Advances in neurology, vol. 19. New York: Raven Press, 1978.
2. Farwell JR, Dohrmann, GJ, Flannery JT. Medulloblastoma in childhood: an epidemiological study. J Neurosurg 1984; 61:657–664.
3. Schoenberg BS, Christine BW, Whisnant JP. The resolution of discrepancies in the reported incidence of primary brain tumors. Neurology 1978; 28:817–823.
4. Albright AL, Price RA, Guthkelch AN. Brain stem gliomas of children: a clinicopathological study. Cancer 1983; 52:2313–2319.
5. Post F. Dementia, depression and pseudodementia. In: Benson DF, Blumer D, eds. Psychiatric aspects of neurologic disease. New York: Grune & Stratton, 1975: 99–120.
6. Blumer D, Benson DF. Personality changes with frontal and temporal lobe lesions. In: Benson DF, Blumer D, eds. Psychiatric aspects of neurologic disease. New York: Grune & Stratton, 1975.
7. Robinson RG, Szetela B. Mood change following left hemisphere brain injury. Ann Neurol 1981; 9:447–453.
8. Diamond S, Medina JL. Headaches. Clin Symp 1981; 33:25–28.
9. Lundberg N. Continuous recording and control of ventricular fluid pressure in neurosurgical practice. Acta Psychiatr Scand (Suppl) 1960; 36(149):1–193.
10. Matsuda M, Yoneda S, Handa H, et al. Cerebral hemodynamic changes during plateau waves in brain-tumor patients. J Neurosurg 1979; 50:483–488.
11. Ketz E. Brain tumors and epilepsy. In: Vinken PJ, Bruyn GW, eds. Handbook of clinical neurology, vol. 16. Amsterdam: North-Holland, 1974:254–269.
12. Hughes JR, Zak SM, EEG and clinical changes in patients with chronic seizures associated with slowly growing brain tumors. Arch Neurol 1987; 44:540–543.
13. Cairncross JG, Posner JB. Radiation therapy of brain metastases. Ann Neurol 1980; 7:529–541.
14. Plum F, Posner JB. The diagnosis of stupor and coma. 3rd ed. Philadelphia: Davis, 1980.
15. Van Crevel H. Papilledema, CSF pressure, and CSF flow in cerebral tumors. J Neurol Neurosurg Psychiatry 1979; 42:493–500.
16. Huber A. Eye symptoms in brain tumors. 2nd ed. St. Louis: C. V. Mosby, 1971.
17. Gassel MM. False localizing signs. Arch Neurol 1961; 4:526–554.
18. Shapiro WR. Treatment of neuroectodermal brain tumors. Ann Neurol 12:231–237, 1982.
19. Wood JR, Green SB, Shapiro WR. The prognostic importance of tumor size in malignant gliomas: a computed tomographic scan study by the Brain Tumor Cooperative Group. J Clin Oncol 1988; 6:338–343.

20. Salcman M. The morbidity and mortality of brain tumors: a perspective on recent advances in therapy. Neurol Clin 1985; 3:1–29.
21. Walker MD, Alexander E, Hunt WE, et al. Evaluation of BCNU and/or radiotherapy in the treatment of anaplastic gliomas: a cooperative clinical trial. J Neurosurg 1978; 49:333–343.
22. Walker MD, Green SB, Byar DP, et al. Randomized comparisons of radiotherapy and nitrosoureas for the treatment of malignant glioma after surgery. N Engl J Med 1980; 303:1323–1329.
23. Walker MD, Strike TA, Sheline GE. An analysis of dose-effect relationship in the radiotherapy of malignant gliomas. Int J Radiat Oncol Biol Phys 1979; 5:1725–1731.
24. Shapiro WR, Green SB, Burger PC, et al. Randomized trial of three chemotherapy regimens and two radiotherapy regimens in postoperative treatment of malignant glioma: Brain Tumor Cooperative Group Trial 8001. J Neurosurgery 1989; 71:1–9.
25. Gutin PH, Prados MD, Phillips TL, Wara WM, Larson DA, Leibel SA, Sneed PK, Levin VA, Weaver KA, Silver P, Lamborn K, Lamb S, Ham B. External irradiation followed by an interstitial high activity iodine-125 implant "boost" in the initial treatment of malignant gliomas: NCOG study 6G-82-2. Int J Radiat Oncol Biol Phys 1991; 21:601–606.
26. Imperato JP, Paleologos NA, Vick NA. Effects of treatment on long-term survivors with malignant astrocytomas. Ann Neurol 1990; 28:818–822.
27. Asai A, Matsutani M, Kohno T, Nakamura O, Tanaka H, Fujimaki T, Funada N, Matsuda T, Nagata K, Takakura K. Subacute brain atrophy after radiation therapy for malignant brain tumor. Cancer 1989; 63:1962–1974.
28. Blasberg RG, Groothuis DR. Chemotherapy of brain tumors: physiological and pharmacokinetic considerations. Semin Oncol 1986; 13:70–82.
29. Shapiro JR. Biology of gliomas. Heterogeneity, oncogenes, growth factors. Semin Oncol 1986; 13:4–15.
30. Barranco SC, Humphrey RM. The effects of BCNU on survival and cell progression in Chinese hamster cells. Cancer Res 1971; 31:191–195.
31. Shapiro WR, Green SB. Neurosurgical Forum, Letter to the editor: Reevaluating the efficacy of intra-arterial BCNU. J Neurosurg 1987; 66:313–315.
32. Neuwelt EA, Frenkel EP, Diehl JT, et al. Monitoring of methotrexate delivery in patients with malignant brain tumors after osmotic blood-brain barrier disruption. Ann Intern Med 1981; 94:449–454.
33. Neuwelt EA, Howieson J, Frenkel EP, et al. Therapeutic efficacy of multiagent chemotherapy with drug delivery enhancement by blood-brain barrier modification in glioblastoma. Neurosurgery 1986; 19:573–582.
34. Shapiro WR, Voorhies RM, Hiesiger EM, et al. Pharmacokinetics of tumor cell exposure to [$^{14}$C] methotrexate after intracarotid administration without and with hyperosmotic opening of the blood-brain and blood-tumor barriers in rat brain tumors: a quantitative autoradiographic study. Cancer Res 1988; 48:694–701.
35. Cairncross JG, Posner JB. Neurological complications of systemic cancer. In: Yarbro JW, Bornstein RS, eds. Oncologic emergencies. New York: Grune & Stratton, 1981:73–96.
36. Mattson RH. General principles: selection of antiepileptic drug therapy. In: Levy R,

Mattson R, Meldrum B, Penry JK, Dreifuss FE, eds. Antiepileptic drugs. 3rd ed. New York: Raven Press, 1989:103–115.
37. Yung WA, Horton BC, Shapiro WR. Meningeal gliomatosis: a review of 12 cases. Ann Neurol 1980; 8:605–608.
38. Delattre JY, Walker RW, Rosenblum MK. Leptomeningeal gliomatosis with spinal cord or cauda equina compression: a complication of supratentorial gliomas in adults. Acta Neurol Scand 1989; 79:133–139.
39. Chamberlain MC, Sandy AD, Press GA. Leptomeningeal metastasis: a comparison of gadolinium-enhanced MR and contrast-enhanced CT of the brain. Neurology 1990; 40:435–438.
40. Liwnicz BH, Rubinstein LJ. The pathways of extraneural spread in metastasizing gliomas. Hum Pathol 1979; 10:453–467.
41. Macdonald DR, O'Brien RA, Gilbert JJ, Cairncross JG. Metastatic anaplastic oligodendroglioma. Neurology 1989; 39:1593–1596.
42. Ruff RL, Posner JB. The incidence of systemic venous thrombosis and the risk of anticoagulation in patients with malignant gliomas. Trans Am Neurol Assoc 1981; 16:1–3.
43. Sawaya R, Cummins CJ, Kornblith PL. Brain tumors and plasmin inhibitors. Neurosurgery 1984; 15:795–800.
44. Olin JW, Young JR, Graor RA, Ruschhaupt WF, Beven EG, Bay JW. Treatment of deep vein thrombosis and pulmonary emboli in patients with primary and metastatic brain tumors. Arch Intern Med 1987; 147:2177–2179.

# 6
# Cerebrovascular Complications of Cancer

**Lisa R. Rogers**

*Wayne State University School of Medicine, Detroit, Michigan*

Cerebrovascular disease is the second most common central nervous system (CNS) abnormality found at autopsy in patients with cancer. In an autopsy study by Graus et al. (1), cerebrovascular disease was present in 500 (14.6%) of 3426 patients who died of systemic cancer. Of these, 255 patients, or 7.4% of the total autopsy series, experienced clinical symptoms related to the cerebrovascular disease. Cerebral hemorrhages and infarctions were equal in frequency, but hemorrhages were more frequently symptomatic.

Cerebrovascular disease in the cancer patient presents a challenge to the clinician. The strokes are often multifocal and can be difficult to distinguish from encephalopathy. Cerebrovascular disease must, therefore, be considered in cancer patients who become encephalopathic.

The etiology of cerebrovascular disease is often unique to the cancer patient. Table 1 shows the etiologies of cerebrovascular disease in the series by Graus et al. (1). The risk factors considered significant for stroke in patients without cancer, such as age, hypertension, coronary artery disease, and diabetes mellitus, are overshadowed by pathophysiological effects of cancer or its treatment, such as brain metastases, coagulation disorders, infections, and antineoplastic treatments.

The clinical recognition of cerebrovascular disease in the cancer patient is important because therapy directed to the cause of stroke may reduce neurological morbidity and prevent further vascular events. In addition, cerebrovascular events

**Table 1** CNS Vascular Disorders Found at Autopsy in Patients with Cancer

|  | Number of patients | | |
|---|---|---|---|
|  | 1970–75 | 1976–81 | 1970–81 |
| Cerebral hemorrhage | 118 (80) | 126 (58) | 244 (138) |
| Intracerebral hematoma | | | |
|   Intratumoral | 28 (22) | 32 (25) | 60 (47) |
|   Secondary to coagulopathy | 42 (35) | 46 (22) | 88 (57) |
|   Hypertensive | 9 (8) | — | 9 (8) |
| Primary subdural hematoma | 28 (9) | 35 (7) | 63 (16) |
| Primary subarachnoid hemorrhage | 11 (6) | 13 (4) | 24 (10) |
| Cerebral infarction | 126 (59) | 130 (58) | 256 (117) |
| Atherosclerosis | 31 (7) | 42 (10) | 73 (17) |
| Intravascular coagulation | 15 (13) | 24 (15) | 39 (28) |
| NBTE | 23 (17) | 19 (15) | 42 (32) |
| Septic embolus | 18 (13) | 15 (9) | 33 (22) |
| Tumor embolus | 6 (3) | 6 (1) | 12 (4) |
| Venous occlusion | 19 (2) | 14 (4) | 33 (6) |
| Miscellaneous | 14 (4) | 10 (4) | 24 (8) |
| Total | 244 (139) | 256 (116) | 500 (255) |

( ) No. of symptomatic patients.
Source: Ref. 1; copyright ©1985 by the Williams & Wilkins Co.

are sometimes the presenting sign of cancer and investigation of the cerebrovascular disorder may lead to the diagnosis of cancer.

## I. INTRACEREBRAL HEMORRHAGE

Intracerebral hemorrhage in cancer patients is usually caused by cerebral metastases, coagulation abnormalities, or a combination of these. It occurs more commonly in leukemia than in lymphoma or solid tumors. Hemorrhage usually occurs into the brain parenchyma, but parenchymal hemorrhage can be associated with subdural or subarachnoid hemorrhage. Isolated subdural or subarachnoid hemorrhage is less common (see Table 1). In the absence of severe thrombocytopenia or leptomeningeal metastasis, isolated subarachnoid hemorrhage is sufficiently rare in cancer patients that cerebral angiography should be performed to search for congenital aneurysms.

### A. Tumor-Related Hemorrhage

#### 1. Intratumoral Hemorrhage

Hemorrhage into metastatic brain tumor(s) is the most common cause of brain hemorrhage in patients with solid tumors (1). It occurs most commonly in metastatic melanoma, germ cell tumors (especially choriocarcinoma), and lung cancer, but has been reported in a wide variety of tumors (1,2). The mechanism of intratumoral brain hemorrhage is multifactorial, including tumor necrosis, rupture of thin-walled neoplastic vessels, and the effects of tumor growth on the surrounding brain tissue and blood vessels (3). Symptoms of intratumoral brain hemorrhage are usually acute and include headache, obtundation, or seizure. These symptoms often are accompanied by focal neurological signs. The acute symptoms of intratumoral hemorrhage may be the first clinical manifestation of metastatic brain tumor (1,2) or they may be superimposed on the chronic neurological symptoms of brain metastasis (3). Rarely, cerebral symptoms associated with intratumoral hemorrhage are chronic and indistinguishable from those caused by brain metastasis without hemorrhage (1).

Clues to intratumoral hemorrhage visible on computed tomography (CT) or magnetic resonance imaging (MRI) brain scans include a multiplicity of hemorrhages, locations other than those usually found with hypertensive hemorrhage, and early edema and enhancement adjacent to the hemorrhage. Spin-echo MRI can distinguish neoplastic from nonneoplastic hematomas, because neoplastic hematomas more often have a heterogeneous signal intensity pattern with delayed or atypical patterns of evolution and they lack the well-defined complete hemosiderin rim visible on MRI that is characteristic of nonneoplastic hematomas (4). However, hemorrhagic neoplasms can be confused with occult vascular malformations on MRI. If the MRI scan findings are equivocal, a CT scan can help to distinguish between these. If intratumoral brain hemorrhage is suspected, but the patient is not known to have cancer, biopsy of the hematoma wall is indicated to establish the diagnosis. Survival with intratumoral hemorrhage is generally poor, although some patients with a single hemorrhage benefit from evacuation of the hematoma (2).

## 2. Neoplastic Aneurysm

A rare cause of intracerebral hemorrhage is rupture of a neoplastic aneurysm. Cerebral neoplastic aneurysms occur most commonly in patients with cardiac myxoma, choriocarcinoma, and lung carcinoma (1). Such aneurysms usually develop from a tumor embolus that invades the cerebral arterial wall and produces focal destruction of the internal elastic lamina. Neoplastic aneurysms also may be caused by direct arterial invasion from an adjacent brain metastasis, may be single or multiple and located in distal arterial branches, typically of the middle cerebral artery (5). Intraparenchymal hemorrhages are typical, but subarachnoid or ventricular hemorrhage also may occur, depending upon the location of the aneurysm. The sensitivity of cerebral angiography in detecting neoplastic aneurysms is not known. Angiography may reveal filling defects, fusiform or saccular aneurysms, and occluded vessels, but in some instances the hemorrhage obliterates the aneurysm and angiography is normal. There is no evidence that aneurysm resection is clinically beneficial. Brain irradiation is indicated in neoplastic brain aneurysms that arise from metastatic carcinoma along with antineoplastic therapy directed to the underlying cancer to prevent further embolization. Removal of the cardiac tumor is indicated in patients with cardiac myxoma.

## 3. Dura/Arachnoid Metastasis

Cerebral dural metastasis from carcinoma (especially gastric or prostate carcinoma), leukemia (especially acute lymphocytic leukemia [ALL]), and lymphoma can result in cerebral subdural hemorrhage (1,6). Neoplastic infiltration of the dura results from hematogenous metastasis to the dural vessels or from direct extension of a skull metastasis. The mechanism of hemorrhage may be tumoral hemorrhage or dilatation and rupture of the capillaries of the inner dural layer because the vessels of the outer layer are obstructed by tumor (7). In other patients there may be an effusion from tumor in the dura. In the study by Graus et al. (1), each of 27 carcinoma patients with subdural hematoma had tumor infiltration of the dura at autopsy. Minette and Kimmel (8) reported head trauma and anticoagulant use to be common causes of subdural hemorrhage in patients with carcinoma, but the incidence of dural metastasis was likely underestimated in that study. In leukemia, thrombocytopenia or other coagulation disorders often underlie subdural hemorrhage (see Sec. I.B) and neoplastic infiltration of the dura is less common.

The symptoms of subdural hemorrhage secondary to dural metastasis are usually acute, typically confusion and lethargy. Focal neurological signs are less common. Computed tomography and MRI scans can show acute or chronic subdural hematomas and adjacent skull metastasis. There also may be dural enhancement after contrast injection. However, dural enhancement is not specific for dural metastasis. Histological examination of the dural membrane or cytological examination of subdural fluid is necessary to establish the diagnosis if a dural metastasis is not otherwise evident. Figure 1 shows bilateral subdural fluid collections and dural enhancement on a brain MRI scan of a patient with prostate carcinoma and dural metastasis. Biopsy of the dura and cytological examination of the subdural fluid in this patient revealed carcinoma. Treatment of dural metastasis is palliative and includes drainage of the subdural fluid and brain irradiation.

Leptomeningeal metastases produce intraparenchymal hemorrhage when infiltration of tumor cells in the Virchow-Robin spaces ruptures brain capillaries. Leptomeningeal metastases also can result in subarachnoid hemorrhage, especially if there is a coagulation disorder or thrombocytopenia.

## 4. Parenchymal Leukemic Infiltration

Coagulopathy is the most common cause of brain hemorrhage in patients with leukemia (see Sec. I.B). In a smaller percentage of patients with leukemia, intracerebral hemorrhage is associated with extreme elevation of the peripheral blast count (hyperleukocytosis), usually above 100,000 cells/mm$^3$. Intracranial hemorrhage associated with hyperleukocytosis is most common in acute myelogenous leukemia (AML), especially acute monocytic leukemia (9), and occurs more

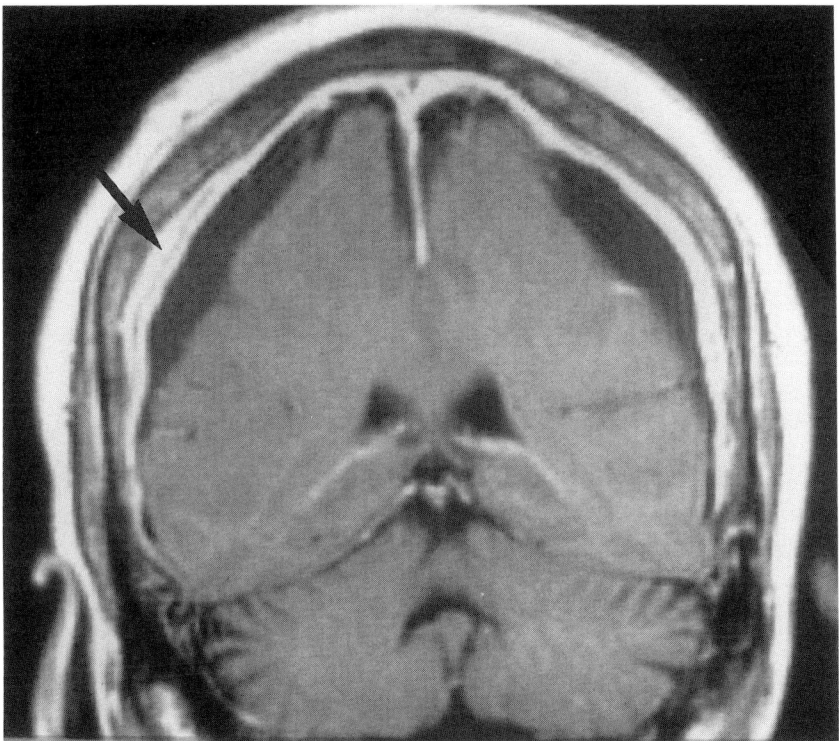

**Figure 1** Bilateral subdural fluid collections in a patient with dural metastasis from prostate carcinoma. The dura overlying the cerebral convexities is thickened and enhances with gadolinium (*arrow*). Reprinted with permission from Ref. 55.

commonly at the diagnosis of leukemia than does hemorrhage from coagulopathy. Coagulation disorders, including thrombocytopenia, may contribute but are not essential to the pathogenesis of hemorrhage associated with hyperleukocytosis. Table 2 shows the clinical factors associated with intracranial hemorrhage and hyperleukocytosis in the series by Graus et al. (1).

The hemorrhages are usually multiple and intraparenchymal, but there may be associated intraventricular or subarachnoid hemorrhage. Postmortem examination invariably reveals parenchymal CNS leukemic nodules and plugging of thin-walled cerebral vessels by leukemic blasts (leukostasis) (10). The mechanism of brain hemorrhage is uncertain but likely is a combination of infiltration with rupture of cerebral blood vessels by the leukemic nodules and hypoxic endothelial damage due to hyperviscosity from leukostasis. The incidence of brain hemorrhage associated with hyperleukocytosis has declined in recent years because of

**Table 2** Factors Leading to Intracerebral Hemorrhage in Patients with Leukemia

|  | Hemorrhage without CNS leukemic infiltration | Hemorrhage with CNS leukemic infiltration | |
|---|---|---|---|
|  |  | Parenchymal infiltrates with leukostasis | Arachnoidal infiltrates without leukostasis |
| Number of patients | 50 | 13 | 6 |
| Number symptomatic* | 38 (76%) | 8 (61.5%) | 3 (50%) |
| Histological type |  |  |  |
| ALL | 5 (2) | 3 (2) | 1 (1) |
| AML | 19 (16) | 2 (1) | 3 (1) |
| CML | 5 (5) | 3 (2) | 1 |
| APL | 9 (7) | — | 1 (1) |
| Other | 12 (8) | 5 (3) | — |
| Hemorrhage at time of diagnosis of leukemia | 7 (18.4%) | 5 (62.5%) | — |
| Fever | 68.4% | 37.5% | 100% |
| WBC (/mm$^3$) | 8,000<br>100–104,000 | 26,000<br>70,000–730,000 | 36,000<br>1,000–97,000 |
| Platelets (/mm$^3$) | 13,500<br>2,000–52,000 | 36,000<br>10,000–50,000 | 32,000<br>3,000–65,000 |
| Multiple hematomas | 12% | 62.5% | 16.6% |

( ) No. of symptomatic patients.
*ALL: Acute lymphoblastic leukemia, AML: Acute myelogenous leukemia, CML: Chronic myelogenous leukemia, APL: Acute promyelocytic leukemia.
Source: Ref. 1; copyright ©1985 by the Williams & Wilkins Co.

effective means to lower the peripheral blast count, including leukapheresis and antimetabolites (11).

## B. Coagulopathy and Thrombocytopenia

Systemic cancer is frequently associated with abnormalities of hemostasis. There are several mechanisms by which malignancies produce hemostatic abnormalities, including neovascularization of tumor by vessels with abnormal endothelial lining, release of necrotic tumor tissue or tumor cell enzymes into the systemic circulation, and fibrinolytic activation. The release of procoagulant material from the cytoplasmic granules of the progranulocytes in acute promyelocytic leukemia (APML), a subtype of AML, can result in acute disseminated intravascular coagulation (DIC). In acute DIC, hemorrhages coexist with small- or large-vessel thrombosis. Most patients with widely metastatic solid tumors have laboratory evidence of coagulation dysfunction, but this rarely causes clinical manifestations. Thrombocytopenia in cancer patients occurs commonly from neoplastic invasion of the bone marrow or from the effects of radiation and chemotherapy on the marrow.

Intraparenchymal brain hemorrhage from coagulopathy is most common in leukemia. Such bleeds typically are symptomatic and often fatal (1). Acute promyelocytic leukemia is frequently associated with intracerebral hemorrhage as a complication of acute DIC, often shortly after beginning treatment. In solid tumors, cerebral hemorrhage from coagulopathy usually occurs as a terminal event.

In leukemias other than APML, intracerebral hemorrhage may be associated with DIC but occurs at relapse or with failure to induce a complete remission. In this setting there is usually superimposed infection, liver failure, and hematologic complications of chemotherapy. Clinically apparent coagulopathy is rare in ALL but can result in intraparenchymal hemorrhage, especially with the T-cell phenotype. Coagulation disorders also can result in subdural hemorrhage, especially in leukemia (12). In the series by Graus et al. (1), thrombocytopenia and sepsis were present in all patients with leukemia who had subdural hematoma, with or without DIC. In contrast, coagulopathy was present in only a few patients with carcinoma who had subdural hematoma. In chronic lymphocytic leukemia and lymphoma, intracranial hemorrhage can be due to thrombocytopenia from autoimmune thrombocytopenic purpura. Although the treatment of solid tumors with chemotherapy can result in significant thrombocytopenia, the incidence of intracerebral hemorrhage in this setting is low.

The symptoms of intracerebral hemorrhage from coagulopathy include headache, vomiting, acutely evolving decline in consciousness and severe focal neurological signs. Computed tomography or MRI brain scans show single or multiple parenchymal or subdural hemorrhages. Patients with acute DIC may have other clinical sites of hemorrhage, including the mucosal surfaces, retinae, gastrointestinal and genitourinary tracts, skin, and venipuncture and bone marrow aspiration sites. No laboratory test is diagnostic of DIC and abnormal coagulation tests must be cautiously interpreted within the clinical context. Useful laboratory tests to diagnose acute DIC include the platelet count, prothrombin time, activated partial thromboplastin time, fibrinogen, fibrin degradation products, D-dimer assay, fibrinopeptide A, and the presence of schistocytes on the peripheral blood smear. In chronic DIC, results of tests of hemostasis are less abnormal and less useful.

Treatment for patients who develop cerebral hemorrhage from coagulopathy should be directed at controlling the tumor, the coagulopathy, and associated medical conditions that may contribute, such as sepsis. Prophylactic heparin with chemotherapy (13,14) and *trans*-retinoic acid (15) are effective in reducing the incidence of intracerebral hemorrhage in APML.

## C. Treatment-Related Hemorrhage

L-Asparaginase, frequently used in the induction therapy of ALL, can cause cerebral hemorrhage or thrombosis. The mechanism for the paradoxical hemostatic effects of this drug is not known, but it is known to produce fibrinolysis and to deplete plasma proteins involved in coagulation. In some instances, intracerebral hemorrhage is correlated with hypofibrinogenemia (16). Although recurrence of intracerebral vascular events with repeated use of L-asparaginase has not been reported, Feinberg and Swenson (17) suggest that prophylactic fresh-frozen plasma be considered to prevent repeated episodes. A syndrome similar to the hemolytic uremic syndrome can complicate chemotherapy, particularly mitomycin (18). It is reported most commonly in patients with gastrointestinal and colorectal carcinomas, possibly reflecting the relative frequency with which these tumors are treated with mitomycin. This syndrome can result in intracerebral hemorrhage, usually as a terminal event.

## D. Miscellaneous

Hypertension is a rare cause of intracerebral hemorrhage in cancer patients; it accounted for only 6% of symptomatic hemorrhages in the series by Graus et al. (1). Another uncommon cause of hemorrhage in the cancer patient is impaired platelet function with chronic myeloproliferative disorders (especially chronic myelogenous leukemia and myelofibrosis) and multiple myeloma. Hemorrhages in this situation may be intraparenchymal, subdural, or subarachnoid and there often is associated systemic bleeding. In polycythemia vera and essential thrombocythemia, intracerebral hemorrhage may coexist with thrombosis (19). Conventional cytoreductive therapy (alkylating agents) and phlebotomy can reduce the rate of thrombohemorrhagic complications in chronic myeloproliferative disorders. Bleeding in patients with multiple myeloma also can occur in the setting of hyperviscosity. Patients with lymphoma may bleed due to idiopathic thrombocytopenic purpura or an acquired form of von Willebrand's disease.

## II. CEREBRAL INFARCTION

Coagulopathy, infection, the direct effects of tumor, and complications of antineoplastic treatment are the most common causes of cerebral infarctions in patients with cancer. Symptomatic cerebral infarctions are more common in lymphoma and carcinoma than in leukemia, where cerebral hemorrhages predominate.

## A. Coagulopathy

### 1. Nonbacterial Thrombotic Endocarditis

Graus and coworkers (1) found cerebral infarction from nonbacterial thrombotic endocarditis (NBTE) to be the most common cause of symptomatic cerebral infarction in cancer patients. Nonbacterial thrombotic endocarditis results from a complex coagulation disorder involving platelets and fibrinogen in which sterile platelet-fibrin vegetations develop on cardiac valves (Fig. 2). It occurs most commonly in adenocarcinomas, especially mucin-producing carcinomas, of the lung or gastrointestinal tract. Nonbacterial thrombotic endocarditis is also a rare complication of autologous or allogeneic bone marrow transplantation in cancer patients. Although NBTE usually occurs in patients with widely disseminated cancer, it may occur at any stage of cancer, and in a few patients, cerebral infarction caused by NBTE is the first sign of malignancy (20). Occlusion of

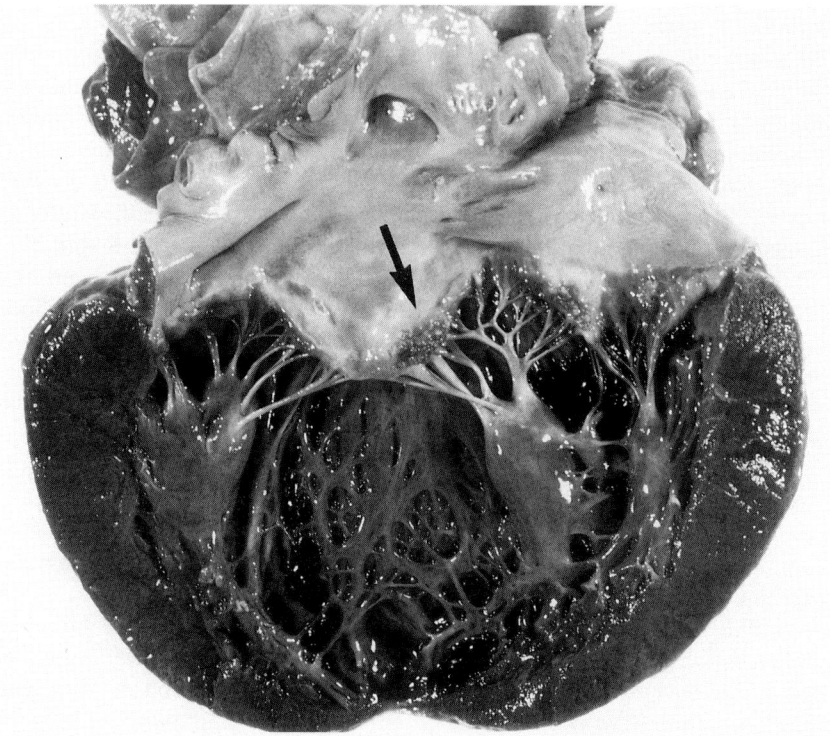

**Figure 2** Mitral valve vegetation of nonbacterial thrombotic endocarditis (NBTE) (*arrow*). (From Ref. 20.)

cerebral vessels in NBTE results from embolization of cardiac vegetations to the brain or from cerebral intravascular thrombosis secondary to the associated coagulation disorder (20,21). Occlusion of small- or medium-sized cerebral vessels is more common than occlusion of large-sized vessels in NBTE (20), resulting in cerebral infarctions that often are multiple and may be hemorrhagic.

Neurological signs with NBTE are usually focal cerebral, most commonly aphasia. Focal signs usually begin abruptly and may be preceded by symptoms suggesting transient ischemic attacks. Focal signs may be accompanied by signs of diffuse encephalopathy or, less commonly, the only neurological sign of NBTE is encephalopathy (20). Focal and diffuse neurological signs are usually progressive, with cumulative neurological dysfunction, but clinical recovery may occur between episodes (20,21).

A clue to the diagnosis of NBTE is evidence of systemic bleeding or thromboembolism, including limb thrombophlebitis or arterial occlusion, pulmonary embolus, or myocardial infarction. In some patients, however, neurological signs are the only clinical evidence of NBTE (20,21) and the diagnosis of NBTE is difficult. A small percentage of patients with NBTE have evidence of DIC by laboratory testing, but in most patients results of coagulation function tests are only mildly abnormal and are indistinguishable from the laboratory abnormalities commonly associated with cancer. New or changing cardiac murmurs are rare and echocardiography is usually not revealing (20), due to the small size of the valve vegetations. Computed tomography or MRI brain scans reveal cerebral infarction(s). In patients who have focal neurological signs, the most specific test for the diagnosis of cerebral infarction from NBTE is cerebral angiography. Rogers et al. (20) reported occlusion of one or more cerebral vessels, most often multiple branch occlusions of the middle cerebral artery, in eight of nine patients with focal neurological signs who underwent angiography (Fig. 3). The usefulness of cerebral angiography in patients who manifest only encephalopathy is unknown.

Therapy of NBTE should be directed to the primary cause of the coagulation disorder, such as the tumor or sepsis. There are no prospective studies of anticoagulation therapy because of the difficulty in establishing the diagnosis of cerebral infarction from NBTE during the patient's lifetime. Heparin can reduce ischemic symptoms in some patients with cerebral ischemia from NBTE (20). Anticoagulation therapy, preferably with intravenous or subcutaneous heparin, may be useful in selected patients. The potential benefit of anticoagulation should be carefully weighed against the risk of systemic or intracerebral bleeding from the coagulation disorder. If anticoagulants are administered. the clinician should be alert to the development of cerebral or systemic thromboembolism when anticoagulants are discontinued (20,22).

## 2. *Intravascular Coagulation*

Thrombotic occlusion of cerebral vessels from coagulopathy in the absence of NBTE (cerebral intravascular coagulation) is the second most common cause of

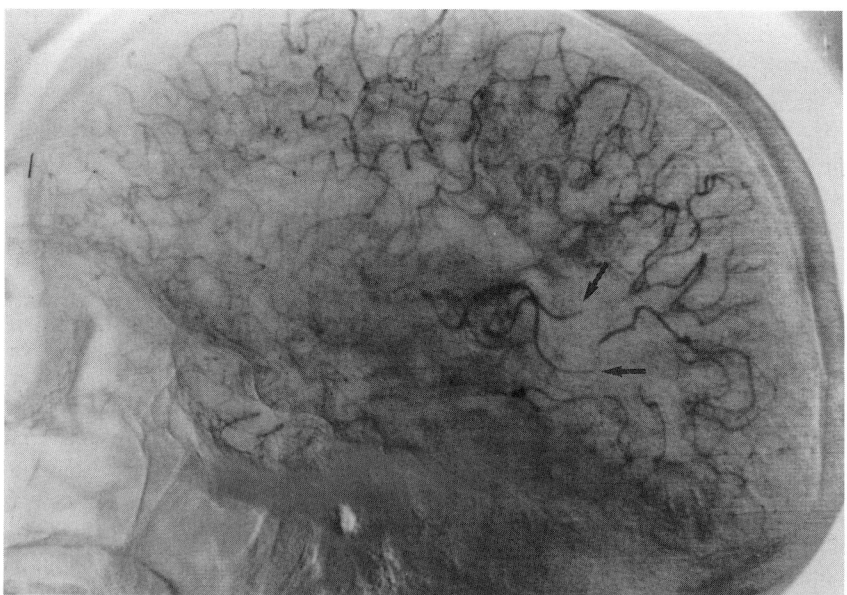

**Figure 3** Cerebral angiography shows branch occlusions of the left middle cerebral artery (*arrows*) in a patient with lung carcinoma and NBTE who experienced aphasia. (From Ref. 20.)

symptomatic cerebral infarction in patients with cancer (1). Cerebral intravascular coagulation probably results from the chronic form of DIC. Symptomatic cerebral intravascular coagulation occurs most commonly in leukemia, breast cancer, and lymphoma, and is usually associated with sepsis and advanced cancer. The neurological signs of cerebral intravascular coagulation usually begin abruptly. In contrast with NBTE, where focal neurological signs predominate, intravascular coagulation typically produces a diffuse encephalopathy. About one-half of patients will have superimposed, often transient, focal signs (23). The clinical course is progressive, but there may be fluctuations in neurological signs. The neuropathological findings are those of cerebral arterial, arteriolar, capillary, and/or venular occlusion by fibrin with adjacent microinfarction or petechiae. Typically, multiple vessels in more than one major vessel territory are thrombosed. Postmortem examination also may show thrombotic occlusions of the microvasculature of systemic organs.

Many patients with cerebral intravascular coagulation have systemic bleeding. Laboratory evidence of classical DIC is rarely found, however, and there is no pathognomonic laboratory test in this disorder. Computed tomography brain scans and angiograms performed in a few patients were normal (1,23). The only definitive way to diagnose this syndrome is by postmortem examination. Appropriate treatment for cerebral intravascular coagulation is not known; a small number of patients treated with heparin did not improve (1,23). The prognosis is very poor and most patients live only a few weeks, death being caused by sepsis, disseminated cancer, or bleeding.

## 3. Venous Occlusion

Occlusion of cerebral venous sinuses or large-sized cortical veins in cancer patients may be metastatic (see Sec. II.C) or nonmetastatic in origin. The superior sagittal sinus is most commonly affected. The clinical incidence of nonmetastatic superior sagittal sinus occlusion is underestimated in autopsy studies, because nonmetastatic sinus occlusions may recanalize. Nonmetastatic venous occlusion is probably related to a coagulation disorder associated with cancer or chemotherapy but, as in other cerebral thromboembolic complications, objective evidence of coagulopathy is difficult to document. Induction therapy with L-asparaginase in ALL can cause cerebral venous thrombosis (17). In lymphoma and solid tumors, nonmetastatic superior sagittal sinus occlusion usually occurs in the setting of widespread metastatic disease (24) but has been reported as a presenting sign in myeloproliferative disorders. Symptomatic, nonmetastatic superior sagittal sinus thrombosis usually presents abruptly with seizures. There also may be focal neurological signs or encephalopathy if there is cerebral infarction. Figure 4 shows bilateral hemorrhagic infarctions secondary to nonmetastatic superior sagittal sinus occlusion in a patient with breast carcinoma.

Magnetic resonance imaging is the method of choice to diagnose cerebral venous occlusion. Spin-echo imaging can document the lack of normal flow void within the occluded sinus and can reveal enlarged medullary or cortical veins and adjacent hemorrhage or infarction (25). In the setting of slow flow or acute/early subacute thrombosis, however, the intraluminal signal may be difficult to interpret. In this setting, magnetic resonance venography (MRV) designed to be sensitive to slow flow may be diagnostic. If MRI or MRV is not available, CT brain scans can be useful. Abnormalities on unenhanced scans include hyperdensity within the sinus from freshly congealed blood, the "cord" sign from thrombosed cortical veins, and adjacent hemorrhage or hemorrhagic venous infarction. Enhanced scans may reveal the "empty delta" sign from a filling defect within the sinus and prominence of collaterals resulting in intense tentorial enhancement (26). When the anterior or midportions of the superior sagittal sinus are occluded, coronal CT sections are needed for adequate visualization.

Many patients with nonmetastatic superior sagittal sinus occlusion show spontaneous recovery, especially when it occurs early in cancer. In patients with widely disseminated disease, however, the chances for recovery are poor. There is evidence that heparin is beneficial in the clinical recovery and survival of patients without cancer who develop superior sagittal sinus thrombosis (27). Patients with

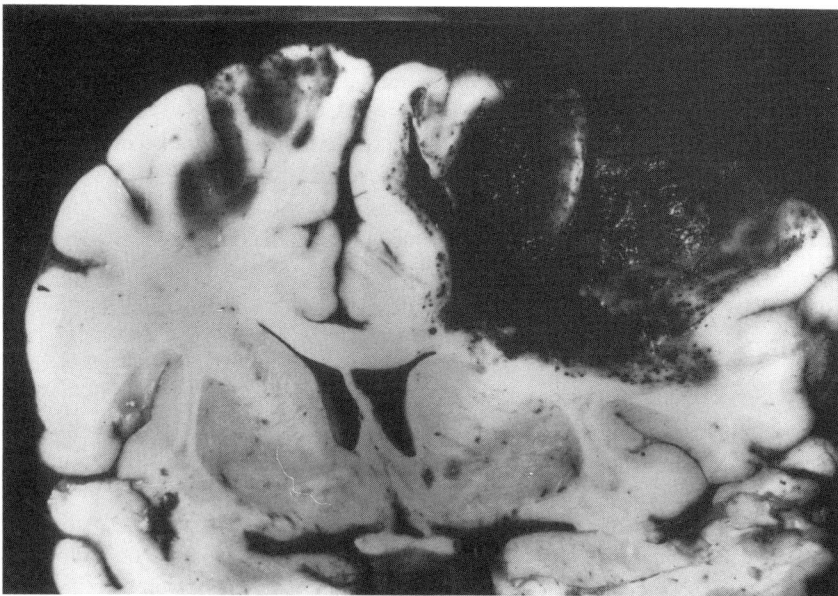

**Figure 4** Bilateral cerebral hemorrhagic infarctions caused by nonmetastatic superior sagittal sinus thrombosis. Reprinted with permission from Ref. 55.

cancer also may benefit from anticoagulation, but this issue has not been adequately studied.

## B. Infection

### 1. Septic Infarction

Septic cerebral infarction occurs more commonly in leukemia than in lymphoma or carcinoma. It is frequently symptomatic (67% in the series by Graus et al. [1]). Septic infarction is usually due to fungal sepsis without meningitis (1,28). Radiation and chemotherapy, broad-spectrum antibiotics, or immunosuppression resulting from the neoplasm, bone marrow transplant, steroids, and other immunosuppressants may make cancer patients susceptible to fungal infection. *Aspergillus* and *Candida* species are the most common fungal organisms causing septic cerebral infarction. Cerebral vascular invasion by the organisms results in thrombosis and infarction. Septic cerebral infarctions are usually multiple and hemorrhagic. The cerebral hemispheres, brainstem, and cerebellum may be involved. The most common port of entry for *Aspergillus* is the lower respiratory tract. In candidiasis, the port of entry is usually the gastrointestinal or genitourinary tract or indwelling venous catheters. Less commonly, cerebral infarction can result from vasculitis due to basilar meningitis from fungal or mycobacterial organisms or to invasion of the brain from a paranasal infection with *Mucor* or *Aspergillus* species.

Neurological symptoms of septic cerebral infarction include seizures, sudden focal neurological signs, and progressive encephalopathy. Acute focal symptoms and seizures are more common in aspergillosis and mucormycosis. Encephalopathy is more common in candidiasis. A clue to *Aspergillus* infection is evidence of pulmonary infection. Pulmonary aspergillosis may produce pleuritic pain, nonproductive cough, and hemoptysis. Chest radiographs often reveal pulmonary infiltration, but may be normal early in the course. *Aspergillus* can be isolated from respiratory secretions or open-lung biopsy, but lung biopsy is hazardous in many cancer patients because of thrombocytopenia. Computed tomography and MRI brain scans in septic cerebral infarction may be normal, show infarction, or show ring enhancement if the infection is evolving into an abscess. Fever may be present in fungal sepsis, but blood cultures are usually negative. Hemorrhagic CSF may be a clue to aspergillosis, but in the absence of meningitis, the CSF examination in septic cerebral infarction reveals only mild pleocytosis and protein elevation. The prognosis in fungal cerebral infarction is extremely poor, even when patients are appropriately treated for fungal infection (28).

Bacterial sepsis is uncommon in patients with cancer, except those who are neutropenic from chemotherapy. In this setting, cerebral infarction can occur from vascular invasion of *Staphylococcus aureus*, *Escherichia coli*, or *Streptococcus fecalis* (29). Encephalopathy, rather than focal neurological signs, usually occurs with bacterial septic brain infarction.

### 2. Herpes Zoster Vasculopathy

Herpes zoster is a common viral infection in cancer patients who are immunosuppressed. Cerebral infection with herpes zoster probably occurs by spread of the virus from the trigeminal ganglion and it can be associated with cerebral granulomatous angiitis. The causal relationship between herpes zoster and granulomatous angiitis is not clear, however, because a similar type of granulomatous angiitis (described in Sec. II.F) occurs without evidence of herpes zoster infection in some patients with lymphoma or leukemia. The syndrome of herpes zoster ophthalmicus followed by contralateral hemiplegia is rare in cancer patients. In this setting, the large proximal branches of the circle of Willis, usually ipsilateral to the site of herpes zoster infection, are thrombosed. Abrupt focal neurological signs or encephalopathy occur and angiography characteristically shows single or multiple segmental narrowings in the proximal pericallosal or middle cerebral artery (30). Postmortem examination suggests that cerebrovascular invasion by the virus results in thrombosis without significant inflammation (31).

## C. Tumor-Related Cerebral Infarction

### 1. Venous Occlusion

Metastatic cerebral venous occlusion is due to skull or dural tumor infiltrating or compressing the sinus producing stasis and thrombosis. The metastatic type of venous occlusion is found more often at autopsy than the nonmetastatic type. Metastatic venous occlusion occurs most commonly in neuroblastoma, lung cancer, and lymphoma, but it can occur in a variety of tumors (1). The symptoms of metastatic superior sagittal sinus occlusion (headache, vomiting, and papilledema) are usually subacute and result from increased intracranial pressure. Focal neurological signs, and less commonly encephalopathy, may result if there is cerebral infarction.

The neuroimaging of superior sagittal sinus occlusion is described in Section II.A. In patients with metastatic superior sagittal sinus occlusion, skull radiographs may also reveal adjacent skull metastases and CT or MRI brain scans may reveal dural or skull metastases. Figure 5 shows the MRV in a patient with neoplastic superior sagittal sinus occlusion. Metastatic superior sagittal sinus occlusion should be treated with brain irradiation. The value of anticoagulation in this disorder is not known.

### 2. Tumor Embolism

Cerebral infarction from embolism of a tumor fragment to the brain is rare. It occurs in patients with solid tumors, usually those with cardiac or lung metastasis that provide the source of cerebral embolism. In patients with primary or metastatic lung tumor, surgical manipulation of the lung at thoracotomy can dislodge tumor emboli (1,32,33). Tumor embolic infarction can also be the presenting sign of cardiac myxoma or carcinoma of unknown origin. Neurological manifestations of tumor embolic infarction include the abrupt onset of focal signs, usually involving the carotid circulation, or occasionally, diffuse encephalopathy accompanied by focal signs. Sometimes the infarction is preceded by transient ischemic attacks (33).

The diagnosis of tumor embolic infarction can be suspected by cerebral infarction(s) on CT scan and embolic occlusions on angiography (33–35). However, these findings are not specific and a definitive diagnosis can be established only by histological examination of a simultaneous peripheral arterial embolus. Congestive heart failure, pericardial effusion, rapid cardiac enlargement, or arrhythmias unresponsive to digitalis are clues to cardiac metastasis underlying cerebral tumor embolism. Echocardiography may reveal cardiac tumor. Clinical studies suggest that cerebral tumor growth is rare in myxoma (35,36), but patients with systemic cancer suspected of having cerebral tumor embolic infarction should undergo follow-up CT or MRI brain scans to check for tumor growth. A

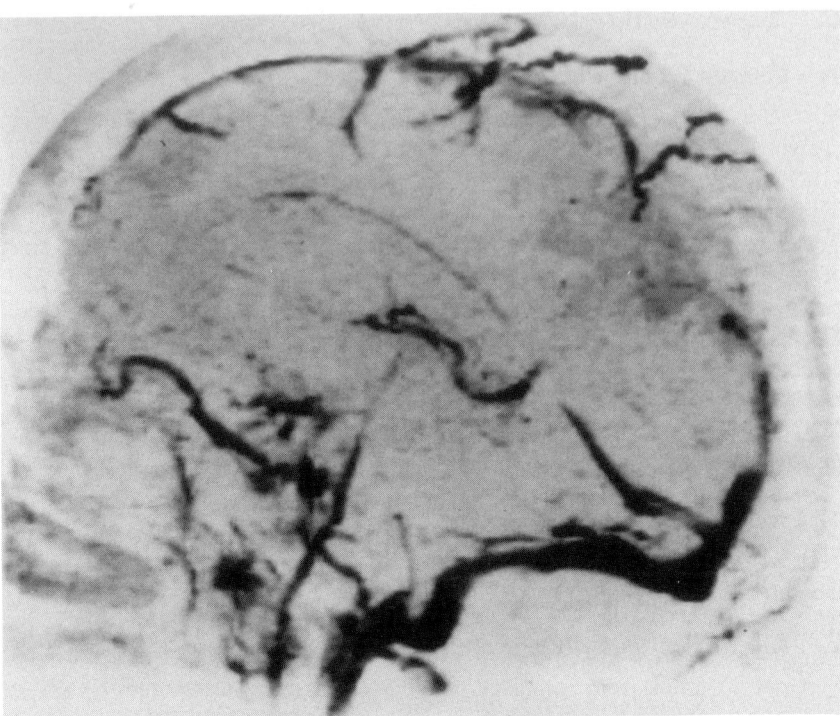

**Figure 5** Sequential two-dimensional magnetic resonance venography shows nonfilling of the posterior superior sagittal sinus which is caused by tumor compression. There is dilation of the collateral cortical and emissary scalp veins. Reprinted with permission from Ref. 55.

rare cause of embolic infarction is embolization of mucinous material from mucin-producing carcinomas. This can be difficult to distinguish pathologically from thrombosis due to coagulopathy (37).

### 3. Leptomeningeal Metastasis

In a small percentage of patients with leptomeningeal metastasis, symptomatic cerebral infarction occurs because of occlusion of the penetrating cerebral vessels in the Virchow-Robin spaces by tumor cells. Computed tomography or MRI brain scans may reveal multifocal infarctions. Angiography may be normal or may reveal focal arteriolar narrowing at the base of the brain or over the cerebral convexities (38). Definitive diagnosis can be established only by demonstration of malignant cells in CSF or on leptomeningeal biopsy.

## D. Treatment-Related Cerebral Infarction

Therapies for cancer can result in cerebral infarction when they cause coagulopathy or direct toxicity to the extra- or intracranial cerebral vessels. Neck irradiation, especially when administered for head and neck cancers and lymphoma, can produce extracranial carotid stenosis or occlusion. Histological analysis of the diseased arteries suggests that radiation produces or accelerates atherosclerosis. Carotid occlusion has been reported after standard radiation, usually greater than 50 Gy doses, but a variety of doses and types of radiation are associated with radiation-induced carotid artery disease. The interval from radiation to carotid occlusive disease varies widely. In a recent review, Murros and Toole (39) reported a range of 6 months to 57 years (mean, 19 years) between radiation therapy and extracranial vascular disease. Symptoms include cerebral hemispheric transient ischemic attacks or infarctions, amaurosis fugax, or seizures. Angiography usually reveals occlusion or extensive stenosis of the common carotid artery (less commonly the internal carotid artery) confined to the field of radiation. Optimal therapy for radiation-induced carotid occlusive disease has not been determined. No prospective medical trials are reported. Although technically more difficult than in nonirradiated patients, the results of endarterectomy in a small number of patients were favorable (40). Successful results also can be achieved with vessel bypass.

Carotid artery rupture can occur following resection of head and neck tumors and neck irradiation and is usually associated with unintentional orocutaneous fistulas, necrosis of the skin flap, and infection. The mortality of carotid artery rupture is high because it may lead to exsanguination. If the carotid rupture is detected and the artery ligated, there is a risk of cerebral infarction and death (41,42). The risk of infarction is reduced in some patients by the administration of low-dose heparin (43).

The mechanism of cerebrovascular complications of chemotherapy is not well understood (44). Possible causes of cerebral thrombosis include endothelial cell damage, vasospasm, coagulation abnormalities, or a chemotherapy-induced syndrome similar to the hemolytic uremic syndrome. Systemic and cerebral venous and arterial thromboembolic complications are observed with increasing frequency in women receiving multi-agent chemotherapy for breast cancer, especially early in treatment. In this setting, cerebral infarction can be fatal (45). There also is an association between combination chemotherapy administered for other solid tumors, especially those containing cisplatin, and cerebral infarction (46). Leukemia patients receiving induction therapy with L-asparaginase may experience cerebral infarction or cerebral venous thrombosis (see Sec. II.A.3). The prognosis for recovery from L-asparaginase–induced cerebral infarction is good. A rare cause of cerebral infarction associated with chemotherapy is cerebral embolization from a ventricular mural thrombus caused by cardiomyopathy from adriamycin (47). Transient focal neurological symptoms, suggesting transient ischemic attacks, can occur during interleukin-2 therapy (48).

## E. Atherosclerosis

Graus et al. (1) found atherosclerosis to be the most common cause of cerebral infarction in cancer patients examined at autopsy, but it represented only 14.5% of symptomatic infarctions. Cancers of the head and neck and lung are most frequently associated with atherosclerotic brain infarction. Several prospective studies have shown an association between low serum cholesterol levels and cancer mortality, particularly in men, but the significance of lower serum cholesterol levels is not known. The inverse relationship between serum cholesterol levels and cancer may be due to a metabolic effect of the preclinical cancer on serum cholesterol.

## F. Miscellaneous

Granulomatous angiitis in the absence of herpes zoster infection is a rare cause of cerebral infarction in cancer patients (49,50). It occurs in Hodgkin's disease and leukemia and it also may affect the spinal cord. The clinical manifestations include headache, fever, confusion, seizures, hemiparesis, coma, and paraparesis if there is spinal cord involvement. The disease progresses gradually, although there may be transient improvement in symptoms. Cerebrospinal fluid examination may reveal pleocytosis and elevated protein. Computed tomography brain scans may be normal or reveal contrast-enhancing masses, hematomas, or nonhemorrhagic infarctions (50). In some patients cerebral angiography shows a classic vasculitic beading pattern but the diagnosis is difficult to establish without brain biopsy. The angiitis often responds to treatment directed to the underlying tumor or to steroids and cytotoxic drugs administered for the vasculitis.

Cerebral thromboembolism can complicate chronic myeloproliferative disorders when there is extreme thrombocytosis. Thrombotic complications are most common in polycythemia vera and essential thrombocythemia and are correlated with older age (51). Cerebral symptoms in patients with polycythemia vera and essential thrombocythemia commonly are hard to localize, such as dizziness, unsteadiness, dysarthria, and blurred vision, and may be accompanied by headache. Occlusion of large and small cerebral vessels in thrombocythemia is believed to be due to inherent alterations of platelet function as well as the high platelet count. There also may be associated systemic thromboembolism, including deep vein thrombosis and myocardial infarction. Antiplatelet aggregating agents and cytoreductive therapy are effective in thrombocytosis (52).

Episodic neurological dysfunction, clinically resembling transient ischemic attacks, has been reported in patients who are in remission or cured of Hodgkin's disease (53). The pathogenesis of this syndrome is unknown and the clinical course is benign. A rare complication of diagnostic testing is cerebral lipid embolism occurring in lymphoma patients undergoing lymphangiography (54). Symptoms of diffuse encephalopathy, sometimes associated with mild focal neurological signs, develop hours after the procedure. There also may be clinical signs of pulmonary embolism. Most patients recover completely.

# REFERENCES

1. Graus F, Rogers LR, Posner JB. Cerebrovascular complications in patients with cancer. Medicine 1985; 64:16–35.
2. Little JR, Dial B, Bélanger G, et al. Brain hemorrhage from intracranial tumor. Stroke 1979; 10:283–288.
3. Kondziolka D, Bernstein M, Resch L, et al. Significance of hemorrhage into brain tumors: clinicopathological study. J Neurosurg 1987; 67:852–857.
4. Atlas SW, Grossman RI, Gomori JM, et al. Hemorrhagic intracranial malignant neoplasms: spin-echo MR imaging. Radiology 1987; 164:71–77.
5. Noterman J, Verhest A, Baleriaux D, et al. A ruptured cerebral aneurysm from choriocarcinomatous origin—a case report and a review. Neurosurg Rev 1989; 12: 71–74.
6. Pitner SE, Johnson WW. Chronic subdural hematoma in childhood acute leukemia. Cancer 1973; 32:185–190.
7. Russell DS, Cairns H. Subdural false membrane or hematoma (pachymeningitis interna hemorrhagica) in carcinomatosis and sarcomatosis of the dura mater. Brain 1934; 57:32–48.
8. Minette SE, Kimmel DW. Subdural hematoma in patients with systemic cancer. Mayo Clin Proc 1989; 64:637–642.
9. Creutzig U, Ritter J, Budde M, et al. Early deaths due to hemorrhage and leukostasis in childhood acute myelogenous leukemia. Cancer 1987; 60:3071–3079.
10. Freireich EJ, Thomas LB, Frei E, et al. A distinctive type of intracerebral hemorrhage associated with "blastic crisis" in patients with leukemia. Cancer 1960; 13: 146–154.
11. Hug V, Keating M, McCredie K, et al. Clinical course and response to treatment of patients with acute myelogenous leukemia presenting with a high leukocyte count. Cancer 1983; 52:773–779.
12. Belmusto L, Regelson W, Owens G, et al. Intracranial extracerebral hemorrhages in acute lymphocytic leukemia. Cancer 1964; 8:1079–1088.
13. Drapkin RL, Gee TS, Dowling MD, et al. Prophylactic heparin therapy in acute promyelocytic leukemia. Cancer 1978; 41:2484–2490.
14. Gralnick HR, Bagley J, Abrell E. Heparin treatment for the hemorrhagic diathesis of acute promyelocytic leukemia. Am J Med 1972; 52:167–174.
15. Castaigne S, Chomienne C, Daniel MT, et al. All-trans retinoic acid as a differentiation therapy for acute promyelocytic leukemia: I, Clinical results. Blood 1990; 76:1704–1709.
16. Urban CH, Sager W. Intracranial bleeding during therapy with L-asparaginase in childhood acute lymphocytic leukemia. Eur J Pediatr 1981; 137:323–327.

17. Feinberg WM, Swenson MR. Cerebrovascular complications of L-asparaginase therapy. Neurology 1988; 38:127–133.
18. Sheldon R, Slaughter D. A syndrome of microangiopathic hemolytic anemia, renal impairment, and pulmonary edema in chemotherapy-treated patients with adenocarcinoma. Cancer 1986; 58:1428–1436.
19. Buss DH, Stuart JJ, Lipscomb GE. The incidence of thrombotic and hemorrhagic disorders in association with extreme thrombocytosis: an analysis of 129 cases. Am J Hematol 1985; 20:365–372.
20. Rogers LR, Cho E, Kempin S, et al. Cerebral infarction from non-bacterial thrombotic endocarditis. Am J Med 1987; 83:746–756.
21. Reagan TJ, Okazaki H. The thrombotic syndrome associated with carcinoma. Arch Neurol 1974; 31:390–395.
22. Sack GH, Levin J, Bell WR. Trousseau's syndrome and other manifestations of chronic disseminated coagulopathy in patients with neoplasms: clinical, pathophysiologic, and therapeutic features. Medicine (Baltimore) 1977; 56:1–37.
23. Collins RC, Al-Mondhiry H, Chernik NL, et al. Neurologic manifestations of intravascular coagulation in patients with cancer. Neurology 1975; 25:795–806.
24. Sigsbee B, Deck MDF, Posner JB. Nonmetastatic superior sagittal sinus thrombosis complicating systemic cancer. Neurology 1979; 29:139–146.
25. Sze G, Simmons B, Krol G, et al. Dural sinus thrombosis: verification with spin-echo techniques. AJNR 1988; 9:679–686.
26. Rao KCVG, Knipp HC, Wagner EJ. Computed tomographic findings in cerebral sinus and venous thrombosis. Radiology 1981; 140:391–398.
27. Einhaupl KM, Villringer A, Meister W, et al. Heparin treatment in sinus venous thrombosis. Lancet 1991; 338:597–600.
28. Walsh TJ, Hier DB, Caplan LR. Aspergillosis of the central nervous system: clinicopathological analysis of 17 patients. Ann Neurol 1985; 18:574–582.
29. Lukes SA, Posner JB, Nielsen S, et al. Bacterial infections of the CNS in neutropenic patients. Neurology 1984; 34:269–275.
30. MacKenzie RA, Forbes, GS, Karnes WE. Angiographic findings in herpes zoster arteritis. Ann Neurol 1981; 10:458–464.
31. Eidelberg D, Sotrel A, Horoupian DS, et al. Thrombotic cerebral vasculopathy associated with herpes zoster. Ann Neurol 1986; 19:7–14.
32. Lefkovitz NW, Roessmann U, Kori SH. Major cerebral infarction from tumor embolus. Stroke 1986; 17:555–557.
33. O'Neill BP, Dinapoli RP, Okazaki H. Cerebral infarction as a result of tumor emboli. Cancer 1987; 60:90–95.
34. Marazuela M, Garcia-Merino A, Yebra M, et al. Magnetic resonance imaging and angiography of the brain in embolic left atrial myxoma. Neuroradiology 1989; 31:137–139.
35. Roeltgen DP, Weimer GR, Patterson LF. Delayed neurologic complications of left atrial myxoma. Neurology 1981; 31:8–13.
36. Sandok BA, von Estorff I, Giuliani ER. Subsequent neurological events in patients with atrial myxoma. Ann Neurol 1980; 8:305–307.
37. Amico L, Caplan LR, Thomas C. Cerebrovascular complications of mucinous cancers. Neurology 1989; 39:522–526.

38. Klein P, Haley EC, Wooten GF, et al. Focal cerebral infarctions associated with perivascular tumor infiltrates in carcinomatous leptomeningeal metastases. Arch Neurol 1989; 46:1149–1152.
39. Murros KE, Toole JF. The effect of radiation on carotid arteries. Arch Neurol 1989; 46:449–455.
40. Atkinson JLD, Sundt TM, Dale AJD, et al. Radiation-associated atheromatous disease of the cervical carotid artery: report of seven cases and review of the literature. Neurosurgery 1989; 24:171–178.
41. McCready RA, Hyde GL, Bivins BA, et al. Radiation-induced arterial injuries. Surgery 1983; 93:306–312.
42. Razack MS, Sako K. Carotid artery hemorrhage and ligation in head and neck cancer. J Surg Oncol 1982; 19:189–192.
43. Leikensohn J, Milko D, Cotton R. Carotid artery rupture: management and prevention of delayed neurologic sequelae with low-dose heparin. Arch Otolaryngol 1978; 104:307–310.
44. Doll DC, Ringenberg QS, Yarbro JW. Vascular toxicity associated with antineoplastic agents. J Clin Oncol 1986; 4:1405–1417.
45. Wall JG, Weiss RB, Norton L, et al. Arterial thrombosis associated with adjuvant chemotherapy for breast carcinoma: a Cancer and Leukemia Group B study. Am J Med 1989; 87:501–504.
46. Kukla LJ, McGuire WP, Lad T, et al. Acute vascular episodes associated with therapy for carcinomas of the upper aerodigestive tract with bleomycin, vincristine, and cisplatin. Cancer Treat Rep 1982; 66:369–370.
47. Schachter S. Transient ischemic attack and adriamycin cardiomyopathy. Neurology 1982; 32:1380–1381.
48. Bernard JT, Ameriso S, Kempf RA, et al. Transient focal neurologic deficits complicating interleukin-2 therapy. Neurology 1990; 40:154–155.
49. Lowe J, Russell NH. Cerebral vasculitis associated with hairy cell leukemia. Cancer 1987; 60:3025–3028.
50. Inwards DJ, Piepgras DG, Lie JT, et al. Granulomatous angiitis of the spinal cord associated with Hodgkin's disease. Cancer 1991; 68:1318–1322.
51. Jabaily J, Iland HJ, Laszlo J, et al. Neurologic manifestations of essential thrombocythemia. Ann Intern Med 1983; 99:513–518.
52. Michiels JJ, Koudstaal PJ, Mulder AH, vanVliet HDDM. Transient neurologic and ocular manifestations in primary thrombocythemia. Neurology 1993; 43:1107–1110.
53. Feldmann E, Posner JB. Episodic neurologic dysfunction in patients with Hodgkin's disease. Arch Neurol 1986; 43:1227–1233.
54. Anderson OF, Fogelberg MG, Rosencranz NM, Weinfeld UA, Westin JE. Post lymphographic cerebral lipid embolization in the vena cava superior syndrome. Cancer 1977; 39:79–84.
55. Rogers LR. Cerebrovascular complications in cancer patients. Oncology 1994; 8: 23–30.

# 7
# Nervous System Infections

**Neil E. Anderson and Mark G. Thomas**

*Auckland Hospital, Auckland, New Zealand*

## I. INTRODUCTION

Central nervous system (CNS) infections occur more frequently in patients with cancer than in immunocompetent patients. Furthermore, they are caused by a different spectrum of organisms, they are often more difficult to diagnose, and, in general, they have a worse prognosis. Infections of the CNS in patients who have cancer are uncommon compared with other neurological complications of malignancy. Central nervous system infections were diagnosed in no more than 0.2% of the admissions to a large cancer hospital (1,2). The highest incidence of CNS infections is seen in association with lymphoma, leukemia, and surgery for tumors involving the head or spine (1,2). Central nervous system infections are much less common in patients with other tumors.

The spectrum of organisms responsible for CNS infections is similar to that seen in other immunocompromised patients (1,3). Meningitis due to *Neisseria meningitidis* or *Hemophilus influenzae* is rare, as is brain abscess caused by anaerobic organisms. In contrast, *Cryptococcus neoformans* and *Listeria monocytogenes* are the most common causes of meningitis, and enteric gram-negative bacilli, *Aspergillus* and *Zygomycetes* are the most common causes of brain abscess (1).

An inadequate host response to the infection is frequently responsible for an atypical clinical presentation. Fever and a change in mental state are the most consistent clinical signs, but neck stiffness is uncommon (1,4). Frequently the symptoms and signs of the CNS infection are wrongly ascribed to concurrent metastatic, vascular, or metabolic insults to the brain or a septic encephalopathy. A CNS infection should be suspected if neurological symptoms and signs are associated with a fever.

Complications of the malignancy or its treatment may hinder or prevent diagnostic procedures. Lumbar puncture can cause a spinal subdural hematoma in patients with thrombocytopenia or other coagulation defects. Poor wound healing, coagulopathies, and general disability may discourage biopsy of lesions in the brain or other organs. Laboratory evidence of infection may be less obvious than in immunocompetent patients. Many of the organisms that cause CNS infections in patients with cancer are difficult to demonstrate and do not grow readily in cultures. Others may be wrongly regarded as contaminants.

Treatment is more difficult and less successful in patients with cancer than in other patients. In one study, 67% of the neutropenic patients with bacterial meningitis were receiving antibiotics appropriate for the offending organism when the CNS infection was diagnosed and 85% of the patients died despite appropriate treatment (4).

## II. PATHOPHYSIOLOGY

The deficits in host defenses which lead to the development of a CNS infection may be due to the cancer itself or to its treatment (Table 1). Disruption of skin or mucous membrane barriers by tumor, chemotherapy-induced mucositis, surgical wounds, or vascular cannulae may provide a portal of entry for microorganisms. Defects in the circulating immune system may inhibit eradication of the organism or may allow a previously suppressed organism to cause disease. Patients with neutropenia due to infiltration of the bone marrow by tumor, bone marrow suppression by radiotherapy or chemotherapy, or following bone marrow transplantation (5), are prone to infection by conventional bacteria and *Candida*. Disorders of cell-mediated immunity following treatment with corticosteroid or immunosuppressive drugs, in allogeneic bone marrow transplant patients, and in patients with lymphoma or chronic lymphocytic leukemia can lead to infection by viruses or atypical organisms such as *L. monocytogenes* and *C. neoformans*. Abnormal B-lymphocyte function and deficient immunoglobulin production in patients with multiple myeloma and chronic lymphocytic leukemia can lead to infection with encapsulated bacteria, especially *Streptococcus pneumoniae* and *H. influenzae* (6). The spleen removes nonopsonized bacteria from the bloodstream. Serotypes of *S. pneumoniae* and *H. influenzae* to which an individual has had no prior contact can cause fulminant infections after a splenectomy. Barriers protecting the CNS may be compromised by tumor infiltration, surgery, intraventricular

**Table 1** Pathogenesis of CNS Infections in Patients with Cancer

|  | Neutropenia | Decreased CMI | Deficient Ig | Splenectomy | Barrier disruption |
|---|---|---|---|---|---|
| Setting | Leukemia<br>Lymphoma<br>Radiotherapy<br>Chemotherapy<br>BMT | Lymphoma<br>CLL<br>Steroids<br>Cyclophosphamide<br>Azathioprine<br>BMT | Myeloma<br>CLL | Splenectomy<br>Hyposplenism | Head, spine surgery<br>CSF shunt<br>Ventricular reservoir |
| Main pathogens | Enteric GNB<br>Candida | L. monocytogenes<br>C. neoformans<br>Viruses | S. pneumoniae<br>H. influenzae | S. pneumoniae<br>H. influenzae | S. aureus<br>S. epidermidis<br>Enteric GNB |

*Abbreviations*: CMI = cell-mediated immunity; Ig = immunoglobulin; CLL = chronic lymphocytic leukemia; BMT = bone marrow transplantation; GNB = gram-negative bacilli.

reservoirs, and ventricular shunts. These patients have an increased risk of infection with staphylococci and enteric gram-negative bacilli.

## III. PATTERNS OF INFECTION

Meningitis, brain abscess, and encephalitis are the most common types of CNS infection in cancer patients. A spinal epidural abscess occasionally appears during a disseminated bacterial or fungal infection and viruses, especially herpes simplex virus and varicella-zoster virus, may cause a myelitis. Infections of peripheral nerves usually are caused by varicella zoster or herpes simplex.

### A. Meningitis

Seventy percent of CNS infections in patients with cancer take the form of meningitis (1). Most patients have fever and an altered mental state early in the course of the illness but neck stiffness is present initially in only 20% of patients and 60% never develop neck stiffness (1). Focal neurological signs and seizures are uncommon early features.

The cerebrospinal fluid (CSF) typically has a pleocytosis, a high protein content, and a low glucose concentration. However, it is not uncommon to find very few leukocytes in the CSF. Fifty percent of patients with a peripheral leukocyte count of less than 3000/mm$^3$ have fewer than 5 leukocytes/mm$^3$ in the CSF despite the presence of untreated bacterial or fungal meningitis (1). Gram's stain and culture of CSF are often positive, even in patients who are receiving antibiotics for other reasons. *C. neoformans*, *L. monocytogenes*, enteric gram-negative bacilli, *Staphylococcus aureus* and *S. pneumoniae* are the most common pathogens (1,3) (Table 2).

In postmortem studies of neutropenic patients with bacterial meningitis, neutrophilic inflammatory exudates are usually absent from the leptomeninges (4). Cerebral and meningeal vasculitis is unusually prominent and may explain the severity of the encephalopathy associated with meningitis in neutropenic cancer patients (4).

### 1. Cryptococcal Meningitis

*Cryptococcus neoformans* is a yeastlike fungus which causes a chronic meningoencephalitis in patients with Hodgkin's disease, chronic lymphocytic leukemia, and, less commonly, non-Hodgkin's lymphoma or acute leukemia (7). Corticosteroids and chemotherapy also predispose these patients to develop cryptococcal meningitis.

Symptoms usually begin insidiously over several weeks or months but an onset over 1 to 2 weeks can occur. The early symptoms are often mild and include headache, nausea, unsteady gait, and an alteration in behavior and mental state. Seizures are uncommon until the last stages. The examination may show an altered

**Table 2** Meningitis in Patients with Cancer

|  | Lymphoma | Leukemia | Head, spine surgery | CSF shunt | Splenectomy myeloma |
|---|---|---|---|---|---|
| Frequency of meningitis | Common | Uncommon | Common | Common | Common |
| Common pathogens | *C. neoformans* | Enteric GNB | Enteric GNB | *S. aureus* | *S. pneumoniae* |
|  | *L. monocytogenes* | *Candida* | Staphylococci | *S. epidermidis* | *H. influenzae* |

*Abbreviations:* GNB = gram-negative bacilli.

mental state, papilledema, cranial nerve palsies, ataxia, hyperreflexia, or areflexia. Fever and neck stiffness may be absent and focal neurological signs are uncommon.

The chest radiograph may show pulmonary infiltrates. The computed tomography (CT) scan either is normal or shows hydrocephalus and enhancing cortical nodules. The CSF may be normal but usually there is a lymphocytic pleocytosis, high protein level, or low glucose concentration. Cryptococci are visible in centrifuged CSF sediment in about 50% of patients. Cryptococcal antigen is detectable in the CSF in more than 90%. *Cryptococcus neoformans* usually grows in CSF cultures, but multiple, large-volume specimens may be needed. The organism may be isolated from blood and urine, even when there is no clinical evidence of infection at these sites.

Immunocompromised patients with cryptococcal meningitis are usually treated with intravenous amphotericin B and oral flucytosine for at least 6 weeks (Table 3) (8). Alterations in the doses are often necessary to avoid serious renal or hematological toxicity. Combined intraventricular and intravenous amphotericin B may be curative in severe cryptococcal meningitis. In patients who have cancer, cryptococcal meningitis has a mortality rate of about 50% (1) and relapses are common among survivors. Maintenance treatment with fluconazole to prevent a relapse should be considered if cell-mediated immunity is persistently impaired.

## 2. Listeria Monocytogenes

*Listeria monocytogenes* is an aerobic gram-positive bacillus which tends to cause infections in patients with depressed cell-mediated immunity, especially patients with lymphoma (9). Meningitis due to *L. monocytogenes* is the most common bacterial infection of the CNS in patients with cancer (1). The symptoms typically develop over 2 to 10 days but a fulminant course can occur. Headache, low-grade fever, and an altered mental state are the most common manifestations. Neck stiffness is uncommon and focal neurological signs are usually absent. *Listeria* also can cause an infection of the brainstem, which is characterized by cranial nerve palsies, nystagmus, and ataxia. A cerebral abscess or focal cerebritis are rare manifestations.

Neutrophils are often predominant in the CSF but a lymphocytic pleocytosis is not uncommon. The CSF glucose concentration may be normal or low. *Listeria* often cannot be seen with a Gram's stain or may be mistaken for diphtheroids and incorrectly regarded as contaminants. *Listeria* usually grows from CSF and blood cultures (10).

*Listeria* infections are treated with either intravenous ampicillin or penicillin for at least 3 weeks (Table 3). Some authors recommend the addition of intravenous or intrathecal gentamicin. Trimethoprim and sulfamethoxazole are used if the patient is allergic to penicillin, but third-generation cephalosporins are inactive against *Listeria*.

**Table 3** Recommended Antibiotic Regimens for the Treatment of Meningitis

| Organism | Drug | Route | Total daily dose | Dose frequency | Minimum duration of treatment |
| --- | --- | --- | --- | --- | --- |
| C. neoformans | Amphotericin B | IV | 0.3 mg/kg | Daily | 6 weeks |
| | + | | | | |
| | Flucytosine | Oral | 150 mg/kg | 6 hourly | 6 weeks |
| L. monocytogenes | Penicillin G | IV | 250,000 units/kg | 4 hourly | 3 weeks |
| | or | | | | |
| | Ampicillin | IV | 200 mg/kg | 6 hourly | 3 weeks |
| S. pneumoniae | Penicillin G | IV | 250,000 units/kg | 4 hourly | 7 days |
| Methicillin-sensitive staphylococci | Nafcillin | IV | 150 mg/kg | 4 hourly | 2 weeks |
| | or | | | | |
| | Oxacillin | IV | 150 mg/kg | 4 hourly | 2 weeks |
| Methicillin-resistant staphylococci | Vancomycin[a] | IV | 30 mg/kg | 6 hourly | 2 weeks |
| H. influenzae (beta-lactamase −) | Ampicillin | IV | 200 mg/kg | 6 hourly | 7 days |
| H. influenzae (beta-lactamase +) | Ceftriaxone | IV | 100 mg/kg | 12 hourly | 7 days |
| E. coli[b] | Ceftriaxone | IV | 100 mg/kg | 12 hourly | 3 weeks |
| P. aeruginosa[b] | Ceftazidime | IV | 200 mg/kg | 12 hourly | 3 weeks |
| Enterobacter[b] and K. pneumoniae[b] | Amikacin[a] | IV | 15 mg/kg | 8 hourly | 3 weeks |
| | + | | | | |
| | Ceftriaxone | IV | 100 mg/kg | 12 hourly | 3 weeks |
| | Amikacin[a] | IV | 15 mg/kg | 8 hourly | 3 weeks |

[a]Check peak and trough levels
[b]Selection of agent dependent on in vitro minimum inhibitory concentration (MIC) testing

## 3. Conventional Bacteria

The infecting organisms, clinical features, and response to treatment differ depending on the underlying immune deficit (Tables 1,2). Patients who have undergone splenectomy or have impaired immunoglobulin production are prone to develop overwhelming infections due to encapsulated bacteria, particularly *S. pneumoniae* and *H. influenzae* (6). In these patients, meningitis is often a component of a community-acquired disseminated infection which presents with the rapid onset of fever and shock. Headache is common but the majority do not have neck stiffness (3). Most patients have a low glucose level, raised protein concentration, and a polymorphonuclear pleocytosis in the CSF, but the CSF may not have any cellular or chemical abnormality (3). A Gram's stain frequently reveals large numbers of bacteria in the CSF and the pathogen usually grows from CSF and blood cultures. Death usually occurs within hours despite appropriate therapy.

Patients with neutropenia are prone to infection with enteric gram-negative bacilli, especially *Pseudomonas aeruginosa*, *Escherichia coli*, and *Klebsiella pneumoniae* (1,4). In these patients meningitis is usually acquired in the hospital and it develops during bacteremia or by local spread from an adjacent site of infection. The pathogen often can be seen on Gram's stain and is readily grown from the CSF (1,4). Less than 20% of patients with cancer and a CNS infection due to enteric gram-negative bacilli survive (2). Survival largely depends on recovery of normal neutrophil counts.

In patients who have had a ventricular shunt or reservoir inserted, meningitis is usually caused by *Staphylococcus aureus*, *Staphylococcus epidermidis*, or other skin organisms (11). In these patients meningitis usually develops within 2 months of the operation. The clinical features may be insidious, with a change in mental state and low-grade fever, but usually there is no headache or neck stiffness. Cellular and chemical abnormalities in the CSF may be wrongly attributed to the surgery (12). In shunt-associated meningitis, the pathogen is more commonly found in CSF aspirated from the shunt reservoir than in the lumbar CSF. Meningitis following other neurosurgical procedures is commonly due to enteric gram-negative bacilli (13). Meningitis in these patients frequently develops within a few weeks of surgery. It is usually clinically obvious and readily diagnosed by visualization of organisms in the CSF.

Initial empiric treatment is influenced by the clinical setting in which meningitis occurs. Third-generation cephalosporins are very active against *S. pneumoniae*, *H. influenzae*, and most enteric gram-negative bacilli, but they are not reliably active against staphylococci. When staphylococcal meningitis is a possibility, nafcillin, oxacillin, or vancomycin also should be used. In selected patients, intrathecal vancomycin may be a useful adjunct to systemic therapy. Identification of the pathogen will allow a definitive antibiotic regimen to be selected (Table 3). Cure of shunt-associated meningitis usually requires at least temporary removal of the shunt.

## 4. Strongyloidiasis

*Strongyloides stercoralis* is a nematode which causes a chronic, benign bowel infection in the immunocompetent host. In patients with lymphoma or leukemia and in patients treated with corticosteroids or other immunosuppressive drugs, larvae can spread by the bloodstream to other organs (14). Hematogenous larval invasion of the CNS can cause multiple cerebral microinfarcts, but the most common neurological complication of disseminated strongyloidiasis is bacterial meningitis. Gram-negative bacilli and other enteric microorganisms are transported to the bloodstream by larvae and cause recurrent bacteremia and meningitis. Disseminated strongyloidiasis should be considered if a patient has unexplained gastrointestinal symptoms, an atypical pneumonia, or a gram-negative bacillary bacteremia or meningitis. Larvae can be detected in feces, duodenal aspirates, and sputum and, rarely, in the CSF. Mortality is often due to secondary bacterial infections. Oral thiabendazole 25 mg/kg/day for 5–15 days may be beneficial and antibiotics are required if there is a bacterial meningitis.

## 5. The Clinical Approach

In patients with cancer, meningitis is often rapidly progressive and antimicrobial therapy must be started before the infecting organism has been identified. A presumptive diagnosis frequently can be made from a knowledge of the underlying disease, the duration of the neurological symptoms, and the CSF microscopy, protein and glucose (Table 4). A diagnosis of cryptococcal meningitis usually can be confirmed rapidly by detection of cryptococcal antigen in CSF or serum. Other organisms that cause meningitis, with the exception of *Listeria*,

**Table 4** Clues to the Cause of Meningitis in Patients with Cancer

|   | Underlying condition | Duration of illness | Visible organisms in CSF | Special features |
|---|---|---|---|---|
| *C. neoformans* | Lymphoma Leukemia | Weeks– months | 50% (india ink or nigrosin) | CSF cryptococcal antigen |
| *L. monocytogenes* | Lymphoma Leukemia | Days | Uncommon | ± Brainstem signs |
| *S. pneumoniae* | Splenectomy Myeloma | Days | Common | Fulminant course Shock |
| Enteric gram-negative bacilli | Leukemia Neutropenia Postsurgical | Days | Common | — |
| Staphylococci | Ventricular shunt, reservoir | Weeks– months | Common (shunt CSF) | — |

often are visible in the CSF with a Gram's stain. Bacterial pathogens, including *Listeria*, usually are isolated from blood or CSF.

## B. Abscess and Other Focal Intracranial Infections

The incidence of brain abscess relative to that of meningitis is much higher in patients with cancer than in the general hospital population (1). Brain abscesses account for about 25% of the CNS infections in a cancer hospital (1) and they occur most commonly in patients with leukemia and following neurosurgery or bone marrow transplantation. Patients typically present with fever, headache, reduced level of consciousness, seizures, and, in some cases, focal neurological signs. The CSF is normal or shows a pleocytosis and a high protein content. The most common pathogens are enteric gram-negative bacilli, *Aspergillus fumigatus*, *Candida albicans*, *Zygomycetes*, *Nocardia asteroides*, and *Toxoplasma gondii* (Table 5).

### 1. Aspergillosis

Disease due to species of the genus *Aspergillus*, most frequently *A. fumigatus*, is more common in patients with leukemia than in patients with other malignancies (15). Neutropenia, bone marrow transplantation, treatment with broad-spectrum antibiotics, and corticosteroid therapy predispose patients with leukemia to develop invasive aspergillosis.

Cerebral aspergillosis commonly follows hematogenous dissemination from a distant site of infection which is usually in the lung (16). *Aspergillus* tends to invade blood vessels, leading to multiple hemorrhagic infarcts or subarachnoid hemorrhage. Other patients have multiple cerebral abscesses or microabscesses. The most common presentation is with abrupt onset of focal neurological signs, seizures, headache, fever, and obtundation. Cranial CT scans may show subtle low

**Table 5** Brain Abscess in Patients with Cancer

|  | Lymphoma | Leukemia | Head, spine surgery | CSF shunt | Splenectomy, myeloma |
|---|---|---|---|---|---|
| Frequency of brain abscess | Uncommon | Common | Uncommon | Rare | Rare |
| Common pathogens | *N. asteroides* *T. gondii* | Enteric GNB *Aspergillus* *Zygomycetes* *Candida* | Enteric GNB | *S. aureus* *S. epidermidis* | — |

*Abbreviations*: GNB = gram-negative bacilli.

attenuation areas without contrast enhancement or mass effect, hemorrhagic lesions, or, in the late stages, ring-enhancing abscesses (16). Granulomatous infections in the orbit and paranasal sinuses may spread by direct extension into the intracranial cavity, leading to a chronic meningitis or a granulomatous mass in the frontal lobe.

The laboratory confirmation of invasive aspergillosis is difficult. The CSF protein may be raised and red blood cells and leukocytes may be present, but the CSF is often normal.

*Aspergillus* is rarely isolated from the CSF or blood. Despite the frequent association between pulmonary disease and CNS aspergillosis, *Aspergillus* is isolated from sputum in less than 50% of patients. Tests for antibodies to *Aspergillus* and *Aspergillus* antigens are not reliable methods of detecting invasive disease. The usual method of confirming the diagnosis is by identification of hyphae in pus or tissue, but *Aspergillus* usually does not grow from these specimens.

The treatment of cerebral aspergillosis is rarely successful, but surgical drainage of abscesses and high doses of amphotericin B (1.0–1.5 mg/kg/day) may be beneficial. Treatment should be continued until 1 month after the resolution of neutropenia.

## 2. *Nocardia*

*Nocardia asteroides* and, less commonly, other *Nocardia* species are bacteria which occasionally cause disease in patients with hematological malignancies and patients receiving corticosteroids or chemotherapy (17). Infection usually begins in the lungs with hematogenous spread to the CNS. Single or multiple brain abscesses, which appear as ring-enhancing lesions in the CT scan, are the most common neurological complications. Occasionally meningitis occurs in association with cerebral abscesses. The CSF may show a lymphocytic pleocytosis, high protein content, and low glucose concentration. The organism may be isolated from CSF but it is more consistently identified in pus or necrotic tissue. Approximately 50% of patients with *Nocardia* infections of the CNS have pulmonary disease; in these patients, identification of *Nocardia* in sputum is a convenient method of confirming the diagnosis.

Trimethoprim 10–20 mg/kg/day and sulfamethoxazole 50–100 mg/kg/day for up to 1 year is the most widely recommended treatment (17). Surgical drainage of pus may be necessary to confirm the diagnosis but its therapeutic role is uncertain. Patients receiving corticosteroids or other immunosuppressive drugs have mortality rates as high as 80%.

## 3. *Zygomycosis (Mucormycosis)*

Members of the *Zygomycetes* class of fungi, most commonly *Rhizopus*, *Absidia*, and *Mucor*, may cause fulminant, often fatal infections in patients with acute leukemia or lymphoma (18). Diabetes mellitus, acidosis, neutropenia, and chronic steroid therapy increase the risk of zygomycosis.

In patients with leukemia and lymphoma, zygomycosis most commonly occurs as a disseminated disease. Neurological symptoms may be caused by cerebral abscesses, subarachnoid hemorrhage from rupture of a mycotic aneurysm, or thrombotic cerebral infarcts due to infiltration of blood vessels. Focal neurological signs, seizures, obtundation, and coma are the usual manifestations.

Rhinocerebral infection begins in the paranasal sinuses and spreads by blood vessel invasion or direct extension to the orbit and intracranial cavity. The early clinical manifestations are periorbital pain, fever, facial swelling, facial numbness, a black palatal eschar, and nasal discharge. Orbital infection is heralded by proptosis, ophthalmoplegia, and visual loss. Intracranial extension leads to meningitis, cavernous sinus thrombosis, carotid artery thrombosis with cerebral infarction, or cerebral abscess.

Computed tomography and magnetic resonance imaging (MRI) scans show the extent of the infection in the sinuses and orbits, cerebral infarcts, and abscesses. The CSF often has a mild pleocytosis and a raised protein concentration, but special stains and cultures are unhelpful. Histological examination and culture of infected tissue are required to confirm the diagnosis.

Zygomycosis should be treated with intravenous amphotericin B 0.7–1.0 mg/kg/day (19). In rhinocerebral zygomycosis, this should be combined with surgical debridement. However, cerebral zygomycosis is rapidly progressive and, in spite of treatment, death usually occurs within 2 weeks of the onset.

### 4. Toxoplasmosis

*Toxoplasma gondii* is a relatively uncommon cause of brain abscess in patients with lymphoma or leukemia (20). Cerebral toxoplasmosis usually presents with the gradual onset of headache, fever, impaired consciousness, seizures, and focal neurological signs. It usually is not associated with ocular toxoplasmosis. The CSF may show a raised protein level and a mild pleocytosis. *Toxoplasma* cannot be seen in the CSF and there is no readily available method of culturing the organism. Serological tests may indicate that the patient has previously been infected with *Toxoplasma*, but they do not distinguish between asymptomatic and active infection. Computed tomography scans typically show single or multiple ring-enhancing lesions in the gray matter (Fig. 1). The diagnosis may be confirmed by biopsy and histological examination of an abscess.

Patients with cerebral toxoplasmosis are treated with pyrimethamine 25–50 mg/day and sulfadiazine 1.0–1.5 g four times daily. Treatment frequently causes anemia, neutropenia, or thrombocytopenia, but folinic acid or folic acid may ameliorate toxicity to bone marrow precursor cells. Pyrimethamine plus clindamycin 600–1200 mg four times daily is an alternative regimen for patients who cannot tolerate sulfadiazine. The treatment of cerebral toxoplasmosis is often

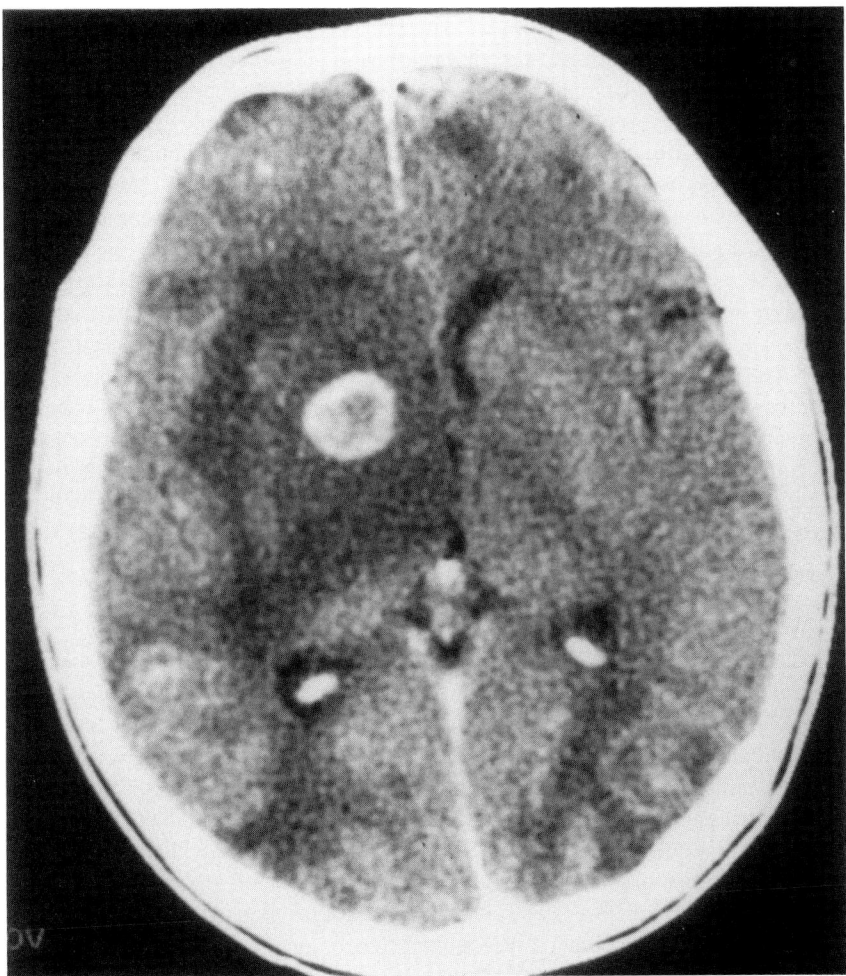

**Figure 1** Cerebral toxoplasmosis. Contrast-enhanced computed tomography scan of the brain: multiple ring-enhancing lesions.

effective, but therapy should be continued for at least 4 to 6 weeks after clinical recovery. Maintenance treatment should be considered for patients with a persistent impairment of cell-mediated immunity.

## 5. Candida

*Candida albicans* and other *Candida* species are increasingly common pathogens in immunocompromised patients. Bone marrow transplantation, neutropenia, corticosteroids, prolonged treatment with broad-spectrum antibiotics, recent major surgery, and indwelling foreign bodies such as intravenous or urinary catheters increase the risk of developing invasive candidiasis (21).

The CNS is involved in about 50% of patients with systemic candidiasis (22). *Candida* most commonly causes multiple microabscesses, although meningitis, macroabscesses, noncaseating granulomata, thrombotic cerebral infarction, and mycotic aneurysms may occur (22). Patients usually have a fever and headache. Seizures, focal neurological signs, and change in consciousness are uncommon. The CSF is not diagnostic in patients with cerebral abscesses. Patients with meningitis may have a polymorphonuclear or mononuclear pleocytosis, low glucose level, and high protein content in the CSF. Yeasts may be seen in the centrifuged CSF sediment and culture is usually positive. Identification of *Candida* from blood is uncommon other than in terminally ill patients, but isolation from urine, the oropharynx, or skin lesions may be a useful clue to the presence of disseminated disease (22). Treatment is with intravenous amphotericin B 0.6–1.0 mg/kg/day and oral flucytosine 100–150 mg/kg/day in four divided doses for at least 6 weeks. Solitary large abscesses should be drained.

## 6. Conventional Bacteria

Conventional bacteria, especially enteric gram-negative bacilli, may cause macroabscesses in neutropenic patients, most commonly patients receiving treatment for leukemia. Infection usually arises in the gastrointestinal tract or urinary tract and is followed by bacteremic spread to the brain. Most patients have a depressed level of consciousness, headache, fever, and focal neurological signs. Seizures are not uncommon (1). Computed tomography and MRI scans confirm the presence of an abscess but cannot distinguish these infections from those due to more unusual organisms. Frequently there is no CSF pleocytosis and the CSF glucose is usually normal (1). The organism is often isolated from blood cultures. The usual management of brain abscesses is with surgical excision or aspiration followed by prolonged antibiotic therapy. If the number, size, or location of the abscesses or the patient's condition prevent surgical drainage, treatment should be with empiric antimicrobial therapy.

## 7. Clinical Approach

In many patients with brain abscess the pathogen is not readily identified. Enteric gram-negative bacilli and staphylococci may be isolated from blood cultures and *Nocardia* may be found in sputum, but confirmation that a brain abscess is caused by *Toxoplasma*, *Aspergillus*, or *Zygomycetes* usually requires biopsy of the brain lesion. Computer-assisted stereotactic techniques have reduced the morbidity of brain biopsy and improved the yield of diagnostic information. If a biopsy is not feasible, the patient's underlying condition, the duration of the neurological symptoms, and the presence of infection in other organs will often be a guide to the etiology of a brain abscess (Table 6).

## Nervous System Infections

**Table 6** Clues to the Cause of Brain Abscess in Patients with Cancer

| | Underlying condition | Duration of illness | Associated disease | Number of lesions | Special features |
|---|---|---|---|---|---|
| *Aspergillus* | Leukemia<br>BMT | Days | Lungs<br>Orbit<br>Sinuses | Often multiple | Hemorrhagic infarct<br>Subarachnoid hemorrhage |
| *Nocardia* | Leukemia<br>Lymphoma | Days | Lungs | Often multiple | — |
| *Zygomycetes* | Leukemia<br>Lymphoma<br>Diabetes<br>Acidosis | Days | Sinuses<br>Orbit | Single (rhinocerebral)<br>Multiple (disseminated) | Hemorrhage, infarction |
| *Toxoplasma* | Lymphoma<br>Leukemia | Weeks | — | Often multiple | — |
| *Candida* | Leukemia<br>Lymphoma<br>BMT<br>Antibiotics<br>Foreign body | Days | Urinary tract<br>Skin<br>GI tract | Usually multiple | CT may be normal |
| Enteric gram-negative bacilli | Leukemia | Days | GI tract<br>Urinary tract | Single or multiple | |

*Abbreviations*: BMT = Bone marrow transplant; GI = Gastrointestinal.

Multiple microabscesses in the CNS are most commonly due to *S. aureus* or *C. albicans* (23). Patients with leukemia and lymphoma are especially prone to develop microabscesses. Antemortem diagnosis is difficult. These patients usually have a fluctuating level of consciousness and intermittent focal neurological signs. The EEG shows diffuse slowing of the background activity, but the CSF and CT scans usually are normal. Magnetic resonance imaging of the brain may be a more effective method of demonstrating disseminated microabscesses. The diagnosis should be suspected if there is a source of infection in the lungs, heart, gastrointestinal tract, or a wound, and if *S. aureus* of *C. albicans* grow from blood cultures.

## C. Viral Infections and Encephalitis

### 1. *Varicella-Zoster Virus*

Patients with cancer have an increased incidence of varicella-zoster virus (VZV) infections. The incidence of herpes zoster infection is greatest among patients with Hodgkin's disease, but it is also raised in patients with chronic lymphocytic leukemia, non-Hodgkin's lymphoma, acute leukemia, and bone marrow transplants.

Several factors can trigger the development of herpes zoster infection in patients with cancer. Radiotherapy may activate a latent VZV infection in dorsal root ganglia causing herpes zoster infection in the irradiated dermatome (24). Spinal metastases occasionally seem to reactivate VZV and herpes zoster infection arises in the corresponding dermatome before signs of spinal cord compression appear.

Disseminated herpes zoster with CNS involvement is more common in patients with cancer than in immunocompetent hosts (24). Neurological symptoms usually appear within 2 or 3 weeks of the onset of the rash but they may precede the skin lesions. In uncomplicated herpes zoster infection, the CSF typically shows a lymphocytic pleocytosis and a raised protein concentration. Similar but usually more severe CSF abnormalities occur in patients with neurological complications.

Meningoencephalitis is the most common CNS complication of herpes zoster infection. Headache, vomiting, fever, altered mental state, and neck stiffness are the usual manifestations, while focal neurological signs and seizures are uncommon. The electroencephalogram (EEG) shows diffuse slowing and the CT scan is usually normal. Varicella-zoster virus has been found in the CSF and brain tissue of some of these patients. Fatalities can occur, but most survivors make a complete recovery.

In patients with cancer, VZV can cause a progressive, eventually fatal leukoencephalopathy which is characterized by multifocal neurological symptoms and signs, focal seizures, and altered mental state (25). This rare disorder develops several months after the episode of herpes zoster infection. Focal white matter attenuation and cortical and subcortical hemorrhages are visible on CT scans. At postmortem there are areas of demyelination in the cerebral white matter and intranuclear inclusions in oligodendrocytes, astrocytes, and neurons, but there are minimal inflammatory changes.

Myelitis is probably caused by spread of VZV from the dorsal root ganglion to the adjacent spinal cord (26). A unilateral or bilateral, asymmetric myelopathy evolves over hours to weeks. It may be accompanied by meningoencephalitis. Residual neurological deficits are common.

A vasculitis in meningeal and cerebral arteries can develop after herpes zoster ophthalmicus. It is probably caused by viral invasion of blood vessels (27). Patients present with transient ischemic attacks or strokes and CT shows multiple infarcts ipsilateral to the zoster rash. Segmental narrowing in branches of the internal carotid artery is visible on angiography (Fig. 2).

Segmental motor weakness may develop in the muscles innervated by the nerve root affected by herpes zoster, but in about 10% of patients the weakness is distant to the rash. Weakness and hyporeflexia are most obvious when the limb muscles or sphincters are affected. The cranial nerves, especially the facial and oculomotor nerves, may be affected in the same way. Of these patients, 50–60% recover completely and another 25% have a significant improvement.

Early treatment with acyclovir accelerates healing of the skin lesions and reduces the incidence of disseminated infection. It may decrease the frequency of some of the neurological complications, but it does not affect the incidence of postherpetic neuralgia. Acyclovir is often administered to patients who have neurological complications, but its efficacy is unknown.

## 2. *Herpes Simplex Virus*

The incidence of herpes simplex encephalitis is not increased in patients with cancer, but the clinical and neuropathological findings are often modified. In bone marrow transplant recipients and patients with cancer, herpes simplex encephalitis can have a slow, progressive course (5,28). At postmortem there is widespread neuronal destruction and numerous Cowdry's type A inclusion bodies, but inflammatory cell infiltrates and hemorrhagic necrosis are absent (28).

## 3. *Cytomegalovirus*

A diffuse meningoencephalitis is a rare complication of disseminated cytomegalovirus infection in bone marrow transplant patients. Cytomegalovirus infections may be acquired by leukocyte transfusion or reactivation of latent infection. Cytomegalovirus meningoencephalitis presents with a change in mental state and an altered level of consciousness, but focal neurological signs are uncommon (29). Symptoms and signs of systemic infection often accompany the meningoencephalitis. Cytomegalovirus usually cannot be found in the CSF but the diagnosis can be confirmed by isolation of the virus from urine, saliva, or buffy coat leukocytes, or by a rise in serum antibody titers.

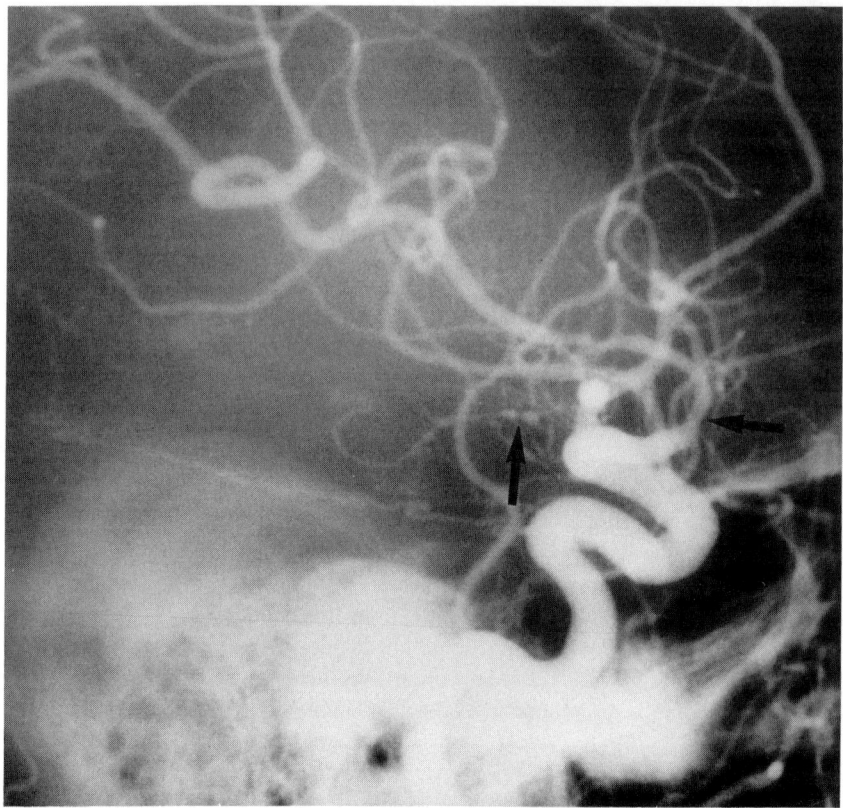

**Figure 2** Cerebral vasculitis following herpes zoster ophthalmicus. Right carotid angiogram, lateral view: multifocal arterial narrowing (*horizontal arrow* indicates focal narrowing of proximal middle cerebral artery) and arterial beading (*vertical arrow*). Note hypertrophied tentorial branch supplying dural arteriovenous malformation.

## 4. Adenovirus

Adenovirus can cause a fatal encephalitis in patients with lymphoma and acute leukemia and in bone marrow transplant recipients (30). Adenovirus encephalitis is characterized by confusion, focal seizures, and progressive obtundation. At postmortem there is a focal hemorrhagic encephalitis with intranuclear neuronal inclusions.

## 5. Measles

A subacute, progressive encephalitis which differs clinically and pathologically from subacute sclerosing panencephalitis can appear several months after a primary measles infection in children with acute lymphocytic leukemia or other childhood tumors (31) and in adults with Hodgkin's disease. In some patients there is no preceding clinically apparent measles illness. Typically there is a progressive encephalopathy, myoclonus, seizures, and focal motor and sensory signs, leading to coma and death within a few months of the onset. The CSF and CT scan usually are normal, but the EEG shows generalized slowing of the background activity. Pathologically there is an encephalitis and neuronal inclusions which contain viral particles and antigens. Inflammation may be absent or prominent.

## 6. Progressive Multifocal Leukoencephalopathy (PML)

With few exceptions, PML develops in patients with impaired cell-mediated immunity, including those with lymphomas, acute leukemia, and myeloproliferative disorders (32). In most patients PML is caused by activation of a dormant polyoma JC virus infection.

Characteristically there is an insidious onset of an altered mental state and signs of focal brain lesions. Fever, neck stiffness, and signs of raised intracranial pressure do not occur and headache and seizures are rare. Most patients die within 4 to 6 months of the onset, but occasionally there is a spontaneous remission or stabilization. Computed tomography and MRI scans show multiple lesions in the

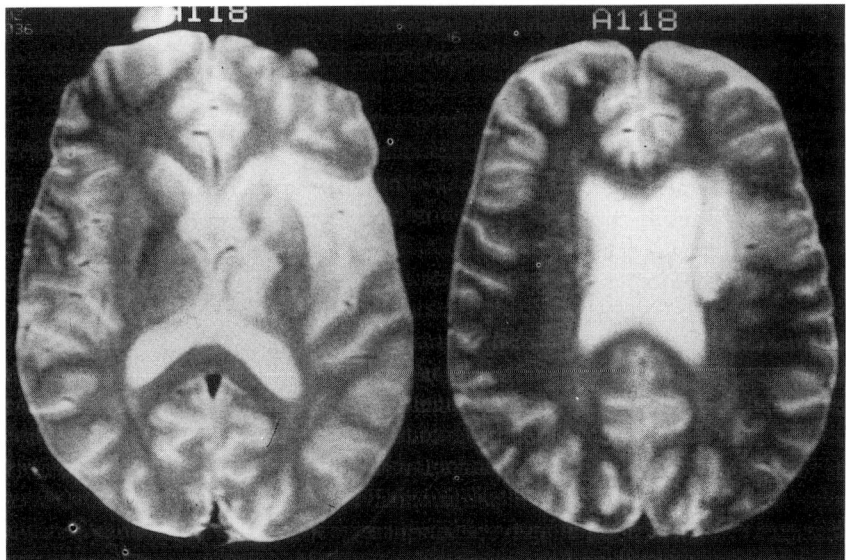

**Figure 3** Progressive multifocal leukoencephalopathy. $T_2$-weighted magnetic resonance imaging scan: Multifocal areas of increased signal in the corona radiata, internal capsule, and thalamus.

cerebral, cerebellar, and brainstem white matter (Fig. 3). The lesions do not have mass effect. The CSF is usually normal but the protein content may be mildly elevated. The EEG shows focal or diffuse slowing. Serological investigations are unhelpful.

The diagnosis usually can be based on the clinical and radiological findings but a brain biopsy is required for confirmation. Pathological examination of the brain shows multiple demyelinating lesions, eosinophilic inclusions in oligodendroglial nuclei, and bizarre, hyperchromatic astrocytic nuclei. There is little or no inflammatory reaction. Polyoma virus virions are present in oligodendroglial nuclei and JC virus antigens can be demonstrated with immunofluorescent techniques.

Treatment is usually ineffective. Remission can occur after administration of intravenous arabinosylcytosine or intrathecal interferon, but the possibility of spontaneous improvement prevents interpretation.

## IV. FUTURE TRENDS AND DEVELOPMENTS

The next decade is certain to bring major changes in the management of CNS infections in patients with cancer. The introduction of new chemotherapeutic agents and regimens may lead to an increase in the number of patients who suffer temporary or prolonged immunosuppression. The increasing use of brachytherapy, surgically implanted vascular cannulae, and other devices will provide organisms with more portals of entry. Antimicrobial prophylaxis to prevent disease by common pathogens may result in more infections due to unusual organisms.

The expanding list of organisms which may cause disease in immunosuppressed patients increases the challenges faced by laboratory staff and clinicians. Fortunately, new diagnostic techniques will enable many infections to be identified with greater accuracy. The polymerase chain reaction should be a rapid and reliable method of diagnosing many CNS infections. New antimicrobial agents such as azithromycin for *Toxoplasma* infection, fluconazole for cryptococcal and other fungal infections, and ganciclovir for cytomegalovirus infection may provide more effective or less toxic treatment. Immunomodulating agents are a major advance in the management of severe infections. Infusion of centoxin, a monoclonal antibody to bacterial lipopolysaccharide, improves the prognosis of patients with gram-negative septicemia (33). Antibodies to tumor necrosis factor (TNF) and other cytokines may benefit some patients with severe sepsis.

Novel methods of preventing infection will be of even greater importance. Administration of hemopoietic growth factors can shorten the duration of neutropenia following chemotherapy and reduce the risk of infection (34). Prophylactic treatment with ganciclovir in bone marrow transplant recipients reduces the risk of infection due to cytomegalovirus (35), and vaccination with an attenuated strain of VZV reduces the incidence of herpes zoster infection in children who have leukemia (36).

## REFERENCES

1. Chernik NL, Armstrong D, Posner JB. Central nervous system infections in patients with cancer. Medicine 1973; 52:563–581.
2. Chernik NL, Armstrong D, Posner JB. Central nervous system infections in patients with cancer: changing patterns. Cancer 1977; 40:268–274.
3. Hooper DC, Pruitt AA, Rubin RH. Central nervous system infection in the chronically immunosuppressed. Medicine 1982; 61:166–188.
4. Lukes SA, Posner JB, Nielsen S, Armstrong D. Bacterial infections of the CNS in neutropenic patients. Neurology 1984; 34:269–275.
5. Patchell RA, White CL, Clark AW, Beschorner WE, Santos GW. Neurologic complications of bone marrow transplantation. Neurology 1985; 35:300–306.
6. Armstrong D, Wong B. Central nervous system infections in immunocompromised hosts. Annu Rev Med 1982; 33:293–308.
7. Kaplan MH, Rosen PP, Armstrong D. Cryptococcosis in a cancer hospital: clinical and pathological correlates in forty-six patients. Cancer 1977; 39:2265–2274.
8. Dismukes WE, Cloud G, Gallis HA, et al. Treatment of cryptococcal meningitis with combination amphotericin B and flucytosine for four as compared with six weeks. N Engl J Med 1987; 317:334–341.
9. Louria DB, Hensle T, Armstrong D, Collins HS, Blevins A, Krugman D, Buse M. Listeriosis complicating malignant disease: a new association. Ann Intern Med 1967; 67:261–281.
10. Pollock SS, Pollock TM, Harrison MJG. Infection of the central nervous system by *Listeria monocytogenes*: a review of 54 adult and juvenile cases. Q J Med 1984; 53:331–340.
11. Schoenbaum SC, Gardner P, Shillito J. Infections of cerebrospinal fluid shunts: epidemiology, clinical manifestations, and therapy. J Infect Dis 1975; 131:543–552.
12. Ross D, Rosegay H, Pons V. Differentiation of aseptic and bacterial meningitis in postoperative neurosurgical patients. J Neurosurg 1988; 69:669–674.
13. Lefrock JL, Smith BR. Gram-negative bacillary meningitis in adults. In: Vinken PJ, Bruyn GW, Klawans HL, Harris AA, eds. Handbook of clinical neurology, Vol. 52: Microbial disease. New York: Elsevier, 1988:103–115.
14. Cook GC. *Strongyloides stercoralis* hyperinfection syndrome: how often is it missed? Q J Med 1987; 64:625–629.
15. Fisher BD, Armstrong D, Yu B, Gold JWM. Invasive aspergillosis: progress in early diagnosis and treatment. Am J Med 1981; 71:571–577.
16. Walsh TJ, Hier DB, Caplan LR. Aspergillosis of the central nervous system: clinicopathological analysis of 17 patients. Ann Neurol 1985; 18:574–582.
17. Mandell W, Neu HC. Nocardial infections. In: Vinken PJ, Bruyn GW, Klawans HL, Harris AA, eds. Handbook of clinical neurology, Vol. 52: Microbial disease. New York: Elsevier, 1988:445–453.

18. Meyer RD, Rosen P, Armstrong D. Phycomycosis complicating leukemia and lymphoma. Ann Intern Med 1972; 77:871–879.
19. Lehrer RI, Howard DH, Sypherd PS, Edwards JE, Segal GP, Winston DJ. Mucormycosis. Ann Intern Med 1980; 93:93–108.
20. Carey RM, Kimball AC, Armstrong D, Lieberman PH. Toxoplasmosis. Clinical experiences in a cancer hospital. Am J Med 1973; 54:30–38.
21. Parker JC, McCloskey JJ, Lee RS. Human cerebral candidosis—a postmortem evaluation of 19 patients. Hum Pathol 1981; 12:23–28.
22. Lipton SA, Hickey WF, Morris JH, Loscalzo J. Candidal infection in the central nervous system. Am J Med 1984; 76:101–108.
23. Pendlebury WW, Perl DP, Munoz DG. Multiple microabscesses in the central nervous system: a clinicopathologic study. J Neuropathol Exp Neurol 1989; 48:290–300.
24. Dolin R, Reichman RC, Mazur MH, Whitley RJ. Herpes zoster–varicella infections in immunosuppressed patients. Ann Intern Med 1978; 89:375–388.
25. Horten B, Price RW, Jimenez D. Multifocal varicella-zoster virus leukoencephalitis temporally remote from herpes zoster. Ann Neurol 1981; 9:251–266.
26. Devinsky O, Cho E-S, Petito CK, Price RW. Herpes zoster myelitis. Brain 1991; 114:1181–1196.
27. Eidelberg D, Sotrel A, Horoupian DS, Neumann PE, Pumarola-Sune T, Price RW. Thrombotic cerebral vasculopathy associated with herpes zoster. Ann Neurol 1986; 19:7–14.
28. Price R, Chernik NL, Horta-Barbosa L, Posner JB. Herpes simplex encephalitis in an anergic patient. Am J Med 1973; 54:222–228.
29. Bale JF. Human cytomegalovirus infection and disorders of the nervous system. Arch Neurol 1984; 41:310–320.
30. Davis D, Henslee PJ, Markesbery WR. Fatal adenovirus meningoencephalitis in a bone marrow transplant patient. Ann Neurol 1988; 23:385–389.
31. Pullan CR, Noble TC, Scott DJ, Wisniewski K, Gardner PS. Atypical measles infections in leukaemic children on immunosuppressive treatment. Br Med J 1976; 1:1562–1565.
32. Walker DL. Progressive multifocal leukoencephalopathy. In: Vinken PJ, Bruyn GW, Klawans HL, Koetsier JC, eds. Handbook of clinical neurology; Vol. 47: Demyelinating diseases. New York: Elsevier, 1985:503–524.
33. Ziegler EJ, Fisher CJ, Sprung CL, et al. Treatment of Gram-negative bacteremia and septic shock with HA-1A human monoclonal antibody against endotoxin. A randomized, double-blind, placebo-controlled trial. N Engl J Med 1991; 324:429–436.
34. Crawford J, Ozer H, Stoller R, et al. Reduction by granulocyte colony-stimulating factor of fever and neutropenia induced by chemotherapy in patients with small-cell lung cancer. N Engl J Med 1991; 325:164–170.
35. Schmidt GM, Horak DA, Niland JC, et al. A randomized, controlled trial of prophylactic ganciclovir for cytomegalovirus pulmonary infection in recipients of allogeneic bone marrow transplants. N Engl J Med 1991; 324:1005–1011.
36. Hardy I, Gershon AA, Steinberg SP, et al. The incidence of zoster after immunization with live attenuated varicella vaccine: a study in children with leukemia. N Engl J Med 1991; 325:1545–1550.

# 8

# Management of Paraneoplastic Neurological Syndromes

**Francesc Graus**

*University of Barcelona, Barcelona, Spain*

**Josep O. Dalmau**

*Memorial Sloan-Kettering Cancer Center, New York, New York*

## I. INTRODUCTION

Paraneoplastic syndromes of the nervous system are defined as neurological disorders of unknown cause that are usually associated with cancer (1). Some paraneoplastic neurological syndromes occur almost exclusively in patients with cancer. In other syndromes, the association occurs in a variable percentage of patients. In these cases, coincident diagnosis of both disorders, along with a higher than expected incidence of cancer and improvement of the neurological syndrome with treatment of the tumor, suggest that the neoplasm may induce the neurological syndrome. Alternatively, a common cause may be responsible for both the neurological disorder and the underlying tumor.

The incidence of paraneoplastic syndromes is low. In series of patients with cancer, mild or subclinical neurological paraneoplastic syndromes are found in 10–20% of patients. However, clinically significant paraneoplastic syndromes occur in less than 1% of patients with cancer. Neurological paraneoplastic syndromes may affect almost any structure of the central or peripheral nervous system. Typically, the paraneoplastic syndromes occur before or immediately after the tumor is diagnosed, but there is increasing evidence that severe syndromes may appear at any time after the diagnosis of the neoplasm. In this setting, the diagnosis of a paraneoplastic complication must be made after an extensive study to rule out other more common causes of neurological dysfunction. In patients

**Table 1** Neurological Syndromes That Suggest a Paraneoplastic Origin

Lambert-Eaton myasthenic syndrome
Subacute pancerebellar syndrome
Subacute involvement of the limbic system
Subacute lower brainstem dysfunction
Subacute sensory neuropathy
Subacute retinopathy
Opsoclonus-myoclonus
Chronic intestinal pseudo-obstruction
Acute necrotizing myopathy
Dermato/polymyositis[a]
"Atypical" motor neuron disease

[a]In older patients

without known cancer, there are several neurological syndromes that should suggest a paraneoplastic origin and indicate the search for an underlying neoplasm (Table 1). Some of these syndromes are associated with specific neoplasms.

The recent discovery of antineuronal antibodies in some cases has been helpful in defining the neurological disorder as paraneoplastic and directing a search for underlying tumor (2) (Tables 2–4). More than 95% of tumors are diagnosed within 3 years after the onset of the paraneoplastic syndrome. During this time, studies to

**Table 2** Paraneoplastic Syndromes of the Central Nervous System

| Syndrome | Associated tumor(s) |
|---|---|
| Cerebellar degeneration | |
| Anti-Yo positive | Ovary, breast |
| Anti-Yo negative | Lung, Hodgkin |
| Encephalomyelitis | |
| Anti-Hu positive | SCLC[a] |
| Anti-Hu negative | Other than SCLC |
| Opsoclonus-myoclonus | |
| Anti-Ri positive[b] | Breast |
| Anti-Ri negative | SCLC, neuroblastoma |
| Retinopathy | SCLC |
| Necrotizing myelopathy | Lymphoma, lung |

[a]SCLC: Small-cell lung cancer
[b]Opsoclonus not present in all patients (see text)

**Table 3** Paraneoplastic Syndromes of the Central Nervous System

| Syndrome | Associated tumor(s) |
|---|---|
| Motor neuron disease | Lymphoma, kidney, lung |
| Subacute motor neuronopathy | Lymphoma |
| Subacute sensory neuronopathy | SCLC[a] |
| Sensorimotor neuropathy | |
|     Acute polyneuritis | Hodgkin's disease |
|     Subacute/chronic neuropathy | Lung, lymphoma |
|     Associated with paraproteinemia | Osteosclerotic myeloma |
| Multineuritis with vasculitis | Prostate, kidney, lymphoma |
| Autonomic neuropathy | SCLC |
| Neuromyotonia | SCLC, thymoma |

[a]SCLC: Small-cell lung cancer

diagnose the suspected neoplasm should be repeated every 3 months, particularly in the first year. After 3 years the syndrome should not be considered paraneoplastic, and later diagnosis of a neoplasm should be strongly considered as coincidental.

## II. PARANEOPLASTIC SYNDROMES OF THE CENTRAL NERVOUS SYSTEM

### A. Paraneoplastic Cerebellar Degeneration

Paraneoplastic cerebellar degeneration (PCD) is a well-characterized paraneoplastic syndrome. Typically, symptoms develop rapidly, over weeks or months, evolving to a severe pancerebellar dysfunction. The pathological hallmark of the

**Table 4** Paraneoplastic Syndromes of the Neuromuscular Junction and Muscle

| Syndrome | Associated tumor(s) |
|---|---|
| Lambert-Eaton myasthenic syndrome | Small-cell lung carcinoma |
| Myasthenia gravis | Thymoma |
| Dermato/polymyositis | Lung, breast, GI tract |
| Acute necrotizing myopathy | GI tract, lung, breast |
| Carcinomatous neuromyopathy | Lung, breast, GI tract |

GI: Gastrointestinal

disorder is an extensive loss of Purkinje neurons, sometimes accompanied by a proliferation of Bergmann astrocytes and microglia in the molecular layer and loss of granule cells. Inflammatory infiltrates in the deep cerebellar nuclei can also be found in some patients. Paraneoplastic cerebellar degeneration has been reported in association with most types of neoplasms, but gynecological tumors, breast cancer, lung cancer, and lymphomas are the most common (3). The etiology of PCD is unknown, but an autoimmune basis has been suggested by the discovery of anti–Purkinje cell antibodies in the serum and cerebrospinal fluid (CSF) of a subgroup of patients with PCD (1,2).

Paraneoplastic cerebellar degeneration can be subdivided into several disorders that can be distinguished clinically and immunologically and differ in their prognosis and type of tumor association. A distinct group of female patients who develop opsoclonus and ataxia in association with a tumor (usually breast cancer) and the presence of an antineuronal antibody called anti-Ri will be discussed later with other paraneoplastic opsoclonus syndromes. Furthermore, predominant cerebellar symptoms may be the form of presentation of a more widespread paraneoplastic encephalomyelitis (PEM) which is usually associated with small-cell lung carcinoma (SCLC) and the presence of an antineuronal antibody called anti-Hu. Anti-Hu–associated PEM is described separately in this chapter.

## 1. Anti-Yo–Associated Paraneoplastic Cerebellar Degeneration

The most common and best-characterized PCD is defined by the subset of patients who harbor an anti–Purkinje cell antibody called anti-Yo (4,5) (Fig. 1). The anti-Yo antibody immunoreacts specifically with protein antigens of 34 and 62 kd molecular mass, expressed in the cytoplasm of Purkinje cells and in the tumors of patients with paraneoplastic symptoms (5). The Yo antigens have recently been cloned by several investigators (6,7). The usual clinical picture is that of a female with no previous history of cancer who acutely (hours) or subacutely (weeks) develops truncal and appendicular ataxia, dysarthria, and nystagmus. After a few months symptoms stabilize, leaving the patient profoundly disabled. The patient is unable to feed herself, walk without assistance, and has difficulty communicating due to severe dysarthria and abnormal writing. Reading or watching TV can be difficult due to oscillopsia.

Ataxia is initially asymmetric in 40% of the patients, becoming symmetric as the disease progresses. Most of the patients have horizontal nystagmus, and half of them also have rotatory or vertical nystagmus. The presence of a downbeating nystagmus and skew deviation have been found to be more common in the anti-Yo PCD group than in some antibody-negative subtypes of PCD. Signs and symptoms of involvement of other areas of the neuraxis are common but usually mild. Emotional lability and memory deficits are found in about 20% of the patients, and 50% have extensor plantar responses. Hyporeflexia or mild distal sensory loss are also described (8,9). In two-thirds of the patients, the neurological symptoms develop before the diagnosis of the tumor. Most have cancer of the ovary (46%),

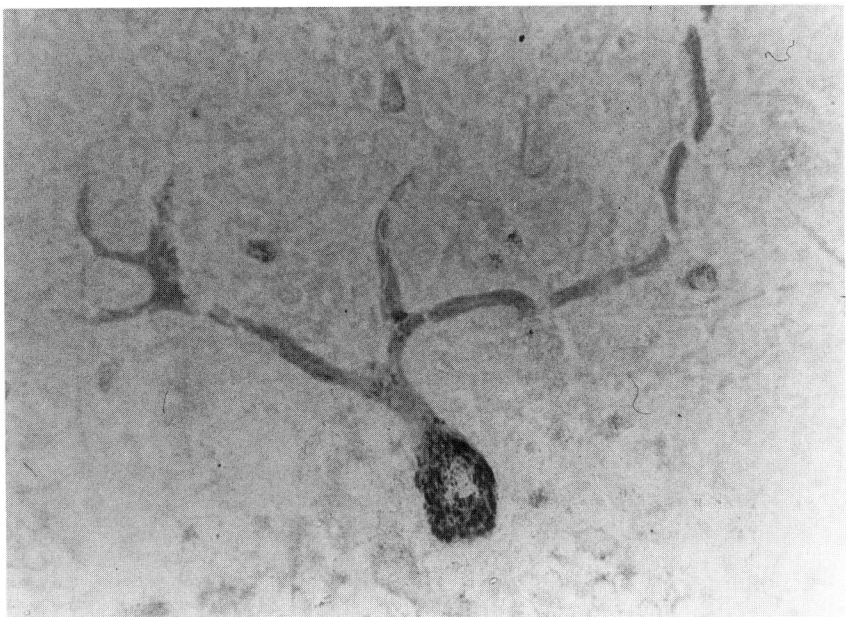

**Figure 1** Immunohistochemical pattern of the anti-Yo antibody. There is a granular staining on the cytoplasm of the Purkinje cell. (Avidin-biotin immunoperoxidase method, without counterstain ×400.)

breast (24%), or other gynecological malignancies (including endometrial, Fallopian, or mesovarian). In 11% the neoplasm is an adenocarcinoma of unknown origin, of which half present with disease in axillary lymph nodes, suggesting a primary breast origin. Tumor is not detected in 5% of patients.

The most important diagnostic test is the presence of the anti-Yo antibody in serum and CSF. The most specific study is Western blot analysis using recombinant Yo antigen or proteins from Purkinje cell neurons. Immunohistochemistry should be complemented with Western blot analysis (5,6), particularly in the setting of a patient with unknown neoplasm. Identifying the antibody as anti-Yo should direct an aggressive search for a gynecological or breast cancer. Atypical anti–Purkinje cell antibodies, with similar immunohistochemical reactivity but different Western blot findings, do not have such a specific tumor type association and indicate a more general but less aggressive diagnostic approach (8).

The study of CSF serves to exclude more common cancer complications such as leptomeningeal metastases. Cerebrospinal fluid demonstrates inflammatory changes in more than 50% of the patients, including lymphocytic pleocytosis (usually <100 white blood cells [WBC]/mm$^3$) and elevated proteins (usually <150 mg/dl). The presence of oligoclonal bands is common, and the ratio of CSF to serum IgG is elevated in most of the patients, suggesting intrathecal synthesis of IgG. Computed tomography (CT) and magnetic resonance imaging (MRI) studies are normal and demonstrate cerebellar atrophy, particularly in the latter stages of the disease (8,9).

## 2. Paraneoplastic Cerebellar Degeneration Not Associated with the Anti-Yo Antibody

These patients include two well-defined subtypes of PCD. One is characterized by the association with Hodgkin's disease (PCD-HD) and the other by the association with SCLC and Lambert-Eaton myasthenic syndrome (PCD-LEMS). Additionally, PCD has been found with a variety of other tumors including SCLC (10). When PCD alone or PCD-LEMS is associated with an SCLC, the anti-Hu or other type of antineuronal antibodies is not present or the anti-Hu is present in low titers, similar to the 16% of patients with SCLC without neurological paraneoplastic syndromes. For all forms of PCD without the anti-Yo antibody, the presentation and development of cerebellar symptoms are similar to those of the anti-Yo group (8,9).

## 3. Paraneoplastic Cerebellar Degeneration and Hodgkin's Disease (PCD-HD)

Hodgkin's disease and PCD have been reported in isolated cases by several authors (8,9,11). A review of these patients along with a recent study of 21 new cases (12) disclosed several clinical features that are characteristic of this paraneoplastic cerebellar disorder. Unlike the anti-Yo–associated PCD, in which all the patients are women, PCD-HD predominates in men. In the study of Hammack and associates (12), men outnumbered women by a ratio of six to one. Furthermore, patients were younger (age: 20–40 years) than the anti-Yo–positive patients (median age: 54 years), probably reflecting the age distribution of the underlying tumor. Cerebellar symptoms usually developed after the diagnosis of Hodgkin's lymphoma, sometimes heralding a tumor recurrence, but occasionally during a prolonged and complete remission of the lymphoma. Diagnostic tests, including head CT and MRI scans and routine CSF studies, do not differentiate PCD-HD from anti-Yo–positive patients. Various antineuronal antibodies have been sporadically reported in PCD-HD patients but a characteristic anti–Purkinje cell antibody has yet to be identified (13,14). Spontaneous remissions of the cerebellar symptoms or remissions after treatment with clonazepam were observed in occasional patients (12).

## 4. Paraneoplastic Cerebellar Degeneration and Lambert-Eaton Myasthenic Syndrome (PCD-LEMS)

The coexistence of PCD and LEMS in several reports (9,15,16) and in a series of six patients (Clouston, unpublished data) suggests an association between the two disorders. Typically, patients develop neurological symptoms, either of LEMS or cerebellar dysfunction, before the tumor is diagnosed. Proximal muscle weakness and cerebellar symptoms may present similarly, and unless LEMS symptoms develop first, the diagnosis may be overlooked. Sometimes, an electrophysiological test to study the loss or reduction of reflexes in a patient with cerebellar symptoms leads to the diagnosis of LEMS. Cerebellar symptoms are progressive, pancerebellar, and stabilize when the patient is very disabled. Search for a neoplasm almost always demonstrates an SCLC. One patient (Clouston, personal communication) had small-cell carcinoma of the prostate and another a non-Hodgkin's lymphoma. When a tumor is not found, the association of severe constitutional symptoms, such as weight loss, is common, suggesting an underlying malignancy. Routine tests, including head CT or MRI scans, are normal or show cerebellar atrophy. Cerebrospinal fluid analysis may disclose inflammatory changes. Several authors have looked for the presence of antineuronal antibodies, but the results, in general, are negative. Two patients with SCLC, LEMS, and PCD harbored antineuronal antibodies with reactivity similar to the anti-Hu antibody (16,17). In one of them, the autopsy showed severe loss of Purkinje cells and mild loss of neurons in the dentate nucleus and brainstem (17). In the other patient, the neuropathological changes were restricted to the cerebellum, without inflammatory infiltrates (16). These findings, and the finding that 16% of SCLC patients without paraneoplastic symptoms had low titer of anti-Hu antibody in their sera (18), suggest that the cerebellar symptoms of these patients were probably part of the PCD-LEMS association. The low titer of anti-Hu was coincidental.

## 5. Diagnostic Approach to Subacute Cerebellar Degeneration

In the setting of no known neoplasm and after exclusion of other causes of acute cerebellar disease, every woman who develops acute or subacute cerebellar symptoms should be studied for the presence of the anti-Yo antibody. The detection of the antibody guarantees the presence of an underlying tumor and directs the search to a few organs. The diagnostic approach should include a breast and pelvis examination, mammography, pelvic CT, and measurement of ovarian tumor antigen CA-125. If no malignancy is revealed, repeat mammography, pelvic examination under anesthesia, and uterine dilation and curettage (D&C) are recommended. If there is still no cancer evident, surgical exploration and removal of pelvic organs may be considered, particularly in the postmenopausal woman. If the anti-Yo antibody is not detected or the patient with subacute cerebellar symptoms is male, the serum and CSF should be studied for presence of anti-Hu antibody. Detection of anti-Hu antibody indicates that cerebellar dysfunction is a component of PEM, and the tumor search should be directed to the lung. If the anti-Yo and anti-Hu antibodies are negative or the patient has symptoms suggesting LEMS, a careful workup for SCLC should be recommended. When the patient has no antineuronal antibodies and is a young man (age 20–40), an underlying Hodgkin's lymphoma should be suspected. A female patient with predominant truncal ataxia and opsoclonus must be tested for the anti-Ri antibody. If the antibody is present the patient most likely has breast cancer or, in rare instances, a gynecological malignancy or SCLC. Finally, if the patient cannot be included in any of the previous groups but has a subacute development of truncal and appendicular ataxia associated with early development of dysarthria and nystagmus, a paraneoplastic origin should be suspected and a general workup for malignancy is indicated.

If the patient already has a known neoplasm, acute or subacute cerebellar symptoms are most likely secondary to leptomeningeal or cerebellar metastasis or neurological complications of chemotherapy. In this setting, anti-Yo or anti-Ri antibodies may confirm the paraneoplastic origin of the disorder. A high titer of anti-Hu antibody in serum and CSF is always associated with PEM. These patients can present with a cerebellar syndrome, but eventually they develop signs of major involvement of other areas of the nervous system. When the tumor is not one typically associated with the anti-Yo (i.e., ovary, breast), anti-Hu (SCLC), or anti-Ri (breast, gynecological) the search for a second malignancy in the appropriate organs is recommended. A patient with Hodgkin's lymphoma whose tumor has been in prolonged remission and who develops PCD symptoms should be restudied for a recurrence.

## B. Paraneoplastic Encephalomyelitis (PEM)

Paraneoplastic encephalomyelitis describes patients with cancer who develop clinical signs of dysfunction of various parts of the nervous system and postmortem signs of inflammation within the hippocampus, brainstem, spinal cord, dorsal root ganglia, and nerve roots. The distribution of pathological findings along the neuraxis is variable, giving rise to several syndromes that can occur alone or in association. Neurological symptoms of PEM include dementia (limbic encephalopathy), cerebellar degeneration, brainstem encephalopathy, or myelopathy. Patients with PEM frequently have associated symptoms of sensory neuropathy. The pathological findings are most marked in dorsal root ganglia, establishing the disease as a sensory neuronopathy. Paraneoplastic encephalomyelitis has been described in association with virtually all types of tumors, but for most patients (77%) the underlying tumor is an SCLC. The tumor usually remains small and its metastatic spread is limited to regional lymph nodes. In some patients, the tumor cannot be detected until autopsy (19).

A subset of patients with PEM have high titers of an antibody called anti-Hu in their serum and CSF. The anti-Hu antibody reacts with protein antigen(s) of 35–40 kd of molecular mass expressed in neurons and SCLC cells (20). The intrathecal synthesis of the antibody (21) and the detection of deposits of anti-Hu IgG (22) and Hu-specific infiltrating lymphocytes in the nervous system and tumor suggest an immunological origin of the disorder (23). The major antigen (Hu-D) has a high degree of homology to the *Drosophila* proteins Elav and sex-lethal and is likely involved in neuron-specific RNA processing (23).

We have studied 71 patients with PEM (24). Neurological symptoms developed subacutely ($< 8$ weeks) in 71% of the patients. For the majority there was a relentless progression or, more rarely, intermittent progression of the symptoms until stabilization. The neurological disease developed before the diagnosis of the tumor in 83% of the patients. The tumor most commonly associated was an SCLC (80%). Other tumors were an adenocarcinoma of the lung, a chondromyxosarcoma, two prostate carcinomas, and a neuroblastoma. Tumor was not found in nine patients, but in only two was an autopsy performed. Usually the tumors were small and in a number of cases could not be demonstrated until autopsy.

The presenting symptoms were sensory neuropathy (59%), limbic encephalopathy (including generalized or partial seizures, 21%), motor weakness (14%), cerebellar degeneration (13%), brainstem dysfunction (11%), and autonomic dysfunction (10%). Most patients (73%) had signs and symptoms of multifocal involvement of the nervous system. In 39%, two areas, and in 34%, three or more areas were clinically involved.

*Sensory neuropathy* was present in 74% of the patients, but in only 62% was it the predominant (most disabling) symptom. This syndrome is described later in this chapter.

*Motor neuron dysfunction* was a predominant symptom in 20% of patients. None developed a "pure" motor neuron syndrome mimicking amyotrophic lateral sclerosis. All had signs of involvement of other areas of the nervous system. In general, symptoms started with proximal loss of strength affecting lower or upper extremities, sometimes in an asymmetric pattern. Distal involvement of extremities, associated with fasciculations in the extremities and tongue, and muscle atrophy were common. Reflexes were abolished or increased, and some patients had clonus and extensor plantar responses.

*Limbic encephalopathy* predominated in 20% of the patients. Symptoms included confusion, depression, agitation, anxiety, memory disturbance, and dementia. Hallucinations (gustatory, olfactory, and auditory) were associated with symptoms of partial complex seizures or occurred without signs of epileptic activity (visual hallucinations).

Symptoms of *cerebellar degeneration* were present in 25% of the patients, but in only 15% were the predominant symptom. Gait ataxia was the usual presentation. However, most patients eventually developed a pancerebellar syndrome. A distinctive clinical feature of these patients, compared with other types of PCD, is that all the anti-Hu patients eventually had signs of severe involvement of other areas of the nervous system.

*Brainstem encephalopathy* developed in 32% of the patients, but in only 14% was it the predominant finding. The most frequent symptoms included oscillopsia, diplopia, dysarthria, dysphagia, gaze abnormalities—both internuclear or supranuclear (vertical and horizontal—subacute hearing loss, and facial numbness.

The *autonomic nervous system* was affected in 28% of the patients. In 10% this was the predominant symptom(s), including orthostatic hypotension, abnormal pupillary responses, sweating abnormalities, urinary retention, constipation, impotence, and xerophthalmia.

The most important diagnostic test was the detection of the anti-Hu antibody in serum and CSF. This assay needs to be done by Western blot analysis of the recombinant Hu protein or proteins from cerebral cortex neurons. Immunohistochemical studies alone are not enough to characterize the anti-Hu antibody because a similar pattern of immunostaining is also observed with the anti-Ri antibody.

Routine CSF studies showed increased protein concentration or pleocytosis in 80% of the patients. The ratio of CSF to serum IgG was elevated in most. On nerve conduction studies the most frequent finding was reduction or absence of sensory evoked potentials, suggesting dorsal root ganglia involvement. In some patients signs of motor denervation were also present, which, as demonstrated at autopsy, were secondary to anterior horn involvement. Only a minority of patients with PEM had head MRI abnormalities. They include atrophy of cerebellum and, in some patients with limbic encephalopathy, an increased signal on $T_2$-weighted images usually affecting both temporal lobes. In these patients, consecutive MRI studies showed that the high-signal abnormalities can revert to normal, leaving only atrophic changes (25).

We have studied the autopsy findings of 17 patients with anti-Hu–associated PEM. The neuropathological changes, including loss of neurons, gliosis, and inflammatory infiltrates, were always severe and multifocal. Lesions predominated in lower brainstem, temporal (limbic)lobes, dorsal root ganglia, cerebellum, spinal cord (anterior horns), and peripheral sympathetic nerves. In 69% the tumor was too small and localized to be responsible for the patient's death. Respiratory or autonomic failure due to severe neurological dysfunction was the principal cause of death for the majority of the patients (24).

## C. Opsoclonus-Myoclonus Syndrome

Opsoclonus is a rare disorder of ocular motility that can be diagnosed at the bedside by the presence of spontaneous, arrhythmic, large-amplitude conjugate saccades occurring in all directions of gaze without a saccadic interval. When the back-to-back saccades without a saccadic interval are limited to the horizontal direction, the disorder is called ocular flutter. Ocular flutter and dysmetria can be observed in the recovery phase of opsoclonus. Opsoclonus has been described as a result of congenital, viral, toxic, and metabolic encephalopathies. In oncological patients opsoclonus can result from brain tumors and as a paraneoplastic syndrome (26). Three groups of patients develop paraneoplastic opsoclonus: (1) pediatric patients with opsoclonus and neuroblastoma; (2) women with opsoclonus, paraneoplastic ataxia, and the anti-Ri antibody, whose underlying tumor is usually breast cancer; and (3) patients with opsoclonus, paraneoplastic ataxia, and encephalopathy not associated with the anti-Ri antibody, in which cases the tumor most commonly associated is SCLC.

## 1. Paraneoplastic Opsoclonus-Myoclonus and Neuroblastoma

Although opsoclonus is rarely a presenting symptom of neuroblastoma, nearly 50% of reported children with opsoclonus-myoclonus had neuroblastoma. Opsoclonus develops with myoclonus of limbs and trunk, hypotonia, and irritability and cannot be clinically differentiated from other nonparaneoplastic syndromes. The disease does not progress but has a prolonged course with frequent fluctuations of symptoms. In half of the patients opsoclonus precedes identification of the neuroblastoma (27). Patients with opsoclonus have a better prognosis of the neuroblastoma than patients without paraneoplastic symptoms. This observation is not explained by disease stage or as a result of early detection of the tumor. An autoimmune protective factor may be present but so far has not been demonstrated. The presence of a single copy of the N-myc oncogene in the neuroblastomas of patients with opsoclonus, compared with multiple copies in tumors of patients without opsoclonus, has been considered a better prognostic factor for the former group (28). Treatment of neuroblastoma results in improvement of the opsoclonus-myoclonus in one-third of the patients. Sometimes there is spontaneous resolution of opsoclonus-myoclonus. Responses to steroids are common, but relapses with steroid withdrawal or recurrent infections are also frequent (27).

## 2. Paraneoplastic Ataxia, Opsoclonus, and Anti-Ri Antibody

The distinctive clinical features of this group of patients are the subacute onset of ataxia and eye movement abnormalities (29). Ataxia predominates in the trunk and may cause severe gait difficulty and frequent falls. Although fine movements of the hands may be limited by the presence of ataxia or tremor, patients usually retain the ability to write and feed themselves. Opsoclonus is present in 75% of the patients. Other oculomotor findings include ocular flutter, nystagmus, abnormal visual tracking, blepharospasm, and abnormal vestibulo-ocular reflexes. In addition, some patients may present with nausea, dizziness, dysarthria, dysphagia, diplopia, decreased hearing, and proximal muscle weakness. The onset of the neurological symptoms is usually rapid, with symptoms reaching their peak in 1 week to 4 months. In half of the patients the neurological symptoms develop before the diagnosis of the tumor, which almost always is adenocarcinoma of the breast.

One patient had a Fallopian tube tumor and another an SCLC (Darnell, personal communication).

The serum and CSF contain a high titer of an antibody, called anti-Ri, that immunoreacts with the nuclei and, to a lesser degree with the cytoplasm of neurons and tumor cells. This pattern of neuronal immunostaining is identical to that of the anti-Hu antibody (Fig. 2), but on Western blot analysis of cortical neuron proteins, the anti-Ri antibody identifies two novel neuronal antigens of 55 and 80 kd (29) (Fig. 3). In half of the patients, routine CSF studies show mild lymphocytic pleocytosis and a mildly elevated protein concentration. Head MRI studies are usually normal, but one patient had a small area of hyperintensity in the dorsal midbrain on $T_2$-weighted images. In another patient, who developed dementia in addition to the oculomotor and ataxic symptoms, the MRI showed signs of cerebral and cerebellar atrophy. The neurological symptoms of two out of four Ri patients appeared to improve after administration of steroids. However, the spontaneous remission of other paraneoplastic or nonparaneoplastic opsoclonus casts doubts on a true response to the steroids. At autopsy, the brain of one patient had widespread inflammatory infiltrates resembling those of PEM patients (Rosenblum, unpublished data).

## 3. Paraneoplastic Opsoclonus, Ataxia, and Encephalopathy Not Associated with the Anti-Ri Antibody

The clinical picture of this paraneoplastic syndrome is a rapid onset of opsoclonus associated with vertigo, nausea, vomiting and ataxia. Gait and truncal ataxia are predominant, with the patient unable to walk or sit without support (30). Unlike the anti-Ri patients, in whom myoclonus and alterations of mental status are rare, two-thirds of these patients have limb or truncal myoclonus and encephalopathy. Patients are usually lethargic and confused, and the clinical course can lead to a relentless progression to stupor and coma (in one-fourth of the patients), to a spontaneous remission, or to a remitting and relapsing course. In two-thirds of the patients neurological symptoms precede diagnosis of the tumor. The tumor most commonly associated is SCLC. Anecdotal reports of other associated tumors include carcinoma of uterus, Fallopian tube, breast, bladder, and thyroid, and chondrosarcoma (26,30,31). Cerebrospinal fluid may show mild inflammatory changes and oligoclonal bands. Head CT and MRI scans are usually normal. Electroencephalogram (EEG) may be normal or demonstrate generalized slowing of the background activity, without epileptiform activity.

There have been clinical responses to immunosuppressants, clonazepam, thiamine, or treatment of the tumor, but interpretation of these results is confounded by the possibility of spontaneous remissions. The majority of autopsy studies show a normal or slightly reduced number of Purkinje cells, proliferation of microglia and gliosis of the cerebellar white matter, and mild inflammatory infiltrates in the leptomeninges or subarachnoidal spaces overlaying the brainstem.

There are reports of a few patients with severe and widespread pathological changes, resembling those of the PEM patients. The study of serum and CSF of three patients with paraneoplastic opsoclonus and mild pathological changes was negative for the presence of antineuronal antibodies (30).

## D. Cancer-Associated Retinopathy

The presenting symptoms of cancer-associated retinopathy include episodes of bizarre visual obscurations, light-induced glare, photosensitivity, and progressive visual loss. Symptoms may begin unilaterally, involving the other eye within days or weeks, and usually precede the diagnosis of the tumor. Examination shows peripheral and ringlike scotomata, impaired visual acuity and color vision, and retinal arteriolar narrowing (32). The electroretinogram demonstrates reduced or flat photopic and scotopic responses, suggesting a dysfunction of cones and rods. Latencies of visually evoked responses are usually normal. A CSF pleocytosis may be observed in some patients. Head CT and MRI scans are normal, but these studies along with the CSF examination serve to exclude other more common complications of cancer such as compressive or infiltrative optic neuropathy. For most patients the underlying tumor is SCLC. In a few instances, other tumor types, including melanoma or gynecological cancers, were believed to be the malignancies related to photoreceptor degeneration. Treatment of the tumor usually does not change the course of the paraneoplastic disease, but steroids can improve or stabilize the loss of vision.

The most common pathological findings in the few reported patients include loss of photoreceptor cells, infiltrative macrophages with melanin granules, and mild inflammatory infiltrates in the retinal arterioles. The optic nerves and tracts are usually preserved (33). Sera from these patients contain antibodies that identify several retinal and SCLC protein antigens, three of which co-migrate electorphoretically with neurofilament proteins. The principal antigen involved in the paraneoplastic degeneration of the retina seems to be a calcium-binding protein of 26 kd present in the photoreceptor cells (34).

## E. Necrotizing Myelopathy

Necrotizing myelopathy is a syndrome that has been associated with several conditions, particularly postinfectious and vascular diseases. A few patients with necrotizing myelopathy have or will develop a malignancy, but the extreme rarity of this association prevents any firm conclusion on the role of the tumor in the pathogenesis of the myelopathy. The syndrome has been associated with lymphomas and adenocarcinomas of the lung or other organs (35,36). Necrotizing myelopathy has an acute or subacute clinical course characterized by an ascending paralysis with sphincter dysfunction and involvement of all modalities of sensation. The CSF is usually acellular with elevated protein levels. Myelograms are

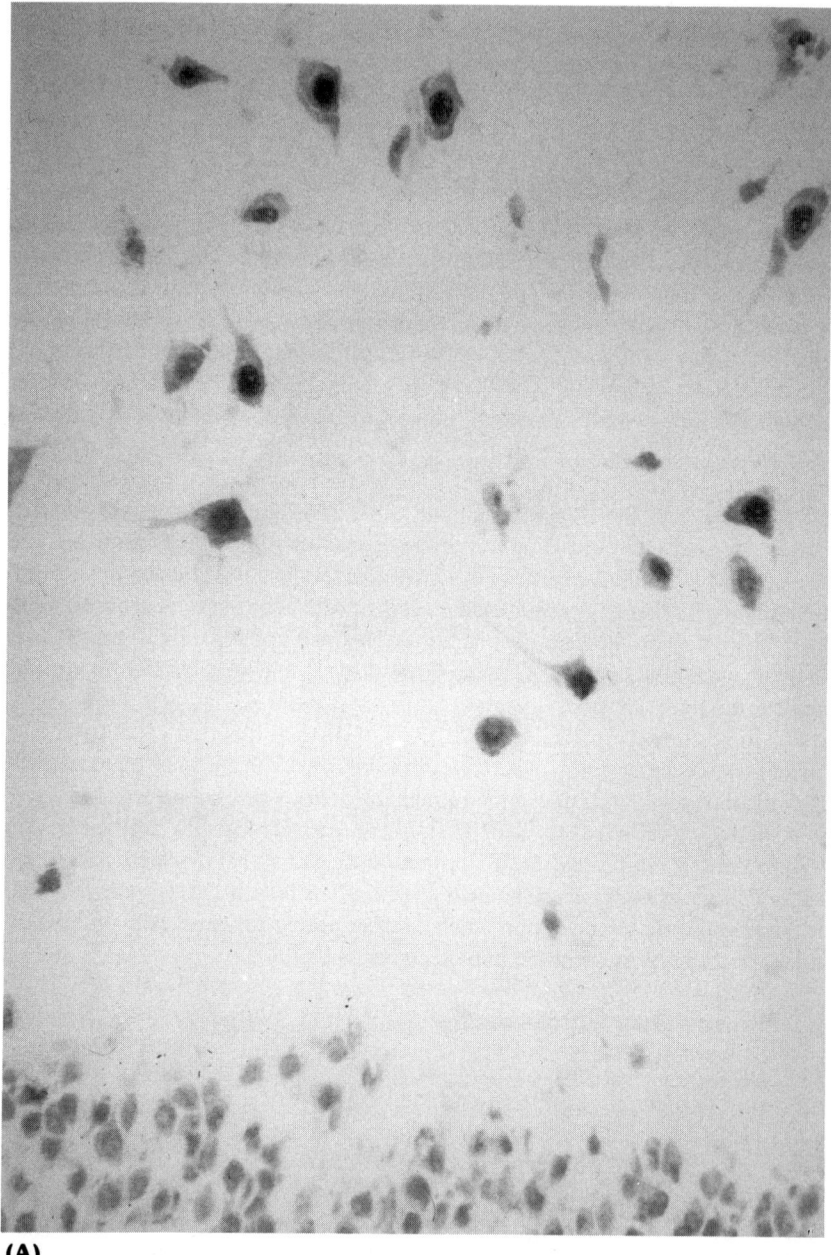

**(A)**

**Figure 2** Consecutive frozen sections of normal hippocampus incubated with anti-Hu antibody (A) and anti-Ri antibody (B). The neuronal nuclear staining is identical with both antibodies. (Avidin-biotin immunoperoxidase technique, without counterstain. ×200.)

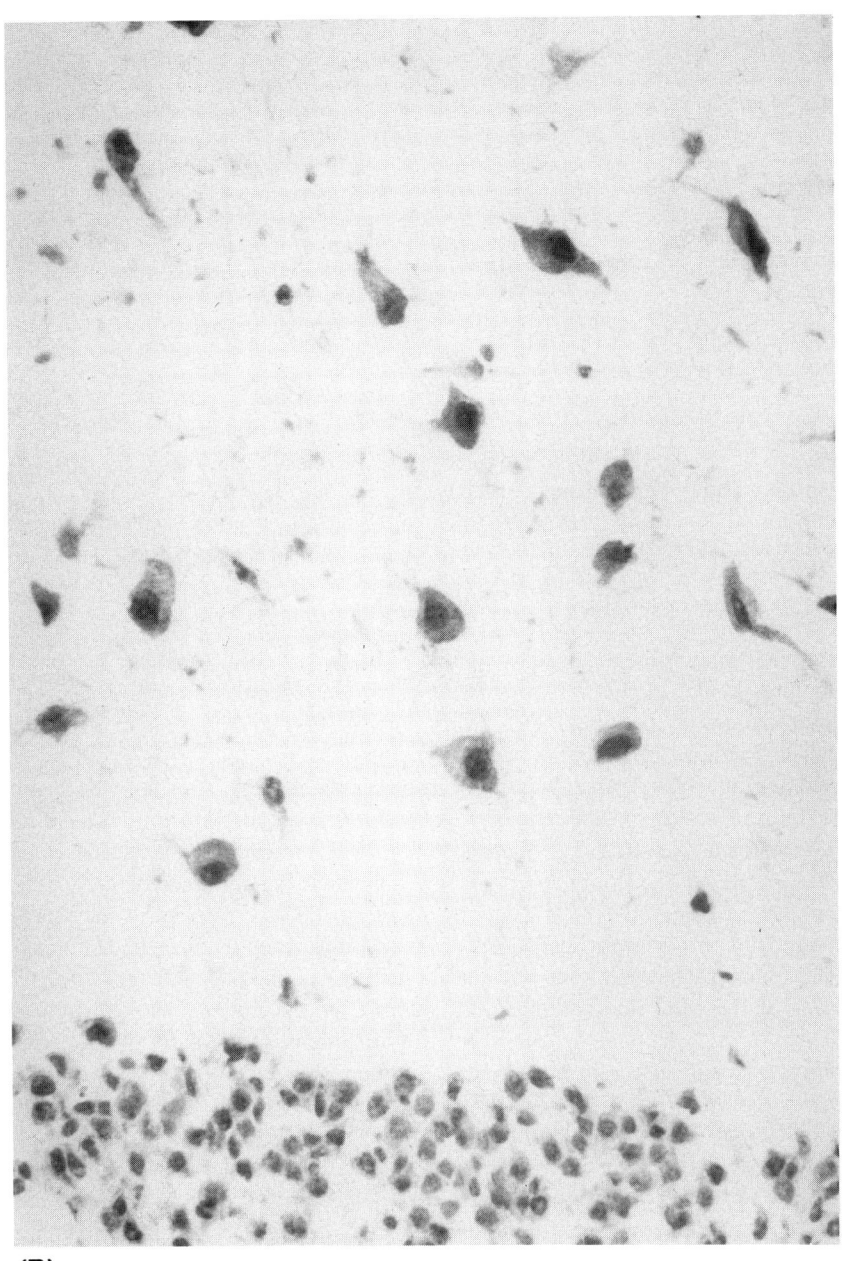

(B)

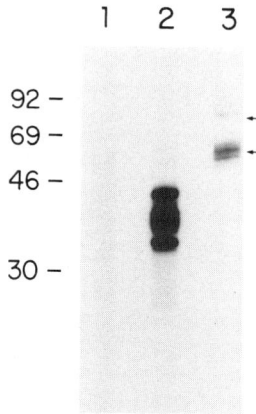

**Figure 3** Western blot of cerebral cortex neurons incubated with normal serum (lane 1), anti-Hu–positive serum (lane 2), and anti-Ri–positive serum (lane 3). The anti-Hu antibody identifies a set of antigens of 35–40 kd molecular mass, whereas the anti-Ri recognizes different antigens of 55 kd and 80 kd molecular mass (*arrows*).

normal or may show unspecific swelling of the spinal cord. Magnetic resonance imaging studies of this syndrome are lacking. In patients with a postinfectious necrotizing myelopathy the MRI may be normal. This was observed in one of our patients with a chronic lymphocytic leukemia.

The diagnosis of paraneoplastic necrotizing myelopathy is made by exclusion of other causes of acute ascending myelopathy. In patients with solid tumors the syndrome may be identical to that caused by the intramedullary metastasis. In the latter, MRI with gadolinium may show an enhancing intramedullary nodule. However, because the MRI features of intramedullary metastasis have been reported in only a few patients and there is no information on the MRI features of the paraneoplastic syndrome, one must be cautious of making the diagnosis on the basis of the MRI findings alone. In patients with lymphoma or leukemia an identical syndrome may be caused by viral infections, particularly of the herpes group, as a side effect of intrathecal chemotherapy or radiation therapy, or more rarely by septic infarcts or intramedullary granulomas. A definitive clinical diagnosis of these etiologies cannot be made in many instances, and the MRI features are nonspecific or not well defined. Therefore, the definitive diagnosis of paraneoplastic necrotizing myelopathy cannot be accepted without a postmortem study. In patients with solid tumors, if the diagnosis of an intramedullary metastasis cannot be ruled out, treatment with radiation therapy should be attempted to stop the progression of the myelopathy.

## III. PARANEOPLASTIC SYNDROMES OF THE PERIPHERAL NERVOUS SYSTEM

### A. Motor Neuron Diseases

Patients with cancer and neurological syndromes that involve the motor neurons can be separated into three groups: (1) those with typical motor neuron disease or amyotrophic lateral sclerosis; (2) those with subacute motor neuronopathy; and (3) those with motor neuron dysfunction in the setting of PEM. As described above, the clinical presentation of PEM may resemble motor neuron disease. However, these patients almost always present or develop in their clinical course symptoms of involvement of other areas of the nervous system that rule out the diagnosis of motor neuron disease.

Epidemiological studies have not demonstrated a higher incidence of cancer in patients with amyotrophic lateral sclerosis. However, there are a few reports of patients with motor neuron disease that improve after treatment of the underlying tumor (37). In these patients the neoplasm appeared closely associated with the diagnosis of the neurological syndrome and was usually a lung or renal cell tumor. Younger and coworkers (38) described nine patients with amyotrophic lateral sclerosis and lymphoma. These patients often presented with paraproteinemia, high protein levels and oligoclonal bands in the CSF, and conduction blocks in peripheral nerves. Treatment of the lymphoma led to improvement of the motor neuron disease in only one patient.

*Subacute motor neuronopathy* (39) is an unusual but well-defined paraneoplastic syndrome associated with Hodgkin's disease or lymphoma. Patients present with proximal, sometimes asymmetric, muscle weakness that is more prominent in the lower extremities. Pain, fasciculations, or upper motor neuron signs are absent. The syndrome usually appears after treatment of the tumor, has an independent, rarely severe, clinical course, and sometimes stabilizes or improves without any specific treatment. Result of CSF examination is normal or shows a mildly elevated protein, and electromyographic studies are compatible with lower motor neuron dysfunction. The preservation of the bulbar muscles, absence of prominent fasciculations and upper motor neuron signs, and the clinical course separates this syndrome from amyotrophic lateral sclerosis. Patients treated with radiation therapy that includes the spinal cord may present with lower motor neuron dysfunction in the irradiated segments. The distribution of the weakness is typically distal and no cases of spontaneous improvement have been reported (see Chap. 10).

When should the neurologist consider the possibility of a paraneoplastic origin in the evaluation of a patient with motor neuron disease? In patients with "atypical" motor neuron disease, particularly those with a subacutely progressive course and development of symptoms involving other areas of the nervous system, the possibility of paraneoplastic encephalomyelitis must be considered. The presence of the anti-Hu antibody in the serum should be evaluated in these patients. Patients who have typical motor neuron disease but who also show the presence of paraproteinemia, oligoclonal bands or high protein levels in the CSF, or nerve conduction blocks should be screened for an underlying lymphoma (see Chaps. 20 and 21). Finally, in patients with typical motor neuron disease who have a tumor diagnosed within a few months after the onset of the neurological disorder, aggressive treatment of the tumor should be recommended despite the dim prognosis of the amyotrophic lateral sclerosis. Careful follow-up of the neurological symptoms would help better define the clinical characteristics of those patients that may improve or stabilize with the successful treatment of the cancer.

## B. Subacute Sensory Neuronopathy

Subacute sensory neuronopathy is considered a particular manifestation of PEM (19). The clinical course is subacute and progressive in weeks. The main complaints are pain and paresthesias in the upper or lower limbs with clumsiness in the hands and gait ataxia. At the onset, pain and paresthesias may be very asymmetric, involving only one limb, and may lead to the misdiagnosis of radiculopathy or multiple neuropathies. In a few patients the neuronopathy remains stable for months, with mild functional deficits; for the majority, however, symptoms progress rapidly, leaving the patient bedbound in a few weeks. Neurological examination reveals involvement of all modalities of sensation, with severe impairment of joint position and vibratory senses that causes pseudoathetotic movements of the hands and sensory gait ataxia. Deep tendon reflexes are abolished. In severe cases the cranial nerves are also involved, with sensorineural deafness, loss of taste, and numbness of the face. Some patients have an isolated subacute sensory neuronopathy, but muscle weakness is common and should not exclude the diagnosis. More than 70% of patients with this syndrome develop symptoms of involvement of other areas of the nervous system, fulfilling the diagnosis of PEM. In this setting muscle weakness reflects the concomitant damage to the motor neurons in the spinal cord (19,24).

The diagnosis of subacute sensory neuronopathy should be considered in those patients with a pure or mostly sensory neuropathy with predominant involvement of kinesthetic and proprioceptive senses. The asymmetric distribution and early involvement of the arms and face are important clinical clues to the diagnosis of neuronopathy rather than neuropathy due to axonal or myelin damage. The CSF usually shows elevated protein levels and a variable pleocytosis, mostly mononuclear cells, and usually less than 100 cells/dl. Electromyographic studies are helpful in confirming selective damage of the sensory pathways. Usually, motor nerve and F wave studies are normal and there are no signs of denervation. Action potentials of sensory nerves and somesthetic evoked potentials are small or absent, particularly in the clinically affected limbs.

In patients with known cancer, if the clinical onset of the sensory neuronopathy is very asymmetric or restricted to one limb, the syndrome can be confused with a metastatic infiltration of the plexus or epidural space. Neuroradiological studies and clinical progression usually rule out these diagnoses. On the other hand, a very similar sensory neuropathy occurs in patients treated with cisplatin or taxol. In the latter, the onset of the neuropathy is usually acute within a few days after the first treatment. With taxol, as in the paraneoplastic syndrome, the arms may be involved first. Patients treated with cisplatin may present with a sensory neuropathy and severe impairment of proprioceptive sensation. The sensory neuropathy usually appears after several courses of the drug. The neuropathy is symmetric with a distal distribution. An important feature is that the neuropathy may appear or progress for several weeks after cisplatin has been stopped, making the distinction from paraneoplastic neuropathy more difficult.

In patients without a known cancer, the differential diagnosis of paraneoplastic sensory neuronopathy has to consider several syndromes. A pure sensory neuropathy of acute or chronic onset has been described in patients that never develop a malignancy (40,41). One group of patients has nerve conduction velocity studies typical of a demyelinating neuropathy and probably represents a sensory variant of the chronic inflammatory demyelinating polyneuropathy. In other patients the neuropathy develops in association with high doses of pyridoxine or with several autoimmune disorders, such as Sjögren's syndrome, primary biliary cirrhosis, or monoclonal gammopathy of undetermined significance. Pathological studies in a few cases demonstrate a severe loss of neurons in dorsal root ganglia.

The clinical setting, such as previous intake of megadoses of pyridoxine or a previous diagnosis of Sjögren's syndrome, and the findings of neurophysiological studies are helpful to orient the diagnosis in some patients. However, in many others there are no definite clinical or electromyographical clues to differentiate the subacute sensory neuronopathy from other sensory neuropathies not associated with cancer. The new onset of signs or symptoms that suggest involvement of other areas of the nervous system, particularly the brainstem, cerebellum, or temporal lobes, strongly suggests the diagnosis of paraneoplastic sensory neuronopathy. These additional features may occur late in the clinical course. At least 20% of patients never develop dysfunction except of the dorsal root ganglia (24). At the present time, the detection of the anti-Hu antibody is the only test that will identify the sensory neuropathies that are associated with a tumor, usually an SCLC. A small percentage of patients whose sensory neuropathy is associated with tumors other than SCLC may not harbor the anti-Hu antibody. No patient with sensory neuropathy, positive anti-Hu antibodies, and a follow-up of more than 3 years without cancer has been reported, supporting the concept that the presence of anti-Hu antibodies reliably identifies patients with paraneoplastic neuropathy.

## C. Sensorimotor Neuropathy

Mild peripheral neuropathies are common in patients with advanced solid tumors and lymphoma. These neuropathies are more frequent in patients with significant weight loss but rarely progress to have a significant impact on quality of life. On the other hand, clinically significant neuropathies antedating the diagnosis of cancer are uncommon, occurring in less than 1% of patients with cancer. In patients with peripheral neuropathies of undetermined causes an underlying neoplasm was found in nine of 91 consecutive patients. Cases of sensory neuronopathy were included in the study (42).

Paraneoplastic sensorimotor neuropathies may have an acute (days) or chronic clinical course; some patients improve spontaneously. Exceptionally, some neuropathies have a remitting and relapsing course. The different clinical features coupled with the diverse electrophysiological and pathological findings indicate that these neuropathies are due to a variety of pathogenetic mechanisms.

### 1. Guillain-Barré Syndrome

A higher incidence of typical Guillain-Barré syndrome is described in patients with Hodgkin's disease, probably due to the susceptibility of these patients to repetitive viral infections or a propensity to develop autoimmune disorders (43). The association of Guillain-Barré syndrome with solid tumors has been considered coincidental. However, the analysis of paraneoplastic neuropathies of acute onset and rapid clinical course reported in patients with solid tumors suggests that these neuropathies had clinical, electrophysiological, and pathological features identical to those seen in the Guillain-Barré syndrome (44). Without definitive laboratory "markers," we cannot rule out the possibility that at least some acute neuropathies reported as paraneoplastic were in fact Guillain-Barré syndrome. A sensory variant of Guillain-Barré has been described in patients with lung cancer and lymphoma. The clinical picture resembles a subacute sensory neuronopathy but the neurographic studies usually show features of a demyelinating neuropathy, the anti-Hu antibody is negative, and the neuropathy usually improves.

In patients with SCLC, a syndrome simulating an acute polyneuritis may be caused by a paraneoplastic encephalomyelitis with predominant involvement of dorsal root ganglia and motor neurons (24). The presence of a positive anti-Hu antibody will aid in the correct diagnosis. In patients with lymphoma, an acute polyneuropathy may be due to diffuse lymphomatous infiltration of peripheral nerves. Malignant cells are sometimes identified in the CSF or sural nerve biopsies (45).

### 2. Multineuritis and Vasculitis

Paraneoplastic vasculitides are usually limited to the small vessels of the skin and are more frequently associated with lymphomas and leukemias. In a few patients, the paraneoplastic vasculitis is found in muscle and nerves without clinical or pathological evidence of systemic vasculitis (46,47). The syndrome is rare and has been reported in only a few patients. The incidence of tumors in series of patients with peripheral nerve vasculitis ranges from 0% to 6% (47). Unlike cutaneous paraneoplastic vasculitis, nerve vasculitis has been more frequently reported in older patients with solid tumors, particularly prostate, kidney, and lung, and the neuropathy antedates the diagnosis of cancer in only half the patients. The clinical course is characterized by a progressive, initially asymmetric, painful sensorimotor neuropathy. Typical mononeuritis multiplex is almost never described. Some patients also complain of proximal muscle weakness probably due to a coincident muscle vasculitis. Neurophysiological studies usually show features of an axonal polyneuropathy, and CSF examination discloses elevated protein levels. The diagnosis is made by histological demonstration of vasculitis. Combined biopsy of nerve and muscle is indicated because it increases the chances of finding the vasculitis.

For patients without known cancer, the diagnosis of paraneoplastic vasculitis should be considered in those older than 50 years who have elevated protein levels in the CSF. In this subset of patients, a screening for malignancy is indicated if the cause of the vasculitis is undetermined. Two reported patients had nerve vasculitis occurring in the setting of paraneoplastic encephalomyelitis and small-cell lung cancer, suggesting that the determination of the anti-Hu antibody is indicated in patients presenting with paraneoplastic vasculitis.

For patients with known cancer, the correct diagnosis of paraneoplastic vasculitis is important because it may improve with treatment. The syndrome should be suspected in those patients presenting with multineuritis or asymmetric, usually painful, neuropathies with or without proximal muscle weakness.

## *3. Chronic Sensorimotor Neuropathies*

Sensorimotor peripheral neuropathies may antedate the diagnosis of cancer. The clinical features are not different from neuropathies due to other causes, with a progressive clinical course over weeks or months. Spontaneous relapses and remissions occur in a few cases. In patients with solid tumors, sensorimotor neuropathies are usually associated with lung cancer but they have been reported with other neoplasms (44). The electrophysiological and pathological studies disclose an axonal neuropathy, but in some patients the neuropathy cannot be differentiated from chronic inflammatory demyelinating polyneuritis.

Chronic sensorimotor peripheral neuropathy is also associated with lymphoma. The clinical features and pathological findings are similar to those of mixed neuropathies complicating solid tumors. However, direct infiltration of the nerves by the lymphoma is increasingly recognized as a cause of sensorimotor neuropathy in these patients (45). In some cases, the clinical picture is caused by lymphomatous infiltration of the spinal roots and CSF examination may disclose malignant cells, but there are well-documented cases of direct infiltration of the peripheral nerves without evidence of lymphomatous meningitis. In these patients, malignant cells are demonstrated in peripheral nerve biopsies. Sensorimotor neuropathies due to neoplastic infiltration of peripheral nerves has been reported in B-cell and T-cell lymphomas or leukemias and angiotropic (previously called malignant angioendotheliosis) lymphomas (see Chap. 21). Pathological studies have disclosed extensive demyelination that could not be attributable to simple compression of the nerve fibers by the malignant cells. This discordance suggests that demyelination may be caused by cytokines or immune mechanisms triggered by the invading lymphomatous cells.

In plasma cell dyscrasias (see also Chap. 22), paraneoplastic sensorimotor neuropathies are heterogeneous and their incidence varies depending on the underlying disease. A peripheral neuropathy is described in 5% of patients with Waldenström's macroglobulinemia. In 40% of these patients the neuropathy antedates the diagnosis of the hematological disease, sensory involvement is prominent, and the monoclonal IgM reacts against myelin-associated glycoprotein. In contrast, patients whose monoclonal IgM lacks activity against this myelin antigen typically develop neuropathy after the diagnosis of Waldenström's disease (48).

Paraneoplastic sensorimotor neuropathies are rare in osteolytic multiple myeloma and resemble the mild terminal axonal neuropathy seen in patients with solid tumors and advanced disease. On the other hand, more than 40% of patients with osteosclerotic myeloma present with a peripheral neuropathy. Motor weakness is usually more prominent than the sensory complaints and the clinical, electrophysiological, and pathological features are similar to those of chronic idiopathic polyneuritis (48). These patients may have a solitary or a few bony lesions, with normal serum and urine immunoelectrophoresis and bone marrow examination. Therefore, bone scan is mandatory in patients with neuropathies resembling chronic idiopathic demyelinating polyneuritis to rule out an osteosclerotic myeloma.

The diagnosis of a sensorimotor neuropathy is not an indication for an aggressive search of an underlying cancer unless there is some evidence in the routine clinical and laboratory examinations. In patients with the possible diagnosis of chronic idiopathic demyelinating polyneuritis, serum immunoelectrophoresis, bone scan, and CT of the chest and abdomen are recommended to rule out an occult malignancy.

## D. Autonomic Neuropathy

The autonomic nervous system may be involved in several paraneoplastic syndromes. Orthostatic hypotension, impotence, and sweating abnormalities may be the presenting symptoms of PEM. In this setting, signs of sensory neuronopathy or CNS dysfunction will appear during the clinical course. Severe orthostatic hypotension has been also reported in a few patients with lung cancer and sensorimotor neuropathy. An isolated, acute autonomic neuropathy involving both the sympathetic and parasympathetic systems or mostly the former has been described in one patient with SCLC and another with Hodgkin's disease. A chronic intestinal pseudo-obstruction has been associated with small-cell lung cancer. This rare but distinct paraneoplastic syndrome is due to damage of the autonomic neurons of the enteric plexuses (49). There are reports of some patients with signs of sensory neuronopathy (50), presented during the clinical course of their disease or found at postmortem study. This feature, coupled with a recent study (49) that describes in these patients an antineuronal antibody probably identical to the anti-Hu, suggests that paraneoplastic intestinal pseudo-obstruction may be included in the spectrum of PEM.

### E. Neuromyotonia

The syndrome of spontaneous muscle fiber activity characterized by muscle cramping, myokymia, and abnormal muscle relaxation due to peripheral nerve damage has been associated with different clinical situations. The syndrome has received different names such as neuromyotonia, Isaac's syndrome, or pseudo-myotonia and rarely occurs as a remote effect of cancer. Paraneoplastic neuro-myotonia has been reported in a few patients with lung cancer, usually SCLC, and thymoma (51). These patients present with muscle stiffness, cramps, myokymia, and sometimes hyperhidrosis. The neurological examination usually demonstrates signs of an underlying sensorimotor neuropathy. The electromyographic studies disclose sustained muscle activity that is not abolished by sleep, general anesthesia, or proximal nerve block. However, the continuous muscle activity disappears by blocking the neuromuscular junction.

In patients with known cancer the presence of muscle cramps may be due to metabolic disturbances, metastatic compression, or infiltration of peripheral nerves and nerve roots or complications of therapy, either toxic peripheral neuropathies or radiation-induced plexopathies. The clinical history and electro-myographic and neuroradiological studies will identify the correct etiology of the muscle cramps in most cases (52).

## IV. PARANEOPLASTIC SYNDROMES OF THE NEUROMUSCULAR JUNCTION AND MUSCLE

### A. Lambert-Eaton Myasthenic Syndrome

Lambert-Eaton myasthenic syndrome (LEMS) is a paraneoplastic disorder characterized by a defect in the presynaptic quantal release of acetylcholine. The presenting symptoms include leg or generalized weakness, aching and stiffness of muscles, and autonomic dysfunction. Patients have difficulty in walking, rising from a chair, or climbing stairs. In some patients, prolonged exercise increases the muscle discomfort and stiffness and causes fatigability. Symptoms may worsen after a hot bath or in hot weather. Although upper-limb weakness is rarely a presenting symptom, at least three-quarters of the patients eventually develop arm weakness. The majority of patients develop symptoms of autonomic dysfunction (dry mouth, sexual impotence, constipation, blurred vision), and mild or transitory symptoms of cranial nerve dysfunction such as diplopia, eyelid ptosis, and difficulty swallowing or chewing. Numbness and paresthesias of extremities are reported by some patients (53). The neurological examination shows a proximal distribution of muscle weakness associated with loss or reduction of reflexes. Typically, a sustained maximum voluntary contraction for a few seconds results in an increase of strength and in a potentiation of the muscle reflex being tested. Sluggish pupillary responses are a common sign of autonomic dysfunction.

In a review of 50 patients with LEMS (53), 60% of the patients had an underlying tumor, usually an SCLC or a poorly differentiated carcinoma of the lung. In most, the neurological symptoms developed before (70%) or at the same time (25%) as tumor diagnosis. When no tumor was found, the risk of developing cancer decreased after 2 years of LEMS symptoms and became very low after 5 years.

The diagnosis of LEMS is made on the basis of clinical and electrophysiological findings. Sensory and motor conduction velocities are usually normal. Typically, there is a reduced amplitude of the compound muscle action potentials (CMAP). Increases of >100% occur progressively during repetitive supramaximal nerve stimulation or following a short period of maximum voluntary contraction. In a recent study the peak-to-peak amplitude of the CMAP in resting abductor digiti minimi at the time of diagnosis of SCLC correlated with the outcome of the tumor and the response of LEMS to antineoplastic therapy (54). The clinical and electrophysiological findings are similar whether LEMS is paraneoplastic or not.

Although an immune basis has been suggested for a number of paraneoplastic disorders, LEMS is the prototype for which direct evidence of a pathogenic antibody has been demonstrated by passive transfer of the disease to animals (55). Lambert-Eaton myesthenic syndrome can develop in association with other antibody-associated paraneoplastic disorders (anti-Hu PEM) (24) or non–antibody-related disorders (group of patients with LEMS and PCD) (16). The current hypothesis postulates an immune response against component(s) of a voltage gated calcium channel (VGCC). Voltage gated calcium channel is expressed in SCLC. Antibody induced by the tumor cross-reacts with VGCC in the presynaptic neuromuscular junction and is responsible for the neurological dysfunction (56). The antibodies of some LEMS patients immunoprecipitate VGCC prelabeled with the specific subtype of w-conotoxin. This finding has been used as a serological test to determine the presence of antibodies against the presynaptic omega-conotoxin–sensitive VGCC in LEMS patients. However, the specificity and sensitivity of this test are not optimal. Only 44% of LEMS patients had significant levels of antibodies using an immunoprecipitation assay with radioactive omega-conotoxin–labeled VGCC (56). Furthermore, anti-VGCC antibodies were commonly found in patients with systemic lupus erythematosus, rheumatoid arthritis, and myasthenia gravis and in some patients with SCLC without LEMS.

In a recent study (Rosenfeld, personal communication) the screening of a human fetal brain expression library with the serum of a patient with LEMS has resulted in the isolation of cDNA clones encoding antigens that have been called myasthenic syndrome antigen A and B (MysA, MysB). Proteins derived from these clones are specifically recognized by LEMS sera but not by the sera from normal individuals or from patients with other paraneoplastic or oncological disorders, including SCLC without LEMS. The predicted amino acid sequence of these clones shows high homology to the beta-subunit of the rabbit skeletal muscle calcium channel. The current purification of MysA and MysB proteins will determine the sensitivity of the assay for detection of specific LEMS antibodies. Furthermore, the immunization of animals with MysA and MysB may determine the role of these antigens in the pathogenesis of the disease.

## B. Myopathic Syndromes

One of the first neurological syndromes considered a remote effect of cancer included muscle weakness restricted to or predominant in the proximal muscles, particularly of the lower extremities, with variable degrees of muscle wasting and normal or depressed deep tendon reflexes. The clinical syndrome was initially defined as "carcinomatous neuromyopathy" to emphasize the uncertain site and nature of the lesion. Later, it became clear that there were several different, and probably unrelated, neurological syndromes. Lambert-Eaton myasthenic syndrome was soon recognized as a separate entity. Patients with Lambert-Eaton myasthenic syndrome may present with proximal weakness without clear evidence of fatigability or autonomic dysfunction. This feature, along with the finding of "myopathic" changes in the EMG, may delay or cause one to overlook the diagnosis unless repetitive stimulation is included as part of the neurophysiological workup.

*Polymyositis* was another disorder separated from the initial concept of "neuromyopathy." Older patients with polymyositis or dermatomyositis have a 20% incidence of cancer. The most frequent tumors are lung, ovary, stomach, and breast (57). The association between these two syndromes and cancer and the opinion that tumors are more frequent in dermatomyositis than in polymyositis have not been accepted by all the authors. However, there is enough evidence in the literature to recommend a nonaggressive search for an underlying tumor in patients over the age of 40 with dermatomyositis. No clinical or laboratory clues, other than older age, identify those patients with an associated tumor.

An *acute necrotizing myopathy* has been described in a few patients with lung, gastrointestinal, breast, and bladder carcinomas (58). The muscle weakness is usually more generalized and rapidly progressive than that seen in polymyositis. Muscle biopsy discloses severe necrotic changes with no or sparse inflammatory infiltrate. This syndrome may represent a particularly severe form of polymyositis, but this hypothesis is not universally accepted. A recent study suggests that the cause of the necrosis could be an immune-mediated microangiopathy different from that observed in dermatomyositis (59).

Nowadays, the term carcinomatous neuromyopathy is still used to describe those patients that present with proximal muscle weakness and sometimes diminished deep tendon reflexes. They have normal or mildly elevated muscle enzyme levels and a combination of "myopathic" and "neuropathic" signs on electrophysiological studies and muscle biopsy. This syndrome is almost always described in patients with known solid tumors, particularly lung cancer. The incidence of carcinomatous neuromyopathy varies depending on the criteria used for the diagnosis. Subclinical evidence of the syndrome may be found in more than 20% of patients with solid tumors but clinically significant symptoms occur in less than 2% of patients. The observation of this syndrome in well-nourished patients distinguishes it from the more common cachectic myopathy seen in late stages of the neoplasm. Muscle enzyme levels are normal and electrophysiological studies disclose small polyphasic motor unit potentials compatible with a primary muscle dysfunction with or usually without features of denervation. Pathological studies were not done in most of the series of carcinomatous neuromyopathy. Barron and Heffner (60) studied eight muscle biopsies of patients with carcinomatous neuromyopathy and they found features of denervation in all. Electron microscopy disclosed degeneration of the intramuscular motor nerves. This distal lesion would explain the "myopathic" electromyographic pattern.

## V. TREATMENT AND PROGNOSIS OF PARANEOPLASTIC SYNDROMES

### A. Natural History

Most neurological paraneoplastic syndromes have a subacute, progressive, unremitting course that causes profound disability and sometimes death. Spontaneous improvement of the neurological disorder has been reported in a few patients with opsoclonus-myoclonus (30,31), subacute motor neuronopathy (39), and sensorimotor neuropathies (43,44). In the latter, the electrophysiological or pathological features are those of a primary demyelinating disease and some of the neuropathies fulfill the criteria of acute or chronic Guillain-Barré syndrome. Although PCD has an unremitting course, there are exceptional case reports of spontaneous improvement when the cerebellar syndrome is associated with Hodgkin's disease (12).

Progression to severe disability is uncommon in the neuromuscular disorders that occur after the diagnosis of the neoplasia, such as some sensorimotor neuropathies or carcinomatous neuromyopathy. A few patients with PEM or PCD, particularly those without anti-Yo antibodies, may spontaneously stabilize when the neurological deficit is still mild.

## B. Effect of Antineoplastic Therapy

In general, neurological paraneoplastic syndromes run a clinical course independent of the underlying neoplasm, suggesting that the pathophysiological mechanisms of the neurological syndrome, presumably triggered by the tumor, become independent of the neoplasm. Occasional examples of improvement after treatment of the tumor have been reported in almost all the neurological paraneoplastic syndromes. However, the effectiveness of antineoplastic therapy or other treatments is difficult to assess due to the following: (1) the incidence of these syndromes is low and the natural history is not uniform; (2) the neoplasm may not have an effective treatment; and (3) some paraneoplastic syndromes are characterized by irreversible neuronal damage. In these cases a beneficial treatment might not lead to clinical improvement but only to stabilization of the syndrome. In spite of these objections, aggressive treatment of the underlying tumor must be recommended in all cases because (1) there are occasional reports of improvement and (2) paraneoplastic syndromes, such as opsoclonus-myoclonus (30) or LEMS (54), respond to immunosuppression along with treatment of the tumor, resulting in improved prognosis.

## C. Immunosuppressive Therapies

Several immunosuppressive therapies have been used in those paraneoplastic syndromes thought to be immune mediated. Paraneoplastic syndromes with a well-established autoimmune pathogenesis include LEMS, acute and chronic inflammatory demyelinating polyneuropathies, multineuritis with vasculitis, and dermato/polymyositis. In these syndromes the targets of the immune attack may regenerate, so a clinical improvement can be expected after treatment. There is the impression that immunosuppressive treatment is not as effective when the same syndromes are not associated with cancer. Corticosteroids, with or without plasmapheresis, is the most frequent treatment used in these syndromes. The possible synergistic effect of antineoplastic treatment is unclear. In patients with LEMS effective treatment of the tumor clearly improves the beneficial effect of the immunosuppressive therapy (54). It is unclear if the chemotherapy protocols should avoid drugs that are potentially neurotoxic.

A second group of paraneoplastic syndromes that present some features that suggest autoimmune pathogenesis includes PCD, PEM, cancer-associated retinopathy, opsoclonus-myoclonus syndrome, and chronic intestinal pseudo-obstruction. Approximately 60% of children with opsoclonus and neuroblastoma improve, at least transiently, with corticosteroids (27). In adult patients with opsoclonus and SCLC or breast cancer, the response to corticosteroid treatment is much less satisfactory and treatment of the tumor seems to be more important than the immunosuppressive treatment (29,30). Except for opsoclonus-myoclonus, this group of paraneoplastic syndromes is characterized by irreversible neuronal damage. Treatment with corticosteroids or plasmapheresis has almost always been unsuccessful. The only exceptions are a few patients with limbic encephalitis who have improved with corticosteroids (24). We retrospectively evaluated the effect of treatment with immunosuppressants, treatment of the tumor, or combination of both therapies in 16 patients with PEM or PCD with anti-Hu or anti-Yo antibodies (61). No patient improved, but two patients treated with plasmapheresis and antineoplastic therapy and three that only received treatment of the tumor remained stable for at least 6 months. Unlike patients that did not improve, four of the five patients with a stable course started the treatment when the neurological deficit was mild, suggesting that early diagnosis improves the chance of responding to treatment.

Patients with PEM, PCD, or retinopathy with severe disability that have been stable for weeks before their diagnosis should not be treated with immunosuppressants, only antineoplastic therapy at the time the tumor is discovered. However, patients with these paraneoplastic syndromes and clear evidence of progression at the time of diagnosis, particularly those with mild or moderate neurological dysfunction, should be treated with immunosuppressive therapy. The value of specific treatments such as plasmapheresis, corticosteroids, or pulses of cyclophosphamide need to be reevaluated by prospective studies; these must include an aggressive search for neoplasm in order to start treatment of the tumor as soon as possible.

## ACKNOWLEDGMENTS

We thank Dr. Myrna Rosenfeld for her helpful criticisms in the review of the manuscript and Dr. Kendra Peterson for clinical aspects of anti-Yo patients.

## REFERENCES

1. Posner JB. Paraneoplastic syndromes. Curr Neurol 1989; 9:245–278.
2. Posner JB, Furneaux HM. Paraneoplastic syndromes. In: BH Waksman, ed. Immunologic mechanisms in neurologic and psychiatric disease. New York: Raven Press: 1990:187–219.

3. Henson RA, Urich H. Cortical cerebellar degeneration. In: Henson RA, Urich H, eds. Cancer and the nervous system. Oxford: Blackwell Scientific Publications, 1982: 314–345.
4. Greenlee JE, Brashear HR. Antibodies to cerebellar Purkinje cells in patients with paraneoplastic cerebellar degeneration and ovarian carcinoma. Ann Neurol 1983; 14: 609–613.
5. Furneaux HM, Rosenblum MK, Dalmau J, Wong E, Woodruff P, Graus F, Posner JB. Selective expression of Purkinje-cell antigens in tumor tissue from patients with paraneoplastic cerebellar degeneration. N Eng J Med 1990; 322:1844–1851.
6. Fathallah-Shaykh H, Wolf S, Wong E, Posner JB, Furneaux HM. Cloning of a leucine zipper protein recognized by the sera of patients with antibody-associated paraneoplastic cerebellar degeneration. Proc Natl Acad Sci U S A 1991; 88:3451–3454.
7. Sakai K, Mitchell DJ, Tsukamoto T, Steinman L. Isolation of a complementary DNA clone encoding an autoantigen recognized by an anti-neuronal cell antibody from a patient with paraneoplastic cerebellar degeneration. Ann Neurol 1990; 28:692–698.
8. Anderson NE, Rosenblum MK, Posner JB. Paraneoplastic cerebellar degeneration: clinical-immunological correlations. Ann Neurol 1988; 24:559–567.
9. Hammack JE, Kimmel DW, O'Neill BP, Lennon VA. Paraneoplastic cerebellar degeneration: a clinical comparison of patients with and without Purkinje cell cytoplasmic antibodies. Mayo Clin Proc 1990; 65:1423–1431.
10. Jaeckle KA, Graus F, Houghton A, Cordon-Cardo C, Nielsen SL, Posner JB. Autoimmune response of patients with paraneoplastic cerebellar degeneration to a Purkinje cell cytoplasmic protein antigen. Ann Neurol 1985; 18:592–600.
11. Brazis PW, Biller J, Fine M, Palacios E, Pagano RJ. Cerebellar degeneration with Hodgkin's disease: computed tomographic correlation and literature review. Arch Neurol 1981; 38:253–256.
12. Hammack JE, Kotanides H, Rosenblum MK, Posner JB. Paraneoplastic cerebellar degeneration. II. Clinical and immunologic findings in 21 patients with Hodgkin's disease. Neurology 1992; 42:1938–1943.
13. Trotter JL, Hendin BA, Osterland K. Cerebellar degeneration with Hodgkin's disease. Arch Neurol 1976; 33:660–661.
14. Unger JW, Reisinger PWM, Huppert D. Purkinje cell antibodies in a patient with cerebellar disorder: detection of responsible antigenic proteins. J Neurol 1991; 238: 288–292.
15. Satoyoshi E, Kowa H, Fukunaga N. Subacute cerebellar degeneration and Eaton-Lambert syndrome with bronchogenic carcinoma. Neurology 1973; 23:764–768.
16. Blumenfeld AM, Recht LD, Chad DA, DeGirolami U, Griffin T, Jaeckle KA. Coexistence of Lambert-Eaton myasthenic syndrome and subacute cerebellar degeneration: differential effects of treatment. Neurology 1991; 41:1682–1685.
17. Tsukamoto T, Yamamoto H, Iwasaki Y, Yoshie O, Terunuma H, Suzuki H. Antineural autoantibodies in patient with paraneoplastic cerebellar degeneration. Arch Neurol 1989; 46:1225–1229.
18. Dalmau J, Furneaux HM, Gralla RJ, Kris MG, Posner JB. Detection of the anti-Hu antibody in the serum of patients with small cell lung cancer—a quantitative Western blot analysis. Ann Neurol 1990; 27:544–552.
19. Henson RA, Urich H. Encephalomyelitis with carcinoma. In: Henson RA, Urich H,

eds. Cancer and the nervous system. Oxford: Blackwell Scientific Publications, 1989: 314–345.
20. Graus F, Elkon KB, Cordon-Cardo C, Posner JB . Sensory neuronopathy and small cell lung cancer: antineuronal antibody that also reacts with the tumor. Am J Med 1986; 80:45–52.
21. Furneaux HM, Reich L, Posner JB. Autoantibody synthesis in the central nervous system of patients with paraneoplastic syndromes. Neurology 1990; 40:1085–1091.
22. Dalmau J, Furneaux HM, Rosenblum MK, Graus F, Posner JB. Detection of the anti-Hu antibody in specific regions of the nervous system and tumor from patients with paraneoplastic encephalomyelitis/sensory neuronopathy. Neurology 1991; 41:1757–1764.
23. Szabo A, Dalmau J, Manley G, Rosenfeld MR, Wong E, Henson J, Posner JB, Furneaux HM. HuD, a paraneoplastic encephalomyelitis antigen, contains RNA-binding domains and is homologous to Elav and sex-lethal. Cell 1991; 67:325–333.
24. Dalmau J, Graus F, Rosenblum MK, Posner JB. Anti-Hu associated paraneoplastic encephalomyelitis/sensory neuronopathy: a clinical study of 71 patients. Medicine 1992; 71:59–72.
25. Dirr LY, Elster AD, Donofrio PD, Smith M. Evolution of brain MRI abnormalities in limbic encephalitis. Neurology 1990; 40:1304–1306.
26. Dropcho E, Payne R. Paraneoplastic opsoclonus-myoclonus: association with medullary thyroid carcinoma and review of the literature. Arch Neurol 1986; 43:410–415.
27. Dyken P, Kolar O. Dancing eyes, dancing feet: infantile polymyoclonia. Brain 1968; 91:305–320.
28. Cohn SL, Salwen H, Herst CV, et al. Single copies of the N-myc oncogene in neuroblastomas from children presenting with the syndrome of opsoclonus-myoclonus. Cancer 1988; 62:723–726.
29. Luque FA, Furneaux HM, Ferziger R, et al. Anti-Ri: an antibody associated with paraneoplastic opsoclonus and breast cancer. Ann Neurol 1991; 29:241–251.
30. Anderson NE, Budde-Steffen C, Rosenblum MK, et al. Opsoclonus, myoclonus, ataxia, and encephalopathy in adults with cancer: a distinct paraneoplastic syndrome. Medicine 1988; 67:100–109.
31. Digre KB. Opsoclonus in adults: report of three cases and review of the literature. Arch Neurol 1986; 43:1165–1175.
32. Jacobson DM, Thirkill CE, Tipping SJ. A clinical triad to diagnose paraneoplastic retinopathy. Ann Neurol 1990; 28:162–167.
33. Buchanan TAS, Gardiner TA, Archer DB. An ultrastructural study of retinal photoreceptor degeneration associated with bronchial carcinoma. Am J Ophthalmol 1984; 97:277–287.
34. Polans AS, Buczylko J, Crabb J, Palczewski K. A photoreceptor calcium binding protein is recognized by autoantibodies obtained from patients with cancer-associated retinopathy. J Cell Biol 1991; 112:981–989.
35. Gray F, Hauw JJ, Escourolle R, Castaigne P. Myelopathies necrosantes et pathologie neoplasique. Rev Neurol 1980; 136:235–246.
36. Mancall EL, Rosales RK. Necrotizing myelopathy associated with visceral carcinoma. Brain 1964; 87:639–659.

37. Rosenfeld MR, Posner JB. Paraneoplastic motor neuron disease. In: Lewis P. Rowland, ed., Advances in neurology, vol. 56: Amyotrophic lateral sclerosis. New York: Raven Press, 1991:445–459.
38. Younger DS, Rowland LP, Latov N, et al. Lymphoma, motor neuron diseases and amyotrophic lateral sclerosis. Ann Neurol 1991; 29:78–86.
39. Schold SC, Cho ES, Somasundaram M, Posner JB. Subacute motor neuronopathy: a remote effect of lymphoma. Ann Neurol 1979; 5:271–287.
40. Windebank AJ, Blexrud MD, Dyck PJ, Daube JR, Karnes JL. The syndrome of acute sensory neuropathy: clinical features and electrophysiologic and pathologic changes. Neurology 1990; 40:584–591.
41. Dalakas MC. Chronic idiopathic ataxic neuropathy. Ann Neurol 1986; 19:545–554.
42. Prineas J. Polyneuropathies of undetermined cause. Act Neurol Scand 1970; 46(Suppl 40):1–72.
43. Lisak RP, Mitchell M, Zweiman, Orrechio E, Asbury AK. Guillain-Barré syndrome and Hodgkin's disease: three cases with immunological studies. Ann Neurol 1977; 1:72–78.
44. Croft PB, Urich H, Wilkinson M. Peripheral neuropathy of sensorimotor type associated with malignant disease. Brain 1967; 90:31–36.
45. Vital C, Vital A, Julien J, et al. Peripheral neuropathies and lymphoma without monoclonal gammopathy: a new classification. J Neurol 1990; 237:177–185.
46. Oh SJ, Slaughter R, Harrell L. Paraneoplastic vasculitic neuropathy: a treatable neuropathy. Muscle Nerve 1991; 14:152–156.
47. Vincent D, Dubas F, Hauw JJ, et al. Nerve and muscle microvasculitis in peripheral neuropathy: a remote effect of cancer? J Neurol Neurosurg Psychiatry 1986; 49:1007–1010.
48. Kelly JJ. Peripheral neuropathies associated with monoclonal proteins: a clinical review. Muscle Nerve 1985; 8:138–150.
49. Lennon VA, Sas DF, Busk MF, et al. Enteric neuronal autoantibodies in pseudo-obstruction with small-cell lung carcinoma. Gastroenterology 1991; 100:137–142.
50. Lhermitte F, Gray F, Lyon-Caen O, Pertuiset BF, Bernard P. Paralyse du tube digestif avec lesions des plexus myenteriques: nouveau syndrome paraneoplasique possible. Rev Neurol 1980; 136:825–836.
51. Garcia-Merino A, Cabello A, Mora JS, Liaño H. Continuous muscle fiber activity, peripheral neuropathy, and thymoma. Ann Neurol 1991; 29:215–218.
52. Steiner I, Siegal T. Muscle cramps in cancer patients. Cancer 1989; 63:574–577.
53. O'Neill JH, Murray NMF, Newsom-Davis J. The Lambert-Eaton myasthenic syndrome: a review of 50 cases. Brain 1988; 111:577–596.
54. Chalk CH, Murray NMF, Newsom-Davis J, O'Neill JH, Spiro SG. Response of the Lambert-Eaton myasthenic syndrome to treatment of associated small-cell lung carcinoma. Neurology 1990; 40:1552–1556.
55. Lang B, Newsom-Davis J, Wray D, Vincent A, Murray N. Autoimmune aetiology for myasthenic (Eaton-Lambert) syndrome. Lancet 1981; 2:224–226.
56. Leys K, Lang B, Johnson I, Newsom-Davis J. Calcium channel autoantibodies in the Lambert-Eaton myasthenic syndrome. Ann Neurol 1991; 29:307–314.
57. Barnes B. Dermatomyositis and malignancy. Ann Intern Med 1976; 84:68–76.

58. Brownell B, Hughes JT. Degeneration of muscle in association with carcinoma of the bronchus. J Neurol Neurosurg Psychiatry 1975; 38:363–370.
59. Emslie AM, Engel AG. Necrotizing myopathy with pipestem capillaries, microvascular deposits of the complement membrane attack complex (MAC) and minimal cellular infiltration. Neurology 1991; 41:936–939.
60. Barron SA, Heffner RR. Weakness in malignancy: evidence for a remote effect of tumor on distal axons. Ann Neurol 1978; 4:268–274.
61. Graus F, Vega F, Delattre JY, et al. Effect of plasmapheresis and antineoplastic treatment in CNS paraneoplastic syndromes with antineuronal autoantibodies. Neurology 1992; 42:536–540.

# 9

# Use of Glucocorticoids in Neuro-Oncology

**Charles J. Vecht**

*Daniel den Hoed Cancer Center, Rotterdam, The Netherlands*

**H. B. C. Verbiest**

*I.C. Hospital the Baronie, Breda, The Netherlands*

## I. GENERAL ASPECTS

### A. Introduction

Use of glucocorticoids in medicine is widespread. In cancer, glucocorticoids are used for many indications, including palliative treatment of pain, emesis, hypercalcemia, as part of chemotherapy, or as a supportive drug in terminal cancer. In neuro-oncological patients, primary indications for glucocorticoids are brain edema associated with primary and secondary brain tumors and metastatic spinal cord compression. In this chapter, we will discuss first general aspects of glucocorticoids, including bioavailability, mechanisms of action, and clinical use for tumor-associated brain and spinal cord edema, followed by side effects, drug interactions, suppression of the pituitary-adrenal axis, and discontinuation of therapy.

### B. Actions of Glucocorticoids

Corticosteroids are hormones produced by the adrenal cortex and include glucocorticoids, mineralocorticoids, and androgenic hormones. Glucocorticoids influence carbohydrate, protein, and fat metabolism and exert anti-inflammatory actions. Mineralocorticoids like aldosterone influence water and electrolyte balance. Glucocorticoids inhibit the secretion of corticotropin-releasing factor

(CRH) in the hypothalamus which normally stimulates corticotropin secretion from the anterior pituitary gland (1).

Therefore, apart from therapeutic actions, glucocorticoids also cause suppression of the hypothalamic-pituitary-adrenalcorticoid (HPA) axis, leading to decreased secretion of adrenocorticosteroids from the adrenal gland. Termination of glucocorticoid administration may be followed by a period of inadequate adrenal secretion of corticosteroids. The degree of adrenal suppression depends on dose, duration of administration, and dose regimens of cortisol or synthetic glucocorticosteroids (2).

Physical and emotional stress induce secretion of CRH and subsequently of corticotropin, leading to an increase in plasma-cortisol levels. The maximal cortisol output under stress conditions is estimated at 300 mg daily. Glucocorticoids are lipophilic and are able to cross the blood-brain barrier. They can be administered orally, intravenously, intramuscularly, and intrathecally. For parenteral use most synthetic glucocorticoids are administered as esters to make them hydrophilic. In the body, the steroid is liberated from the ester by liver esterases.

## C. Bioavailability

Peak levels of dexamethasone appear between 1 and 2 h following oral administration and within 5 min after intravenous injection (3). The half-life of dexamethasone in controls is 3–4 h for males and 2–3 h for females (4) (see Table 1). The half-life of administered glucocorticoids as measured in plasma has a poor relation to the duration of its action. The biological half-life is determined by the duration of corticotropin suppression after a single dose of glucocorticoids and is grouped into short (cortisol), intermediate (prednisone, methylprednisolone), and

**Table 1** Equivalent Dose of Different Glucocorticoids, Administered Orally or Intravenously

| | Glucocorticoid potency | Equivalent glucocorticoid dose (mg) | Plasma half-life (min) | Biologic half-life (h) | Physiological replacement dose (mg/day) |
|---|---|---|---|---|---|
| Cortisol (hydrocortisone) | 1 | 20 | 80–115 | 8–12 | 30 |
| Cortisone | 0.8 | 25 | 30 | 8–12 | 37.5 |
| Prednisone | 4 | 5 | 200 | 12–36 | 7.5 |
| Prednisolone | 4 | 5 | 120–200 | 12–36 | 7.5 |
| Methylprednisolone | 5 | 4 | 80–180 | 12–36 | 6 |
| Dexamethasone | 25–30 | 0.75 | 110–300 | 36–54 | 0.5–0.75 |

Source: Refs. 2 and 66.

long-acting (dexamethasone) effects of steroids (Table 1), but different actions of one glucocorticoid can be unequal in duration. Methylprednisolone and dexamethasone are extensively bound to plasma proteins and only the small unbound fraction is biologically active. In disorders associated with decreased albumin concentrations in serum, the clearance, the biological effect, and the toxicity of glucocorticoids are usually enhanced (5).

## II. BRAIN TUMOR EDEMA

### A. Actions of Glucocorticoids on Brain Tumor Edema

Brain edema secondary to intracranial tumors consists of an increased content of water, sodium, and albumin in and around the tumor. This edema is predominantly vasogenic, indicating that damage to the blood-brain barrier and vascular endothelium causes increased permeability of vessels. The rate and extent of peritumoral brain edema depends on the transcapillary hydrostatic and osmotic pressure gradient, the hydraulic conductivity of bulk flow through the extracellular compartment, and the rate at which the edema can be resorbed. The effect of dexamethasone and other corticosteroids on cerebral edema include actions on water permeability of the blood-brain barrier and on cerebral blood flow (CBF). Water permeability is increased in brain tumors compared with normal brain tissue with intact blood-brain barrier (6). Administration of dexamethasone or other glucocorticoids produces a reduction in water permeability in experimental brain tumors (6,7). This effect is probably caused by a stabilizing effect on the endothelial cell membrane with decreased permeability of the blood-brain barrier in capillary and arterial segments of brain tissue and can be observed within a few hours after dexamethasone administration (7,8). Reduced delivery of water-soluble methotrexate to brain tissue adjacent to tumor following dexamethasone administration also indicates decreased water permeability (9). Tissue concentrations of dexamethasone at 60 min after intravenous injection are high in the periphery of the tumor, adjacent cortex, and white matter, but low in the center of the tumor and remote normal cortex, suggesting that dexamethasone acts primarily around the tumor rim (10,11). Regional CBF is impaired in a variety of experimental brain tumors (6,12). Also, in edematous areas surrounding brain tumors, regional blood flow is reduced together with an impairment of vascular autoregulation (13). Steroids may influence CBF by affecting the vascular endothelium or by modifying aminergic or peptidergic systems that influence the blood-brain barrier. They may also cause vasoconstriction by inhibiting the release of prostacyclin from vascular endothelial cells (14).

Following dexamethasone administration, changes in blood flow have been observed within brain metastasis (15). Initially impaired vasomotor responses to changes in arterial $P_{CO_2}$ and blood pressure improve remarkably and suggest that dexamethasone restores directly or indirectly vaso-autonomic control (13). Until now, human studies on the effect of dexamethasone on CBF have produced inconclusive results. With single photon emission computed tomography (SPECT) using $^{99m}$Tc HM-PAO (hexamethylpropylene amine oxime), a reduced CBF has been observed within gliomas (16). With Xenon-133 no change was seen the first 2 days of treatment with high-dose dexamethasone, but after 7 days an ipsilateral increase in CBF was found (13,15). Using PET (positron-emission tomography) scanning, conflicting results have been observed for changes in CBF, which were interpreted as being reduced following a standard dose of dexamethasone of 16 mg/day in primary and metastatic brain tumors (17).

Recently a vascular permeability factor has been discovered, which is produced by glial cells, and it may well be that this factor is at least partially responsible for the formation of pathogenic brain edema associated with brain tumors (18). It is a polypeptide with a molecular weight of 46–56 kilodaltons and can be distinguished from other inducers of microvascular permeability such as histamine, serotonin, polyamines, leukokinines, and lymphokines. The action of vascular permeability factor is possibly based upon inflammatory reactions via the prostaglandin pathway induced by activation of phospholipase $A_2$ (18). This factor seems capable of inducing increased vascular permeability by direct action upon vascular endothelial cells and can be inhibited by pretreatment with dexamethasone or by binding to heparin. Dexamethasone reduces the expression of this vascular permeability factor in cultured malignant glial cells (18), suggesting that dexamethasone may also exert its protective effect on the development of vasogenic edema of brain tumors by inhibiting synthesis of this vascular permeability factor. Whether there exists more than one permeability-inducing factor is as yet unknown (19).

## B. Steroid Receptors in Brain Tumors

The presence of steroid hormone receptors has been determined in different types of primary brain tumors, including low- and high-grade gliomas and meningiomas. In very low concentrations, tumor growth in vitro was stimulated by the addition of dexamethasone (20). Higher dexamethasone doses induced a decrease in tumor growth, independent of tumor glucocorticoid receptor status. In one controlled trial, high-dose methylprednisolone had no effect on survival of patients with high-grade gliomas whether or not combined with systemic chemotherapy (21).

## C. Clinical Use of Glucocorticoids for Brain Tumor Edema

Glucocorticoids have been used for more than 30 years for the treatment of brain edema associated with primary brain tumors or brain metastasis (22). Glucocorticoids are effective in reducing neurological symptoms in more than 70% of patients with brain tumors. Prospective data are not available, but one early review indicated that 50% of patients enjoy almost complete relief, about 15% have moderate relief, and the others have minimal or no relief of central nervous system symptoms following glucocorticoid administration (23). The often impressive clinical effects of glucocorticoids on neurological signs are probably caused by action on surrounding brain edema and not on the tumor itself. The onset of action is rapid and becomes clinically evident within 24 to 48 h, but without further antitumor treatment the original neurological symptoms usually recur within 1 or 2 months. The use of glucocorticoids is particularly effective in patients with cerebral lymphoma. Following administration, clinical remission and complete resolution on computed tomography (CT) or magnetic resonance imaging (MRI) may follow in up to 40% of patients (24). This response usually continues a few months and occasionally for periods of 2 years or more (25). The disappearance of contrast-enhancing lesions on neuro-imaging studies may mask appropriate sites for stereotactic biopsy or surgery and create technical difficulties in obtaining a tissue diagnosis. It is therefore advisable in case of suspicion of primary cerebral lymphoma to postpone administering glucocorticoids until the diagnosis has been confirmed (26).

No differences in efficacy have been observed between the various glucocorticosteroids for the treatment of brain edema associated with brain tumors. Commonly dexamethasone is used because of absence of mineralocorticoid effect. The conventional starting dose of dexamethasone is 16 mg per day, often given as a first bolus of 10 mg intravenously, followed by 4 mg four times daily (q.i.d.) per os or intravenously (22). Some patients may benefit from higher doses if 16 mg gives insufficient clinical response.

No prospective randomized studies have been performed to determine the ideal dose for glucocorticosteroids for tumor-associated brain edema. However, it has been demonstrated that the toxicity of glucocorticoid administration is dependent on dose and on duration of administration. One would therefore prefer to administer the lowest possible dose necessary. A pilot study of 20 patients has shown that a starting dose of 16 mg daily, followed by 8 mg daily for 4 days, and then 4 mg daily until the last day of radiation therapy, is well tolerated (27). In this study, dexamethasone was well tolerated when given twice daily. Despite a plasma half-life of 2–5 h for dexamethasone, its biological half-life of 36–54 h explains why twice daily instead of four times daily dosing is fully justified and may have the advantage of lessening adrenal suppression (28). In one prospective trial it has now been established that 4 mg per day is as efficacious as the standard dose of 16 mg per day (Fig. 1), but leads to significantly fewer side effects (Fig. 2) (29). Based on these findings, we favor a starting dose of 4 mg per day. For patients with decreased consciousness or signs of impending tentorial or cerebellar herniation, a higher starting dose of 16 mg per day may be used, but in the great majority, an

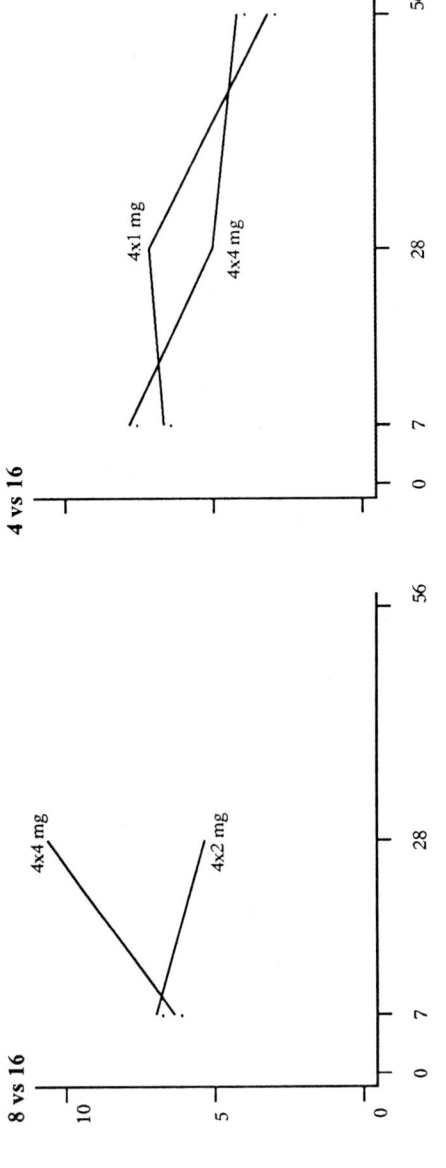

**Figure 1** Time course of Karnofsky score in two double-blind series, comparing 8 mg versus 16 mg dexamethasone in the first and 4 mg versus 16 mg in the second series. There were no significant differences in Karnofsky scores between 4, 8, or 16 mg at Day 7 (endpoint) or later. The differences at day 28 between 8 and 16 mg in the left panel are explained by withdrawal of dexamethasone after day 7 during a shorter time period in the 8 mg group at a time not all patients had already received or completed radiation therapy.

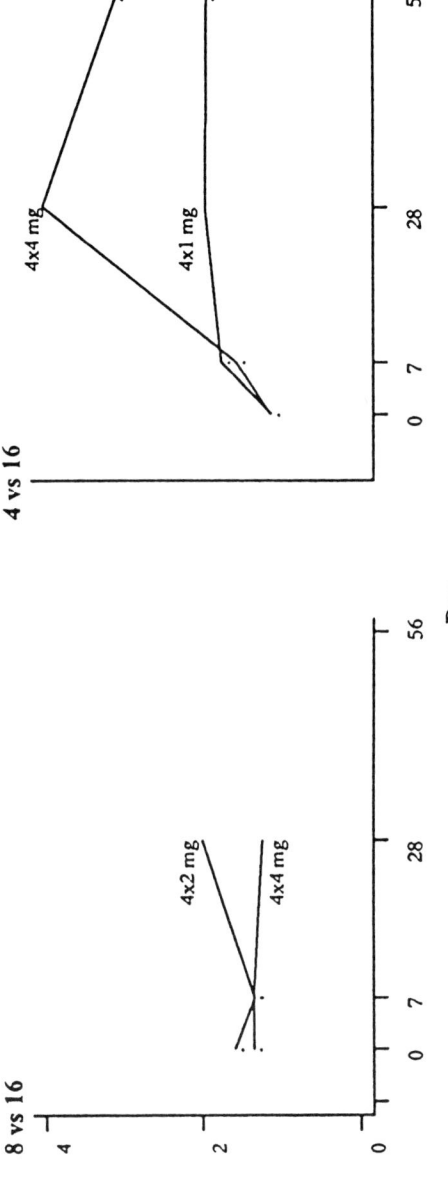

**Figure 2** Time course of mean number of side effects in two double-blind series, comparing 8 mg versus 16 mg and 4 mg versus 16 mg dexamethasone. In the first series, dexamethasone withdrawal was started at Day 7, in the second series at Day 28. This explains the remarkable difference in number of side effects with 16 mg dexamethasone between the first and second series at Day 28. Also note the significant difference in number of side effects between 4 mg and 16 mg in the second series at Day 28.

oral dose of 4 mg per day as a starting dose can be given until the end of radiation therapy, followed by tapering the dose over a period of about 4 weeks.

Under certain circumstances, it has been noted that increasing the dose in deteriorating patients with brain tumors can be effective. Doubling or increasing the dose from 16 to 32 and later up to 64 or 96 mg can result in a significant clinical benefit, although usually for limited periods of time (30).

Similar experiences have been reported with the use of methylprednisolone at doses of 200–2000 mg/day (equivalent to 40–4000 mg of dexamethasone per day). In eight of 11 patients with inoperable brain tumors and deterioration on conventional doses, neurological improvement could be maintained for a median period of 4 weeks (31). Doses higher than 1000 mg methylprednisolone per day gave no additional improvement.

The first signs of action of glucocorticoids on brain edema become apparent within 24 h after administration. In one study with methylprednisolone at a dose of 160 mg, clinical signs improved significantly after 24 h, with further progressive improvement over the succeeding 2 days (32). In another study, a high dose of methylprednisolone (500 mg/day for 7 days) resulted in clinical improvement within 24–48 h of therapy. Mean reduction of peritumoral edema volume was 30% and tumor volume decreased 15% after 7 days of methylprednisolone therapy (33). Under conditions associated with intracranial hypotension, the intracranial pressure and volume-pressure response clearly improve after 24 h of steroid therapy (32,34). Intraventricular pressure measurements have revealed that the compliance of the intracranial cavity improves after 24 h of treatment and that intracranial pressure is reduced within 48 h. Other studies using continuous lumbar measurement of cerebrospinal fluid pressure showed that intracranial pressure decreased 6 h after start of treatment in 7 of 10 investigated patients (32). Plateau waves of increased intracranial pressure are reduced in height, frequency, and duration within 24 h following high-dose dexamethasone administration (32). Clinical signs of improvement often start within 4–6 h after treatment (35). These effects, however, cannot easily be confirmed with imaging studies. In most instances, decrease in brain edema or brain displacement as observed with CT or MRI scan appears not earlier than 1 or 2 weeks after starting glucocorticoid treatment (36,37).

## III. METASTATIC SPINAL CORD COMPRESSION

### A. Actions of Glucocorticoids on Spinal Cord Compression

Edema associated with spinal cord compression by tumor may differ from brain tumor edema because the responsible lesion lies outside the nervous tissue from which it is separated by the dura. This suggests that different pathogenic mechanisms are involved in causing spinal cord edema and likewise glucocorticoids may exert their effect through different actions than in peritumoral brain edema. Nevertheless, vasogenic spinal cord edema has been shown in experimental models of tumor compression. Transcapillary leakage of both horseradish peroxidase and Evans blue dye occurs together with histological evidence of edema (38,39). In patients, one can observe vascular congestion, hemorrhage, and edema (40). Vasogenic edema may result from direct mechanical compression by the tumor with or without simultaneous obstruction of the epidural venous plexus. However, cytotoxic edema also may play a role. $N$-methyl-D-aspartate receptor antagonists such as MK-801 and ketamine were able to reduce water content but had no effect on dye extravasation or on prostaglandin synthesis in animal studies of spinal cord compression (39,41).

An impressive amount of experimental work has been devoted to the effect of glucocorticoids, particularly on their protective or healing effects in traumatic, ischemic, or neoplastic lesions of the spinal cord. The spinal cord contains a high concentration of glucocorticoid-binding sites, but it is not certain if the mechanisms of action of glucocorticoids in separate pathological conditions are similar. Glucocorticoid effects include facilitation of neuronal excitability and nerve transmission, an increase in spinal blood flow due to vasodilatation by β-receptor activation, and impairment of vasoconstriction by inhibition of prostaglandin and thromboxane synthesis (42). Another possibly important mechanism of glucocorticoid protection against spinal cord injury is the preventing or lessening of lipid peroxidation of neuronal cell membranes (43). Lipid peroxidation probably is an important mechanism of damage to the nervous system that results from peroxidation of nervous membranes by oxygen-free radicals (44). Methylprednisolone can prevent these free-radical reactions (43,45). Also, inhibition of prostaglandin synthesis by the action of glucocorticoids on phospholipase can result in reduced lipid hydrolysis. Decreased formation of eicosanoid (prostaglandin $F_{2\alpha}$ and thromboxane $A_2$) also may lead to a reduction in inflammatory reactions. Other actions of glucocorticoids include prevention of secondary ischemia and protection against increased intracellular calcium. Most of these proposed mechanisms are based on studies of traumatic spinal cord injury (45). It is uncertain whether all these mechanisms also play a role in spinal cord compression by tumor.

## B. Effects in Experimental Animals

There are indications for the existence of a therapeutic window for glucocorticoids. The dose-response relationship may be a biphasic curve, implying that lower or higher doses than optimal are less effective and may even become detrimental. For spinal cord trauma in animals, the optimal dose of methylprednisolone seems to be 30 mg/kg, which is similar to observations in humans. Another factor may be the time at which therapy starts. Only administration within

8 h after acute spinal cord injury seems to be able to improve recovery or prevent further deterioration (46).

Experiments using animal models of compression of the spinal cord showed impaired drainage by the vertebral venous plexus and development of vasogenic edema. These changes are followed by autonomic dysregulation of the spinal circulation, a decrease in spinal blood flow, and finally irreversible cord damage. Use of dexamethasone in a dose of 10 mg/kg in one model of spinal cord compression gave significant but transient improvement in neurological function and reduction of water content of the compressed cord (38,47). Both high- and low-dose dexamethasone administration in rats produced an equally strong improvement in neurological function in a nontumoral model of cord compression when compared to untreated animals, but animal mortality was higher with high-dose dexamethasone because of infectious and gastrointestinal complications (48). In a tumor model, there was significant but modest clinical improvement with high-dose dexamethasone administration (10 mg/kg) together with a clear reduction in blood–spinal cord transport and in water content of the compressed cord (49). Using a similar model, others were unable to demonstrate an effect of high-dose glucocorticoids on water or inhibition of prostaglandin $E_2$ synthesis in the spinal cord (50). Vascular permeability as measured by Evans blue was significantly reduced by dexamethasone, methylprednisolone, and indomethacin (41).

In rats with neoplastic spinal cord compression, deterioration of neurological function was significantly less severe in rats following administration of dexamethasone or indomethacin (50).

## C. Clinical Effects

The results of experimental work in animals on the effect of glucocorticoids on spinal cord compression have provided the rationale for high-dose regimens of dexamethasone in the clinical setting. One retrospective study using 100 mg intravenous (IV) bolus of dexamethasone, followed by 96 mg per day for the first 3 days, followed by a tapering schedule, gave no indication of any better neurological improvement than a conventional regimen but was claimed to show better analgesic effect in 64% of patients within 1 day of treatment (51). In the only randomized prospective trial, a conventional dose of 10 mg IV following demonstration of complete block on myelography was equally as effective for the relief of pain as an initial high dose of 100 mg bolus, followed by 4 mg four times per day orally. Sixty-seven percent of patients had substantial pain relief within 24 h of administration. Also, changes over time in neurological function were approximately the same and there were no differences between the two different doses of dexamethasone on ambulation or bladder function. After 1 week, 54% of patients with conventional regimen and 55% of patients with high-dose dexamethasone were able to walk (52). In another study, 28 consecutive patients received high-dose dexamethasone with 100 mg as loading dose and decreasing doses to zero within 2 weeks. There was a 14% incidence of serious side effects, which included three patients with gastrointestinal perforation and one with rectal bleeding. In a subsequent series of 38 patients receiving 16 mg daily, with dosage reduced to zero in 14 days, there were significantly fewer side effect (8%) and none was serious. Ambulation after treatment was similar, with 57% of patients walking following high-dose dexamethasone and 58% following conventional dose of dexamethasone (53).

It is useful to realize that a conventional dose of dexamethasone of 16 mg daily is not a low dose and is equivalent to 100 mg prednisone or 400 mg hydrocortisone daily. Given the absence of convincing positive effects for high-dose regiments, and the observed toxicity, we favor a conventional schedule with an initial bolus of 10 mg dexamethasone IV followed by 16 mg daily for patients with metastatic spinal cord compression.

## IV. TOXICITY OF GLUCOCORTICOIDS

### A. Direct Side Effects

The use of corticosteroids can induce a multitude of side effects (listed in Table 2). Occurrence of side effects is dependent on dose and duration of treatment, cumulative dose, and dose regimen (Table 3). In neuro-oncological patients, the reported incidence of steroid-induced toxicities differ greatly. Following high-dose corticosteroid administration (16 mg of dexamethasone or higher), the incidence of major complications was only 2.4% in a total of 121 patients who had undergone major surgery, although the duration of treatment was not reported (54). Another study reported little serious toxicity from the use of a high-dose, short-term dexamethasone regimen (100 mg IV bolus followed by 96 mg for 3 days, tapering to zero in 2 weeks) for epidural spinal cord compression (50). However, another study in neuro-oncological patients revealed that 51% of patients developed at least one steroid toxicity and 19% of these required hospital admission (55). Frequent complications were hyperglycemia (9%), infections (22%), gastrointestinal signs (14%), proximal myopathy (19%), and peripheral edema (8%). The majority of side effects occurred in patients who received dexamethasone for longer than 3 weeks or who were given a cumulative dose greater than 400 mg. One-third of patients with toxicity developed their first toxic event within 3 weeks of starting treatment. Patients with toxicity more often had low serum albumin concentration (mean of 3.0 g/dl) (50). This is in agreement with earlier observations that showed serum albumin levels of 2.5 g/dl lead to twice as high a frequency of steroid-related toxicity (5). Although peptic ulcer perforation occurs infrequently in neuro-oncological patients, it is a particular serious complication, with a high mortality in patients older than 50 years of age.

**Table 2** Side Effects of Glucocorticoids

| | |
|---|---|
| *Neuropsychiatric* | *Gastrointestinal* |
| Euphoria | Peptic ulcer disease |
| Increased appetite | Intestinal perforation |
| Insomnia | Pancreatitis |
| Depression | *Cardiovascular* |
| Anxiety | Hypertension |
| Psychosis | Congestive heart failure |
| Benign intracranial pressure (pseudotumor cerebri) | Hypokalemic alkalosis |
| *Musculoskeletal* | Sodium retention |
| Myopathy | *Ophthalmic* |
| Osteoporosis, vertebral compression, and other spontaneous fractures | Cataract |
| | Glaucoma |
| Avascular bone necrosis | Exophthalmos |
| Spinal epidural lipomatosis | *Dermatologic* |
| Poststeroid pseudorheumatism | Facial erythema |
| *Endocrine-metabolic* | Thin skin |
| Obesity | Petechiae and ecchymoses |
| Moon face, supraclavicular and posterior cervical fat deposition | Striae |
| | Impaired wound healing |
| Acne, hirsutism, impotence, or menstrual irregularities | Panniculitis |
| | *Immune system* |
| Retardation of growth in children | Susceptibility to infections |
| Hyperglycemia and diabetes mellitus | Neutrophilia, monocytopenia, lymphocytopenia |
| Hyperosmolar, nonketotic coma | |
| Diabetic ketoacidosis | Impaired wound healing |
| Hyperlipoproteinemia | |
| Negative balance of nitrogen, potassium, and calcium | |
| Secondary adrenal insufficiency | |

Source: Ref. 2.

A relatively low dose dexamethasone regimen—starting first at 16 mg/day for 4 days followed, by 8 mg/day for four days, followed by 4 mg per day until the last day of radiotherapy—resulted in mild toxicity in six of 20 treatment patients; this consisted of either hyperglycemia, candida esophagitis, steroid pseudo-rheumatism, or signs of withdrawal syndrome. Only two episodes of toxicity were recorded in patient receiving steroids for less than 21 days (27). The severity of complications is greater in long term treated patients. In 11 patients receiving very high daily doses of methylprednisolone (200–2000) for longer periods of time, all developed toxicities, including three cases of serious bacterial infections and six cases of candida pharyngitis; all had features of hyperadrenocorticoism (31). A frequent but peculiar and harmless side effect which follows intravenous adminis-

**Table 3** Frequency of Side Effects (at 4-mg, 8-mg, and 16-mg doses)

| Side effects | Day 0 | Day 28 | | |
|---|---|---|---|---|
| | | 4 mg | 8 mg | 16 mg |
| Number of patients observed | 94 | 22 | 16 | 34 |
| Raised glucose | 22% | 18% | 25% | 21% |
| Raised blood pressure | 24% | 45% | 12% | 26% |
| Infectious disease | 0% | 9% | 6% | 9% |
| Gastrointestinal complaints | 15% | 18% | 6% | 24% |
| Mental changes | 30% | 14% | 19% | 21% |
| Ankle edema | 1% | 14% | 13% | 26% |
| Moon face | 2% | 32% | 69% | 65% |
| Proximal muscle weakness | 18% | 14% | 38% | 38% |

Source: Ref. 29.

tration of dexamethasone is a transient burning sensation, particularly felt around the anus and genitalia (51).

Glucocorticoids can induce psychiatric symptoms in up to 50% of patients. However, severe psychiatric conditions occur in only about 5% of patients (56). These include affective disorders (depression or mania), psychosis, and cognitive disturbances. Neuropsychiatric signs include tremor or tremulousness, hyperkinesia, and insomnia. Euphoria is a well-known side effect of glucocorticosteroids, occurring in up to 40% of patients, and can be viewed as helpful in cancer patients, although it may progress to hypomania. Usually these disturbances occur within the first 2 weeks of steroid treatment. Most psychiatric signs are dose related and occur more frequently with high doses.

Reduction, discontinuation, or division of the doses over the day may help to alleviate symptoms. On the other hand, withdrawal or particularly rapid tapering may induce psychiatric symptoms such as depression, anxiety, or psychosis. Slowly tapering or briefly increasing the dose may lead to disappearance of withdrawal effects. If symptoms persist and glucocorticosteroids cannot be withdrawn, symptomatic therapy with neuroleptics, including haloperidol, may be indicated.

## B. Drug Interactions

The primary pathway for elimination of glucocorticosteroids is hepatic biotransformation to water-soluble glucuronides followed by renal excretion. Hydroxylation of glucocorticosteroids take place by liver microsomal cytochrome

P-450 enzymes and may thus interact with other drugs metabolized through this pathway. Several anticonvulsants are also metabolized via this route, a clinically relevant consideration because many patients with primary or secondary brain tumors have concomitant epilepsy. Phenytoin accelerates conjugation of microsomal liver enzymes (57) and induces a fourfold increase in the clearance of dexamethasone, reducing the half-life to 1.7 h (58). Vice versa, phenytoin also is more rapidly metabolized due to induction of the liver microsomal enzymes by action of glucocorticoids. This implies that for either of these groups of drugs, concentrations and pharmacological effects can easily become insufficient if one is added to the other. Thus, phenytoin administration should be increased if glucocorticoids are added. When initiating therapy, a higher than usual maintenance dose of phenytoin should be administered. However, precise information on how much the dose should be increased is not available.

An immunological interaction may occur with the simultaneous use of dexamethasone, phenytoin, and cranial irradiation, which can lead to the development of erythema multiforme (Stevens-Johnson syndrome) (59).

Other potent inducers of hepatic microsomal metabolism are barbiturates, although these are now becoming obsolete for treatment of epilepsy. Clearance of methylprednisolone is increased fourfold and prednisolone twofold if used together with phenobarbital (60). Another primary anticonvulsant for symptomatic or partial epilepsy is carbamazepine (61), which also induces metabolism of glucocorticoids by cytochrome P-450 enzymes. However, little information is available on the degree of interaction of carbamazepine with glucocorticoids and any clinical implications. Controlled trials have suggested that sodium valproate is effective for partial epilepsy. An important advantage for using it in neuro-oncological patients may be its apparent lack of interaction with glucocorticoids.

## C. Pituitary-Adrenal Suppression

A major problem in administering glucocorticoids is suppression of the hypothalamic pituitary-adrenal axis. In general, the degree of adrenal suppression depends on dose level and duration of administration (62). The concentration of plasma cortisol may be either normal or lowered after corticosteroid treatment and gives no reliable information on the degree of adrenal suppression. Almost half of patients with normal basal cortisol levels after discontinuation of glucocorticoid therapy have impaired pituitary-adrenal function. Therefore, stimulation tests are usually required to assess pituitary-adrenal function. Measuring plasma cortisol concentration after administration of corticotropin-releasing factor (CRF test) has the advantage of being safer than the insulin hypoglycemia test. There is an unpredictable correlation between duration of glucocorticoid administration, the daily dose, and the cumulative dose with the extent of pituitary-adrenal dysfunction (62). This implies that for neuro-oncological patients in whom glucocorticoids have been withdrawn, supplementation with glucocorticoids is advised if clinical stress conditions recur. Ideally, a CRF test is performed first, but in practice this is often omitted, and in cases of acute complications there is no time to do this. Generally one assumes a duration of hypothalamic-pituitary-adrenalcorticoid (HPA) suppression of about 12 months following previous glucocorticoid therapy of more than a few weeks (63). On the other hand, adrenal failure seems to be relatively rare in neuro-oncological patients despite relatively high doses (64).

The syndrome of steroid withdrawal should be distinguished from HPA suppression as such. This syndrome may occur during or after tapering, particularly following longer periods of use of high-dose glucocorticoids. It is characterized by fatigue, weakness, weight loss, nausea, orthostatic dizziness and postural hypotension, dyspnea, hypoglycemia, and occasionally fever. Tapering may also induce arthralgia (post-steroid pseudo-rheumatism) that consists of bilateral pain in the joints, often involving the knees. Withdrawal symptoms can occur despite normal cortisol levels and normal HPA responsiveness (2). Occasionally systemic infections, for example by *Pneumocystis carinii*, become activated during or after withdrawal of glucocorticoids (65).

## D. Discontinuation of Therapy

Dose and duration of glucocorticoid steroid therapy depend on the nature and severity of the underlying disorder. With high-dose steroid therapy for short periods (less than 2 weeks), there is a small risk of adverse effects, and steroid administration can be discontinued instantly. For longer periods of therapy, careful withdrawal of medication is required in order to avoid signs of adrenal insufficiency caused by HPA suppression. If the condition of the underlying disease permits withdrawal of glucocorticoids, the first phase of tapering the drug can be performed rather quickly until the physiological dose of glucocorticoids is reached (see Table 1). From then on, further tapering of the dose should proceed slowly and cautiously (66). In order to improve recovery of HPA suppression, the dose is then best taken once daily, preferably in the morning. One may also switch to alternate-day therapy, using glucocorticoids with a biological half-life of short or intermediate duration of action (66). However, in brain tumor patients this is often poorly tolerated (67). In case of recurrence of clinical signs of the underlying disease, of withdrawal symptoms, or of adrenal insufficiency, obviously the dose may have to be raised or restarted.

## ACKNOWLEDGMENTS

The authors thank Dr. M. J. van den Bent and Dr. J. G. M. Klijn for critical review and Janet van Vliet for her assistance in preparing the manuscript.

# REFERENCES

1. Müller OA, Von Werder K. Corticotropin-releasing hormone: basic and clinical aspects. In Motta M, ed. Brain endocrinology, 2nd Ed. New York: Raven Press, 1991:351–375.
2. Axelrod L. Glucocorticoids. In: Kelley, WN, Harris ED, Ruddy S, Sledge CB, eds. Textbook of Rheumatology. Philadelphia: Saunders, 1989, 845–860.
3. Brophy T, McCafferty J, Tyrer JH, Eadie MJ. Bioavailability of oral dexamethasone during high dose steroid therapy in neurological patients. Eur J Clin Pharmacol 1983; 24:103–108.
4. Brady ME, Sartiano GP, Rosenblum SL, Zaglama NE, Bauguess CT. The pharmacokinetics of single high doses of dexamethasone in cancer patients. Eur J Clin Pharmacol 1987; 32:593–596.
5. Lewis GP, Jusko WJ, Burke CW, Graves L. Prednisone side-effects and serum protein levels. Lancet 1971; 2:778–781.
6. Hossman KA, Hurter T, Oschlies U. The effect of dexamethasone on serum protein extravasation and edema development in experimental brain tumors of cat. Acta Neuropathol (Berl) 1983; 223–231.
7. Shapiro WR, Hiesiger EM, Cooney GA, Basler GA, Lipschutz LE, Posner JB. Temporal effects of dexamethasone on blood-to-brain and blood-to-tumor transport of $^{14}$C-alpha-aminoisobutyric acid in rat $C_6$ glioma. J Neurooncol 1990; 8:197–204.
8. Nakagawa H, Groothuis DR, Owens ES, Fenstermacher JD, Patlak CS, Blasberg RG. Dexamethasone effects on [$^{125}$I] albumin distribution in experimental RG-2 gliomas and adjacent brain. J Cereb Blood Flow Metab 1987; 7:687–701.
9. Neuwelt EA, Barnett PA, Bigner DD, Frenkel EP. Effects of adrenal cortical steroids and osmotic blood-brain barrier opening on methotrexate delivery to gliomas in the rodent. Proc Natl Acad Sci USA 1982; 79:4420–4423.
10. Shapiro WR, Posner JB . Corticosteroid hormones: effects in an experimental brain tumor. Arch Neurol 1974; 30:217–221.
11. Yamada K, Bremer AM, West ChR. Effects of dexamethasone on tumor-induced brain edema and its distribution in the brain of monkeys. J Neurosurg 1979; 50:361–367.
12. Blasberg RG, Shapiro BR, Molnar P, Patlat CS, Fenstermachter JP. Local blood-to-tissue transport in Walker 256 metastatic brain tumors. J Neurooncol 1984; 2: 205–218.
13. Reulen HJ, Hadjidimos A, Schürmann K. The effect of dexamethasone on water and electrolyte content and on rCBF in perifocal brain edema in man. In: Reulen HJ, Schürmann K, eds. Steroids and brain edema. Berlin: Springer Verlag, 1972: 239–252.
14. Picard JD. Role of prostaglandins and arachidonic acid derivatives in the coupling of cerebral blood flow to cerebral metabolism. J Cereb Blood Flow Metab 1981; 1: 361–384.
15. Weinstein JD, Toy FJ, Jaffe ME, Goldberg HI. The effect of dexamethasone on brain edema in patients with metastatic brain tumors. Neurology 1973; 23:121–129.
16. Lindegaard MW, Skretting A, Hager B, Watne K, Lindegaard KF. Cerebral and cerebellar uptake of 99 mTc HM PAO in patients with brain tumors studied by SPECT. Eur J Nucl Med 1986; 12:417–420.

17. Leenders KL, Beaney RP, Brooks DJ, et al. Dexamethasone treatment of brain tumor patients: effects on regional cerebral blood flow and oxygen utilization. Neurology 1985; 35:1610–1616.
18. Criscuolo GR, Lelkes PI, Rotrosen D, Oldfield EH. Cytosolic calcium changes in endothelial cells induced by a protein product of human gliomas containing vascular permeability factor activity. J Neurosurg 1989; 71:884–891.
19. Ohnishi T, Sher PB, Posner JB, Shapiro WR. Increased capillary permeability in rat induced by factors secreted by cultured $C_6$ glioma cells: role in peritumoral brain edema. J Neurooncol 1991; 10:13–25.
20. Paoletti P, Butti G, Zibera C, Scerrati M, Gibelli N, Roselli R, Magrassi L, Sica G, Rossi G, Robustelli G. Characteristics and biological role of steroid hormone receptors in neuroepithelial tumors. J Neurosurg 1990; 73:736–742.
21. Green SB, Byar DP, Walker MD. Comparison of carmustine, procarbazine and high-dose methylprednisolone as additions to surgery and radiotherapy for the treatment of malignant gliomas. Cancer Treat Rep 1983; 67:121–137.
22. French LA, Galicich JH. The use of steroids for control of cerebral edema. Clin Neurosurg 1962; 10:212–223.
23. Ruderman NB, Hall TC. Use of glucocorticoids in the palliative treatment of metastatic brain tumors. Cancer 1965; 18:298–306.
24. Hochberg FH, Miller DC. Primary central nervous system lymphoma. J Neurosurg 1988; 68:835–853.
25. Bent van den MJ, Vanneste JAL, Ansink BJJ. Prolonged remission of primary central nervous system lymphoma after discontinuation of steroid therapy. J Neurooncol 1992; 13:257–259.
26. DeAngelis LM. Primary central nervous system lymphoma: a new clinical challenge. Neurology 1991; 41:619–621.
27. Weissman DE, Janjan NA, Erickson B, Wilson FJ, Greenberg M, Ritch PS, Anderson T, Hansen RM, Chitambar CR, Lawton CA, Rousey SR. Twice-daily tapering dexamethasone treatment during cranial radiation for newly diagnosed brain metastases: clinical study. J Neurooncol 1991; 11:235–239.
28. Vick NA, Wilson CB. Total care of the patient with a brain tumor: with consideration of some ethical issues. In: Vick NA, Bigner DD, Eds. Neurologic clinics, symposium on neuro-oncology. Philadelphia: Saunders, 1985; 705–710.
29. Vecht ChJ, Hovestadt A, Verbiest HBC, Van Vliet JJ, Van Putten WLJ. Dose-effect relation of dexamethasone on brain tumor edema: a randomized study with 16 mg, 8 mg and 4 mg per day. Neurology 1994; 44:675–680.
30. Renaudin J, Fewer D, Wilson ChB, Boldrey EB, Calogero J, Enot KJ. Dose dependency of Decadron in patients with partially excised brain tumors. J Neurosurg 1973; 39:302–305.
31. Lieberman R, Lebrun Y, Glass D, Goodgold A, Lax W, Wise A, Ransohoff J. Use of high dose corticosteroids in patients with inoperable brain tumors. J Neurol Neurosurg Psychiatry 1977; 40:678–682.
32. Miller JD, Sakalas R, Ward JD, Young HF, Adams WE, Vries JK, Becker DP. Methylprednisolone treatment in patients with brain tumors. Neurosurgery 1977; 1: 114–117.

33. Hatam A, Bergström M, Yu ZY, Granholm L, Berggren BM. Effect of dexamethasone treatment on volume and contrast enhancement of intracranial neoplasms. J Comput Assist Tomogr 1983; 7:295–300.
34. Miller JD, Leech P. Effects of mannitol and steroid therapy on intracranial volume-pressure relationships in patients. J Neurosurg 1975; 42:274–281.
35. Alberti A, Hartmann A, Schütz HJ, Schreckenberger F. The effect of large doses of dexamethasone on the cerebrospinal fluid pressure in patients with supratentorial tumors. Neurology 1978; 217:173–181.
36. Bell BA, Smith MA, Kean DM, et al. Brain water measured by magnetic resonance imaging. Lancet 1987; i:66–69.
37. Cairncross JG, MacDonald DR, Pexman JHW, Ives FJ. Steroid-induced CT changes in patients with recurrent malignant glioma. Neurology 1988; 38:724–726.
38. Ushio Y, Posner R, Posner JB, Shapiro W. Experimental spinal cord compression by epidural neoplasms. Neurology 1977; 27:422–429.
39. Siegal T, Siegal Tz, Shohami E, Lossos F. Experimental neoplastic spinal cord compression: effect of ketamine and MK-801 on edema and prostaglandins. Neurosurgy 1990; 26:963–966.
40. Aguello F, Baggs RB, Duerst RE, Johnstone L, McQueen K, Frantz CN. Pathogenesis of vertebral metastasis and epidural spinal cord compression. Cancer 1990; 65:98–106.
41. Siegal T, Siegal Tz, Lossos F. Experimental neoplastic spinal cord compression: effect of anti-inflammatory agents and glutamate receptor antagonists on vascular permeability. Neurosurgy 1990; 26:967–970.
42. Hall ED, Braughler JM. Glucocorticoid mechanisms in acute spinal cord injury: a review and therapeutic rationale. Surg Neurol 1982; 18:320–327.
43. Hall ED, Braughler JM. Role of lipid peroxidation in post-traumatic spinal cord degeneration: a review. Cent Nerv Syst Trauma 1986; 3:281–294.
44. Demopoulos HB, Flamm ES, Seligman ML, et al. Further studies on free-radical pathology in the major central nervous system disorders: effects of very high doses of methylprednisolone on the functional outcome, morphology and chemistry of experimental spinal cord impact injury. Can J Physiol Pharmacol 1982: 60:1415–1424.
45. Hall ED. The neuroprotective pharmacology of methylprednisolone. J Neurosurg 1992; 76:13–22.
46. Bracken MB, Shepard MJ, Collins WF, Holford TR, Baskin DS, Eisenberg M, Flamm E, Leo-Summers L, Maroon JC, Marshall LF, Perot PL, Piepmeier J, Sonntag VKH, Wagner FC, Wilberger JL, Winn R, Young W. Methylprednisolone or naloxone treatment after acute spinal cord injury: 1 year follow-up data. J Neurosurg 1992; 76:23–31.
47. Ushio Y, Posner R, Kim JH, Shapiro WR, Posner JB. Treatment of experimental spinal cord compression caused by extradural neoplasms. J Neurosurg 1977; 47:380–390.
48. Delattre JY, Arbit E, Rosenblum MK, Thaler HT, Lau N, Galicich JH, Posner JB. High dose versus low dose dexamethasone in experimental epidural spinal cord compression. Neurosurgy 1988; 22:1005–1007.

49. Delattre JY, Arbit E, Thaler HT, Rosenblum MK, Posner JB. A dose-response study of dexamethasone in a model of spinal cord compression caused by epidural tumor. J Neurosurg 1989; 70:920–926.
50. Siegal T, Shohami E, Shapira Y, Siegal Tz. Indomethacin and dexamethasone treatment in experimental neoplastic spinal cord compression: Part 2, Effect on edema and prostaglandin synthesis. Neurosurgy 1988; 22:334–339.
51. Greenberg HS, Kim JH, Posner JB. Epidural spinal cord compression from metastatic tumor: results with a new treatment protocol. Ann Neurol 1980; 8:361–366.
52. Vecht ChJ, Haaxma-Reiche H, Van Putten WLJ, De Visser M, Vries EP, Twijnstra A. Initial bolus of conventional versus high-dose dexamethasone in metastatic spinal cord compression. Neurology 1989; 39:1255–1257.
53. Heimdal K, Hirschberg H, Slettebø H, Watne K, Nome O. High incidence of serious side effects of high-dose dexamethasone treatment in patients with epidural spinal cord compression. J Neurooncol 1992; 12:141–144.
54. Marshall LF, King J, Langfitt TW. The complications of high-dose corticosteroid therapy in neurosurgical patients: a prospective study. Ann Neurol 1977; 1:201–203.
55. Weissman D, Dufer D, Voge V, Abeloff MD. Corticosteroid toxicity in neuro-oncology patients. J Neurooncol 1987; 5:125–128.
56. Stiefel FC, Breitbart WS, Holland JC. Corticosteroids in cancer: neuropsychiatric complications. Cancer Invest 1989; 7:479–491.
57. Jubiz W, Meikle AW, Levinson RA, Mizutani S, West CD, Tyler FH. Effect of diphenylhydantoin on the metabolism of dexamethasone: mechanism of the abnormal dexamethasone suppression in humans. N Engl J Med 1970; 283:11–14.
58. Chalk JB, Ridgeweay K, Brophy T, Yelland JDN, Eadie MJ. Phenytoin impairs the bioavailability of dexamethasone in neurological and neurosurgical patients. J Neurol Neurosurg Psychiatry 1984; 47:1087–1090.
59. Delattre JY, Safai B, Posner JB. Erythema multiforme and Stevens-Johnson syndrome in patients receiving cranial irradiation and phenytoin. Neurology 1988; 38:194–198.
60. Bartozek M, Brenner AM, Szefler SJ. Prednisolone and methylprednisolone kinetics in children receiving anticonvulsant therapy. Clin Pharmacol Ther 1987; 42:424–432.
61. Mattson RH, Cramer JA, Collins JF, Smith DB, Delgado-Escueta AV, Browne TR, Williamson PD, Treiman DM, McNamara JO, McCatchen CB, Homan RW, Crill WE, Lubozynshi MF, Rosenthal NP, Mayersdorf A. Comparison of carbamazepine, phenobarbital, phenytoin and primidone in partial and secondarily generalized tonic-clonic seizures. N Engl J Med 1985; 313:145–151.
62. Schlaghecke R, Kornely E, Santen RT, Ridderskamp P. The effect of long-term glucocorticoid therapy on pituitary-adrenal responses to exogenous corticotropin-releasing hormone. N Engl J Med 1992; 326:226–230.
63. Livanou T, Ferriman D, James VHT. Recovery of hypothalamo-pituitary-adrenal function after corticosteroid therapy. Lancet 1967; 2:856–859.
64. Brophy T, Chalk JB, Ridgeway K, Tyrer JH, Eadie MJ. Cortisol production during high dose dexamethasone therapy in neurological and neurosurgical patients. J Neurol Neurosurg Psychiatry 1984; 47:1081–1086.

65. Henson JW, Jalai JK, Walker RW, Stover DE, Fels AO. Pneumocystis carinii pneumonia in patients with primary brain tumors. Arch Neurol 1991; 48:406–409.
66. Helfer EL, Rose LI. Corticosteroids and adrenal suppression. Characterizing and avoiding the problem. Drugs 1989; 38:838–845.
67. Selker RG. Corticosteroids: their effect on primary metastatic brain tumors. In: Walker MD, ed. Oncology of the nervous system. Boston: Martinus Nijhoff, 1983.

# 10

# Neurological Complications of Radiotherapy

**Mark T. Jennings**

*Vanderbilt University School of Medicine, Nashville, Tennessee*

The challenges in radiotherapy of central nervous system (CNS) tumors arise from the biology of CNS neoplasms and their origin within a critical organ. For example, most patients with newly diagnosed brain tumors have a tumor volume of 30–60 g. This represents $3-6 \times 10^{10}$ cells within the mass, which typically infiltrate into adjacent brain. Depending on the location of the lesion, the neurosurgeon may resect 20–90% of it. The "best case" postoperative scenario is a residual tumor burden of $3-6 \times 10^{9}$ cells. Conventional external beam radiotherapy (EBRT) may achieve an additional two-log cell kill. Chemotherapy with currently available drugs may produce an additional one-log cytoreduction. Thus, a patient completes multimodality therapy with a $3-6 \times 10^{5}$ repository of malignant cells, which may then be clinically radio- and chemoresistant (1). This chapter reviews newer radiotherapeutic methods for primary and metastatic CNS tumors in the context of their neurological toxicity.

## I. METHODS OF ADMINISTRATION OF RADIOTHERAPY

X-rays generate electrons which are energetic but weakly ionizing due to their small mass. In contrast, alpha particles are ionizing and heavier but of slower velocity. Neutrons possess an ionizing density intermediate between the two. The relative biological effectiveness of particles with high linear energy transfer, such as alpha particles and neutrons, is greater than that of X-ray electrons and gamma rays. Neutron beam radiotherapy has the theoretical advantages of less variation in radiosensitivity at different phases of the cell cycle and impairing the repair of sublethal damage. Toxicity, including carcinogenesis, is influenced by factors such as dosage and fractionation. Neurotoxicity may be ameliorated by increasing the number of daily fractionated doses and decreasing the amount of each dose, in order to exploit the difference in repair capacity of sublethal damage between normal and malignant tissues (reviewed by 2).

## A.  External Beam Radiotherapy

Cushing was the first to prescribe EBRT for the treatment of medulloblastoma (MBL) in 1919. By 1930, he was using whole-brain radiotherapy (3). Radiation therapy has emerged as the nonsurgical mainstay of treatment for CNS malignancies, although this was not acknowledged until the 1970s. The Brain Tumor Cooperative Group trial 6901 proved, for the first time, the efficacy of EBRT for the treatment of adult malignant gliomas (MG) (reviewed by 4,5). The conventional radiotherapeutic prescription for MG usually consists of fractions of 2 Gray (Gy) per day, 5 days/week to achieve total dosages of 40–60 Gy (1 Gy equals 100 rad). Current recommendations for primitive neuroectodermal tumors and MBL (PNET/MBL) are 50–55 Gy to the primary tumor with 36–45 Gy to the neuraxis (6,7). The dose-response of MG to megavoltage EBRT has encouraged the use of hyperfractionated radiotherapy (HF-EBRT) to escalate total dosages to 64–80 Gy (8, reviewed by 6).

## B.  Interstitial Radiotherapy

Interstitial radiation therapy (IRT) (brachytherapy) of primary CNS tumors has long been practiced in Europe (reviewed by 9). Preliminary results using IRT for supratentorial MG and metastases in North America are encouraging (reviewed by 10). The intratumoral application of encapsulated radioisotopes results in maximal radiation doses (34–130 Gy) to the tumor, while delivering lower doses to surrounding normal tissues. The rapid fall-off of dose beyond the implanted volume is determined by (1) the inverse square relationship between the intensity of radiation and the distance from the source; (2) the energy and type of radiation emitted from the isotope; and (3) attenuation of the radiation by intervening tissues. The surgical inaccessibility of certain tumors and their complex geometry limit the usefulness of this technique. Development of computer tomographic (CT) and magnetic resonance (MR) imaging–assisted stereotactic placement of isotopes addresses this problem. Multifocal tumors, multiple metastases, lesions with ill-defined borders, transcallosal involvement, or subependymal spread are considered inappropriate candidates for IRT. Brainstem and cerebellar tumors are not implanted due to the limited radiobiologic reserve of these tissues (11).

## C. Stereotactic Radiosurgery

Computerized stereotactic radiosurgery (CSR) is the destruction of a precisely defined intracranial target by ionizing beams of focused radiation delivered externally in a limited number of fractions. Radiosurgery may be used to obliterate a lesion that is inaccessible, unsuitable for open surgical approaches, or at risk of iatrogenic dissemination via the subarachnoid space. With respect to therapeutic principles, CSR has little in common with conventional radiotherapy. There is no attempt to preserve nonmalignant cells within the lesion by taking advantage of a differential biological sensitivity to radiation, which is the basic principle of EBRT. The technique uses a precisely collimated beam of ionizing radiation as a surgical tool to destroy all cells within a defined volume, rather than preserve the matrix of normal tissue containing the disease, as is done with IRT (12).

The basic concept and theoretical advantage of CSR is the focused administration of a large amount of ionizing radiation to a very circumscribed target. The energies of both the "gamma knife" and the linear accelerator (LINAC) as well as their photon absorption characteristics are similar. The source of the gamma ray radiation is the decay of a $^{60}$Co atom, which produces two photons with an average energy of 1.25 MeV. The LINAC unit generates photons through the slowing of high energy electrons. With microwave power, the LINAC accelerates electrons to energies of 4-15 MeV and focuses them upon a high atomic number alloy. The interaction of electrons with this heavy metal slows the electrons, resulting in the loss of energy through collisional and radiation losses. The radiation losses produce x-ray photons outside of the nucleus. The effective energies of these x-rays are approximately one-third of their maximum energy. In tissue of uniform density, a $^{60}$Co beam will lose approximately 5% of its intensity per centimeter, whereas a 6-MeV LINAC beam will lose approximately 4% of its intensity per centimeter. Since this loss is constant, after a small initial build-up depth, photon beams possess no special properties that allow any significant concentration of energy over a target volume. The gamma knife consists of 201 separate $^{60}$Co sources which are focused upon the target. The LINAC-based CSR unit accomplishes volume focusing through the application of radiation over multiple noncoplanar arcs. The specific clinical difference relates to the precision of targeting rather than the physics of radiation administration. The Brown-Roberts-Well, Leksell frame or other stereotactic apparatus are used for angiographic, CT, or MR localization (reviewed by 13), and CSR.

## II. RADIATION INJURY OF THE BRAIN

### A. External Beam Radiotherapy

#### 1. Acute and Intermediate Effects

Clinicians have historically distinguished between early, intermediate, and late CNS neurotoxicity of radiotherapy. As many as 49% of carefully observed patients may demonstrate some toxicity following EBRT. The *early effects* (within hours–days) of EBRT are related to the fractionation and dosage. The mechanism appears to be mediated by acute cerebral edema secondary to a capillary endothelial insult (see below, Sec. II.F). Single radiation exposures in excess of 100 Gy produce acute ataxia, lethargy, agitation, seizures, and shock culminating in death. Single doses of 7.5–10 Gy may elicit headache, nausea, vomiting, fever, and cerebral herniation (the older literature is reviewed by 14). The use of lower fractions and "prophylactic" doses of corticosteroids have largely reduced this clinical problem. *Intermediate* symptoms may follow EBRT by weeks to months and are usually transient. These include the "somnolence syndrome," which is characterized by hypersomnia, lethargy, and anorexia (15). When this occurs coincident with the initiation of chemotherapy, it may be mistaken for a toxic effect or progressive disease. While the somnolence syndrome resolves without specific treatment, low doses of steroids are effective in symptomatic relief. Little is known of the neuropathology of intermediate complications, which are hypothesized to represent transient demyelination (14,16). Patchy demyelination, necrosis, and minute hemorrhages are found in the irradiated portal among severe cases, usually following high fractionation and/or dosages (17).

#### 2. Intellectual Sequelae

Increasing survival rates among pediatric and adult patients have heightened concern regarding the long-term sequelae of their treatment. Adult survivors of MG and brain metastases experience a spectrum of late morbidity from radiation therapy and systemic chemotherapy. In one series, 30% of survivors suffered from dementia and died without evidence of recurrence. Another 22% were afflicted with short-term memory loss and other neurological deficits, such as gait apraxia. Only 30% continue to function independently (18). Memory loss, confusion, depression, and personality alterations may be disabling due to the loss of employment and self-sufficiency. While psychometric testing may remain consistent with premorbid function, diffuse cortical dysfunction is usually manifest by poor problem solving and adaptability (19). Similar problems are reported among long-term survivors of small-cell lung cancer, who have been treated with chemotherapy and smaller doses of EBRT (reviewed in Chap. 11).

Among pediatric patients, whose prognosis is better, the controversy regarding radiation injury to the developing CNS resulted from reliance on retrospective analyses, lack of appropriate controls, and varying criteria as to what constitutes

**Table 1** Clinical Syndromes Associated with Radiation Therapy (in Terms of Diagnostic Criteria)

| Disorder | Symptoms, signs | Diagnosis | Associated radiotherapy |
|---|---|---|---|
| Acute encephalopathy | Headache, vomiting, fever, cerebral edema, shock, death | Clinical | Immediate following fractions of 7:5–10 Gy of EBRT |
| Somnolence syndrome | Lethargy, somnolence, anorexia | Clinical | Weeks-months following conventional EBRT; steroid responsive |
| Dementia | Amnesia, gait apraxia, confusion, behavioral change | Clinical, intracranial calcifications | Long-term sequelae of conventional EBRT at doses ≥ 24 Gy |
| Stroke | Focal neurological deficit | Clinical, angiographic, MRI | Carotid and cerebral arterial thrombosis |
| Radionecrosis | Encephalopathy, seizures, focal neurological deficit, intracranial hypertension | Clinical, MRI, PET | EBRT doses of > 70 Gy, fractions > 2.5 Gy, NEURET doses > 14.5 Gy; IRT, CSR |
| Chronic progressive myelopathy | Transverse myelopathy | Clinical, MRI, PET | EBRT doses > 55 Gy |
| Growth failure | Hypothyroidism, panhypopituitarism | Clinical | EBRT, CSR to head and neck |
| Radiation-induced second malignancy | Neurilemomas, meningiomas, gliomas, fibrosarcomas | Clinical, MRI, PET | EBRT > 2.5 Gy, survival > 2 yr |

Abbreviations: CSR = Computerized stereotactic radiosurgery; EBRT = External beam radiotherapy; IRT = Interstitial radiation therapy; MRI = Magnetic resonance imaging; NEURET = Neural equivalent therapy; PET = Positron-emission tomography.

quality of life (see 20,21 for taxonomic classifications). Recent prospective evaluation of PNET/MBL patients who received whole-brain EBRT demonstrates progressive loss in intelligence. There is a mean fall of 14 points in full-scale intelligence quotient (FSIQ) during the 2 years after treatment ($p = 0.001$). The decline in FSIQ is inversely related to age ($p < 0.02$). Children less than 7 years at time of diagnosis have a median FSIQ of 82 (range 50–98), compared to 103 (range 92–133) for the older children. Children less than 5 years of age suffer a mean decline of 25 in FSIQ (22). Hirsch et al. (23) note that only 12% of MBL survivors have IQs above 90, while 93% display behavioral disorders. Losses as severe as 47 points following EBRT are documented (23–26). The severity of such deficits appears to correlate with early age of irradiation and adjuvant chemotherapy (22,24,27–29, see below). Patients with anterior cerebral and midline tumors also do worse. It is controversial whether hydrocephalus influences intellectual outcome (24,28–30). Although the frequency and etiology of intellectual deficits of this magnitude are disputed, it is conceded that pediatric brain tumor patients suffer from learning disabilities consequent to therapeutic irradiation (31–33). Radiotherapy cannot be proven to be the sole cause of this damage. However, the clinical impression of many workers is that EBRT is the major contributor (18). Analogous deficits are not seen among children with posterior fossa astrocytomas who receive only surgical therapy (23,25,27).

A similar controversy exists regarding the neurotoxicity of prophylactic CNS irradiation for childhood leukemia. Meadows and coworkers (34) found that 24 Gy of cranial EBRT and intrathecal methotrexate (MTX) (6 doses) is associated with significant deterioration in psychometric test scores. The severity of this effect correlates with earlier age of treatment. The average IQ loss is 14 points among children aged 2.7–3.25 years, 21 points for children aged 3.75–5.25 years, and 7 points in children older than 6 years. Notably, the complication is not evident until 3 or more years after therapy. These changes were not seen among patients who received only MTX prophylaxis (34). Ochs (35) notes that 50% of children less than 5 years old at the time of cranial radiotherapy, with or without MTX, require special education, as compared with 26% of the total group treated. In a literature review of the neuropsychological sequelae of cranial EBRT for leukemia, 13/20 studies report the adverse effect of age upon toxicity (36). Prophylactic cranial EBRT for leukemia may be associated with ataxia, perceptual-motor abnormalities, seizures, and CT abnormalities, also worse among children less than 5 years of age ($p < 0.008$) (37).

Notwithstanding the above, the contribution of radiotherapy to the intellectual decline of leukemic children who receive prophylactic cranial EBRT remains controversial (reviewed by 36). More recent work finds comparable neuropsychological deficits among patients receiving prophylactic MTX alone (reviewed by 38,39). The severity of the radiographic abnormalities (atrophy, parenchymal calcifications) is related to the dose of MTX or arabinosylcytosine (40). Leukoencephalopathy and mineralizing microangiopathy with attendant dementia and focal neurological deficits constitute a well-characterized entity seen in children treated for CNS leukemia with EBRT and MTX, administered intravenously and/or intrathecally (reviewed by 41).

### 3. Cerebrovascular Disease

Another late sequela of EBRT recognized among children is stroke. The latency for ischemic complications may range between 2 and 24 years (42). This appears related to radiation-induced thrombosis of the carotid and intracranial arteries which may present as transient ischemic attacks or infarction (reviewed by 43,44).

### 4. Radiation Necrosis

Of the long-term effects, radiation necrosis has been the most impressive and receives the greatest attention. Radionecrosis is progressive, irreversible, dose-dependent, and potentially fatal. It occurs in about 3–14% of EBRT-treated patients; the incidence is increasing as duration of survival and imaging techniques improve. The latency interval is 6–36 months in 78% of cases (range 2 months–19 years). Clinical features include focal seizures, encephalopathy, dementia, signs of increased intracranial pressure, and new focal neurological deficits. Angiography may reveal an avascular mass, while CT and MR show an enhancing lesion with surrounding edema which is indistinguishable from recurrent tumor (43). Positron-emission tomography (PET) is the best diagnostic test currently available for distinguishing radionecrosis from recurrent neoplasm (45).

### 5. Complications of Altered Fractionation Schedules

The theoretical basis for administration of HF-EBRT is to allow escalating tumor doses without an attendant increase in neurotoxicity (see above). Early neurological toxicity may include transient neurological deterioration, intratumoral hemorrhage, intralesional necrosis (in 5%) or cyst formation, and chronic steroid dependence. Toxicity appears to be dose related, being greater among patients treated in excess of 70.2 Gy (46,47). An unexplained associated finding has been protracted lymphopenia with opportunistic infections (48). Late toxicity has not been appreciated among brainstem glioma patients; however, survival of this population is limited (47,48). Statistical differences in toxicity between conventional versus HF-EBRT have not been demonstrated, although certain workers have had the impression that increasing the fractionation is associated with earlier deterioration (49). In contrast, a MR study found fewer leukoencephalopathic changes among patients treated with HF-EBRT than with conventional EBRT. This suggests that the morbidity is lessened with the smaller dose fractions despite total doses in excess of 70 Gy (50). The recent interest in accelerated fractionation (2 Gy fractions to 60 Gy over 26 days) is associated with a relative increase in the incidence of the somnolence syndrome and chronic steroid dependence (51).

## B. Interstitial Radiotherapy

Brachytherapy with removable, high-activity $^{125}$I sources (57.4–120 Gy) was used initially in the United States for the treatment of recurrent malignant brain tumors. Perioperative complications included headache, fever, seizure, catheter malposition, acute cerebral edema, abscess, bacterial meningitis, wound dehiscence, radiation-induced calvarial resorption, intracranial hemorrhage, and aggravated neurological deficits in 8–24% (52,53). One series reports that 49% of survivors required reoperation about 29 weeks (range 3–105 weeks) following IRT. This subgroup of patients experiences progressive focal neurological deficits related to radionecrosis and mass effect at the implantation site. While selected patients maintain their Karnofsky performance scores, the majority remain steroid-dependent for as long as 18 months after brachytherapy (53). Among newly diagnosed MG patients treated with EBRT, chemotherapy, and IRT, the reoperation rate is 38%, on the average 42 weeks later (range 7–113 weeks) (10). Reoperation is associated with significantly prolonged survival among recurrent glioma patients, although there is no correlation with the amount of tumor or necrosis in the resected specimen (53). Among patients needing postimplantation re-resection, 90% or more have residual/recurrent disease in addition to radionecrosis. However, the viability of these nests of anaplastic astrocytes within the radionecrotic lesion is controversial (10,52,54). Stereotactic interstitial radiotherapy is also performed for recurrent metastatic brain tumors. Temporary high activity [$^{125}$I] implants are used to deliver dosages of 34.4–130 Gy. In one small series, 22% of patients with metastases required reoperation for symptomatic radionecrosis (10,55). In conclusion, the combination of EBRT and IRT delivers total doses of 110–120 Gy, which may be adequate to arrest the progression of an MG. The limiting toxicity is focal radionecrosis, which should be regarded as an anticipated complication requiring surgical intervention (10).

## C. Stereotactic Radiosurgery

Treatment of intracranial arteriovenous malformations with CSR affords sufficient experience to discuss its central neurotoxicity. Gamma knife stereotactic radiosurgery of more than 600 patients, aged 4–70 years, treated in Stockholm and Buenos Aires has been summarized (56,57). In 3% of cases, radiation-associated injury is noted after a latency of 3–11 months. Symptoms may be transient, static, or progressive but typically consist of a focal neurological deficit with increased intracranial pressure. Focal necrosis, mass effect, and leukoencephalopathy correlate with clinical localization and CT hypodense abnormalities (57,58). The development of radionecrosis is likely to be fraction size and total dose dependent, as adverse effects have been associated with dosages of 75–125 Gy (59,60).

Few brain tumor patients have been treated with CSR, administered to total doses of 32–40 Gy in staged fractions of 10–25 Gy. In one of six patients followed about 6%. These include radiation injury to the hypothalamus, visual loss, leakage of radioisotope, parenchymal or subarachnoid hemorrhage, meningitis, and death (72; see also 73).

## F. Mechanisms of Radiation Neurotoxicity

The exact mechanism of the CNS damage following therapeutic ionizing radiation remains controversial. Radiotherapy elicits a predictable response among cells progressing through the cell cycle. The initial mitotic delay results in an accumulation of cells in $G_2$ phase. Following entry into M phase, treated cells experience death at the first or later division, as a function of EBRT dose (74). The cells within the CNS most vulnerable to radiation injury are those capable of replication, the glial elements and endothelia. The historical and functional importance of the capillary endothelial cell in radionecrosis has been previously reviewed (43,75; see also 76). Demyelination may result from the sensitivity of oligodendroglia to EBRT. The neuropathological appearance of the radiation-associated injury includes necrosis, especially within the white matter, vascular proliferation, and astrocytic atypia. There may be distinctive zones of coagulative and fibrinoid necrosis, telangiectasias, fibrous thickening, calcification, reactive gliosis, and edema (77).

The literature emphasizes the occurrence of radionecrosis at fractionation schedules greater than 250 cGy, total doses exceeding 70 Gy, neurad equivalent therapy (NEURET) doses of 1450–1800 cGy (2100–2600 ret), and large treatment volumes (14,78–81). The lowest recorded dosage to produce radionecrosis is 20 Gy (82). Thus, it can occur in patients receiving an appropriate radiotherapy prescription (83, reviewed by 81). Sheline (11) concludes that the tolerance of the CNS for radiotherapy is dependent upon the number of fractions rather than the overall treatment time. There are regional differences in vulnerability to radionecrosis; the upper dose limit for the brainstem and posterior fossa has been suggested to be 55–60 Gy in fractions of less than 2 Gy (84). Therapy of CNS radionecrosis is limited to the administration of corticosteroids or surgical debulking of the necrotic debris in an attempt to control the associated mass effect. Anticoagulant therapy has not been widely accepted (85).

## III. RADIATION INJURY OF THE SPINAL CORD

Several broad syndromes of spinal cord radiotoxicity have been delineated, which include (1) an early transient effect; (2) chronic radiation myelitis; (3) a rare anterior horn cell syndrome; and (4) a radiation-associated vascular compromise of the spinal cord (reviewed by 86). An early-intermediate effect of EBRT on the spinal cord is *Lhermitte's sign*, which is typically self-limited. This consists of paresthesias or electric shocks over the spine induced with cervical spine flexion. In some patients it is sufficiently severe to be described as a "white-hot bolt down for more than 6 months, an enlarging hypodense area around the tumor developed without change in the neoplasm itself (61). No significant complications occurred among six previously irradiated CNS tumor patients with LINAC-CSR (62). In a series of solitary CNS metastases, recurrent following conventional EBRT, LINAC-CSR was administered as a single fraction with a mean dose of 15.5 Gy (0.9–25 Gy). Twenty-two percent (4/18) developed deep white matter lesions with cerebral edema, which required steroid therapy after 2–6 months. No new permanent neurological deficits were observed (63). In another series of 40 patients with metastatic disease, one patient with a cerebellar metastasis was treated and subsequently died from tonsillar herniation (64).

Caution is advised regarding the interpretation of neuroradiographic abnormalities following CSR. A temporal pattern has been identified which consists of an apparent absence of change during the first 6 months, followed by a gradual increase in mass size with the development of a ring-enhancing lesion. This corresponds to the original target volume treated. Subsequently, over the next 12–24 months, progressive shrinkage may occur (52,65). Similar observations have been made following brachytherapy with [$^{125}$I] sources, where altered blood-brain barrier function and necrosis produce mass effect, cerebral edema, and demyelination (10,66).

## D. Heavy Particle Beam Therapy

The relative efficacy of heavy particle beam therapy for CNS neoplasms has been compared in several series, which utilize neutron beam, mixed neutron and $^{60}$Co irradiation, and neutron versus photon radiotherapy. In one series of patients, 14 of 15 autopsies reveal coagulative necrosis at the site of the primary tumor. Diffuse gliosis and leukoencephalopathic changes are found remote to the treated lesion and implicated as the proximate cause of death (67). Recent studies correlate these pathological changes with the evolution of a progressive dementia (reviewed by 6). Permanent neurological deficits and radiographic lesions may develop in 5–25% of arteriovenous malformation patients treated with helium ion beams (68–70). Unfortunately, no therapeutic advantage is derived from dosage escalation or various types of ion beam administration (reviewed by 6). The Radiation Therapy Oncology Group trials 76–11 and 80–07 actually note a higher mortality rate among anaplastic astrocytoma patients receiving photons with a neutron boost than in historical controls treated with conventional EBRT (71), apparently due to a toxic effect of the therapy.

## E. Intracavitary Irradiation

Stereotactic installation of beta- and mixed beta/gamma–emitting radioisotopes such as [$^{90}$Y], [$^{32}$P], and [$^{186}$Re]sulfide have been used for the ablation of craniopharyngiomas and tumor cysts. Treatment-related complications occur in my back" (reviewed by 87). Radiation-induced Lhermitte's sign usually abates without treatment in 2–36 weeks (88; for review of older literature, see 14). Glucocorticoid therapy may provide symptomatic relief. This syndrome is hypothesized to represent transient demyelination of sensory fiber tracts and should be distinguished from late-onset progressive radiation myelopathy (88).

While much less frequent than Lhermitte's sign, *chronic progressive myelopathy* is the most common form of permanent radiation-induced injury. It may present as discrete sensory deficits and progress to a transverse myelopathy, with an average latency of 14 months to onset. The initial deterioration is often rapid but may later stabilize. Radiation myelitis occurs in as many of 6% (0.6–12.5%) of patients treated with spinal cord doses of more than 55 Gy (reviewed by 76,89,90). Both dosage and fractionation appear important, as smaller fractionated doses may be less toxic (90). The PET may have diagnostic utility among patients with cervical myelopathy in distinguishing radionecrosis from a parenchymal tumor (R. Wiley, personal communication). The neuropathological changes found with progressive postradiation myelopathy are similar to those seen in the cerebrum. These consist of lymphocytic infiltrates, perivascular and microvascular changes, thickened vascular endothelium, secondary thrombi, telangiectasias, and capillary hemorrhages. Over time, the lesions may progress to demyelination, calcification, and liquefactive necrosis. It is unusual for the myelopathy to present as an expansile lesion such as may occur with radionecrosis in the brain (76). In the rare anterior horn cell syndrome, the clinical deficit is usually restricted to the lower extremities after lumbar irradiation (91). Acute paraplegia or quadriplegia may also result from infarction in the distribution of the anterior spinal artery (92).

## IV. RADIATION INJURY OF THE CRANIAL AND PERIPHERAL NERVES

### A. External Beam Radiotherapy

Radiotherapy of the basicranium for the management of pituitary adenomas, meningiomas, craniopharyngiomas, acoustic neuromas, malignant schwannomas, glomus jugulare tumors, chondrosarcomas, and other head and neck cancers may produce cranial neuropathies. Radiation injury to the cranial and peripheral nerves may be acute or chronic. The former tends to be transient, whereas the latter may be progressive and disabling. Visual loss may ensue following radiotherapy of the optic nerve and chiasm; both fractionation ($> 2.0$ Gy) and dosage ($> 60$ Gy) are felt to be important (reviewed by 81). This may manifest as bitemporal hemianopsia, monocular blindness, slowly progressive visual loss, or sudden blindness. The latency is approximately 16.8 months (range 5 months–7 years). Hearing loss, ear pain, and tinnitus have been reported following posterior fossa EBRT (93). The pathological appearance of the lesion is that of an obliterating endarteritis in the region of the cochlea (94). Vestibular injury is said to be uncommon (95). There may be an interaction between EBRT and ototoxic chemotherapy with cisplatin in potentiating eighth cranial nerve toxicity (reviewed by 96).

Brachial and lumbosacral plexopathies may be attributable to EBRT; the clinical problem is often that of distinguishing this from recurrent metastatic disease. The relative incidence of brachial plexopathy secondary to radionecrosis may be as low as 1%, whereas disease dissemination accounts for 78% of cases (97,98). Among patients with radiation-associated brachial plexopathy, risk factors appear to include use of a posterior boost and adjuvant chemotherapy (99). Lumbosacral plexopathy secondary to EBRT is a less well described uncommon lesion (100). This is discussed more fully in Chapter 10.

## B. Stereotactic Radiosurgery

Computerized stereotactic radiosurgery may be administered with both LINAC and gamma-knife units to treat extra-axial skull base neoplasms, as single- (50 Gy maximal target dose with 25 Gy to the 50% isodose curve) or multiple-fraction (15–25 Gy) treatments (101). Steiner (57) (1988) reviewed Noren's experience with 115 acoustic neuromas (110 patients) treated with the gamma knife and followed for a mean of 4.0 years (0.5–12.8 years). There has been no surgical mortality related to the treatment (102). The major toxicity is cranial neuropathies adjacent to the target or cochlear dysfunction. Among acoustic neuroma patients, frank deafness occurs in 20%. About 27% retain hearing within 5 dB of baseline. The remaining patients experience a slow decline in hearing, hypothesized due to ischemia of the cochlea. One patient with bilateral neurinomas suffered sudden and irreversible deafness within 24 h of the treatment. Seventh cranial nerve neuropathies occur in 15% of patients within 4–15 months of treatment but often improve later. A dose-response relationship is evident, with neurotoxicity following total doses of 40 Gy but not with doses of less than 27 Gy. Hypesthesia in the distribution of the fifth cranial nerve is observed in 18% of the acoustic neuroma cases, 6–9 months posttreatment. The hypesthesia was severe, irreversible, and associated with a deafferentation pain syndrome among the initially treated patients. Peritumoral edema causes varying degrees of cerebellar symptoms in 5% of the cases of acoustic neuroma treated by radiosurgery, which subsides 6–12 months after the onset (57,102).

## V. NEUROENDOCRINE EFFECTS OF CRANIAL AND CRANIOSPINAL RADIOTHERAPY

### A. External Beam Radiotherapy

Radiotherapy portals which include the hypothalamus, pituitary, or thyroid carry the risk of long-term hormonal insufficiency. Basicranial EBRT is associated with some degree of hypopituitarism in as many as 43–55% of adult patients so treated (81,103). Children treated with craniospinal EBRT are at risk for growth failure secondary to growth-hormone deficiency, or primary, secondary, or tertiary hypothyroidism (28,104–106). Growth-hormone deficiency is the most common form of pituitary insufficiency to follow radiotherapy to the hypothalamic-pituitary axis. This may be evident as suboptimal responses to provocative testing or low spontaneous nocturnal secretion (107). Among children receiving 24 Gy for craniospinal prophylaxis for leukemia, growth-hormone deficiency may be self-limited 6–12 months after treatment (108). Thyroid insufficiency may develop years following EBRT to the head and neck. Chemical evidence of hypothyroidism may occur in 25–50% of patients, although not all will be symptomatic. This may be a progressive process which requires replacement years following EBRT (109). Growth retardation due to vertebral arrest following neuraxis EBRT is not treatable (110). Infertility may be caused by pelvic EBRT, although the dose required varies with age and gender. Older women are sterilized by 6 Gy. Girls and younger women may retain function up to dosages of 20 Gy (reviewed by 111). The sterilizing dose for males is lower, on the order of 5–9.5 Gy, although these patients may not express chemical evidence of endocrinologic castration (112).

## B. Stereotactic Radiosurgery

"Gamma knife" application of a single dose of radiation of 70–100 Gy (60 Gy in children) for Cushing's disease is associated with pituitary deficiency in 50% of adult patients. The latency period is 4 months–7 years posttreatment. Pituitary failure begins with loss of corticotropin function, followed by hypothyroidism and FSH-LH deficiency. Questions exist regarding the precision of the original localization in the series cited, because many patients have required retreatment. The complication rate may improve with better targeting technique (113,114).

## VI. RISK OF SECOND MALIGNANCY RELATED TO CNS RADIOTHERAPY

Neuroectodermal tissue is sufficiently vulnerable to the carcinogenic effects of radiation to permit an animal model of radioneuro-oncogenesis (115). The clear association between EBRT and development of CNS or parameningeal neoplasms is exemplified among patients irradiated in childhood for *tinea capitis* (reviewed by 116). Of 10,834 subjects treated between 1948–1960, there is a 8.4-fold higher incidence of neural tumors of the head and neck relative to untreated siblings and the general population. A strong dose-response relationship exists as higher EBRT levels ($\geq$ 2.5 Gy) are associated with a 20-fold increased carcinogenic potential. Neurilemomas, meningiomas, and gliomas are the most commonly reported tumors (116). Prophylactic or therapeutic doses of cranial EBRT ($>$ 10 Gy) may be complicated by the development of a second CNS tumor in as many as 1.8–5% of patients who survive more than 2 years (reviewed by 28,81; see also 117–122). The latency of postradiation neuro-oncogenesis may range from 4 to 30 years) (123–125). Fibrosarcomas are the most common second malignancy, followed by malignant gliomas (reviewed by 81).

Leukemia, usually acute nonlymphocytic, is associated with EBRT for Hodgkin's disease, non-Hodgkin's lymphoma, Wilm's tumors, and skeletal neoplasms (126–129). There is also an association between therapeutic radiotherapy with the development of soft tissue and mesenchymal tumors, such as thyroid tumors, sarcomas, breast and colon cancer, and renal carcinomas (130–134). The cumulative probability of a second neoplasm is 12% within 5–24 years following EBRT treatment, in contrast to age-matched controls whose risk is less than 1% (124,127,130). A synergistic oncogenic interaction between EBRT and chemotherapy is evident among patients with Hodgkin's disease (129). It is not known whether radiation functions as a permissive or competence-transforming event in the molecular pathogenesis of these diseases.

## VII. CONCLUSIONS

No "safe" dose of EBRT, IRT, or stereotactic radiotherapy has been established. Ionizing radiation is both toxic and oncogenic to neuroectodermal tissues. Unanticipated interactions include Stevens-Johnson syndrome among patients receiving whole-brain EBRT and phenytoin (135). Nevertheless, radiotherapy remains the most effective nonsurgical modality of antineoplastic therapy available for most solid tumors, especially those of the CNS. The challenge for the clinician is to balance the risk/benefit ratio for the patient, which is influenced by the age, functional state, and prognosis of the patient.

## ACKNOWLEDGMENTS

This work was supported by the National Institutes of Neurological Disorders and Stroke (1 K08 NS00986), National Institutes of Health BRSG, and Vanderbilt University Research Council. The author wishes to thank Dr. Michael Smith for his helpful comments.

## REFERENCES

1. Shapiro WR. Treatment of neuroectodermal brain tumors. Ann Neurol 1982; 12: 231–237.
2. Fry RJM. Principles of cancer biology: physical carcinogenesis. In: DeVita VT, Hellman S, Rosenberg SA, eds. Cancer: principles and practice of oncology. 2nd ed. Philadelphia: JB Lippincott Co., 1985:101–112.

3. Cushing H. Experiences with cerebellar medulloblastoma—a critical review. Acta Pathol Microbiol Scand 1930; 7:1–86.
4. Sheline GE. Radiation therapy of brain tumors. Cancer 1977; 39:873–881.
5. Shapiro WR. Therapy of adult malignant brain tumors: what have the clinical trials taught us? Semin Oncol 1986; 13:38–45.
6. Sheline GE. Radiotherapy for high grade gliomas. Int J Radiat Oncol Biol Phys 1990; 18:793–803.
7. Karlsson JL, Leibel SA, Wallner K, et al. Brain. In: Perez CA, Brady LW, eds. Principles and practice of radiation oncology. 2nd ed. Philadelphia: JB Lippincott Co., 1992:515–563.
8. Walker MD, Strike TA, Sheline GE. An analysis of dose-effect relationship in the radiotherapy of malignant gliomas. Int J Radiat Oncol Biol Phys 1979; 5:1725–1731.
9. Mundiger F. Rationale and methods of interstitial Ir 192 brachcurietherapy and Ir 192 and I 125 protracted long term irradiations. In: Szikla G, ed. Stereotactic cerebral irradiations. Amsterdam: Elsevier, 1979:101–117.
10. Leibel SA, Gutin PH, Sneed PK, et al. Interstitial irradiation for the treatment of primary and metastatic tumors. Principles Practice Oncology 1989; 3(7):1–11.
11. Sheline GE. Radiotherapy of adult primary cerebral neoplasms. In: Walker MD, ed. Oncology of the nervous system. Boston: Martinus Nijhoff, 1983:223–245.
12. Winston KR, Lutz W. Linear accelerator as a neurosurgical tool for stereotactic radiosurgery. Neurosurg 1988; 22:454–464.
13. Friedman WA, Bova FJ. Stereotactic radiosurgery. Contemp Neurosurg 1989; 11:1–7.
14. Sheline G. Irradiation injury of the human brain: a review of clinical experience. In: Gilbert HA, Kagan AR, eds. Radiation damage to the nervous system. New York: Raven Press, 1980:39–58.
15. Druckmann A. Schlafsucht als Folge der Rontgenbestrahlung: Beitrag zur Strahlenempfindlichkeit des Gehirns. Strahlenther Onkol 1929; 33:382–384.
16. Hoffman WF, Levin VA, Wilson CB. Evaluation of malignant glioma patients during the postirradiation period. J Neurosurg 1979; 50:624–628.
17. Lampert P, Tom MI, Rider WD. Disseminated demyelination of the brain following $Co^{60}$ (gamma) radiation. Arch Pathol 1959; 68:322–330.
18. Imperato JP, Paleologos NA, Vick NA. Effects of treatment on long-term survivors with malignant astrocytomas. Ann Neurol 1990; 28:818–822.
19. Hochberg FH, Slotnick B. Neuropsychologic impairment in astrocytoma survivors. Neurology 1980; 30:172–177.
20. Bloom HJG, Wallace ENK, Hank JM. The treatment and prognosis of medulloblastoma in children. Am J Roentgenol 1969; 105:43–62.
21. Bouchard J, Pierce B. Radiation therapy in the management of neoplasms of the central nervous system with a special note in regard to children: twenty years experience, 1939–1958. Am J Roentgenol 1960; 84:610–628.
22. Packer RJ, Sutton LN, Atkins TE, et al. A prospective study of cognitive function in children receiving whole brain radiotherapy and chemotherapy: 2-year results. J Neurosurg 1989; 70:707–713.

23. Hirsch JF, Reiner D, Czernichew R, et al. Medulloblastoma in childhood: survival and functional results. Acta Neurochir (Wien) 1979; 48:1–15.
24. Ellenberg L, McComb JG, Siegel SE, Stowe, S. Factors affecting intellectual outcome in pediatric brain tumor patients. Neurosurgery 1987; 21:638–644.
25. Riva D, Pantaleoni C, Milani N, Belani FF. Impairment of neuropsychological functions in children with medulloblastomas and astrocytomas in the posterior fossa. Childs Nerv Syst 1989; 5:107–110.
26. Hoppe-Hirsch E, Renier D, Lellouch-Tubiana A, et al. Medulloblastoma in childhood: progressive intellectual deterioration. Childs Nerv Syst 1990; 6:60–65.
27. Raimondi AJ, Tomita T. The disadvantages of prophylactic whole CNS postoperative radiation therapy for medulloblastoma. In: Paoletti P, Walker MD, Butti G, Knerich R, eds. Multidisciplinary aspects of brain tumor therapy. Amsterdam: Elsevier/North Holland, 1979:209–218.
28. Danoff BF, Cowchock FS, Marquette C, et al. Assessment of the long-term effects of primary radiation therapy for brain tumors in children. Cancer 1982; 49:1580–1586.
29. Duffner PK, Cohen ME, Parker MS. Prospective intellectual testing in children with brain tumors. Ann Neurol 1988; 23:575–579.
30. Brookshire B, Copeland DR, Moore BD, Ater J. Pretreatment neuropsychological status and associated factors in children with primary brain tumors. Neurosurgery 1990; 27:887–891.
31. Spunberg JJ, Chang CH, Goldman M, et al. Quality of long-term survival following irradiation for intracranial tumors in children under the age of two. Int J Radiat Oncol Biol Physi 1981; 7:727–736.
32. Kun LE, Mulhern RK. Neuropsychologic function in children with brain tumors: II, Serial studies of intellect and time after treatment. Am J Clin Oncol 1983; 6:651–656.
33. Mulhern RK, Kun LE. Neuropsychologic function in children with brain tumors: III, Interval changes in the six months following treatment. Med Pediatr Oncol 1985; 13:318–324.
34. Meadows AT, Gordon J, Massari DJ, et al. Declines in IQ scores and cognitive dysfunctions in children with acute lymphoblastic leukaemia treated with cranial irradiation. Lancet 1981; 2:1015–1018.
35. Ochs JJ. Proceedings of controversies in paediatric and adolescent hematology and oncology, 1981.
36. Williams JM, Davis KS. Central nervous system prophylactic treatment of childhood leukemia: neuropsychological outcome studies. Cancer Treat Rev 1986; 13:113–127.
37. Carli M, Perilongo G, Laverda AM, et al. Risk factors in long-term sequelae of central nervous system prophylaxis in successfully treated children with acute lymphocytic leukemia. Med Pediatr Oncol 1985; 13:334–340.
38. Ochs JJ, Mulhern R, Fairclough D, et al. Comparison of neuropsychologic functioning and clinical indicators of neurotoxicity in long-term survivors of childhood leukemia given cranial radiation or parenteral methotrexate: a prospective study. J Clin Oncol 1991; 9:145–151.
39. Mulhern RK, Fairclough D, Ochs J. A prospective comparison of neuropsychologic

performance of children surviving leukemia who received 18-Gy, 24-Gy, or no cranial irradiation. J Clin Oncol 1991; 9:1348–1356.
40. McIntosh S, Tischer DB, Rothman RT, et al. Intracranial calcifications in childhood leukemia: an association with systemic chemotherapy. J Pediatr 1977; 91:909–913.
41. Bleyer WA, Griffin TW. White matter necrosis, mineralizing microangiopathy, and intellectual abilities in survivors of childhood leukemia: associations with central nervous system irradiation and methotrexate therapy. In: Gilbert HA, Kagan AR, eds. Radiation damage to the nervous system. New York: Raven Press, 1980: 155–174.
42. Painter MJ, Chutorian AM, Hilal SK. Cerebrovasculopathy following irradiation in childhood. Neurology 1975; 25:189–194.
43. Rottenberg DA, Chernik NL, Deck MDF, et al. Cerebral necrosis following radiotherapy of extracranial neoplasms. Ann Neurol 1977; 1:339–357.
44. Mitchell WG, Fishman LS, Miller JH, et al. Stroke as a late sequela of cranial irradiation for childhood brain tumors. J Child Neurol 1991; 6:128–133.
45. Di Chiro G, Oldfield E, Wright DC, et al. Cerebral necrosis after radiotherapy and/or intrarterial chemotherapy for brain tumors: PET and neuropathologic studies. Am J Radiol 1988; 150:189–197.
46. Packer RJ, Allen JC, Goldwein JL, et al. Hyperfractionated radiotherapy for children with brainstem gliomas: a pilot study using 7,200 cGy. Ann Neurol 1990; 27: 167–173.
47. Freeman CR, Krischer J, Sanford RA, et al. Hyperfractionated radiation therapy in brain stem gliomas. Cancer 1991; 68:474–481.
48. Edwards MSB, Wara WM, Urtasun RC, et al. Hyperfractionated radiation therapy for brain-stem glioma: a phase I-II trial. J Neurosurg 1989; 70:691–700.
49. Keim H, Pothoff PC, Schmidt K, et al. Survival and quality of life after continuous accelerated radiotherapy of glioblastomas. Radiother Oncol 1987; 9:21–26.
50. Constine KS, Konski A, Ekholm S, et al. Adverse effects of brain irradiation correlated with MR and CT imaging. Int J Radiat Oncol Biol Phys 1988; 15: 219–220.
51. Shenouda G, Souhami L, Freeman CR, et al. Accelerated fractionation for high-grade cerebral astrocytomas. Cancer 1991; 67:2247–2252.
52. Willis BK, Heilbrun MP, Sapozink MD, McDonald PR. Stereotactic interstitial brachytherapy of malignant astrocytomas with remarks on postimplantation computed tomographic appearance. Neurosurgery 1988; 23:348–354.
53. Larson DA, Gutin PH, Leibel SA, et al. Stereotaxic irradiation of brain tumors. Cancer 1990; 65:792–799.
54. Malkin MG, Arbit E, Fass DE, et al. Stereotactic implantation of removable, high-activity iodine-125 sources for the treatment of malignant glioma. Neurology 1989; 39(Suppl 1):263.
55. Prados M, Leibel S, Barnett CM, et al. Interstitial brachytherapy for metastatic brain tumors. Cancer 1989; 63:657–660.
56. Steiner L. Radiosurgery in cerebral arteriovenous malformations. In: Fein JM, Flamm ES, eds. Cerebrovascular surgery. New York: Springer-Verlag, 1984; 4: 1161–1215.

57. Steiner L. Stereotactic radiosurgery with the cobalt 60 gamma unit in the surgical treatment of intracranial tumors and arteriovenous malformations. In: Schmidek HH, Sweet WH, eds. Operative neurosurgical techniques: indications, methods and results. Orlando: Grune and Stratton, 1988:515–529.
58. Steiner L. Treatment of arteriovenous malformations by radiosurgery. In: Wilson CB, Stein BM, eds. Intracranial arteriovenous malformations. Baltimore: Williams & Wilkins, 1984:295–313.
59. Steiner L, Greitz T, Backlund EO, et al. Radiosurgery of arteriovenous malformations of the brain. In: Szikla G, ed. Stereotactic cerebral irradiation. Amsterdam: Elsevier/North Holland, 1979; 12:257–269.
60. Betti OO, Manari C, Rosler R. Stereotactic radiosurgery with the linear accelerator: treatment of arteriovenous malformations. Neurosurgery 1989; 24:311–321.
61. Colombo F, Benedetti A, Pozza F, et al. External stereotactic irradiation by linear accelerator. Neurosurgery 1985; 16:154–160.
62. Loeffler JS, Rossitch E Jr, Siddon R, et al. Role of stereotactic radiosurgery with a linear accelerator in treatment of intracranial arteriovenous malformations and tumors in children. Pediatrics 1990; 85:774–782.
63. Loeffler JS, Kooy HM, Wen PY, et al. The treatment of recurrent brain metastases with stereotactic radiosurgery. J Clin Oncol 1990; 8:576–582.
64. Sturm V, Kober B, Hover KH, et al. Stereotactic percutaneous single dose irradiation of brain metastases with a linear accelerator. Int J Radiat Oncol Biol Phys 1987; 13:279–282.
65. Pozza F, Colombo F, Benedetti A, et al. In: Karim ABMF, ed. Proceedings of the fifth Varian European users meeting. Zug: Varian, 1987:93–95.
66. Ostertag CB, Groothuis D, Kleihues P. Effects on tumour and brain: experimental data on early and late morphologic effects of permanently implanted gamma and beta sources (iridium-192, iodine-125 and yttrium-90) in the brain. Acta Neurochir Suppl (Wien) 1984; 33:271–280.
67. Laramore GE, Griffin TW, Gerdes AJ, Parker RG. Fast neutron and mixed (neutron/photon) beam teletherapy for grades III and IV astrocytomas. Cancer 1978; 42:96–103.
68. Hosobuchi Y, Fabrikant J, Lyman J. Stereotactic heavy-particle irradiation of intracranial arteriovenous malformations. Appl Neurophysiol 1987; 50:248–252.
69. Marks MP, Delapaz RL, Fabrikant JI, et al. Intracranial vascular malformations: imaging of charged-particle radiosurgery; II: Complications. Radiology 1988; 168:457–462.
70. Fabrikant JI, Levy RP, Frankel KA, et al. Stereotactic helium-ion radiosurgery for the treatment of intracranial arteriovenous malformations. In: Heikkinen E, Kiviniitty K, eds. Proceedings of the international workshop on proton and narrow proton beam therapy. Oulu: University of Oulu Press, 1989:33–37.
71. Laramore GE, Martz KL, Nelson JS, et al. RTOG survival data on anaplastic astrocytoma of the brain: does a more aggressive form of treatment adversely impact survival? Int J Radiat Oncol Biol Phys 1988; 15:195.
72. Sturm V, Wowra B, Clorius J, et al. Intracavitary irradiation of cystic craniopharyn-

giomas. In: Lunsford LD, ed. Modern stereotactic neurosurgery. Boston: Martinus Nijhoff, 1988:229–233.
73. Pollack IF, Lunsford LD, Slamovits TL, et al. Stereotaxic intracavitary irradiation for cystic craniopharyngiomas. J Neurosurg 1988; 68:227–233.
74. Denekamp J. Changes in the rate of proliferation in normal tissues after irradiation. In: Nysgaard O, Adler HI, Sinclair WK, eds. Radiation research: biomedical chemical and physical perspectives. New York: Academic Press, 1975:810–825.
75. Caveness WF. Experimental observations: delayed necrosis in normal monkey brain. In: Gilbert HA, Kagan AR, eds. Radiation damage to the nervous system. New York: Raven Press, 1980:1–37.
76. Jellinger K, Sturm KW. Delayed radiation myelopathy in man: report of twelve necropsy cases. J Neurol Sci 1971; 14:389–408.
77. Burger PC, Mahaley MS Jr, Dudka L, Vogel FS. The morphologic effects of radiation administered therapeutically for intracranial gliomas: a postmortem study of 25 cases. Cancer 1979; 44:1256–1272.
78. Kramer S. The hazards of therapeutic irradiation of the central nervous system. Clin Neurosurg 1968; 15:301–318.
79. DiLorenzo N, Nolletti A, Palma L. Late cerebral radionecrosis. Surg Neurol 1978; 10:281–290.
80. Marks JE, Baglan RJ, Prassad SC, Blank WF. Cerebral radionecrosis: incidence and risk in relation to dose, time, fractionation and volume. Int J Radiat Oncol Biol Phys 1981; 7:243–252.
81. Al-Mehty O, Kersh JE, Routh A, Smith RR. The long-term side effects of radiation therapy for benign brain tumors in adults. J Neurosurg 1990; 73:502–512.
82. Boellaard JW, Jacoby W. Rontgenspatschaden des gehirns. Acta Neurochir (Wien) 1962; 10:533–564.
83. Grigsby PW, Simpson JR, Stokes S, et al. Results of surgery and irradiation or irradiation alone for pituitary adenomas. J Neurooncol 1988; 6:129–134.
84. Kramer S, Lee KF, Complications of radiation therapy: the central nervous system. Semin Roentgenol 1974; IX:75–83.
85. Rizzoli HV, Pagnanelli DM. Treatment of delayed radiation necrosis of the brain: a clinical observation. J Neurosurg 1984; 60:589–594.
86. Reagan TJ, Thomas JE, Colby MY Jr. Chronic progressive radiation myelopathy: its clinical aspects and differential diagnosis. JAMA 1968; 203:106–110.
87. Ventafridda V, Caraceni C, Martini C, et al. On the significance of Lhermitte's sign in oncology. J Neurooncol 1991; 10:133–137.
88. Jones A. Transient radiation myelopathy (with reference to Lhermitte's sign of electrical paresthesia). Br J Radiol 1964; 37:727–744.
89. Wara WM, Phillips TL, Sheline GE, et al. Radiation tolerance of the spinal cord. Cancer 1975; 35:1558–1562.
90. Jeremic B, Djuric L, Mijatovic L. Incidence of radiation myelitis of the cervical spinal cord at doses of 550 cGy or greater. Cancer 1991; 68:2138–2141.
91. Maier JG, Perry RH, Saylor W, Sulak, MH. Radiation myelitis of the dorsolumbar spinal cord. Radiology 1969; 93:153–160.

92. Boden G. Radiation myelitis of the brain stem. J Fac Radiol 1950; 2:79–94.
93. Leach W. Irradiation of the ear. J Laryngoscopy 1965; 79:870–880.
94. Borsanyi S, Blanchard CL. Ionizing radiation and the ear. JAMA 1962; 181: 958–961.
95. Moskovskaya NU. Effects of ionizing radiation on the functioning of the vestibular analyser. Vestn Otorinolaringol 1960; 21:59–62.
96. Kretschmar CS, Warren MP, Lavally BL, et al. Ototoxicity of preradiation cisplatin for children with central nervous system tumors. J Clin Oncol 1990; 8:1191–1198.
97. Kori SH, Foley KM, Posner JB. Brachial plexus lesions in patients with cancer: clinical findings in 100 cases. Neurology 1979; 29:583.
98. Thomas JE, Colby MY. Radiation-induced or metastatic brachial plexopathy? A diagnostic dilemma. JAMA 1972; 222:1392–1395.
99. Kinsella TJ, Weichselbaum RR, Sheline GE. Radiation injury of cranial and peripheral nerves. In: Gilbert HA, Kagan AR, eds. Radiation damage to the nervous system. New York: Raven Press, 1980:145–153.
100. Klaya M. Radiogenic peripheral neuropathies following cobalt radiation to the abdominal cavity. Radiobiol Radiother (Berl) 1974; 15:459–464.
101. Lunsford LD, Flickinger J, Lindner G, Maitz A. Stereotactic radiosurgery of the brain using the first United States 201 Cobalt-60 source gamma knife. Neurosurgery 1989; 24:151–159.
102. Noren G, Arndt J, Hindmarsh T, Hirsch A: Stereotactic radiosurgical treatment of acoustic neuromas. In: Lunsford LD, ed. Modern stereotactic neurosurgery. Boston: Martinus Nijhoff, 1988:481–489.
103. Ross DA, Wilson CB. Results of transsphenoidal microsurgery for growth hormone-secreting pituitary adenoma in a series of 214 patients. J Neurosurg 1988; 68: 854–867.
104. Samaan NA, Bakdash MM, Caderao JB, et al. Hypopituitarism after external irradiation: evidence for both hypothalamic and pituitary origin. Ann Intern Med 1975; 83:771–777.
105. Richards GE, Wara WM, Grumbach MM, et al. Delayed onset of hypopituitarism: sequelae of therapeutic irradiation of central nervous system, eye and middle ear tumors. J Pediatr 1976; 89:553–559.
106. Shalet SM, Beardwell CG, MacFarland IA, et al. Endocrine morbidity in adults treated with cerebral irradiation for brain tumors during childhood. Acta Endocrinol 1977; 84:673–680.
107. Dickenson WP, Berry DH, Dickenson L, et al. Differential effects of cranial radiation on growth hormone response to arginine and insulin infusion. J Pediatr 1978; 92:754–757.
108. Docou-Voutetekis C, Haidas ST, Zannos-Mariolea L. Radiation and pituitary function in children. Lancet 1975; 2:1206–1207.
109. Nelson DF, Reddy V, O'Mara RE, et al. Thyroid abnormalities following irradiation for Hodgkin's disease. Cancer 1978; 42:2553–2562.
110. Probert JC, Parker BR, Kaplan HS. Growth retardation in children after megavoltage irradiation of the spine. Cancer 1973; 32:634–639.

111. Lushbaugh CC, Casarett GW. The effects of gonadal irradiation in clinical radiation therapy: a review. Cancer 1976; 37:1111–1120.
112. Shalet SM, Beardwell CG, Jacobs HS, et al. Testicular function following irradiation of the human prepubertal testis. Clin Endocrinol 1978; 9:483–490.
113. Rahn T. Stereotactic radiosurgery in Cushing's disease. (Thesis). Stockholm: Sundt Offset, 1980. [cited in 57]
114. Degerblad M, Rahn T, Bergstrand G. Long term results of stereotactic radiosurgery to the pituitary gland in Cushing's disease. Acta Endocrinol 1986; 112:310–315.
115. Traynor JE, Casey HW. Five-year follow-up of primates exposed to 55 Mev protons. Radiat Res 1971; 47:143–148.
116. Ron E, Modan B, Boice JD, et al. Tumors of the brain and nervous system after radiotherapy in childhood. N Engl J Med 1988; 319:1033–1039.
117. Waga S, Handa H. Radiation-induced meningioma, with review of literature. Surg Neurol 1976; 5:215–219.
118. Meadows AT. Late malignant neoplasms. In: Nesbit ME, Duncan W, Ellis H, et al., eds. Late effects in successfully treated children with cancer: Philadelphia: WB Saunders, 1985; Clinics Oncology 4:247–261.
119. Rimm IJ, Li FC, Tarbell NJ, et al. Brain tumors after cranial irradiation for childhood acute lymphoblastic leukemia: a 13-year experience from the Dana-Farber Cancer Institute and The Children's Hospital. Cancer 1987; 59:1506–1508.
120. Kumar PP, Good RR, Skultety FM, et al. Radiation-induced neoplasms of the brain. Cancer 1987; 59:1274–1282.
121. Moss SD, Rockswold GL, Chou SN, et al. Radiation-induced meningiomas in pediatric patients. Neurosurgery 1988; 22:758–761.
122. Palma L, Vagnozzi R, Annino L, et al. Post-radiation glioma in a child: case report and review of the literature. Childs Nerv Syst 1988; 4:296–301.
123. Goldberg MB, Sheline GE, Malamud N. Malignant intracranial neoplasms following radiation therapy for acromegaly. Radiology 1963; 80:465–470.
124. Li FP, Cassady JR, Jaffee N. Risk of second tumors in survivors of childhood cancer. Cancer 1975; 35:1230–1235.
125. Shapiro S, Mealy J Jr, Sartorius C. Radiation-induced intracranial malignant gliomas. J Neurosurg 1989; 71:77–82.
126. Schwartz AD, Lee H, Baum ES. Leukemia in children with Wilm's tumor. J Pediatr 1975; 87:374–376.
127. Li FP. Second malignant tumors after cancer in childhood. Cancer 1977; 40:1899–1902.
128. O'Donnell JF, Brereton HD, Greco FA, et al. Acute non-lymphocytic leukemia and acute myeloproliferative syndrome following radiation therapy for non-Hodgkin's lymphoma and chronic lymphocytic leukemia: clinical studies. Cancer 1979; 44:1930–1938.
129. DeVita VT Jr. The consequences of the chemotherapy of Hodgkin's disease. Cancer 1981; 47:1–13.
130. Li FP. Follow-up of survivors of childhood cancer. Cancer 1977; 39:1776–1778.
131. Andler W, Harvers W, Stambolis CH, et al. Renal cell carcinoma following radiation therapy for an adrenal cortical carcinoma. J Pediatr 1978; 93:634–636.

132. Meadows AT, Strong LC, Li FP, et al. Bone sarcomas as a second malignant neoplasm in children: influence of radiation and genetic predisposition. Cancer 1980; 46:2603–2606.
133. Li FP. Colon cancer after Wilm's tumor. J Pediatr 1980; 96:954–955.
134. Tang TT, Holcenberg JS, Duck SC, et al. Thyroid carcinoma following treatment for acute lymphoblastic leukemia. Cancer 1980; 46:1572–1576.
135. Delattre J-Y, Safai B, Posner JB. Erythema multiforme and Stevens-Johnson syndrome in patients receiving cranial irradiation and phenytoin. Neurology 1988; 38:194–198.

# 11

## Neurological Complications of Chemotherapy

**Peter A. J. Forsyth**

*University of Calgary, Tom Baker Cancer Centre, Calgary, Alberta, Canada*

**Terrence L. Cascino**

*Mayo Clinic, Rochester, Minnesota*

This chapter presents the spectrum of complications of chemotherapy involving the nervous system, with emphasis on clinical toxicity. Table 1 lists the chemotherapeutic agents that are reliably associated with a particular syndrome (Table 1).

Drug-related neurotoxicity is important for several reasons. First, chemotherapeutic drugs can produce major disability, and failure to stop the offending agent may lead to irreversible neurological damage. Second, chemotherapy may affect the nervous system in ways that are clinically indistinguishable from metastatic disease. Knowledge of these syndromes may lead to a timely diagnosis and obviate the need for extensive diagnostic tests. Third, the neurotoxicity of chemotherapy is intriguing and may lead to further understanding of the nervous system and provide models of neurological disease.

Caution should be exercised in accepting some reported complications ascribed to particular drugs because the evidence is often circumstantial. Pathological confirmation is uncommon. There are, however, certain well-known neurological complications of chemotherapy that have been established by clinical experience or pathological confirmation; these are the subject of this chapter.

## I. METHOTREXATE

Methotrexate (MTX) is a folic acid analog whose primary action is inhibition of dihydrofolate reductase, resulting in depletion of intracellular pools of reduced

**Table 1** Neurological Complications of Chemotherapy and Associated Agents

| | |
|---|---|
| Encephalopathy | Peripheral neuropathy |
|   5-Fluorouracil |   Cisplatin |
|   Ara-C (HD) |   Vincristine |
|   Methotrexate (IT) |   Procarbazine |
|   Procarbazine |   Ara-C |
|   Ifosfamide |   Taxol |
|   BCNU (HD,IA) |   Hexamethylmelamine |
|   Asparaginase |   Suramin |
| Acute cerebellar syndrome | Myelopathy with paraparesis |
|   5-Fluorouracil |   Ara-C (IT) |
|   Ara-C (HD) |   Methotrexate (IT) |
| Acute meningeal syndrome |   BCNU (HD) |
|   Methotrexate (IT) |   Thio-TEPA (IT) |
| Encephalopathy with multifocal | Other syndromes |
|     demyelinating cerebral lesions |   Lhermitte's sign |
|   5-Fluorouracil and levamisole |     Cisplatin |
| Cranial neuropathy |   SIADH |
|   Ototoxic |     Vincristine |
|     Cisplatin |   Strokelike syndrome |
|     BCNU (IA) |     Methotrexate |
|   Vestibulopathy |     Cisplatin |
|     Cisplatin |   Cerebral vasculopathy |
|   Extraocular muscle palsies |     Asparaginase (venous) |
|     Vincristine |     Cisplatin (IA) |
| |     BCNU (IA) |

IT = intrathecal; HD = high dose; IA = intra-arterial

folate necessary for thymidylate and purine metabolism; this leads to impaired DNA synthesis (1).

## A. Acute and Subacute Toxicity

### 1. Aseptic Meningitis

This syndrome begins within several hours of intrathecal (IT) administration of the drug and lasts for 12–72 h (2–4). Aseptic meningitis occurs in 10% of patients; it is more common following intraventricular injection than lumbar administration. It is characterized by the abrupt onset of headache, nausea, vomiting, meningismus, lethargy, and fever. It may resemble acute bacterial meningitis with a high fever and massive pleocytosis but occurs too soon after drug administration to be due to bacterial growth. Cerebrospinal fluid (CSF) cultures are negative. The syndrome is self-limited, resolves without sequelae, and does not require specific therapy, though some investigators (5) have pretreated patients with IT hydrocortisone. Rare complications of IT methotrexate may include neurogenic pulmonary edema (6) and sudden death of unknown cause (7,8). Massive intrathecal overdose—which is almost uniformly fatal—has been treated successfully with immediate (within 1 h) ventriculolumbar perfusion via ventricular and lumbar cannulas (9).

## 2. Transverse Myelopathy

This is a rare complication of IT methotrexate (10–16) that usually begins within 30 min to 48 h of IT administration but may be delayed for up to 2 weeks. The first symptoms are leg pain followed by paraplegia, ascending sensory level, and impairment of bowel and bladder function. The degree of recovery is variable. Occasionally the myelopathy may progress to a meningoencephalomyelopathy (15) with stiff neck, progressive lethargy, coma, and death. Pathologically there is necrosis or microvacuolation of the spinal cord without striking inflammatory or vascular changes (11,15,16). The pathogenesis of this syndrome is unknown but may be an idiosyncratic reaction to the drug. This rare complication may be more common in patients with meningeal metastases, in patients receiving concurrent radiotherapy, or in patients given frequent IT methotrexate (13).

## 3. Strokelike Syndromes

This occasionally follows weekly systemic administration of high-dose methotrexate. Walker et al. (17) reported 22 patients with this syndrome 2 or 3 weeks following high-dose methotrexate ($8–9$ g/m$^2$); the syndrome was characterized by encephalopathy and mono- or hemiparesis of acute onset which lasted for 15 min to 72 h and resolved. The focal findings may fluctuate from one side to the other. The methotrexate levels, computed tomography (CT) scans of the head, and CSF examinations are all normal. The electroencephalogram (EEG), however, shows diffuse slowing in all patients. This has also been described in two patients treated with moderately high dose ($2.76$ g/m$^2$) methotrexate and concurrent IT methotrexate (18). These syndromes are rapidly and almost completely reversible and require no specific treatment. Surprisingly, the syndrome usually does not recur with further treatment. The pathogenesis is unknown, but the syndrome may be due to reduced cerebral glucose metabolism (19). A similar syndrome has been described in a patient with acute lymphocytic leukemia with meningeal involvement. Postmortem examination showed neuroaxonal dystrophy in the patient's midbrain (20). Strokelike episodes with corresponding radiographic changes have also been described with low-dose IT methotrexate or triple IT treatment with methotrexate, arabinosylcytosine and hydrocortisone (21).

## B. Delayed Toxicity

### 1. Diffuse Leukoencephalopathy

This is the most devastating delayed complication of methotrexate and follows repeated doses of high-dose intravenous (IV) or IT methotrexate; it has also been reported in patients receiving standard-dose IV methotrexate with cranial irradiation (22–30). Cranial irradiation increases the risk of encephalopathy. Intrathecal methotrexate with defective cerebrospinal fluid dynamics and delayed egress of methotrexate also may result in leukoencephalopathy. The clinical syndrome may begin insidiously or abruptly many months to years following treatment and consists of a change in personality, lethargy, seizures, spasticity, ataxia, hemi- or quadriparesis and occasionally may progress to coma and death. The degree of recovery is variable. Computed tomographic scans of the brain may look normal but often show hypodensity of the periventricular white matter bilaterally as well as atrophy and occasional cortical calcifications. Occasionally there may be areas of enhancement (31,32). Similar radiographic changes may be seen in asymptomatic patients treated with IT methotrexate (33) or cranial irradiation and IT methotrexate (34). Pathologically these lesions usually consist of areas of coagulative and fibrinoid necrosis. In other cases, there is only periventricular necrosis without blood vessel changes (23–26,30,35). One case was reported to show only multifocal axonal degeneration (36). The typical lesions affect both myelin and axons. The CSF examination may show an elevated myelin basic protein (37). The pathogenesis of these lesions is unknown. It is postulated that cranial irradiation may either damage vessels and potentiate the toxic effects of methotrexate or that radiation may disrupt the blood-brain barrier allowing unusually high concentrations of methotrexate to reach normal brain. Cranial irradiation has been reported to increase blood-brain barrier permeability to methotrexate in rodents (38,39).

## II. 5-FLUOROURACIL

5-Fluorouracil (5-FU) is a fluorinated pyrimidine. The related drugs carmofur and ftorafur have also been used. Their main mechanism of action is felt to be inhibition of DNA synthesis by inhibition of thymidylate synthetase. Monkey (40) and rodent (41) studies suggest that 5-FU crosses the blood-brain barrier and that concentrations of the drug are higher in the cerebellum than elsewhere in the brain.

## A. Acute Cerebellar Syndrome

This syndrome (42–45) is characterized by the acute onset of ataxia, dysmetria, nystagmus, and ataxic dysarthria and may be seen in 5% of patients. Onset is weeks to months following the initiation of therapy. Neurological dysfunction resolves completely when 5-FU is stopped. The incidence and severity of the cerebellar syndrome seem to be directly related to the dose and schedule of administration, with most patients developing this syndrome following large doses (1.0 to 3.4 g/m$^2$) given as IV bolus. None developed the syndrome in one series with lower doses (7.5 or 15 mg/kg) (44). The clinical presentation may resemble other conditions, such as a posterior fossa mass, drug intoxication, or a paraneoplastic syndrome, but clears following discontinuation of the 5-FU. The pathophysiology of this syndrome is unknown. There are no relevant pathological studies of patients who experienced the syndrome. Some (46) have suggested that 5-FU toxicity is due to inhibition of the Kreb's cycle by fluoroacetate but this does not explain why the syndrome is predominantly limited to cerebellar dysfunction.

## B. Uncommon Complications

Rarely the drug has been associated with encephalopathy (47), oculomotor disturbances (48), parkinsonian syndrome (49), and optic neuropathy (50).

## C. 5-Fluorouracil and Levamisole: Encephalopathy with Multifocal Demyelinating Cerebral Lesions

This rare syndrome has occurred in patients with colon cancer receiving 5-FU and levamisole (51,52). The symptoms were progressive encephalopathy and ataxia; two patients developed hemiparesis. One patient also had dysarthria. Symptoms improved following the discontinuation of chemotherapy and the administration of corticosteroids. Magnetic resonance imaging of the head in these patients demonstrated multiple gadolinium-enhancing white matter lesions predominantly in a periventricular distribution. Cerebral biopsies in these three patients revealed demyelination and perivascular inflammation similar, if not identical, to that described in patients with multiple sclerosis. The electron microscopic, light microscopic, and cerebrospinal fluid findings suggest an immune-mediated process similar to multiple sclerosis. Similar lesions have been seen in one patient who was asymptomatic. Although an inflammatory demyelinating process may represent the anatomic substrate of 5-FU neurotoxicity, a role for levamisole cannot be excluded. This complication is important clinically since multiple cerebral lesions in a patient with cancer receiving 5-FU and levamisole may be mistakenly assumed to be cerebral metastases and be treated with radiotherapy and continued chemotherapy. The key radiographic feature that differentiates this condition from metastases is the predominance of lesions in the white matter resembling the demyelinating plaques of multiple sclerosis.

## D. 5-Fluorouracil and Other Agents

The coadministration of 5-FU and allopurinol probably increases the neurotoxicity (53,54) over either agent used separately. Interestingly, the neurotoxicity of these two agents produces an encephalopathy as well as a cerebellar syndrome. 5-Fluorouracil and PALA have been reported to result in neurotoxicity (55) with seizures, encephalopathy, cerebellar syndromes, and hallucinations.

### E. Other Fluorinated Antipyrimidines

Reversible encephalopathy and ataxia has been reported in several patients receiving doxifluridine (56,57). Symptoms resolved after discontinuation of therapy. A reversible leukoencephalopathy was reported in two patients after the administration of either of the 5-FU derivatives carmofur or tegafur. Kuzuhara et al. (58) reported three cases of a subacute progressive leukoencephalopathy in patients receiving carmofur and summarized 16 other cases reported in Japan. These patients had progressive dementia, gait ataxia, and somnolence. Neuropathological examination in four patients showed massive demyelination limited to the cerebral hemispheres. The syndrome of progressive leukoencephalopathy clinically and pathologically resembles the leukoencephalopathy seen with 5-FU and levamisole.

## III. CISPLATIN

Cisplatin or cis-diamminedichloroplatinum (CDDP) has a heavy metal base and probably exerts its cytotoxic effects by binding to DNA (59).

### A. Peripheral Neuropathy

This most common and well-described neurological complication of cisplatin (60) follows doses of $400 \text{ mg/m}^2$ or greater and is characterized by the subacute onset of numbness and tingling in the heads and feet. Examination reveals predominantly vibratory sensory loss with decreased or absent deep tendon reflexes. Pin-prick and temperature sensation may be slightly reduced and motor involvement is minimal or absent. As the neuropathy progresses, joint position sense may be impaired and the patient may become severely disabled by a sensory ataxia. The neuropathy may begin or progress (61,62) after the cisplatin administration has stopped (63). The incidence and severity of neurotoxicity is related to both cumulative dose and individual doses (64). Electrophysiological studies and sural nerve biopsies have confirmed it is largely damage to large myelinated sensory fibers; pathological examination shows demyelination and axonal loss (65–68). It is not yet clear whether the damage is to the dorsal root ganglia, sensory nerve, or both. Cisplatin neuropathy may initially be confused with a paraneoplastic neuropathy, but in the latter case all sensory fibers tend to be affected and relentless progression occurs in spite of discontinuing the drug.

Currently, there is no effective, accepted treatment for any of the neurological complications of cisplatin. The compound WR-2721 (ethiofos) has been shown to reduce the incidence and severity of neuropathy in patients treated with this agent (69). The use of an ACTH (4–9) analog, Org 2766, has been shown to reduce or prevent cisplatin neuropathy in patients with ovarian cancer (70). Recently Apfel and coworkers (71) have reported that nerve growth factor prevents cisplatin neuropathy in mice; clinical trials should be under way soon.

## B. Cranial Neuropathies

The most common cranial neuropathy is ototoxicity. Hearing loss occurs mostly in the high frequencies and may be asymptomatic. Melamed et al. (72) found that although 74% of patients had audiometric hearing loss, only 16% of patients were symptomatic. It is usually bilateral, symmetric, gradual in onset, and progressive. Tinnitus is common (68%) and usually accompanies hearing loss (72). High doses can rarely produce acute deafness (73). At a dose of 450 mg/m$^2$ or greater, the risk of significant hearing loss is 10% or more and may be irreversible (74), though one group reported a 26% partial recovery (75). In a prospective study of 24 pediatric patients, McHaney et al. (76) found audiometrically significant hearing loss occurred in 88% of their patients, and no significant recovery of hearing was found in patients at 15 months of follow-up. Animal models suggest that toxicity is due to peripheral receptor (hair cell) loss in the organ of Corti (77). It is likely that cranial irradiation increases the probability of significant hearing loss (74,78). Young children may be more affected than adults (78) but may recover more. Vestibulopathy has also been described, with vertigo and vestibular dysfunction that is usually asymptomatic and found only with electrophysiological testing (79,80).

Visual toxicity has been described. Walsh et al. (81) found papilledema in a child without evidence of increased intracranial pressure. Ostrow et al. (82) reported one patient with papilledema and increased intracranial pressure and one with a diagnosis of retrobulbar neuritis. Retinopathy has been described in patients receiving high doses (200 mg/m$^2$) of cisplatin. Of 13 patients, eight developed blurred vision and 11 had abnormal cone function by electroretinography and color vision testing (83). Visual symptoms developed at a cumulative dose of about 600 mg/m$^2$ and all patients had a concomitant peripheral neuropathy. Despite the visual complaints, the peripheral neuropathy remained the dose-limiting side effect.

## C. Lhermitte's Sign

This symptom is common and has been reported in 21–40% of patients receiving cisplatin. It occurs in patients with symptomatic peripheral neuropathy who have received cumulative doses and resolves over months (61,68,84). Presumably this reflects demyelination of the posterior columns. There is one autopsy study of a child (81) with cisplatin neurotoxicity that showed degeneration and gliosis of the dorsal columns. Although Lhermitte's sign may be associated with epidural cord compression, other neurological symptoms (such as pain) or signs of spinal cord dysfunction are not seen with cisplatin (85).

## D. Uncommon Complications

These include focal cranial neuropathies (86) and lumbosacral plexopathies or mononeuropathies (87) from intra-arterial cisplatin. Seizures occurring in patients who received cisplatin and other chemotherapeutic agents were usually single and didn't require long-term treatment (88) Seizures are unexpected because little cisplatin is present in the CSF of humans following systemic administration (89); however, seizures have been described in frogs several weeks following the administration of cisplatin (90).

Rarely, cisplatin has been associated with focal brain dysfunction or cortical blindness. These may be strokelike syndromes. Doll et al. (91) described one patient with bilateral cerebral infarcts in a distribution typical of small-vessel disease and another patient with a right hemiparesis and a normal magnetic resonance imaging (MRI) scan. Berman and Mann (92) describe a single patient who developed transient cortical blindness and generalized seizures following the administration of cisplatin, vinblastine, and bleomycin. It is unclear what caused this syndrome; it may have been focal ischemia or a post-ictal event. This patient had levels of cisplatin which were as high in the CSF as they were in the serum. Pippitt et al. (93) describe a patient with transient cortical blindness following single-agent therapy with cisplatin. Diamond et al. (94) described a patient with the acute onset of cortical blindness and encephalopathy which persisted as a homonymous hemianopsia several months following the event. Cohen et al. (95) describe a patient receiving cisplatin, vinblastine, and bleomycin who acutely developed encephalopathy, a left homonymous hemianopsia, and a left parietal syndrome who recovered almost completely over several days. In only one of these four studies was CSF cisplatin measured and in all cases results of CT scans of the head were found to be normal. The pathogenesis of these complications remains obscure. There is no histopathology and no MRI studies are reported.

Cisplatin has also been associated with cerebral herniation syndromes (96), though it is likely that the cause of the edema was multifactorial. Ritch et al. (97) report a patient who developed the syndrome of inappropriate antidiuretic hormone secretion (SIADH) accompanied by seizures and somnolence 1 day after finishing cisplatin. Finally, hypomagnesemia and hypocalcemia occur in the majority of patients and are presumably related to cisplatin nephrotoxicity. Hayes et al. (98) reported severe tetany and carpopedal spasms in 4 of 16 pediatric patients receiving cisplatin in spite of 15 of 16 of these patients having hypomagnesemia.

## IV. CARBOPLATIN

This relatively new agent is a structural analog of cisplatin with similar antineoplastic activity but no neurotoxicity. One patient has been described who developed a thrombotic microangiopathy (99) resulting in multiple cortical infarcts that led to coma and death. Intracarotid artery infusion has produced strokelike syndromes and retinal toxicity (100). As experience grows, reports of neurotoxicity may follow but will likely remain much fewer than with cisplatin.

## V. VINCRISTINE (Vinca Alkaloids)

Vincristine and the related compounds vinblastine and vindesine inhibit microtubule assembly, which arrests cell division and interferes with axonal transport and secretory function of the neuron (101,102). This probably forms the basis of its neurotoxicity (103,104). The lower neurotoxicity of vinblastine and vindesine may be related to differences in lipid solubility (105), plasma clearance and terminal half-life (106), and potency in inhibiting fast axoplasmic transport (107).

### A. Peripheral Neuropathy

Most patients receiving vincristine develop peripheral neuropathy with an early loss of ankle jerks and paresthesias in the feet and finger tips. This is related to total dose and duration of therapy. There may be loss of all sensory modalities, though more marked to small fiber modalities, and occasionally muscle weakness may develop. These symptoms may begin after the drug has been discontinued and progress for several months but usually improve. Children recover more quickly and completely than adults. Objective sensory deficits are minor in comparison to symptoms of paresthesias or dysesthesias (108,109) that may be painful. Continued administration of the drug may lead to weakness, especially bilateral foot-drop (110) and less commonly bilateral wrist-drop (109,111). Rarely, vincristine can produce focal mononeuropathies (112). There is no accepted effective treatment of vincristine neuropathy (113–116).

Several factors may enhance the neurotoxic reaction to vincristine, including older age (117), systemic lymphoma (118), and radiation to the peripheral nerves (119). In one report, vincristine may have had a synergistic effect with radiotherapy to the spine in producing a myelitis (120). Preexisting peripheral neuropathy may increase the severity of neurotoxicity. Three patients with Charcot-Marie-Tooth disease have been reported who developed severe polyneuropathy, fatal in one case, after only one or two doses of vincristine (121,122). One patient with a remote history of poliomyelitis developed a transient tetraparesis after a single dose of vincristine (123). However, severe idiosyncratic polyneuropathy has also been reported in patients without prior neuropathy (124,125) and vincristine neuropathy was not debilitating in one patient with a prior diabetic neuropathy

(110). The use of other potentially neurotoxic agents may increase or potentiate the neurotoxicity of vincristine (126,127).

Electrophysiology suggests that vincristine neuropathy is a primarily axonal neuropathy of the dying back type. No abnormalities have been found in the dorsal root ganglia or anterior horn cells (110,128–131). These studies have emphasized that small and large sensory fibers and motor fibers are all affected.

## B. Autonomic Dysfunction

Acute abdominal pain and transient ileus are very common, occurring in up to 46% (109–111) of patients. This usually resolves within days and precedes other signs or symptoms of neurotoxicity. After several weeks some mild abdominal complaints may occur, occasionally with urinary incontinence (132,133) and postural hypotension (134,135) that may reflect a postganglionic lesion of the sympathetic nerves. Reduced heart rate variability during respiration has been reported during vincristine therapy, presumably reflecting autonomic dysfunction (136). In some patients, autonomic symptoms develop without evidence of peripheral neuropathy. A comprehensive study of the putative autonomic neuropathy associated with vincristine is lacking.

## C. Hyponatremia

The syndrome of inappropriate antidiuretic hormone secretion following vincristine (137–139) and vinblastine (140) therapy has been reported. In at least two cases (137,138), the serum antidiuretic hormone was markedly elevated during the period of hyponatremia. The syndrome occurs within days (or hours with very high doses) and in the setting of other signs of neurotoxicity. Stuart et al. (138) demonstrated that the clinical and biochemical criteria of SIADH may recur following rechallenge with vincristine.

## D. Cranial Neuropathies

These are uncommon and include (presumably) laryngeal neuropathies with hoarseness following administration of vincristine (108,111,130,141) and vinblastine (142). There have been no pathological studies, but the presumed lesion is of the recurrent laryngeal nerve as direct laryngoscopy shows vocal cord paresis. Both bilateral (143) and unilateral optic neuropathies have been reported (144). A variety of ocular muscle palsies, ptosis, and seventh and fifth nerve palsies have been described as occurring several weeks after the initiation of vincristine (109, 130,145).

## E. Intrathecal Administration

This is fatal (146–150), with one exception (151), and is characterized by progressive ascending meningoencephalitis, bulbar paresis, and finally coma over a period of several days to weeks. The single case which was nonfatal was treated with aggressive removal of as much CSF as possible via the lumbar route followed by a 24-h continuous infusion of lactated Ringer's solution through a catheter inserted in the lateral ventricle and IV glutamic acid (151). However, this treatment has been reported to be unsuccessful in other cases.

## F. Uncommon Complications

These include coma without hyponatremia (152), seizures without hyponatremia or other discernible cause (153), and a single patient with ataxia and athetosis (154). Transient cortical blindness has been reported in three children receiving vincristine as well as a number of other chemotherapeutic agents but the mechanism is unclear (155). A single instance of permanent blindness has been reported but it is unknown whether this was cortical or ocular dysfunction or an optic neuropathy (156).

It is unclear whether vincristine causes a myopathy. There has been rare histological (130) or electrophysiological (110) documentation of a myopathy produced by vincristine but this is probably not clinically significant. Complaints of jaw and leg pain are common acutely and may be due to a focal cranial neuropathy or myopathy or other cause. In patients receiving vincristine and prednisone, the clinical examination can distinguish between the weakness produced by the proximal myopathy of prednisone from the distal weakness caused by the vincristine neuropathy (157).

## VI. ARABINOSYLCYTOSINE (Ara-C)

Ara-C is a pyramidine analog of cytidine and its mechanism of action is through the inhibition of DNA synthesis. Ara-C must undergo intracellular conversion to Ara-C triphosphate to be cytotoxic. Systemically administered Ara-C is primarily eliminated by metabolism to the inactive compound Ara-U by cytidine deaminase. Cerebrospinal fluid levels of Ara-C are 6–22% of serum concentrations and the CSF half-life is longer than the serum half-life (158). Intrathecal administration produces no level of drug in the serum but very high levels of Ara-C in the CSF, which persist at biologically active levels for at least 24 h (159). When this agent is used in conventional systemic doses, it has no significant neurological side effects.

### A. Aseptic Meningitis, Encephalopathy, and Transverse Myelopathy

Intrathecal administration may cause neurotoxicity similar to that seen with IT methotrexate. There are several reports of paraparesis following IT Ara-C (10,11, 16,160–164). Less commonly reported are encephalopathy, headaches, meningismus, or seizures (165). The onset of the paraparesis may be within hours to several weeks, with leg and back pain, loss of motor and sensory function in the legs, and loss of bladder or bowel control (16,160,164). Pathological examination shows demyelination of the spinal nerve roots as well as in the white matter of the cord, hyalinization of meningeal vessels, and prominent microvascular changes in the cord, including axonal swelling and loss of myelin with scattered fat-laden macrophages. In most cases, patients with paraparesis were also receiving other chemotherapy or had concomitant meningeal disease. At the time of the paraparesis, the spinal fluid may be normal or show increased protein. There is one report of elevated myelin basic protein (16). Interestingly, none of the patients receiving IT Ara-C developed a cerebellar syndrome as is seen with high-dose systemic administration.

## B. Acute Cerebellar Syndrome

This syndrome, seen with high-dose systemic Ara-C therapy (3 g/m$^2$ twice daily [b.i.d.] for 12 doses) (166–174), occurs within several days of beginning drug administration. About 10–20% of patients will experience neurological symptoms. Various risk factors have been proposed, including older age, higher doses (i.e., > 30 g), and hepatic (172) or renal dysfunction (173,174). It is usually reversible unless very large cumulative doses (e.g., > 24 g/m$^2$) are given (166,170). These patients also experience diffuse cerebral symptoms such as somnolence, confusion, seizures, and personality changes. A single patient with an expressive aphasia is also reported (175). At postmortem examination, irreversible cerebellar symptoms correlated with loss of Purkinje cells (168) and degeneration of the dentate nuclei (169). No pathological correlate has been found for the encephalopathy.

## C. Uncommon Complications

These have been reported following high-dose Ara-C and include ocular toxicity (176,171), SIADH (178), peripheral neuropathy (178–180), brachial plexopathy (181), lateral rectus palsy (166,172), and parkinsonism (182).

## VII. ASPARAGINASE

Asparaginase catalyzes the hydrolysis of serum asparagine, which deprives tumor cells of the required amino acid and inhibits protein synthesis. Normal cells are spared because they have the ability to synthesize their own asparagine. Toxicity is usually due to allergic reactions or hepatic or pancreatic damage. In high doses asparaginase may cause liver dysfunction, hyperammonemia, and hepatic encephalopathy (183). In the past, when higher doses were used, encephalopathy was a common complication (184–186). Now cumulative doses are smaller and this complication is less common. More important clinically, thrombosis of the cerebral veins or dural sinuses caused by asparaginase (187–190) may be associated with cerebral hemorrhage. This is usually seen within the first few weeks of therapy but may occur after cessation of treatment. Patients usually present with headache, seizures, hemiparesis, and altered mental status ranging from encephalopathy to coma. Diagnosis is possible with a contrast-enhanced head CT scan (191), which may show an empty "delta sign," but digital subtraction angiography or a head MRI (192,193) is preferable. This complication appears to be due to depletion of plasma proteins involved in coagulation and fibrinolysis. There is no universally accepted treatment. An early suspicion of this disorder should lead to prompt imaging, evaluation of coagulation profiles, and appropriate supportive care. Some have recommended the empiric use of steroids. Careful attention to fluid status and maneuvers to reduce increased intracranial pressure also may be useful.

## VIII. PROCARBAZINE

Procarbazine is a weak monoamine oxidase (MAO) inhibitor that rapidly crosses the blood-brain barrier (194). Its mechanism of antineoplastic activity is unknown and it is currently only given orally. It may produce an encephalopathy ranging from confusion to profound stupor (195) and rarely to manic psychosis (196). Procarbazine potentiates the sedative effects of phenothiazines, barbiturates, and narcotics (197) and these interactions may contribute to the observed encephalopathy. Patients taking procarbazine may develop a "disulfiram-like" syndrome characterized by facial flushing, headache, and diaphoresis following alcohol ingestion. A peripheral neuropathy characterized by paresthesias with decreased or absent deep tendon reflexes occurs and is reversible with discontinuation of the drug (195). Since the drug is a MAO inhibitor, patients should be advised to avoid tyramine-containing foods, tricyclic antidepressants, and other sympathomimetic drugs to avoid acute hypertension.

## IX. IFOSFAMIDE

Ifosfamide is an analog of cyclophosphamide and its major neurotoxicity is encephalopathy, occurring in about 20% of patients (198–201). The encephalopathy begins within hours to days of beginning administration of the drug and usually resolves completely, although altered mental status may persist in some patients (202). There is no specific treatment. Patients at risk for this complication include those with low serum albumin, renal dysfunction, previous encephalopathy from ifosfamide (199), or prior administration of cisplatin (200). Other uncommon neurological abnormalities that have been reported include cerebellar ataxia, weakness, cranial nerve dysfunction, and seizures.

## X. NITROSOUREAS (BCNU AND CCNU)

These agents have been used for many years in a wide variety of applications. Nitrosoureas are lipid-soluble agents that cross the blood-brain barrier. The largest clinical experience is with BCNU, and its neurotoxicity is probably similar to the other nitrosoureas. These drugs are generally not neurotoxic except when administered intra-arterially or in high doses systemically. It is also possible that radiation may enhance the neurotoxicity of nitrosoureas (203).

High-dose systemic BCNU has been used in the setting of autologous bone marrow transplantation. Burger et al. (204) described an encephalomyelopathy that developed over a period of weeks to months following administration of BCNU in three of four patients. Pathological examination showed discrete foci of myelin vacuolization and swollen axis cylinders or large areas in the gray and white matter of fibrinoid necrosis, edema, and fibrin microthrombi.

Optic neuropathy has been reported following nitrosourea administration with cranial irradiation that included the anterior visual system (205). The optic chiasm in these patients showed severe demyelination that may reflect toxic synergy between CCNU and radiation.

Intra-arterial BCNU has been reported to produce severe neurotoxicity in 33–48% of patients. Patients develop an encephalopathy acutely following the infusion and, over several weeks to months, develop progressive deficits such as encephalopathy, hemiparesis, field deficits, or seizures (206–209). Neurological deterioration may be associated with or preceded by severe ocular toxicity. Pathologically, there is a vasculopathy which is similar to radiation necrosis but is confined to the BCNU perfusion territory. Miliary foci of necrosis with mineralizing axonopathy within the perfused arterial distribution also were reported (209). This may be difficult to distinguish from tumor recurrence by CT scan which demonstrates hypodensity of the white matter in the perfused territory with mass effect. There may be enhancement or irregular calcification, persistent white matter hypodensity, or ventricular dilation.

## XI. MISCELLANEOUS AGENTS

### A. VP-16

VP-16 or etoposide has little or no neurotoxicity even in high doses (210). Peripheral neuropathy is rare (211) and mild disorientation seen during administration of high doses may be due to intoxication by the large volumes of ethanol included with the chemotherapy (212).

### B. Taxol

Taxol is a promised new agent which has a dose-limiting neuropathy seen with doses of more than 200 mg/m$^2$. The neuropathy is predominantly sensory, with reduced or absent deep tendon reflexes, small- and large-fiber sensory loss, and occasional burning dysesthesias. Symptoms begin within 1 day to 3 weeks of taxol administration (213) and improve with discontinuation of the drug. Patients may also develop perioral numbness (214), weakness, or an autonomic neuropathy. Taxol likely produces neuropathy through its actions on the microtubules of the dorsal root ganglion cells, axons, and Schwann cells. Nerve growth factor (NGF) prevents taxol neuropathy in mice (215) and trials of NGF in patients receiving taxol will soon be under way.

### C. Suramin

Suramin may be useful in the treatment of refractory prostate cancer. It produces a severe polyneuropathy in 10% of patients in one report (216). These patients developed paresthesias in the face or limbs followed by progressive weakness of the proximal muscles of the legs and arms. Two patients progressed to complete limb and trunk paralysis over several weeks, with bulbar involvement requiring intubation and ventilation. There was evidence of an autonomic neuropathy as well. Two patients developed a syndrome resembling Guillain-Barré syndrome.

### D. Intrathecal Thio-TEPA

Thio-TEPA, although not routinely used at present, has been reported to produce a myelopathy with paraparesis (217).

## REFERENCES

1. Jolivet J, Cowan KH, Curt GA, et al. The pharmacology and clinical use of methotrexate. N Engl J Med 1983;309:1094–1104.
2. Bleyer WA. Neurologic sequelae of methotrexate and ionizing radiation: a new classification. Cancer Treat Rep 1981; 65:89–98.
3. Mott MG, Stevenson P, Wood CBS. Methotrexate meningitis. Lancet 1972; 2:656.
4. Geiser CF, Bishop Y, Jaffe N, et al. Adverse effects of intrathecal methotrexate in children with acute leukemia in remission. Blood 1975; 45:189–195.
5. Sullivan MP, Moon TE, Trueworthy R, et al. Combination intrathecal therapy for meningeal leukemia: two versus three drugs. Blood 1977; 50:471–479.
6. Bernstein ML, Sobel DB, Wimmer RS. Noncardiogenic pulmonary edema following injection of methotrexate into the cerebrospinal fluid. Cancer 1982; 50:866–868.
7. Back EH. Death after intrathecal methotrexate. Lancet 1969; 2:1005.
8. Ten Hoeve RF, Twijnstra A. A lethal neurotoxic reaction after intraventricular methotrexate administration. Cancer 1988; 62:2111–2113.
9. Spiegel RJ, Cooper PR, Blum RH, et al. Treatment of massive intrathecal overdose by ventriculolumbar perfusion. N Engl J Med 1984; 311:386–388.
10. Bagshawe KD, MacGrath IT, Golding PR. Intrathecal methotrexate. Lancet 1969; 2: 1258.
11. Saiki JH, Thompson S, Smith F, Atkinson R. Paraplegia following intrathecal chemotherapy. Cancer 1972; 29:370–374.
12. Luddy RE, Gilman PA. Paraplegia following intrathecal methotrexate. J Pediatr 1973; 83:988–992.

13. Bleyer WA, Drake JC, Chabner BA. Neurotoxicity and elevated cerebrospinal-fluid methotrexate concentration in meningeal leukemia. N Engl J Med 1973; 289:770–773.
14. Gagliano R, Costanzi JJ. Paraplegia following intrathecal methotrexate. Cancer 1976; 37:1663–1668.
15. Skullerud K, Halvorsen K. Encephalomyelopathy following intrathecal methotrexate treatment in a child with acute leukemia. Cancer 1985; 42:1211–1215.
16. Clark AW, Cohen SR, Nissenblatt MJ, et al. Paraplegia following intrathecal chemotherapy. Cancer 1982; 50:42–47.
17. Walker RW, Allen JC, Rosen G, Caparros B. Transient cerebral dysfunction secondary to high-dose methotrexate. J Clin Oncol 1986; 4:1845–1850.
18. Martino RL, Benson AB, Merritt JA, et al. Transient neurologic dysfunction following moderate-dose methotrexate for undifferentiated lymphoma. Cancer 1984; 54:2003–2005.
19. Phillips PC, Dhawan V, Strother SC, et al. Reduced cerebral glucose metabolism and increased brain capillary permeability following high-dose methotrexate chemotherapy: a positron emission tomographic study. Ann Neurol 1987; 21:59–63.
20. Phanthumchinda K, Intragumtorchai T, Kasantikul V. Stroke-like syndrome, mineralizing microangiopathy, and neuroaxonal dystrophy following intrathecal methotrexate therapy. Neurology 1991; 41:1847–1848.
21. Yim YS, Mahoney DH, Oshman DG. Hemiparesis and ischemic changes of the white matter after intrathecal therapy for children with acute lymphocytic leukemia. Cancer 1991; 67:2058–2061.
22. McIntosh S, Aspnes GT. Encephalopathy following CNS prophylaxis in childhood lymphoblastic leukemia. Pediatrics 1973; 52:612–615.
23. Rubinstein LJ, Herman MM, Long TF, Wilbur JR. Disseminated necrotizing leukoencephalopathy: a complication of treated central nervous system leukemia and lymphoma. Cancer 1975; 35:291–305.
24. Price RA, Birdwell DA. The central nervous system in childhood leukemia. Cancer 1978; 42:717–728.
25. Liu HM, Maurer HS, Vongsvivut S, Conwa JJ. Methotrexate encephalopathy. Hum Pathol 1978; 9:635–648.
26. Allen JC, Rosen G, Mehta BM, Horten B. Leukoencephalopathy following high-dose IV methotrexate chemotherapy with leucovorin rescue. Cancer Treat Rep 1980; 64:1261–1273.
27. Ch'ien LT, Aur RJA, Verzosa MS, et al. Progression of methotrexate-induced leukoencephalopathy in children with leukemia. Med Pediatr Oncol 1981; 9:133–141.
28. Ojeda VJ. Necrotising leucoencephalopathy associated with intrathecal/intraventricular methotrexate therapy. Med J Aust 1982; 2:289–293.
29. Cruz-Sanchez FF, Artigas J, Cervos-Navarro J, et al. Brain lesions following combined treatment with methotrexate and craniospinal irradiation. J Neurooncol 1991; 10:165–171.
30. Jacobs P, Rutherford GS, King HS, Vincent M. Methotrexate encephalopathy. Eur J Cancer 1991; 27:1061–1062.
31. Di Chiro G, Arimitsu T, Brooks RA, et al. Computed tomography profiles of

periventricular hypodensity in hydrocephalus and leukoencephalopathy. Radiology 1979; 130:661–665.
32. Shalen PR, Ostrow PT, Glass PJ. Enhancement of the white matter following prophylactic therapy of the central nervous system for leukemia. Radiology 1981; 140:409–412.
33. Duffner PK, Cohen ME, Brecher ML, et al. CT abnormalities and altered methotrexate clearance in children with CNS leukemia. Neurology 1984; 34:229–233.
34. Peylan-Ramu N, Poplack DG, Pizzo PA, et al. Abnormal CT scans of the brain in asymptomatic children with acute lymphocytic leukemia after prophylactic treatment of the central nervous system with radiation and intrathecal 124 Cutting HO. Inappropriate secretion of antidiuretic hormone secondary to vincristine therapy. Am J Med 1971; 51:269–271.
35. Shapiro WR, Chernik NL, Posner JB. Necrotizing encephalopathy following intraventricular instillation of methotrexate. Arch Neurol 1973; 28:96–102.
36. Shibutani M, Okeda R, Hori A, Schipper H. Methotrexate-related multifocal axonopathy. Acta Neuropathol 1989; 79:333–335.
37. Gangji D, Reaman GH, Cohen SR, et al. Leukoencephalopathy and elevated levels of myelin basic protein in the cerebrospinal fluid of patients with acute lymphoblastic leukemia. N Engl J Med 1980; 303:19–21.
38. Griffin TW, Rasey JS, Bleyer WA. The effect of photon irradiation on blood-brain barrier permeability to methotrexate in mice. Cancer 1977; 40:1109–1111.
39. Storm AJ, Van Der Kogel AJ, Nooter K. Effect of X-irradiation on the pharmacokinetics of methotrexate in rats: alteration of the blood-brain barrier. Eur J Cancer Clin Oncol 1985; 21:759–764.
40. Bourke RS, West CR, Chheda G, et al. Kinetics of entry and distribution of 5-fluorouracil in cerebrospinal fluid and brain following intravenous injection in a primate. Cancer Res 1973; 33:1735–1746.
41. Chadwick M, Rogers WI. The physiologic disposition of 5-fluorouracil in mice bearing solid L1210 lymphocytic leukemia. Cancer Res 1972; 32:1045–1056.
42. Riehl J, Brown WJ. Acute cerebellar syndrome secondary to 5-fluorouracil therapy. Neurology 1964; 14:961–967.
43. Moertel CG, Reitemeier RJ, Bolton CF, et al. Cerebellar ataxia associated with fluorinated pyrimidine therapy. Cancer Treat Rep 1964; 41:15–18.
44. Horton J, Olson KB, Sullivan J, et al. 5-fluorouracil in cancer: An improved regimen. Ann Intern Med 1970; 73:897–900.
45. Bagley CM. Single I.V. doses of 5-fluorouracil: A phase 1 study. Proc Am Assoc Cancer Res 1975; 16:12.
46. Koenig H, Patel A. A biochemical basis for 5-fluorouracil neurotoxicity. Arch Neurol 1970; 23:155–160.
47. Lynch HT, Droszcz CP, Albano WA, Lynch JF. Organic brain syndrome secondary to 5-fluorouracil. Dis Colon Rectum 1981; 24:130–131.
48. Bixenman WW, Nichols JV, Warwick OH. Oculomotor disturbances associated with 5-fluorouracil chemotherapy. Am J Ophthalmol 1977; 83:789–793.
49. Bergevin PR, Patwardhan VC, Weissman J, et al. Neurotoxicity of 5-fluorouracil. Lancet 1975; 410.

50. Adams JW, Bofenkamp TM, Kobrin J, et al. Recurrent acute toxic optic neuropathy secondary to 5-FU. Cancer Treat Rep 1984; 68:565.
51. Forsyth PA, Kimmel DW, Hook C, et al. Multifocal inflammatory leukoencephalopathy in patients receiving adjuvant therapy with 5-fluorouracil and levamisole for adenocarcinoma of the colon. Ann Neurol 1991; 30:273.
52. Peterson K, Rosenblum MK, Alvord E, Posner JB. Effect of radiation therapy on demyelinating lesions of the brain. Neurology 1992 (submitted).
53. Campbell TN, Howell SB, Pfeifle CP, et al. High-dose allopurinol modulation of 5-FU toxicity: phase 1 trial of an outpatient dose schedule. Cancer Treat Rep 1982; 66:1723–1727.
54. Howell SB, Pfeifle CE, Wung WE. Effect of allopurinol on the toxicity of high-dose 5-fluorouracil administered by intermittent bolus injection. Cancer 1983; 51: 220–225.
55. Muggia FM, Camacho FJ, et al. Weekly 5-fluorouracil combined with PALA: Toxic and therapeutic effects in colorectal cancer. Cancer Treat Rep 1987; 71:253–256.
56. Heier MS, Fossa SD. Neurologic manifestations in a phase 2 study of 13 patients treated with doxyfluridine. Acta Neurol Scand 1985; 72:171–175.
57. Heier MS, Fossa SD. Wernicke-Korsakoff-like syndrome in patients with colorectal carcinoma treated with high-dose doxyfluridine (5'-dFUrd). Acta Neurol Scand 1986; 73:449–457.
58. Kuzahara S, Ohkoshi N, Hashimoto H, et al. Subacute leucoencephalopathy induced by carmofur, a 5-fluorouracil derivative. J Neurol 1987; 234:365–370.
59. Gormley P, Gangji D, Wood JH, Poplack DG. Pharmacokinetic study of cerebrospinal fluid penetration of cis-diamminedichloroplatinum (2). Cancer Chemother Pharmacol 1981; 5:247–260.
60. Kedar A, Cohen ME, Freeman AI. Peripheral neuropathy as a complication of cis-dichlorodiammineplatinum II treatment: a case report. Cancer Treat Rep 1978; 62: 819–821.
61. Siegal T, Haim N. Cisplatin-induced peripheral neuropathy. Cancer 1990; 66:1117–1123.
62. Grunberg SM, Sonka S, Stevenson LL, Muggia FM. Progressive paresthesias after cessation of therapy with very high dose cisplatin. Cancer Chemother Pharmacol 1989; 25:62–64.
63. Mollman JE, Hogan WM, Glover DJ, McCluskey LF. Unusual presentation of cis-platinum neuropathy. Neurology 1988; 38:488–490.
64. Ozols RF, Ostchega Y, Myers CE, et al. High-dose cisplatin in hypertonic saline in refractory ovarian cancer. J Clin Oncol 1985; 3:1246–1250.
65. Hemphill M, Pestronk A, Walsh T, et al. Sensory neuropathy in cis-platinum chemotherapy. Neurology 1980; 30:429.
66. Roelofs R, Hrushesky W, Rogin J, Rosenberg L. Neurology 1984; 34:934–938.
67. Thompson SW, Davis LE, Kornfeld M, Hilgers RD, Standefer JC. Cisplatin neuropathy: clinical, electrophysiologic, morphologic, and toxicologic studies. Cancer 1984; 54:1269–1275.
68. Ongerboer de Visser BW, Tiessens G. Polyneuropathy induced by cisplatin. Prog Exp Tumor Res 1985; 29:190–196.

69. Mollman JE, Glover DJ, Hogan WM, Furman RE. Cisplatin neuropathy: risk factors, prognosis and protection by WR-2721. Cancer 1988; 61:2192–2195.
70. Gerritsen Van Der Hoop, Vecht CJ, Van Der Burg MEL, et al. Prevention of cisplatin neurotoxicity with an ACTH(4–9) analogue in patients with ovarian cancer. N Engl J Med 1990; 322:89–94.
71. Apfel SC, Lipton RB, Arezzo JC, Kessler JA. Nerve growth factor prevents toxic neuropathy in mice. Ann Neurol 1991; 29:87–90.
72. Melamed LB, Selim MA, Schuchman D. Cisplatin ototoxicity in gynecologic cancer patients. Cancer 1985; 55:41–43.
73. Guthrie TH, Gynther L. Acute deafness: a complication of high-dose cisplatin. Arch Otolaryngol 1985; 111:344–345.
74. Schell MJ, McHaney VA, Green AA, et al. Hearing loss in children and young adults receiving cisplatin with or without prior cranial irradiation. J Clin Oncol 1989; 7:754–760.
75. Aguilar-Markulis NV, Beckley S, Priore R, Mettlin C. Auditory toxicity effects of long-term cis-dichlorodiammineplatinum II therapy in genitourinary cancer patients. J Surg Oncol 1981; 16:111–123.
76. McHaney VA, Thibadoux G, Hayes FA, et al. Hearing loss in children receiving cisplatin chemotherapy. J Pediatr 1983; 102; 314–317.
77. Stadnicki SW, Fleischman RW, Schaeppi U, Merriam P. Cisdichlorodiammine platinum (II) (NSC–119875): hearing loss and other toxic effects in rhesus monkeys. Cancer Chemother Rep 1975; 59:467–480.
78. Granowetter L, Rosenstock JG, Packer RJ. Enhanced cis-platinum neurotoxicity in pediatric patients with brain tumors. J Neurooncol 1983; 1:293–297.
79. Schaeffer SD, Wright CG, Post JD, Frenkel EP. Cis-platinum vestibular toxicity. Cancer 1981; 47:857–859.
80. Black FO, Myers EN, Schramm VL, et al. Cisplatin vestibular ototoxicity: preliminary report. Laryngoscope 1982; 92:1363–1368.
81. Walsh TJ, Clark AW, Parhad IM, Green WR. Neurotoxic effects of cisplatin therapy. Arch Neurol 1982; 39:719–720.
82. Ostrow S, Hahn D, Wiernik PH, et al. Ophthalmologic toxicity after cis-dichlorodiammineplatinum II therapy. Cancer Treat Rep 1978; 62:1591–1594.
83. Wilding G, Caruso R, Lawrence T, et al. Retinal toxicity after high-dose cisplatin therapy. J Clin Oncol 1985; 3:1683–1689.
84. Eeles R, Tait DM, Peckham MJ. Lhermitte's sign as a complication of cisplatin-containing chemotherapy. Cancer Treat Rep 1986; 70:905–907.
85. Ventafridda V, Caraceni A, Martini C, et al. On the significance of Lhermitte's sign in oncology. J Neurooncol 1991; 10:133–137.
86. Pomes A, Frustaci S, Cattaino G, et al. Local neurotoxicity of cisplatin after intra-arterial chemotherapy. Acta Neurol Scand 1986; 73:302–303.
87. Castellanos AM, Glass JP, Yung WKA. Regional nerve injury after intra-arterial chemotherapy. Neurology 1987; 37:834–837.
88. Mead GM, Arnold AM, Green JA, et al. Epileptic seizures associated with cisplatin administration. Cancer Treat Rep 1982; 66:1719–1722.
89. Stewart DJ, Leavens M, Maor M, et al. Human central nervous system distribution

of cis-diamminedichloroplatinum and use as a radiosensitizer in malignant brain tumors. Cancer Res 1982; 42:2474–2479.
90. Blisard KS, Harrington DA. Cisplatin-induced neurotoxicity with seizures in frogs. Ann Neurol 1989; 26:336–341.
91. Doll DC, List AF, Greco FA, et al. Acute vascular ischemic events after cisplatin-based combination chemotherapy for germ-cell tumors of the testes. Ann Intern Med 1986; 105:48–51.
92. Berman IJ, Mann MP. Seizures and transient cortical blindness associated with cis-platinum (II) diamminedichloride (PPD) therapy in a thirty-year old man. Cancer 1980; 45:746–766.
93. Pippit CH, Muss HB, Homesley HD, et al. Cisplatin-associated cortical blindness. Gynecol Oncol 1981; 12:253–155.
94. Diamond SB, Rudolph SH, Lubicz SS, et al. Cerebral blindness in association with cis-platinum chemotherapy for advanced carcinoma of the fallopian tube. Obstet Gynecol 1982; 59:84S–86S.
95. Cohen RJ, Cuneo RA, Cruciger MP, et al. Transient left homonymous hemianopsia and encephalopathy following treatment of testicular carcinoma with cisplatinum, vinblastine, and bleomycin. J Clin Oncol 1983; 1:392–393.
96. Walker RW, Cairncross JG, Posner JB. Cerebral herniation in patients receiving cisplatin. J Neurooncol 1988; 6:61–65.
97. Ritch PS, Cis-dichlorodiammineplatinum II-induced syndrome of inappropriate secretion of antidiuretic hormone. Cancer 1988;61:448–450.
98. Hayes FA, Green AA, Senzer N, Pratt CB. Tetany: a complication of cis-dichlorodiammine platinum II therapy. Cancer Treat Rep 1979; 63:547–548.
99. Walker RW, Rosenblum MK, Kempin SJ, Christian MC. Carboplatin-associated thrombotic microangiopathic hemolytic anemia. Cancer 1989; 64:1017–1020.
100. Stewart DJ. Intraarterial chemotherapy of primary and metastatic brain tumors. In: Rottenberg DA, ed. Neurological complications of cancer treatment. Boston: Butterworth-Heinemann, 1991:143–170.
101. Bunt AA, Lund RD. Vinblastine-induced blockage of orthograde and retrograde axonal transport of protein in retinal ganglion cells. Exp Neurol 1974; 45:288–297.
102. Iqbal Z, Ochs S. Uptake of vinca alkaloids into mammalian nerve and its subcellular components. J Neurochem 1980; 34:59–68.
103. Shelanski ML, Wisniewski H. Neurofibrillary degeneration induced by vincristine therapy. Arch Neurol 1969; 20:199–206.
104. Sahenk Z, Brady ST, Mendell JR. Studies on the pathogenesis of vincristine-induced neuropathy. Muscle Nerve 1987; 10:80–84.
105. Gerzun K, Ochs S, Todd GC. Polarity of vincristine, vindesine and vinblastine in relation to neurologic effects, abstracted. Proc Am Assoc Cancer Res 1979; 20:46.
106. Nelson RL, Dyke RW, Root MA. Comparative pharmacokinetics of vindesine, vincristine and vinblastine in patients with cancer. Cancer Treat Rev 1980; 7(Suppl):17-24.
107. Chan SY, Worth R, Ochs S. Block of axoplasmic transport in vitro by vinca alkaloids. J Neurobiol 1980; 11:251–264.
108. Bohannon RA, Miller DG, Diamond HD. Vincristine in the treatment of lymphomas and leukemias. Cancer Res 1963; 23:613–621.

109. Sandler SG, Tobin W, Henderson ES. Vincristine-induced neuropathy: a clinical study of fifty leukemic patients. Neurology 1969; 19:367–374.
110. Casey EB, Jellife AM, Le Quesne PM, Millet YL. Vincristine neuropathy: clinical and electrophysiologic observations. Brain 1973; 96:69–86.
111. Holland JF, Scharlau C, Gailani S, et al. Vincristine treatment of advanced cancer: A cooperative study of 392 cases. Cancer Res 1973; 33:1258–1264.
112. Levitt LP, Prager D. Mononeuropathy due to vincristine toxicity. Neurology 1975; 25:894–895.
113. Jackson DV, McMahan RA, Pope EK, et al. Clinical trial of folinic acid to reduce vincristine neurotoxicity. Cancer Chemother Pharmacol 1986; 17:281–284.
114. Jackson DV, Pope EK, McMahan RA, et al. Clinical trial of pyridoxine to reduce vincristine neurotoxicity. J Neurooncol 1986; 4:37–41.
115. Jackson DV, Wells HB, Atkins JN, et al. Amelioration of vincristine neurotoxicity by glutamic acid. Am J Med 1988; 84:1016–1022.
116. Di Gregorio F, Favaro G, Panozzo C, Fiori MG. Efficacy of ganglioside treatment in reducing functional alterations induced by vincristine in rabbit peripheral nerves. Cancer Chemother Pharmacol 1990; 26:31–36.
117. Whitelaw DM, Cowan DH, Cassidy FR, Patterson TA. Clinical experience with vincristine. Cancer Chemother Rep 1963; 30:13–20.
118. Watkins SM, Griffin JP. High incidence of vincristine-induced neuropathy in lymphomas. Br Med J 1978; 1:610–612.
119. Cassady JR, Tonnesen GL, Wolfe LC, Sallan SE. Augmentation of vincristine neurotoxicity by irradiation of peripheral nerves. Cancer Treat Rep 1980; 64:963–965.
120. Byfield JE. Ionizing radiation and vincristine: possible neurotoxic synergism. Radiol Clin Biol 1972; 41:129–138.
121. Weiden PL, Wright SE. Vincristine neurotoxicity. N Engl J Med 1972; 286:1369–1370.
122. Hogan-Dann CM, Fellmeth WG, McGuire SA, Kiley VA. Polyneuropathy following vincristine therapy in two patients with Charcot-Marie-Tooth syndrome. JAMA 1984; 252:2862–2863.
123. Miller BR. Neurotoxicity and vincristine. JAMA 1985; 253:2045.
124. Mubashir BA, Bart JB. Vincristine neurotoxicity. N Engl J Med 1972; 287:517.
125. O'Callaghan MJ, Ekert H. Vincristine toxicity unrelated to dose. Arch Dis Child 1976; 51:289–292.
126. Thant M, Hawley RJ, Smith MT, et al. Possible enhancement of vincristine neuropathy by VP-16. Cancer 1982; 49:859–864.
127. Griffiths JD, Stark RJ, Ding JC, Cooper IA. Vincristine neurotoxicity enhanced in combination chemotherapy including both teniposide and vincristine. Cancer Treat Rep 1986; 70:519–521.
128. Tobin W, Sandler SG. Neurophysiologic alterations induced by vincristine (NSC-67574). Cancer Chemother Rep 1968; 52:519–526.
129. McLeod JG, Penny R. Vincristine neuropathy: an electrophysiological and histological study. J Neurol Neurosurg Psychiatry 1969; 32:297–304.
130. Bradley WG, Lassman LP, Pearce GW, Walton JN. The neuromyopathy of vincristine in man: clinical, electrophysiological and pathological studies. J Neurol Sci 1970; 10:107–131.

131. Guiheneuc P, Ginet J, Groleau JY, Rojouan J. Early phase of vincristine neuropathy in man. J Neurol Sci 1980; 45:355–366.
132. Gottlieb RJ, Cuttner J. Vincristine-induced bladder atony. Cancer 1971; 28: 674–675.
133. Raphaelson MI, Stevens JC, Newmwan RP. Vincristine neuropathy with bowel and bladder atony, mimicking spinal cord compression. Cancer Treat Rep 1983; 67: 604–605.
134. Aisner J, Weiss HD, Chang P, Wiernik PH. Orthostatic hypotension during combination chemotherapy with vincristine (NSC-67574). Cancer Chemother Rep 1974; 58: 927–930.
135. DiBella NJ. Vincristine-induced orthostatic hypotension: a prospective clinical study. Cancer Treat Rep 1980; 64:359–360.
136. Hirvonen HE, Salmi TT, Heinonen E, et al. Vincristine treatment of acute lymphoblastic leukemia induces transient autonomic cardioneuropathy. Cancer 1989; 64: 801–805.
137. Suskind RM, Brusilow SW, Zehr J. Syndrome of inappropriate secretion of antidiuretic hormone produced by vincristine toxicity (with bioassay of ADH level). J Pediatr 1972; 81:90–92.
138. Stuart MJ, Cuaso C, Miller M, Oski FA. Syndrome of recurrent increased secretion of antidiuretic hormone following multiple doses of vincristine. Blood 1975; 45: 315–320.
139. Robertson GL, Bhoopalam N, Zelkowitz LJ. Vincristine neurotoxicity and abnormal secretion of antidiuretic hormone. Arch Intern Med 1973; 132:717–720.
140. Ginsgerg SJ, Comis RL, Fitzpatrick AV. Vinblastine and inappropriate ADH secretion. N Engl J Med 1977; 296:941.
141. Whittaker JA, Griffith IP. Recurrent laryngeal nerve paralysis in patients receiving vincristine and vinblastine. Br Med J 1977; 1:1251–1252.
142. Brook J, Schreiber W. Vocal cord paralysis: a toxic reaction to vinblastine (NSC-49842) therapy. Cancer Chemother Rep 1971; 55:591–593.
143. Sanderson PA, Kuwabara T, Cogan DG. Optic neuropathy presumably caused by vincristine therapy. Am J Ophthalmol 1976; 81:146–150.
144. Norton SW, Stockman JA. Unilateral optic neuropathy following vincristine chemotherapy. J Pediatr Ophthalmol Strabismus 1979; 16:190–193.
145. Albert DM, Wong VG, Henderson ES. Ocular complications of vincristine therapy. Arch Ophthalmol 1967; 78:709–713.
146. Schochet SS, Lampert PW, Earle KM. Neuronal changes induced by intrathecal vincristine sulfate. J Neuropathol Exp Neurol 1968; 27:645–658.
147. Shepherd DA, Steuber CP, Starling K, et al. Accidental intrathecal administration of vincristine. Med Pediatr Oncol 1978; 5:85–88.
148. Slyter H, Liwnicz B, Herrick MK, Mason R. Fatal myeloencephalopathy caused by intrathecal vincristine. Neurology 1980; 30:867–871.
149. Gaidys WG, Dickerman JD, Walters CI, et al. Intrathecal vincristine. Cancer 1983; 52:799–801.
150. Williams ME, Walker AN, Bracikowski JP, et al. Ascending myeloencephalopathy due to intrathecal vincristine sulfate. Cancer 1983; 51:2041–2047.

151. Dyke RW. Treatment of inadvertent intrathecal injection of vincristine. N Engl J Med 1989; 321:1270–1271.
152. Whittaker JA, Parry DH, Bunch PC, Weatherall DJ. Coma associated with vincristine therapy. Br Med J 1973; 4:335–337.
153. Johnson FL, Bernstein ID, Hartmann JR, et al. Seizures associated with vincristine sulfate therapy. J Pediatr 1973; 82:699–702.
154. Carpentieri U, Lockhart LH. Ataxia and athetosis as side effects of chemotherapy with vincristine in non-Hodgkins lymphoma. Cancer Treat Rep 1978; 62:561–562.
155. Byrd RL, Rohrbaugh TM, Raney B, Norris DG. Transient cortical blindness secondary to vincristine therapy in childhood malignancies. Cancer 1981; 47:37–40.
156. Awidi AS. Blindness and vincristine. Ann Intern Med 1980; 93:781.
157. DeAngelis LM, Gnecco C, Taylor L, et al. Evolution of neuropathy and myopathy during intensive vincristine/corticosteroid chemotherapy for non-Hodgkin's lymphoma. Cancer 1991; 67:2241–2246.
158. Slevin ML, Piall EM, Aherne GW, et al. Effect of dose and schedule on pharmacokinetics of high-dose cytosine arabinoside in plasma and cerebrospinal fluid. J Clin Oncol 1983; 1:546–551.
159. Zimm S, Collins JM, Miser J, et al. Cytosine arabinoside cerebrospinal fluid kinetics. Clin Pharmacol Ther 1984; 35:826–830.
160. Breuer AC, Pitman SW, Dawson DM, Schoene WC. Paraparesis following intrathecal cytosine arabinoside. Cancer 1977; 40:2817–2822.
161. Wolff L, Zighelboim J, Gale RP. Paraplegia following intrathecal cytosine arabinoside. Cancer 1979; 43:83–85.
162. Mena H, Garcia JH, Velandia F. Central and peripheral myelinopathy associated with systemic neoplasia and chemotherapy. Cancer 1981; 48:1724–1737.
163. Bates SE, Raphaelson MI, Price RA, et al. Ascending myelopathy after chemotherapy for central nervous system acute lymphoblastic leukemia: correlation with cerebrospinal fluid myelin basic protein. Med Pediatr Oncol 1985; 13:4–13.
164. Dunton SF, Nitschke R, Spruce WE, et al. Progressive ascending paralysis following administration of intrathecal and intravenous cytosine arabinoside. Cancer 1986; 57:1083–1088.
165. Eden OB, Goldie W, Wood T. Etcubanas E. Seizures following intrathecal cytosine arabinoside in young children with acute lymphoblastic leukemia. Cancer 1978; 42:53–58.
166. Lazarus HM, Herzig RH, Herzig GP, et al. Central nervous system toxicity of high-dose systemic cytosine arabinoside. Cancer 1981; 48:2577–2582.
167. Grossman L, Baker MA, Sutton DMC, Deck JHN. Central nervous system toxicity of high-dose cytosine arabinoside. Med Pediatr Oncol 1983; 11:246–250.
168. Winkelman MD, Hines JD. Cerebellar degeneration caused by high-dose cytosine arabinoside: a clinical pathological study. Ann Neurol 1983; 14:520–527.
169. Salinsky MC, Levine RL, Aubuchon JP, Schutta HS. Acute cerebellar dysfunction with high-dose Ara-C therapy. Cancer 1983; 51:426–429.
170. Hwang T, Yung A, Estey EH, Fields WS. Central nervous system toxicity with high-dose Ara-C. Neurology 1985; 35:1475–1479.
171. Benger A, Browman GP, Walker IR. Clinical evidence of a cumulative effect of

high-dose cytarabine on the cerebellum in patients with acute leukemia: a leukemia intergroup report. Cancer Treat Rep 1985; 69:240–241.
172. Nand S, Messmore HL, Patel R, et al. Neurotoxicity associated with systemic high-dose cytosine arabinoside. J Clin Oncol 1986; 4:571–575.
173. Herzig RH, Hines JD, Herzig GP, et al. Cerebellar toxicity with high-dose cytosine arabinoside. J Clin Oncol 1987; 5:927–932.
174. Damon LE, Mass R, Linker CA. The association between high-dose cytarabine neurotoxicity and renal insufficiency. J Clin Oncol 1989; 7:1563–1568.
175. Watson PR, Brubaker LH, Yaghmai F. Severe central nervous system toxicity from high-dose cytarabine: expressive aphasia occurring after the second day of treatment. Cancer Treat Rep 1985; 69:313–314.
176. Ritch PS, Hansen RM, Heuer DK. Ocular toxicity from high-dose cytosine arabinoside. Cancer 1983; 51:430–432.
177. Rudnick SA, Cadman EC, Capizzi RL, et al. High dose cytosine arabinoside (HDARAC) in refractory acute leukemia. Cancer 1979; 44:1189–1193.
178. Russell JA, Powles RL. Neuropathy due to cytosine arabinoside. Br Med J 1974; 14: 652–653.
179. Borgeat A, De Muralt B, Stalder M. Peripheral neuropathy associated with high-dose Ara-C therapy. Cancer 1986; 58:852–854.
180. Powell BL, Capizzi RL, Lyerly ES, Cooper MR. Peripheral neuropathy after high-dose cytosine arabinoside, daunorubicin, and asparaginase consolidation for acute nonlymphocytic leukemia. J Clin Oncol 1986; 4:95–97.
181. Scherokman B, Filling-Katz MR, Teil D. Brachial plexus neuropathy following high-dose cytarabine in acute monoblastic leukemia. Cancer Treat Rep 1985; 69: 1005–1006.
182. Luque FA, Selhorst JB, Petruska P. Parkinsonism induced by high-dose cytosine arabinoside. Mov Disord 1987; 2:219–222.
183. Leonard JV, Kay JDS. Acute encephalopathy and hyperammonaemia complicating treatment of acute lymphoblastic leukemia. Lancet 1986; 1:162.
184. Moure JM, Whitecar JP, Bodey GP. Electroencephalogram changes secondary to asparaginase. Arch Neurol 1970; 23:365–368.
185. Land VJ, Sutow WW, Fernbach DJ, et al. Toxicity of L-asparaginase in children with advanced leukemia. Cancer 1972; 30:339–347.
186. Lessner HE, Valenstein S, Kaplan R, et al. Phase 2 study of L-asparaginase in the treatment of pancreatic carcinoma. Cancer Treat Rep 1980; 64:1359–1361.
187. Cairo MS, Lazarus K, Gilmore RL, Baehner RL. Intracranial hemorrhage and focal seizures secondary to use of L-asparaginase during induction therapy of acute lymphocytic leukemia. J Pediatr 1980; 97:829–833.
188. Priest JR, Ramsay NKC, Latchaw RE, Lockman LA, et al. Thrombotic and hemorrhagic strokes complicating early therapy for childhood acute lymphoblastic leukemia. Cancer 1980; 46:1548–1554.
189. Priest JR, Ramsay NKC, Steinherz PG, Tubergen DG, et al. A syndrome of thrombosis and hemorrhage complicating L-asparaginase therapy for childhood acute lymphoblastic leukemia. J Pediatr 1982; 100:984–989.

190. Feinberg WM, Swenson MR. Cerebrovascular complications of L-asparaginase therapy. Neurology 1988; 38:127–133.
191. Zilkha A, Diaz AS. Computed tomography in the diagnosis of superior sagittal sinus thrombosis. J Comput Assist Tomogr 1980; 4:124–126.
192. Macchi PJ, Grossman RI, Gomori JM, et al. High field MR imaging of cerebral venous thrombosis. J Comput Assist Tomogr 1986; 10:10–15.
193. Moots PL, Walker RW, Sze G, Mast J. Diagnosis of dural venous sinus thrombosis by magnetic resonance imaging. Ann Neurol 1987; 22:431–432.
194. Oliverio VT, Denham C, DeVita VT, et al. Some pharmacologic properties of a new antitumor agent, N-isopropyl-alpha-(2-methylhydrazino)-p-toluamide, hydrochloride (NSC-77213). Cancer Chemother Rep 1964; 42:1–7.
195. Weiss HD, Walker MD, Wiernik PH. Neurotoxicity of commonly used antineoplastic agents. N Engl J Med 1974; 291:127–133.
196. Carney MWP, Ravindran A, Lewis DS. Manic psychosis associated with procarbazine. Br Med J 1982; 284:82–83.
197. Lee IP, Lucier GW. The potentiation of barbiturate-induced narcosis by procarbazine. J Pharmacol Exp Ther 1976; 196:586–593.
198. Brade WP, Herdrich K, Varini M. Ifosfamide—pharmacology, safety and therapeutic potential. Cancer Treat Rep 1985; 12:1–47.
199. Meanwell CA, Blake AE, Kelly KA, et al. Prediction of ifosfamide/mesna associated encephalopathy. Eur J Cancer Clin Oncol 1986; 22:815–819.
200. Pratt CB, Goren MP, Meyer WH, et al. Ifosfamide neurotoxicity is related to previous cisplatin treatment for pediatric solid tumors. J Clin Oncol 1990; 8:1399–1401.
201. Weiss RB. Ifosfamide vs cyclophosphamide in cancer therapy. Oncology 1991; 5:67–76.
202. Watkins SM, Husband DJ, Green JA, et al. Ifosfamide encephalopathy: a reappraisal. Eur J Cancer Clin Oncol 1989; 25:1303–1310.
203. Breuer AC, Blank NK, Schoene WC. Multifocal pontine lesions in cancer patients treated with chemotherapy and CNS radiotherapy. Cancer 1978; 41:2112–2120.
204. Burger PC, Kamenar E, Schold SC, et al. Encephalomyelopathy following high-dose BCNU therapy. Cancer 1981; 48:1318–1327.
205. Wilson WB, Perez GM, Kleinschmidt-DeMasters. Sudden onset of blindness in patients treated with oral CCNU and low-dose cranial irradiation. Cancer 1987; 59:901–907.
206. Mahaley MS, Whaley RA, Blue M, et al. Central neurotoxicity following intracarotid BCNU chemotherapy for malignant gliomas. J Neurooncol 1986; 3:297–314.
207. Kleinschmidt-DeMasters BK. Intracarotid BCNU leukoencephalopathy. Cancer 1986; 57:1276–1280.
208. Walker RW, Gargan R, Delattre J, Rosenblum M, Shapiro WR. Complications in intra-arterial (IA) BCNU in the treatment of malignant gliomas. Proc ASCO 1988; 7:84.
209. Rosenblum MK, Delattre J, Walker RW, Shapiro WR. Fatal necrotizing encepha-

lopathy complicating treatment of malignant gliomas with intra-arterial BCNU and irradiation: a pathologic study. J Neurooncol 1989; 7:269–281.
210. Postmus PE, Mulder NH, Sleijfer DT, et al. High-dose etoposide for refractory malignancies: a phase 1 study. Cancer Treat Rep 1984; 68:1471–1474.
211. O'Dwyer PJ, Leyland-Jones B, Alonso MT, et al. Etoposide (VP-16-213): current status of an active anticancer drug. N Engl J Med 1985; 312:692–700.
212. Wolff SN, Fer MF, McKay CM, et al. High-dose VP-16-213 and autologous bone marrow transplantation for refractory malignancies: a phase 1 study. J Clin Oncol 1983; 1:701–705.
213. Lipton RB, Apfel SC, Dutcher JP, et al. Taxol produces a predominantly sensory neuropathy. Neurology 1989; 39:368–373.
214. Rowinsky EK, Cazenave LA, Donehower RC. Taxol: a novel investigational antimicrotubule agent. J Natl Cancer Inst 1990; 82:1247–1259.
215. Apfel SC, Arezzo JC, Lipson L, Kessler JA. Nerve growth factor prevents experimental cisplatin neuropathy. Ann Neurol 1992; 31:76–80.
216. La Rocca RV, Meer J, Gilliatt RW, et al. Suramin-induced polyneuropathy. Neurology 1990; 40:954–960.
217. Gutin PH, Levi JA, Wiernik PH, Walker MD. Treatment of malignant meningeal disease with intrathecal thio-TEPA: a phase 2 study. Cancer Treat Rep 1977; 61:885–887.

# 12
# Neurological Complications of Immunotherapy

**Jean-Yves Delattre, Felipe Vega B, and Qiming Chen**

*Groupe Hospitalier Pitié-Salpêtrière, Paris, France*

Immunotherapy is one of the modalities used in the treatment of cancer. The goal of immunotherapy is to elicit an immune reaction capable of eliminating or retarding tumor growth (Table 1). Promising results have been reported for certain malignancies such as hairy-cell leukemia, lymphoproliferative disorders, renal cell carcinoma, and melanoma. Unfortunately, neurotoxicity is an important limiting factor. Immunotherapy can affect the nervous system directly or indirectly (for example central nervous system [CNS] infection or lymphoma related to the consequences of immunosuppression). The purpose of this chapter is to describe some direct side effects of immunotherapy on the central and peripheral nervous system. The emphasis is on interferon and interleukin-2 (IL-2) which are now widely used in clinical practice. Glucocorticoids are reviewed elsewhere in this volume.

## I. LEVAMISOLE

Levamisole is an antihelmintic drug with immunostimulant properties in both animals and humans. It is mainly used in colon cancer in association with 5-fluorouracil (5-FU) (1). In dogs, treatment with levamisole induced the development of disseminated perivascular cuffing with mononuclear cells throughout the

**Table 1** Classification of Cancer Immunotherapies

Active immunotherapy
  Immune adjuvants (BCG, C parvum, levamisole)
  Interferons
  Interleukin-2
  Immunization with tumor-cell vaccines
Passive immunotherapy
  Antibodies (monoclonal or polyclonal)
    Alone or conjugated with toxins or radiolabels
  Cells
    Lymphokine-actived killer (LAK) cells
    Tumor infiltrating lymphocytes (TIL)
Combination of above approaches

brain and meninges without damage to the neural tissue. In the clinical setting, neurological complications of levamisole are rare. In two studies of 447 and 1179 patients treated with levamisole for cancer, only 1.3–3% of patients developed neurological symptoms (2,3) (Table 2).

An acute encephalopathy with lethargia, insomnia, and sometimes headache and nausea has been described (4,5). These mental status changes are usually mild and discontinuation of treatment is rarely necessary. Recently, Hook and coworkers (2) reported a multifocal inflammatory leukoencephalopathy in three patients treated with 5-FU and levamisole for colon cancer. The patients developed subacute decline in mental status and ataxia or unexplained episodes of loss of consciousness 3–5 months after the onset of chemotherapy. Gadolinium-enhanced magnetic resonance imaging (MRI) demonstrated multifocal enhancing white matter lesions. One patient had a cerebrospinal fluid (CSF) pleocytosis. Cerebral biopsy showed demyelinating lesions with axonal sparing and perivascular lymphocytic infiltrations similar to that described in multiple sclerosis (MS). Patients improved after cessation of chemotherapy and a short course of corticosteroid therapy. Several hypotheses were suggested to explain the pathogenesis of this disorder including exacerbation of a subclinical multiple sclerosis (because neurological deterioration has been reported in clinical trials of levamisole for MS) or direct toxic effect of levamisole and/or 5-FU on the CNS. Other neurological complications of levamisole include dysgeusia with a metallic taste and altered sense of smell; cramps and myalgias with stiffness of proximal muscles; dizziness; tremor; and rarely seizures. Anxiety and depression have also been reported. One patient developed diplopia and vertigo that quickly resolved when levamisole was discontinued (4).

**Table 2** Neurological Complications of Levamisole

| Complication | Signs/symptoms | Laboratory | Treatment/outcome |
|---|---|---|---|
| Acute encephalopathy | Lethargy<br>Confusion<br>Insomnia<br>Headache<br>Nausea | — | Usually no Rx needed<br>Reversible |
| Subacute encephalopathy with 5-FU (3–5 months after starting Rx) | Cognitive decline<br>Ataxia<br>Episodes of LOC | Increased CSF WBC<br>MRI: Multifocal enhancing white matter lesions<br>Biopsy: Demyelinating plaques<br>Perivascular lymphocytic infiltration | Glucocorticoids<br>DC chemotherapy |

Rx: Treatment. DC: Discontinuation. WBC: White blood cells. CSF: Cerebrospinal fluid. LOC: Loss of consciousness. MRI: Magnetic resonance imaging. 5-FU: 5-Fluorouracil.

## II. CYCLOSPORINE

Cyclosporine (CsA) is a potent immunosuppressive agent with little myelotoxicity. It is used in the prevention of graft rejection, including bone marrow transplantation (BMT) for malignancy. The main organs involved during CsA toxicity are the kidney, CNS, and liver. Hypertension is also frequent (6). Neurological complications occur in 10–30% of patients treated with CsA, especially in patients treated with high doses (Table 3). Severe headaches have been rarely reported.

A 10-Hz postural tremor of the extremities that is aggravated by action occurs in at least 20% of patients. In many cases, it diminishes with time or responds to lowering of the cyclosporine level. The pathogenesis of the tremor is unknown but could result from an activation of the sympathetic nervous system (7). Seizures, including untreatable status epilepticus (8), occur in 1.5–5% of patients after BMT (compared to 15–25% after cardiac or liver transplantation). Children are thought to be more susceptible than adults. Whether CsA is responsible for the seizures is not always clear, because these patients have many other reasons to develop seizures, including electrolyte imbalance, hypertension, administration of high-dose methylprednisolone (9), previous chemotherapy, total body irradiation, and impending rejection (10). Nevertheless, when seizures occur in a patient treated with CsA, in the absence of other predisposing factors, an elevated blood

**Table 3** Neurotoxicity of Cyclosporine (CsA)

| Complication | Signs/symptoms | Laboratory | Treatment/outcome |
| --- | --- | --- | --- |
| Encephalomyelopathy[a,b] | Tremor<br>Seizures[c]<br>Deteriorating mental status<br>Confusion/lethargy<br>Anxiety/depression<br>Aphasia/dysarthria<br>Ataxia<br>Quadriparesis | Increased CSF WBC and proteins<br>Brain CT/MRI: normal<br>EEG: focal/diffuse abnormalities<br>Hypomagnesemia<br>High CSF/blood CsA | Decrease or DC CsA<br>Correction of metabolic imbalance |
| Leukoencephalopathy[a,b] | Deteriorating mental status<br>Confusion<br>Lethargy/coma<br>Cortical blindness<br>Seizures<br>Hallucinations<br>Focal signs | Increased CSF WBC and proteins<br>Brain CT/MRI: reversible, focal nonenhancing white matter lesions<br>EEG: focal/diffuse abnormalities<br>Hypomagnesemia<br>High CSF/blood CsA | AED (valproic acid)<br>Improvement, but sequelae are possible |

| | | | |
|---|---|---|---|
| Peripheral neuropathy | Distal acute paresthesias<br>Pain/burning[d]<br>Decreased vibratory and pinprick sensation<br>Quadriparesis<br>Absent deep tendon reflex | EMG: Diffuse axonal neuropathy | Reduce the infusion rate of CsA for acute paresthesias<br>Improvement after DC of CsA |
| Myopathy | Muscular pain<br>Cramps<br>Weakness<br>Proximal atrophy | Muscle biopsy:<br>Type 2 fiber atrophy<br>Large-size mitochondria<br>Cytoplasmic vacuoles | Improvement 2 weeks–2 months after reduction or DC of CsA |

[a]Predisposing factors: previous intrathecal chemotherapy; total body irradiation; association with glucocorticoids; hypercholesterolemia
[b]Dose dependent
[c]Including status epilepticus
[d]Usually during the infusion
WBC: White blood cells. CSF: Cerebrospinal fluid. DC: Discontinuation. AED: Antiepileptic drugs. MRI: Magnetic resonance imaging. CT: Computed tomography. EEG: Electroencephalogram. EMG: Electromyogram.

level of CsA is frequently found. Cyclosporine-induced hypomagnesemia could also be a risk factor for seizures. The treatment consists in reducing the CsA dose, correcting hypomagnesemia, and if necessary giving an anticonvulsant, such as a benzodiazepine or sodium valproate, that does not induce the metabolism of other drugs. Long-term antiepileptic drug therapy is seldom indicated. It is possible that rare reports of transient aphasia with hypomagnesemia during treatment with CsA were due to focal seizures.

A severe encephalopathy is the most feared neurological complication of CsA. Predisposing factors include high concentration of the drug, the use of the intravenous (IV) formulation, previous treatment with intrathecal methotrexate or arabinosylcytosine (Ara-C), total body irradiation, low cholesterol levels (in liver transplants), and advanced liver failure (11). It should be emphasized that the diagnosis of CsA-induced encephalopathy remains a diagnosis of exclusion. Metabolic abnormalities, opportunistic infection, or even hypertensive encephalopathy should always be ruled out when CsA-induced encephalopathy is considered. Mental symptoms most commonly occur within 10 days of beginning the drug, but sometimes they may be delayed several months.

Two main types of encephalopathy may occur during CsA treatment:

1. A subacute encephalomyelopathy, sometimes called "cerebrocerebellar syndrome" characterized by a combination of cerebral, cerebellar, spinal cord, and sometimes extrapyramidal symptoms. This syndrome has been described in 8% of the recipients of human leukocyte antigen (HLA)-identical sibling marrow allografts, mainly for hematological malignancy (10) but also following liver or renal transplantation (12). The symptoms include mental status changes (confusion, aphasia, depression), seizures, akinesia, ataxia, intentional tremor, dysarthria, and sometimes paraparesis or quadriparesis. Cerebrospinal fluid is normal or shows increased protein (up to 661 mg/l) and a mild lymphocytic pleocytosis (10). Computed tomographic (CT) scan of the brain is normal.
2. A leukoencephalopathy with alteration in mental status that may progress to coma (13), sometimes associated with cortical blindness, seizures, hallucinations, or other focal symptoms (14), is the second form of encephalopathy. The electroencephalogram (EEG) demonstrates diffuse slowing and, more rarely, epileptiform activity. The CSF is normal or reveals increased protein concentration. The CT or MRI of the brain shows nonenhancing diffuse white matter damage (hypodensity or T2 prolongation on MRI) (13,15) that predominates in the occipital regions. Cortical abnormalities may also be present in association with the leukoencephalopathy. The blood CsA levels are generally high. Reports of visual hallucination sometimes associated with decreased visual acuity could represent a milder form of this syndrome.

In addition to neurological deterioration, a number of behavioral and psychological complications may occur with CsA treatment, including delirium, generalized anxiety disorder, hallucinosis, and organic mood disorders with depression (12).

In the various forms of encephalopathy, the clinical and radiological symptoms improve with discontinuation or reduction of CsA, but significant residua are possible (12).

A few observations of isolated and severe myelopathy have been reported during CsA therapy after bone marrow transplantation in patients previously treated with intrathecal chemotherapy (16). Postmortem examination showed diffuse myelin and axonal loss in the entire spinal cord.

Distal paresthesias and dysesthesias (burning and pain) occur during drug infusion in about 10% of patients, especially at the onset of treatment. Severity may be reduced by slowing the infusion (9). A polyneuropathy is rare. One observation of a Guillain-Barré-like syndrome (17) and one case of bilateral deltoid paralysis have been reported (18). There are several observations of myopathy including a severe form with muscle pain, cramps, weakness, and rhabdomyolysis (19). In one case, muscle biopsy showed type 2 fiber atrophy, large lipid vacuoles, and abnormally large mitochondria, some with ruptured cristae (18).

The mechanism by which CsA causes neurological complications is unknown. Serum levels of CsA are often high in patients with neurotoxicity, but this is not always the case. The serum level of this drug may vary widely between individuals, and a number of other drugs may interfere with its metabolism, thereby increasing serum levels. Even when the CsA levels are considered "therapeutic," the principal CsA metabolite (M17) may be high in patients with neurological dysfunction. In addition, high levels of CsA may be found in the CSF despite a normal serum level resulting from an alteration of the blood-brain barrier (BBB) (20). A direct toxic effect of CsA on the neurons or on the intracranial vasculature (microvascular damage leading to a disturbance of the BBB) have been suggested (12). The possible role of polyoxyethylated castor oil, the surfactant added to intravenous CsA, has also been suspected.

## III. INTERFERONS

Isaacs and Lindenmann observed that virus-infected cell cultures produced a protein that reacted with cells to render them resistant to infection by many viruses. These proteins that "interfere" with the establishment of a viral infection were named interferons (IFN). Subsequent studies demonstrated that, in addition to their antiviral effect, IFNs profoundly affected cell metabolism and proliferation, immunity, and tumor development (21). Interferons consist of three families of proteins (alpha, beta, gamma) which are synthesized by body cells in response to viral infection, immune stimulation, and a variety of chemical inducers. Useful quantities of recombinant alpha, beta, and gamma IFNs, available for clinical use, are now produced through genetic-engineering techniques. FDA-approved indications for IFNs in oncology are hairy-cell leukemia, Kaposi's sarcoma in AIDS, and basal cell carcinoma. In addition IFNs are being tested in many other neoplasms, including brain tumors. Unfortunately, the development of these treatment programs has revealed that intrathecal or systemic administration of IFNs may have profound effects on the central and, to a lesser extent, the peripheral nervous system (Tables 4, 5).

## A. Neurotoxicity of Intrathecal and Intratumoral IFNs

Intrathecal (IT) or intratumoral IFNs have been used in patients with meningeal and brain tumors (22–24). Trials of IT IFN have also been performed in patients suffering from multiple sclerosis, amyotrophic lateral sclerosis (ALS), and progressive multifocal leukoencephalopathy (PML).

An acute reaction is almost constant following IT IFN-$\alpha$, occurring within hours after the first injection, independently of the dose given (50,000 to 6 million units of IFN-$\alpha$); it consists of headache, nausea, vomiting, fever, and more rarely dizziness (Table 4). The symptoms improve over 12–24 h. These acute changes are not observed with IFN-$\alpha$ or IFN-$\beta$ when the catheter of the Ommaya reservoir is placed in a tumor cavity that does not communicate with the ventricles (22,23). The immediate tolerance of IT IFN-$\beta$ seems better (23), although Jacobs and coworkers (25) reported frequent headache. In MS patients, some studies have found striking acute neurological deterioration following IT IFN-$\alpha$, even with a low dose ($0.3 \times 10^6$ IFN-$\alpha$). A possible explanation is that fever is responsible for the neurological deterioration because MS patients are extremely sensitive to moderate changes in body temperature (neuroelectric block) (26).

A severe encephalopathy occurring within days of the onset of treatment has been reported in 75% of patients who received intraventricular infusions of IFN-$\alpha$ (with doses ranging from $1.5 \times 10^6$ IU daily up to $9 \times 10^6$ IU three times per week) for meningeal tumors (24). This toxicity seems to be dose dependent because a severe encephalopathy has not been reported with repeated intrathecal infusion of low-dose IFN (no more than $1 \times 10^6$ IU twice weekly) to treat MS or PML. Furthermore, Meyers and coworkers (24) found that all patients with a severe neurotoxic reaction had previously received whole-brain radiation therapy, suggesting a synergistic or additive effect of radiation therapy and IFN toxicity. The clinical picture shows worsening lethargy and expressive speech difficulties progressing to a state of "catatonia" resembling akinetic mutism with unresponsiveness to verbal commands and only eye opening to verbal or tactile stimulation.

**Table 4** Neurological Complications of Intrathecal Interferon

| Complication | Signs/symptoms | Laboratory | Treatment/outcome |
|---|---|---|---|
| Influenzalike syndrome[a–c] (hours after infusion of IFN-α) | Headache Fever Nausea Vomiting Dizziness | CSF: slight WBC and protein increase | Acetaminophen or Nonsteroidal anti-inflammatory drugs Spontaneously reversible within 12–24 h |
| Acute encephalopathy[b,d,e] (days after infusion of IFN-α) | Lethargy Speech difficulties Catatonia Akinetic mutism Seizures Parkinsonian syndrome Hearing loss Hiccups | Brain CT: periventricular white matter changes Increased CSF WBC and protein EEG: Frontal and central delta and theta activity with sharp components | If lethargy, DC of IFN needed Improvement over 3 weeks Sequelae are possible |

[a]Not observed with intratumoral administration
[b]Only with IFN-α
[c]Not dose dependent
[d]Dose dependent
[e]Synergistic effect with radiotherapy
CSF: Cerebrospinal fluid. WBC: White blood cells. DC: Discontinuation. CT: Computed tomography. EEG: Electroencephalogram.

Other neurological symptoms and signs may be present, including seizures, parkinsonian syndrome, hearing loss, and hiccups.

The EEG shows frontal and central or diffuse synchronous delta and theta activity with occasional sharp components getting worse with subsequent treatment. The CT scan demonstrates the development of a leukoencephalopathy in 50% of the patients. Cerebrospinal fluid protein levels, if normal on pretreatment studies, become elevated even when the tumor cells disappear (22). There are no data on CSF white blood cell (WBC) counts in encephalopathic patients, but a progressive sterile pleocytosis may occur in the absence of overt toxicity (25). After termination of treatment, symptoms gradually resolve over approximately 3 weeks, but some patients (two out of seven in Meyers and coworkers' study) do not recover before death (24).

Repeated IT infusions of IFN-β for MS and meningeal leukemia seem to be better tolerated and a severe progressive encephalopathy has not been reported in this setting (25,27), although general malaise and lethargy may occur.

**Table 5** Neurological Complications of Systemic IFN

| Complication | Signs/symptoms | Laboratory | Treatment/outcome |
|---|---|---|---|
| Influenzalike syndrome | See Table 4 | — | Acetaminophen or nonsteroidal anti-inflammatory drugs |
| Subacute encephalopathy[a,b] (2–4 weeks after onset of IFN) | Lethargy/coma<br>Hallucinations<br>Anxiety/depression<br>Unsteady gait<br>Paraparesis<br>Pyramidal signs | EEG:[c,d]<br>Slowing of the alpha rhythm<br>Appearance of diffuse slow waves<br>CSF: normal | Recovery over 2–4 weeks after DC of IFN but sequelae are possible<br>Restart IFN with lowest dose possible |
| Chronic encephalopathy[e] | Cognitive changes/dementia<br>Memory/attention deficit<br>Parkinsonian syndrome<br>Psychiatric disorders<br>Coma/death | EEG: diffuse slow activity<br>Brain CT/MRI: cerebral atrophy<br>CSF: normal | DC of IFN<br>Residual deficits are frequent |
| Peripheral neuropathy[b,f] | Oculomotor nerve palsy<br>Sensory/motor polyneuropathy<br>Brachial plexopathy<br>Polyradiculopathy | EMG/biopsy: mixed axonal and demyelinating neuropathy | DC of IFN<br>Usually no sequelae |

[a]Predisposing factors: Concomitant treatment with sedative and analgesics; preexisting neurological abnormalities
[b]Dose dependent
[c]The sequence of EEG abnormalities reach a peak 1–2 weeks after onset of IFN
[d]No correlation with clinical state
[e]Elderly patients are more vulnerable
[f]Predisposing factors: Preexisting polyneuropathy, vitamin $B_{12}$ deficiency, previous chemotherapy with vincristine

DC: Discontinuation. CSF: Cerebrospinal fluid. CT: Computed tomography. MRI: Magnetic resonance imaging. EEG: Electroencephalogram. EMG: Electromyogram.

## B. Neurotoxicity of Systemic IFNs

A variety of acute, subacute, and chronic neurotoxic reactions to systemically administered IFN has been described in patients treated with IFN for cancer, hepatitis, and amyotrophic lateral sclerosis (Table 5). In an analysis of 1403 cancer patients who received IFN-α in clinical trials, neurological side effects were noted in 33%. However, these complications were severe in only 7% (28).

The most frequent reaction associated with systemic IFN-α is the influenzalike syndrome (general malaise, fever, headache, fatigue, myalgias, arthralgia, and anorexia) lasting 4–8 h. This syndrome is experienced by most patients receiving more than $1-2 \times 10^6$ IU/day. Severe dose-related headache, sometimes refractory to narcotics, has also been reported in patients treated with IFN-β and IFN-γ, particularly during continuous infusion (29). The syndrome is usually less severe or even disappears during repeated dosing. Seizures may occur rarely during this period (30) and are possibly related to a reduction of the epileptic threshold by fever.

In order to improve tolerance, it is important to inform the patients of the acute reaction, to deliver treatment in the evening, and to administer acetaminophen or nonsteroidal anti-inflammatory agents systematically (31,32) at the time of IFN treatment.

### 1. Subacute Encephalopathy

As with IT administration, repeated systemic infusions of IFN-α may induce a subacute encephalopathy with behavioral and cognitive changes (33) affecting principally frontal lobe functions (34). Several predisposing factors have been identified, including (1) concomitant treatment with sedatives and analgesics; (2) preexisting neurological abnormalities; and (3) the dose of IFN (35). Almost 100% of patients develop a severe encephalopathy with high doses of IFN-α (100–200 $\times 10^6$ IU/day) (36,37). When doses are reduced to 15–20 $\times 10^6$ IU/day, the incidence of encephalopathy is lower (40–60%) (31). With the commonly used dose of $3 \times 10^6$ IU administered 3 times per week, the incidence of encephalopathy is much lower (4–20%) and the clinical picture less severe. The symptoms appear several days after the onset of treatment, with the peak between the second and fourth week depending on the IFN dose (38). The clinical picture consists of progressive psychomotor slowing, speech difficulties, loss of interest, and lethargy sometimes preceded by a brief period of excitation and hallucination (34,36,37). Occasionally, psychiatric symptoms such as anxiety are prominent. More often, anxiety and suicidal ideation are reduced, reflecting a state of emotional indifference.

On examination, patients are often disoriented, with striking attention disorder, memory loss (33), and sometimes perseveration and visuoconstructional deficiency, although the intelligence test scores may remain unaffected (34). Usually there are no focal neurological manifestations but signs of upper motor neuron lesions (paraparesis, bilateral Babinski sign) have rarely been reported, as well as generalized increase in tone, twitching movements of the extremities, unsteady gait, and lack of coordination of limb movements (31,34,39). When treatment is continued with the same doses, lethargy may become worse (31) or remain stable (33).

On rare occasions, the symptoms may progress rapidly to coma simulating a viral encephalitis, especially when high doses are used (100–200 × $10^6$ IU/day/1 week) (37). A characteristic sequence of EEG abnormalities has been found, reaching a peak between 1 to 2 weeks after the onset of treatment. The EEG abnormalities are not always correlated with the patient's clinical state and they have even been reported in patients without clinical evidence of CNS toxicity. They consist of slowing of the alpha rhythm with gradual loss of attenuation on eye opening, followed by the appearance of diffuse slow waves (theta then delta) then monorhythmic frontal delta bursts (36,38,39) which slowly return to normal after cessation of IFN. However, in some cases the EEG abnormalities may persist after clinical improvement (39).

There are very few data on CSF analysis: Matson and coworkers (38) reported an increase in the proportion of lymphocytes in CSF while others did not find CSF changes (37,39). After discontinuation of IFN, recovery generally follows within 2 weeks (34,38).

The systemic administration of IFN-β, even with high doses, is more rarely associated with clinical or electrophysiological evidence of a severe encephalopathy (35). One case of a transient manic episode has been reported. Yung and coworkers (40) treated recurrent malignant glioma with escalating doses of IV IFN-β ranging from 90–540 × $10^6$ IU three times per week. Only 11% (7/65) had severe but reversible neurotoxicity requiring discontinuation of treatment (headache, encephalopathy). In addition, two had retinal toxicity with decreased visual acuity and retinal changes suggestive of ischemic abnormalities. A severe encephalopathy has been reported with IFN-γ in association with tumor necrosis factor.

## 2. Chronic Encephalopathy

Although most patients with subacute encephalopathy return to normal within 2 weeks after withdrawal of IFN and may tolerate the reintroduction of IFN at a reduced dose (31), some patients do not improve or even get worse for weeks or months despite discontinuation of IFN (41,42). The exact incidence of this complication is unknown, but Meyers and coworkers (42) identified 14 patients with disabling chronic neurobehavioral dysfunction among 1300 individuals treated with IFN-α over a 3-year period. Elderly patients seem particularly vulnerable. There is no clear relationship between the severity of the chronic toxicity and the severity of acute toxicity or the duration of treatment (42).

However, there is a relation between the dose and schedule of IFN-α treatment and the severity of the encephalopathy. Patients who receive daily injections of IFN have much worse delayed toxicity than individuals who receive lower doses or less frequent injections. The clinical picture shows cognitive and psychiatric changes. The cognitive abnormalities are suggestive of subcortical dysfunction, with deficits of memory and attention and impaired problem-solving ability with simple cortical functions intact. Even patients with minor dysfunction are often unable to return to work. Occasionally a frank dementia is observed. Parkinsonism with masked facies, tremor, and rigidity is present in 30% of cases. The main psychiatric symptoms are depression with periods of agitation and anxiety. The EEG shows diffuse, slow activity. Computed tomography or MRI scans are abnormal in more than 50% of the patients, showing cerebral atrophy sometimes associated with white matter changes (41,42). Cerebrospinal fluid is normal (41). The course seems unpredictable; some patients improve over time while others deteriorate progressively to coma and death (41,42). Independent events may affect the course of the disease. There is one report of a patient who progressed from a mild chronic encephalopathy to coma during an intercurrent pulmonary infection (43). There is no treatment. Antidepressant or neuroleptics are sometimes useful to treat psychiatric symptoms, but patients should be carefully followed for the development of extrapyramidal side effects.

*Mechanism.* The pathogenesis of IFN-induced neurotoxicity is unknown. It does not appear to be related to contamination of the IFN. The transport of IFNs across the blood-brain and blood-CSF barrier is very low after systemic administration, and high doses of IFN ($100-200 \times 10^6$ IU) are generally needed to achieve measurable levels in CSF. It is clear that systemic administration of IFN can induce sever CNS neurotoxicity even in the absence of measurable CSF IFN (36). In vitro, IFN increases neuronal excitability (44). Cerebral injection of IFN-α in animals causes catalepsy and decreased spontaneous locomotion. In monkeys, no pathological changes indicative of local toxicity could be demonstrated in CNS after IT IFN. A direct effect of INF on the brain has been incriminated (opiatelike activity) as well as the induction of secondary toxic cytokines, changes in neuroendocrine hormone secretion, and neurotransmitter effects.

## 3. Peripheral Neuropathy

Peripheral nerve injury is a rare and poorly described complication of IFN therapy. Predisposing factors include vitamin $B_{12}$ deficiency, a preexistent polyneuropathy (alcoholism, diabetes) (45), and previous chemotherapy with vincristine (46). The dose of IFN, particularly the cumulative dose of IFN, also appears to be an important factor.

Acute and transient distal paresthesias have been reported in 7% of patients.

More rarely, patients may develop a progressive-chronic neuropathy. The symptoms develop progressively weeks to months after the onset of treatment (46,47). The clinical picture is usually that of a sensory neuropathy with paresthesias or burning dysesthesias in hands and feet (31). On examination, there is no weakness and objective sensory findings are inconstant (38,48). The deep tendon reflexes are normal or reduced in the lower extremities. The CSF is normal. Electromyography and nerve biopsy suggest a mixed axonal and demyelinating neuropathy. An axonal motor or sensorimotor polyneuropathy has also been reported (47). The symptoms disappear within weeks after discontinuation of IFN (46) but they return if IFN is restarted.

A neuropathy resembling neuralgic amyotrophy has been reported by Bernsen and coworkers (45) in a patient who received high doses of IFN ($20-30 \times 10^6$). Except for loss of taste and smell, which has been frequently noted during IFN treatment (38), the cranial nerves are spared. One exception is a report of reversible bilateral oculomotor nerve paralysis in one leukemic patient after 3 months of treatment with IFN ($5 \times 10^6$ $IU/m^2/day$). Laboratory studies were negative (CT scan and MRI of the brain, CSF study, EEG) (49). The ophthalmoplegia disappeared 2½ months after discontinuation of therapy.

## IV. NEUROLOGICAL COMPLICATIONS OF AUTOLOGOUS LAK CELLS AND INTERLEUKIN-2 THERAPY

Clinical tumor immunotherapy was renewed in the 1980s with the description of lymphokine-activated killer (LAK) cells that are capable of killing tumor cells. The LAK cells are produced by the incubation of peripheral blood lymphocytes with interleukin (IL)-2. Clinical studies have shown immunotherapy using autologous LAK cells and recombinant-derived lymphokine IL-2 to be effective against certain metastatic tumors. However, these trials have also shown that many patients developed significant toxicity, mainly related to IL-2. The reported systemic toxicities of IL-2 are dose dependent and generally reversible. They include a capillary leak syndrome with hypotension and fluid retention; renal, hepatic, pulmonary, and cardiac dysfunction; anemia; and constitutional symptoms. Neurological side effects also have been reported frequently.

### A. Neurological Complications of Intratumoral IL-2

Intratumoral LAK cell and/or IL-2 therapy, administered through an Ommaya reservoir, has been used in recurrent malignant gliomas. Preliminary reports suggested that tolerance was good (50), but additional studies have revealed substantial neurotoxicity (Table 6). Apart from scalp inflammation (probably due

**Table 6** Neurological Complications of Treatment with Intratumoral IL-2

| Complication | Signs/symptoms | Laboratory | Treatment/outcome |
| --- | --- | --- | --- |
| Acute encephalopathy (hours/days after onset of IL-2) | Headache Progressive lethargy | Brain CT/MRI: progression of peritumoral edema | Acetaminophen Corticosteroids DC IL-2 Sequelae in 50% of cases |

DC: Discontinuation

to the contact of LAK cells and IL-2 with the scalp wounds), the main complication is fever, headache, and lethargy, in most patients occurring hours to days after the onset of treatment. The development of new focal deficits or worsening of preexisting deficits referable to the region of brain receiving treatment is also frequent when large doses of IL-2 and LAK cells are used (51). Computed tomography scan and MRI show signs of increased cerebral edema and sometimes increase in contrast enhancement suggesting treatment-related vasogenic edema. The symptoms may regress within days after termination of treatment, but in one study more than 50% of patients were left with new permanent deficits (51). The CT changes persist for several weeks (52). The development of hydrocephalus has been reported in a few malignant glioma patients who received intratumoral LAK cells alone or associated with a bispecific monoclonal antibody of murine origin (anti-CD3 and antiglioma) (53).

## B. Neurological Complications of Systemic Treatment with IL-2

### 1. Acute/Subacute Encephalopathy

It is estimated that 30–50% of patients who receive IV bolus of IL-2 alone or combined with LAK cells for metastatic cancer develop behavioral and cognitive changes (54). The incidence may be lower (10%) when IL-2 is administered as a constant infusion (55). The risk of encephalopathy appears to be dose and tumor dependent (Table 7). In Denicoff and coworkers' study (54), cognitive and behavioral changes were twice as frequent in patients with systemic cancer treated with 100,000 U/kg than in patients treated with 30,000 U/kg. In patients with gliomas, treatment with intravenous IL-2 is not tolerated because of increased cerebral edema (56).

Symptoms develop after 5 to 6 days of treatment with IL-2, sometimes later. They are not correlated with the fluid retention syndrome or with a past medical history of psychiatric illness. Lethargy, irritability, and word-finding difficulties

**Table 7** Neurological Complications of Treatment with Systemic IL-2

| Complication | Signs/symptoms | Laboratory | Treatment/outcome |
| --- | --- | --- | --- |
| Acute encephalopathy[a] (5–6 days after onset of IL-2) | Irritability/agitation Anxiety/depression Attention/memory deficits Seizures Lethargy/coma | NR | DC IL-2 Neuroleptics AED Usually no sequelae Constant IV infusion may reduce the risk of toxicity |
| Transient neurological deficits[b] | Monocular blindness Homonymous visual loss | NR | Improvement |
| Leukoencephalopathy[b] | Delirium Ataxia Blindness Coma/death | Autopsy: Perivascular demyelination with lymphocytic infiltration Brain CT: normal | Fatal |
| Brachial plexopathy | Pain and weakness of C5-C6 distribution | EMG Denervation C5-C6 | Treatment: unknown Improvement |

[a]Dose and tumor size dependent
[b]Sporadic cases
DC: Discontinuation. AED: Antiepileptic drugs. EMG: Electromyogram. NR: Not reported.

are early symptoms, followed by more profound neurological and psychiatric alterations. The most frequent behavioral changes consist of agitation, combative behavior and, more rarely, paranoid delusions. The cognitive changes include disorientation, memory loss, and impaired attention and judgment that can be quantified by a substantial drop in various cognitive tests (54). Occasionally, seizures may occur (57) and the lethargy may progress to coma (58). Patients should be informed about potential neuropsychiatric side effects before the administration of IL-2. Neuroleptics are useful in case of severe agitation or paranoid delusions. After discontinuation or reduction of IL-2, the encephalopathy may continue to worsen (59) but full recovery generally occurs over a few days, except for cognitive changes that may be slower to regress. Margolin and coworkers (59) recommend discontinuing IL-2 in patients with evidence of disorientation, inappropriate thought patterns, or paranoid or psychotic ideation. With resolution of neurotoxicity, IL-2 can be cautiously restarted.

The mechanism of neuropsychiatric toxicity is not known. Interleukin-2 seems to be the main offender; it could affect the CNS directly or indirectly by enhancing the accumulation of behaviorally active substances or by increasing the permeability of the BBB (60). Experimental studies have demonstrated that systemic or intracerebral administration of IL-2 (with its excipient) profoundly increased BBB permeability to horseradish peroxidase and endogenous IgG (61). Quantified MRI studies have shown that parenteral IL-2 substantially increased the cerebral gray and white matter water content but no relationship between increased MRI signal intensity and mental status change was found (56).

## 2. Severe Leukoencephalopathy

There is one report of acute fatal leukoencephalopathy after IL-2 therapy. The patient developed delirium, ataxia, and blindness 5 days after the completion of IL-2. Computed tomographic scan of the brain was normal. Subsequently, the patient became comatose and died 17 days after the last dose of IL-2. Microscopically, the brain lesions consisted of multiple perivascular foci of demyelination. Perivascular infiltration by small lymphocytes was also noted. The clinicopathological picture of this case most closely resembles acute perivenous encephalomyelitis that occurs as an allergic or autoimmune response after an infection or a vaccination. It is possible that IL-2 had triggered an immunological reaction involving activated T lymphocytes directed against myelin (62).

## 3. Transient Focal Neurological Deficits

Repeated, stereotyped transient episodes of monocular blindness or homonymous visual loss unassociated with hypotension has been reported during a course of IL-2 therapy. The symptoms resolved after discontinuation of the treatment. In one patient, similar attacks were triggered when IL-2 was restarted on two occasions (57). Bernard and coworkers (63) suggested that these transient neurological deficits were due to the effect of IL-2 on endothelial cells. Other possible mechanisms include focal edema (a restricted form of the vascular leak syndrome in an area of preexisting vascular damage), vasospasm, or hypotension in some cases.

## 4. Peripheral Neuropathy

The occurrence of symptomatic nerve compression related to edema is possible during the vascular leak syndrome (64). A brachial plexopathy, bilateral in one case, has been reported in two patients treated with IL-2 and LAK cells. They developed severe pain in the shoulder and arm in the week following treatment. Examination revealed weakness of the deltoid, supra-, and infraspinatus. Sensory loss in the distribution of the axillary nerves was found in one case. Deep tendon reflexes were normal. Electromyogram demonstrated denervation in C5-C6 innervated muscles predominating in the muscles innervated by the upper brachial plexus. Magnetic resonance imaging of the cervical spine and brachial plexus was normal. Complete clinical recovery occurred over several weeks. In one patient, repeat trial of IL-2 resulted in a relapse of the neurological symptoms (65).

## V. NEUROLOGICAL COMPLICATIONS OF MONOCLONAL ANTIBODY (MoAb) THERAPY

### A. Murine Monoclonal CD3 Antibody Therapy

The murine monoclonal CD3 antibody (OKT3) reacts specifically with the CD3 antigen on human T lymphocytes. OKT3 is used to prevent and reverse refractory allograft rejection following renal, hepatic, and cardiac transplantation. OKT3 has also been used to treat refractory solid tumors (66). Different neurological complications are observed (Table 8).

Headache is a common complication of therapy with OKT3, affecting half the patients. It generally occurs between the second and fifth day of treatment and resolves in 2 to 4 days. Mild analgesic agents could be necessary in this period. Neurotoxicity has not recurred with subsequent treatment. There is one observation of necrotizing temporal arteritis occurring days after the initiation of OKT3 treatment (67).

#### 1. Aseptic Meningitis

An aseptic meningitis occurs in 3–14% of patients treated with OKT3 to prevent graft rejection. The incidence is even higher (up to 54%) in the absence of immunosuppression when OKT3 is used for the treatment of human refractory solid tumors. The symptoms generally start within 72 h of the onset of OKT3 (68–70) but may occur later, up to 16 days after completion of OKT3 therapy (70). The clinical picture shows headache, fever, photophobia, and nuchal rigidity. A sixth nerve palsy may be associated. In some patients, the meningeal symptoms and signs may be quite discrete or absent while changes in mental status (lethargy, impaired attentiveness, loss of memory) dominate. An encephalitic form with stupor and quadriparesis has been reported (71).

Computed tomographic scan of the brain and MRI are normal or show brain edema in the encephalitic form. The opening pressure of the CSF may be elevated (71). Studies of CSF reveal a moderate increase in protein (0.50–0.80 mg/dl), a normal glucose in most cases, and a hyperleukocytosis (up to 500/mm$^3$), often with a dominance of polymorphonuclear neutrophils. Bacterial and viral cultures are sterile (72). The CSF changes may be present in the absence of overt clinical manifestation of meningitis. With pretreatment with steroids, antihistamines, and acetaminophen, the severity of the response to the first dose has been greatly reduced; however, it may be necessary to withhold OKT3 over a few days until improvement. Some patients improve spontaneously while the treatment is continued (71,72); one patient was left with a permanent sixth nerve palsy. The pathogenesis of CNS dysfunction from OKT3 is unknown. It is possible that elimination of opsonized T lymphocytes causes the release of cytokines (tumor

**Table 8** Neurological Complications of Monoclonal $CD_3$ and $14G_{2a}$ Antibodies Therapy

| Complication | Signs/symptoms | Laboratory | Treatment/outcome |
|---|---|---|---|
| Aseptic meningitis (2–16 days after onset of $CD_3$ MAb therapy) | Headache<br>Fever<br>Photophobia<br>Nuchal rigidity<br>Memory/attention deficit<br>Seizures<br>Lethargy/stupor[a]<br>Quadriparesis[a] | Brain CT/MRI normal, but brain edema in encephalitic form<br>CSF:<br>Increased opening pressure<br>Increased WBC and proteins[b] | Temporary DC of MAb<br>Acetaminophen<br>Retreatment possible<br>Improvement |
| Peripheral neuropathy (Related to anti–$GD_2$ MAb $14G_{2a}$ therapy) | Paresthesias:<br>Severe burning and pain[c]<br>Leg weakness<br>Decreased deep tendon reflexes | Biopsy:<br>Demyelination<br>Endoneural and perivascular mononuclear infiltrate<br>$GD_2$ in the nerve fibers<br>EMG: denervation in the proximal and distal muscles | DC of MAb<br>Morphine<br>Recovery over 24 h–6 weeks after DC of MAb but sequelae are possible |

[a] Rare
[b] Up to 500 leukocytes, polymorphonuclear predominance
[c] Usually occurred within 24 h following the third infusion
DC: Discontinuation. MAb: Monoclonal antibody. CSF: Cerebrospinal fluid. WBC: White blood cells. CT: Computed tomography. MRI: Magnetic resonance imaging.

necrosis factor, IL-2, interferon-γ) that induce meningeal inflammation and encephalopathy.

Seizures have been reported in 6% of patients treated with OKT3 but, as with cyclosporine, these patients often have multiple metabolic risk factors for seizures, particularly fever, uremia, hypocalcemia, or hyponatremia.

## B. Neurological Complications of Other Monoclonal Antibodies

Many clinical trials of MoAb therapy for metastatic cancer have been reported. Tolerance is generally excellent but occasionally severe neurotoxin reactions are encountered. In these cases, an unexpected cross-reactivity of the MoAb with nervous system antigens may be found, as illustrated by the following example. Saleh and coworkers (73) treated metastatic melanoma patients with the murine anti-GD2 MoAb 14G2a. GD2 is preferentially expressed on tumors of neuroectodermal origin. Following administration of the MoAb, more than 40% of the patients developed transient severe and burning pain in hands and feet requiring intravenous morphine for control. In addition, 4 of 12 patients developed a severe neuropathy of the lower extremities. Biopsy of the right sural nerve in one case showed demyelination and a mononuclear infiltrate in the endoneural and perivascular space. Immunohistological studies demonstrated GD2 on the nerve fibers of the patient. The neuropathy could have been caused by binding of the MoAb or immune complexes to the peripheral nerves. Such tissue-specific toxicity supports the need for extensive antibody screening of different normal human tissues from multiple patients to exclude cross-reactivity before clinical trials.

## C. Neurological Complications of Intrathecal Radiolabeled MoAb

Intrathecal administration of radiolabeled MoAb is used for the treatment of leptomeningeal tumors. The main complication is an acute aseptic meningitis with pyrexia and a sterile leukocytosis in almost 50% of the patients (74). The symptoms improve over 48 h. Transient paresthesia over sacral dermatomes and seizures, including status epilepticus, have also been reported in a few patients (75).

## VI. Neurological Complications of Immunotoxins

Immunotoxins are a new class of antitumor agents consisting of tumor-selective ligands (generally monoclonal antibodies) linked to highly toxic protein molecules. Toxins used in the construction of immunotoxins include ricin, abrin, *Pseudomonas* exotoxin A, and diphtheria toxin. The major systemic toxicity is a toxin-dependent capillary leak syndrome with hypoalbuminemia, edema, and weight gain (76). The neurotoxicity of immunotoxin is higher than with MoAb alone (Table 9). A diffuse encephalopathy and a myopathy are the most frequently encountered neurological side effects.

About half the patients who received the anti-CD22 Fab' fragment Ab (specific for human B cells) coupled to chemically deglycosylated ricin A chain for advanced refractory B-cell lymphoma (77) developed mild to severe myalgia and sometimes elevated levels of creatine kinase. A rhabdomyolysis occurred in one case; muscle biopsy showed a moderate increase in macrophages between muscle fibers. The mechanism of the myalgia is not understood but a myositis has been found in mice treated with ricin A chain–containing immunotoxins. In addition, 2 of 15 patients had transient aphasia. The authors speculated that cerebral edema associated with the vascular leak syndrome could be responsible for these transient speech difficulties. An encephalopathy with expressive aphasia or seizures and myalgias have also been reported in some patients treated with ricin A chain immunotoxin (791T/36) for metastatic colorectal cancer (78) and antimelanoma antibody–ricin A chain immunotoxin (Xomazyme-mel) in conjunction with cyclophosphamide (79).

A severe neuropathy has been reported in three of five patients with metastatic breast cancer who received continuous infusion of a murine MoAb (260 F9, directed against a breast cancer antigen) conjugated with recombinant ricin A chain (80). Patients developed a diffuse sensorimotor neuropathy which began on the side of previous chest wall and nodal irradiation (i.e., at a site where one

**Table 9** Neurological Complications of Immunotoxins

| Antibody | Toxin | Tumor type | Encephalopathy/ seizure | Peripheral neuropathy | Myopathy |
|---|---|---|---|---|---|
| Anti-CD22 | Ricin A | B-cell malignancy | + | − | ++ |
| Xomazyme + cyclophosphamide | Ricin A | Melanoma | + | − | + |
| 791 T36 | Ricin A | Colon | ++ | − | − |
| 260 F9 | Ricin A | Breast | − | ++ | − |
| OVB 3 | *Pseudomonas* exotoxin | Ovarian | + | − | − |
| Anti-CD5 | Ricin A | GVHD[a] | + | − | +/− |

[a]GVHD: Graft-versus-host disease
+: <25%
++: >25% <50%
Source: Ref. 81.

brachial plexus had received previous irradiation). The symptoms worsened over 2 to 3 months to such an extent that the patients were unable to care for themselves. Improvement of the motor function occurred over the following 6 months but paresthesias persisted. A nerve biopsy in one patient revealed axonal loss and segmental demyelination. The 260 F9 MoAb was found to stain the nerve sheath, suggesting cross-reactivity of the MoAb with Schwann cells or myelin antigens.

Intraperitoneal immunotoxin therapy can also induce severe neurotoxicity. An immunoconjugate between OVB3, a murine MoAb that reacts with human ovarian cancer, and *Pseudomonas* exotoxin was administered intraperitoneally to 23 patients with refractory ovarian cancer (81). The dose-limiting toxicity was neurological, with three patients developing a severe encephalopathy with confusion, apraxia, and dysarthria. Two patients recovered after several months but one of them experienced myoclonus and seizures, became comatose, and eventually died. On follow-up analysis, OVB3 was determined to be weakly reactive with cells in the molecular layer of the cerebellum, suggesting cross-reactivity with a CNS antigen.

As new and more effective forms of immunotherapy are developed, neurotoxicity will be an important consideration. Studies of the pathophysiology of the currently identified neurological complications of immunotherapy may point the way toward strategies for protecting the nervous system and uncover new insights into the biology and interaction between the nervous and immune systems.

## REFERENCES

1. Moertel CG, Fleming TR, Macdonald JS, Haller DG, Laurie JA, Goodman PJ, Ungerleider JS, Emerson WA, Tormey DC, Glick JH, Veeder MH, Mailliard JA. Levamisole and fluorouracil for adjuvant therapy of resected colon carcinoma. N Engl J Med 1990; 322:352–358.
2. Hook CC, Kimmel DW, Kvols LK, Scheithauer BW, Forsyth PA, Rubin J, Moertel CG, Rodriguez M. Multifocal inflammatory leukoencephalopathy with 5-fluorouracil and levamisole. Ann Neurol 1992; 31:262–267.
3. Symoens J, Veys E, Mielants M, Pinals R. Adverse reactions to levamisole. Cancer Treat Rep 1978; 62:1721–1730.
4. Parkinson DR, Jerry LM, Shibata HR, Lewis MG, Cano PO, Capek A, Mansell PW, Marquis G. Complications of cancer immunotherapy with levamisole. Lancet 1977; 1:1129–1132.
5. Smith RB, deKernion J, Lincoln B, Skinner DG, Kaufman JJ. Preliminary report of the use of levamisole in the treatment of bladder cancer. Cancer Treat Rep 1978; 62:1709–1714.
6. Rush DN. Cyclosporine toxicity to organs other than the kidney. Clin Biochem 1991; 24:101–105.
7. Walker RW, Brochstein JA. Neurologic complications of immunosuppressive agents. Neurol Clin 1988; 6:261–278.

8. Velu Th, Debusscher L, Stryckmans PA. Cyclosporin-associated fatal convulsions. Lancet 1985; 1:219.
9. Kennedy MS, Yee GC, Deeg HJ, Storb R, Thomas ED. Pharmacokinetics and toxicity of cyclosporine in marrow transplant patients. Transplant Proc 1983; 15:2416–2418.
10. Atkinson K, Biggs J, Darveniza P, Boland J, Concannon A, Dodds A. Cyclosporine-associated central nervous system toxicity after allogenic bone marrow transplantation. Transplantation 1984; 38:34–38.
11. De Groen PC, Aksamit AL, Rakela J, Forbes GS, Krom RAF. Central nervous system toxicity after liver transplantation. N Engl J Med 1987; 317:861–866.
12. Stein DP, Lederman RJ, Vogt DP, Carey WD, Broughan TA. Neurological complications following liver transplantation. Ann Neurol 1992; 31:644–649.
13. Berden JHM, Hoitsma AJ, Merx JL, Keyser A. Severe central nervous system toxicity associated with cyclosporin. Lancet 1985; 1:219–220.
14. Rubin AM, Kang H. Cerebral blindness and encephalopathy with cyclosporin A toxicity. Neurology 1987; 37:1072–1076.
15. Turwit CL, Denaro CP, Lake JR, DeMarco T. MR Imaging of reversible cyclosporin A-induced neurotoxicity. AJR Am J Roentgenol 1991; 157:851–859.
16. Lind MJ, Mcwilliam L, Scarffe JH, Morgenstern GR, Chang J. Cyclosporin associated demyelination following allogenic bone marrow transplantation. Hematol Oncol 1989; 7:49–52.
17. Palmer BF, Toto RD. Severe neurologic toxicity induced by cyclosporine A in three renal transplant patients. Am J Kidney Dis 1991; 18:116–121.
18. Fernandez-Sola J, Campistol J, Casademont J, Grau JM, Urbano-Marquez A. Reversible cyclosporin myopathy. Lancet 1990; 335:362–363.
19. Goy JJ, Stauffer JC, Deruaz JP, Gillard D, Kaufmann U, Kuntzer T, Kappenberger L. Myopathy as possible side-effect of cyclosporin. Lancet 1989; 1:1446–1447.
20. Gottrand F, Largillière C, Farriaux JP. Cyclosporine neurotoxicity. N Engl J Med 1991; 324:1744–1745.
21. Baron S, Tyring SK, Fleischmann WR, Coppenhaver DH, Niesel DW, Kimpel GR, Stanton GJ, Hughes TK. The interferons: mechanisms of action and clinical applications. JAMA 1991; 266:1375–1383.
22. Obbens EA, Feun LG, Leavens ME, Savaraj N, Stewart DJ, Gutterman JU. Phase I clinical trial of intralesional or intraventricular leukocyte interferon for intracranial malignancies. J Neurooncol 1985; 3:61–67.
23. Fetell MR, Housepian EM, Oster MW, Cote DN, Sisti MB, Marcus SG, Fisher PB. Intratumoral administration of beta-interferon in recurrent malignant gliomas. Cancer 1990; 65:78–83.
24. Meyers CA, Obbens EA, Scheibel RS, Moser RP. Neurotoxicity of intraventriculary administered alpha-interferon for leptomeningeal disease. Cancer 1991; 66:88–92.
25. Jacobs L, O'Malley J, Freeman A, Murawski J, Ekes R. Intrathecal interferon in multiple sclerosis. Arch Neurol 1982; 39:609–615.
26. Ruutiainen J, Panelius M, Cantell K. Toxic effects of interferon administered intrathecally. Br Med J 1983; 286:940.
27. Misset JL, Mathe G. Intrathecal interferon in meningeal leukemia. N Engl J Med 1981; 304:1544.

28. Spiegel RJ. The alpha interferons: clinical overview. Semin Oncol 1987; 14:1–12.
29. Schiller JH, Storer B, Witt PL, Nelson B, Brown RR, Horisberger M, Grossberg S, Borden EC. Biological and clinical effects of the combination of β- and γ-interferons administered as a 5-day continuous infusion. Cancer Res 1990; 50:4588–4594.
30. Abbruzzese JL, Levin B, Ajani JA, Faintuch JS, Pazdur R, Saks S, Edwards C, Gutterman JU. A phase II trial of recombinant human interferon-gamma and recombinant tumor necrosis factor in patients with advanced gastrointestinal malignancies: results of a trial terminated by excessive toxicity. J Biol Response Mod 1990; 9: 522–527.
31. Scott GM, Secher DS, Flowers D, Bate J, Cantell K, Tyrrell DAJ. Toxicity of interferon. Br Med J 1981; 282:1345–1348.
32. Smedley H, Katrak M, Sikora K, Wheeler T. Neurological effects of recombinant human interferon. Br Med J 1983; 286:262–284.
33. Adams F, Quesada JR, Gutterman JU. Neuropsychiatric manifestations of human leukocyte interferon therapy in patients with cancer. JAMA 1984; 252:938–941.
34. Iivanainen M, Laaksonen R, Niemi ML, Färkkilä M, Bergström L, Mattson K, Niiranen A, Cantell K. Memory and psychomotor impairment following high-dose interferon treatment in amyotrophic lateral sclerosis. Acta Neurol Scand 1985; 72:475–480.
35. Liberati AM, Biagini S, Perticoni G, Ricci S, D'Alessandro P, Senatore M, Cinieri S. Electrophysiological and neuropsychological functions in patients treated with interferon-β. J Interferon Res 1990; 10:613–619.
36. Rohatiner AZS, Prior PF, Burton AC, Smith AT, Balkwill FR, Lister TA. Central nervous system toxicity of interferon. Br J Cancer 1983; 47:419–422.
37. Färkkilä M, Iivanainen M, Roine R, Bergström L, Laaksonen R, Niemi ML, Cantell K. Neurotoxic and other side effects of high-dose interferon in amyotrophic lateral sclerosis. Acta Neurol Scand 1984; 69:42–46.
38. Mattson K, Niiranen A, Iivanainen M, Färkkilä M, Bergström L, Holsti RL, Kauppinen HL, Cantell K. Neurotoxicity of interferon. Cancer Treat Rep 1983; 67:958–961.
39. Suter CC, Westmoreland BF, Sharbrough FW, Hermann RC. Electroencephalographic abnormalities in interferon encephalopathy: a preliminary report. Mayo Clin Proc 1984; 59:847–850.
40. Yung WKA, Castellanos AM, Van Tassel P, Moser RP, Marcus SG. A pilot study of recombinant interferon beta (IFN-βser) in patients with recurrent glioma. J Neurooncol 1990; 9:29–34.
41. Merimsky O, Reider-Groswasser I, Inbar M, Chaitchik S. Interferon-related mental deterioration and behavioral changes in patients with renal carcinoma. Eur J Cancer 1990; 26:596–600.
42. Meyers CA, Scheibel RS, Forman AD. Persistent neurotoxicity of systemically administered interferon-alpha. Neurology 1991; 41:672–676.
43. Russo D, Zuffa E, Bandini G, Baccarani M, Tura S. Mental depression, acute infection and coma in a patient treated with interferon-alpha (letter). Haematologica (Pavia) 1989; 74:228.
44. Calvet MC. Interferon enhances the excitability of cultured neurones. Nature 1979; 278:558–560.

45. Bernsen PLJ, Wong-Chung RE, Janssen JTP. Neuralgic amyotrophy and poliradiculopathy during interferon therapy. Lancet 1985; 1:50.
46. Gastineau DA, Habermann TM, Hermann RC. Severe neuropathy associated with low-dose recombinant interferon-alpha. Am J Med 1989; 87:116.
47. Cudillo L, Cantonetti M, Venditti A, Lentini R, Rossini PM, Caramia M, Masi M, Papa G. Peripheral polyneuropathy during treatment with alpha-2 interferon (letter). Haematologica (Pavia) 1990; 75:485–486.
48. Jaubert D, Hauteville D, Pelissier JF, Muzellec Y. Neuropathie périphérique au cours d'un traitement par interféron alpha. Presse Med 1991; 20:221–222.
49. Bauherz G, Soeur M, Lustman F. Oculomotor nerve paralysis induced by alpha II-interferon. Acta Neurol Belg 1990; 90:111–114.
50. Jacobs SK, Wilson DJ, Kornblith PL, Grimm EA. Interleukin-2 and autologous lymphokine-activated killer cells in the treatment of malignant glioma: preliminary report. J Neurosurg 1986; 64:743–749.
51. Barba D, Saris SC, Holder C, Rosenberg SA, Oldfield EH. Intratumoral LAK cell and interleukin-2 therapy of human gliomas. J Neurosurg 1989; 70:175–182.
52. Merchant RE, Grant AJ, Merchant LH, Young HF. Adoptive immunotherapy for recurrent glioblastoma multiforme using lymphokine activated killer cells and recombinant interleukin-2. Cancer 1988; 62:665–671.
53. Nitta T, Sato K, Yagita H, Okumura K, Ishii S. Preliminary trial of specific targeting therapy against malignant glioma. Lancet 1990; 335:368–371.
54. Denicoff KD, Rubinow DR, Papa MZ, Simpson C, Seipp CA, Lotze MT, Chang AE, Rosenstein D, Rosenberg SA. The neuropsychiatric effects of treatment with interleukin-2 and lymphokine-activated killer cells. Ann Intern Med 1987; 107:293–300.
55. West WH, Tauer KW, Yanelli JR, Marshall GD, Orr DW, Thurman GB, Oldham RK. Constant-infusion recombinant interleukin-2 in adoptive immunotherapy of advanced cancer. N Engl J Med 1987; 316:898–905.
56. Saris SC, Patronas NJ, Rosenberg SA, Alexander JT, Frank J, Schwartzentruber DJ, Rubin JT, Barba D, Oldfield EH. The effect of intravenous interleukin-2 on brain water content. J Neurosurg 1989; 71:169–174.
57. Dillman RO, Oldham RK, Tauer KW, Orr DW, Barth NM, Blimenschein G, Arnold J, Birch R, West W. Continuous interleukin-2 and lymphokine-activated killer cells for advanced cancer: a national biotherapy study group trial. J Clin Oncol 1991; 9:1233–1240.
58. Rosenberg SA, Lotze MT, Mull LM, Chang AE, Avis FP, Leitman S, Linehan WM, Robertson CN, Lee RE, Rubin JT, Seipp CA, Simpson CG, White DE. A progress report on the treatment of 157 patients with advanced cancer using lymphokine-activated killer cells and interleukin-2 or high-dose interleukin-2 alone. N Engl J Med 1987; 316:889–897.
59. Margolin KA, Rayner AA, Hawkins MJ, Atkins MB, Dutcher JP, Fisher RI, Weiss GR, Doroshow JH, Jaffe HS, Roper M, Parkinson DR, Wiernik PH, Creekmore SP, Boldt DH. Interleukin-2 and lymphokine-activated killer cell therapy of solid tumors: analysis of toxicity and management guidelines. J Clin Oncol 1989; 7:486–498.
60. Ellison GD, Povlishock JT, Merchant RE. Blood-brain barrier dysfunction in cats following recombinant interleukin-2 infusion. Cancer Res 1987; 47:5765–5770.

61. Delattre JY, Posner JB. The blood-brain barrier: morphology, physiology and its changes in cancer patients. In: Hildebrand J, ed. (European School of Oncology. Monographs. Series ed: Veronesi U) Neurological adverse reactions to anticancer drug. Berlin: Springer-Verlag, 1990: 3–24.
62. Vecht CJ, Keohane C, Menon RS, Punt CJA, Stoter G. Acute fatal leukoencephalopathy after interleukin-2 therapy. N Engl J Med 1990; 323:1146–1147.
63. Bernard JT, Ameriso S, Kempf RA, Rosen P, Mitchell MS, Fisher M. Transient focal neurologic deficits complicating interleukin-2 therapy. Neurology 1990; 40:154–155.
64. Rosenberg SA, Longo DL, Lotze MT. Principles and applications of biologic therapy. In: DeVita VT, Hellman S, Rosenberg SA, eds. Cancer: principles and practice of oncology. Philadelphia: JB Lippincott Co., 1989:301–347.
65. Loh FL, Herskovitz S, Berger AR, Swerdlow ML. Brachial plexopathy associated with interleukin-2 therapy. Neurology 1992; 42:462–463.
66. Richards JM, Vogelzang NJ, Bluestone JA. Neurotoxicity after treatment with muromonab-CD3. N Engl J Med 1990; 323:487–488.
67. Hammond EH, Watson FS, Bristow MR, O'Connell JB, Gilbert EM, Doty DB, Renlund DG. Fibrinoid necrosis of a temporal artery complicating the treatment of refractory cardiac allograft rejection with murine monoclonal CD3 antibody (OKT3). J Heart Transplant 1990; 9:236–238.
68. Martin MA, Massanari RM, Nghiem DD, Smith JL, Corry RJ. Nosocomial aseptic meningitis associated with administration of OKT3. JAMA 1988; 259:2002–2005.
69. Thistlethwaite JR, Stuart JK, Mayes JT, Gaber AO, Woodle S, Buckingham MR, Stuart FP. Monitoring and complications of monoclonal therapy: complications and monitoring of OKT3 therapy. Am J Kidney Dis 1988; 11:112–119.
70. Adair JC, Woodley SL, O'Connell JB, Call GK, Baringer JR. Aseptic meningitis following cardiac transplantation: clinical characteristics and relationship to immunosuppressive regimen. Neurology 1991; 41:249–252.
71. Coleman AE, Norman DJ, OKT3 encephalopathy. Ann Neurol 1990; 28:837–838.
72. Emmons C, Smith J, Flanigan M. Cerebrospinal fluid inflammation during OKT3 therapy (letter). Lancet 1986; 2:510–511.
73. Saleh MN, Khazaeli MB, Wheeler RH, Dropcho E, Liu T, Urist M, Miller DM, Lawson S, Dixon P, Russell CH, LoBuglio AF. Phase I trial of the murine monoclonal anti-GD2 antibody 14G2a in metastatic melanoma. Cancer Res 1992, 52:4342–4347.
74. Lashford LS, Davies G, Richardson RB, Bourne SP, Bullimore JA, Eckert H, Kemshead JT, Coakham HB. A pilot study of $^{131}$I monoclonal antibodies in the therapy of leptomeningeal tumors. Cancer 1988; 61:857–868.
75. Moseley RP, Davies AG, Richardson RB, Zalutsky M, Carrel S, Fabre J, Slack N, Bullimore J, Pizer B, Papanastassiou V, Kemshead JT, Coakham HB, Lashford LS. Intrathecal administration of $^{131}$I radiolabelled monoclonal antibody as a treatment for neoplastic meningitis. Br J Cancer 1990; 62:637–642.
76. Hertler AA, Frankel AE. Immunotoxins: a clinical review of their use in the treatment of malignancies. J Clin Oncol 1989; 7:1932–1942.
77. Vitetta ES, Stone M, Amlot P, Fay J, May R, Till M, Newman J, Clark P, Collins R, Cunningham D, Ghetie V, Uhr JW, Thorpe PE. Phase I immunotoxin trial in patients with B-cell lymphoma. Cancer Res 1991; 51:4052–4058.

78. Byers VS, Rodvien R, Grant K, Durrant LG, Hudson KH, Baldwin RW, Scannon PJ. Phase I study of monoclonal antibody–ricin A chain immunotoxin XomaZyme-791 in patients with metastatic colon cancer. Cancer Res 1989; 49:6153–6160.
79. Spitler LE, del Rio M, Khentigan A, Wedel NI, Brophy NA, Miller LL, Harkonen WS, Rosendorf LL, Lee HM, Mischak RP, et al. Therapy of patients with malignant melanoma using a monoclonal antimelanoma antibody–ricin A chain immunotoxin. Cancer Res 1987; 47:1717–1723.
80. Gould BJ, Borowitz MJ, Groves ES, Carter PW, Anthony D, Weiner LM, Frankel AE. Phase I study of an anti-breast cancer immunotoxin by continuous infusion: report of a targeted toxic effect not predicted by animal studies. J Natl Cancer Inst 1989; 81:775–781.
81. Grossbard ML, Nadler LM. Immunotoxin therapy of malignancy. In: DeVita VT, Hellman S, Rosenberg SA, eds. Important advances in oncology 1992. Philadelphia: JB Lippincott Co., 1992:111–135.

# 13
# Neurological Complications of Lung Cancer

**Karl E. Misulis**

*Vanderbilt University Medical Center, Nashville, and Semmes-Murphey Clinic, Jackson, Tennessee*

**Ronald G. Wiley**

*Vanderbilt University Medical Center and Veterans Affairs Medical Center, Nashville, Tennessee*

## I. INTRODUCTION

Lung cancer is the leading cause of cancer mortality in the United States and the most common cause of central nervous system (CNS) metastases. Lung cancer also can cause a wide variety of other neurological complications. Most direct and indirect neurological complications of systemic neoplasms can be seen in patients with lung cancer (Table 1). A few, such as subacute sensory neuronopathy, Eaton-Lambert syndrome, and Pancoast's syndrome, are almost unique to lung cancer. The incidence of specific neurological complications is related to histological tumor type (41). Management decisions are profoundly influenced by the presence of neurological complications.

## II. EPIDEMIOLOGY OF LUNG CANCER

Each year, more than 150,000 individuals in the United States are diagnosed with primary lung carcinoma (41a). Of these, 60% of small cell and 30–40% of non-small cell patients will have distant metastases at the time of diagnoses (30a), with the CNS being frequently affected (51a).

The typical types and incidence of neurological complications are illustrated by our retrospective study of patients with neurological complications of lung cancer at the Nashville Veterans Affairs Medical Center. Squamous cell was the most

**Table 1** Neurological Complications of Lung Cancer

| Neurological disorder | Signs and symptoms | Associated cancer | Treatment |
|---|---|---|---|
| Brain metastases | | | |
|   Single | Focal dysfunction (e.g., hemianopia) | Adeno > Squam > SCLC | Surgery and RT |
|   Multiple | Encephalopathy or multifocal | SCLC > Adeno > Squam | RT and chemo |
| Epidural spinal cord compression | Back pain<br>Gait change<br>Sensory level | Squam > SCLC > Adeno | Corticosteroids<br>XRT<br>Surgery in selected cases |
| Brachial plexus | Pain<br>Weakness | SCLC > Adeno > Squam | XRT to tumor |
| Cerebellar degeneration (anti-HU) | Ataxia | SCLC | Treat underlying tumor |
| Myasthenic syndrome | Generalized weakness | SCLC | Treat underlying tumor<br>4-Aminopyridine<br>Plasmapheresis |
| Peripheral neuropathy (anti-HU) | Weakness<br>Numbness | SCLC | Treat underlying tumor |

Associated cancer indicates which tissue type is most commonly associated with the complication. Adeno = adenocarcinoma; Squam = squamous cell carcinoma; SCLC = small cell lung cancer.

common tumor histology in the present series. The relative frequencies of the various tissue types are in close agreement with previously published autopsy data when patients with large cell undifferentiated carcinoma are grouped with squamous cell carcinoma patients (41).

The incidence of neurological complications correlates with histological tumor type (Table 2). Adenocarcinoma was relatively overrepresented among neurological complications: 42% of patients with neurological complications had this tumor type but only 25% of patients had this type of tumor (relative risk = 1.68). Neurological complications were less frequent in patients with squamous cell carcinoma (relative risk = 0.70). Neurological complications in patients with small cell lung cancer (SCLC) were proportionate to tumor incidence (relative risk = 0.95). Patients in this study received a variety of treatment regimens including prophylactic cranial irradiation for SCLC that likely decreased the incidence of brain metastases with SCLC. The reason(s) for the greater prevalence of CNS complications in the present retrospective clinical series compared to the autopsy series of Matthews (41) is not readily apparent, but the higher figures, particularly

**Table 2** Epidemiological Data for Neurological Complications (NC) of Lung Cancer

| Parameter | Squamous | Adeno | Small |
|---|---|---|---|
| Prevalence | | | |
| % of all lung Ca | 54 | 25 | 21 |
| % of pts with NC | 38 | 42 | 20 |
| Specific complications (%) | | | |
| Brain metastases | 74 | 81 | 90 |
| Spinal cord compression | 26 | 9 | 14 |
| Neoplastic meningitis | 0 | 7 | 14 |
| Plexopathy | 0 | 5 | 14 |
| Patient summary | | | |
| Number | 39 | 43 | 21 |
| Age at presentation | 59 | 58 | 60 |
| Had NC at presentation (%) | 49 | 37 | 38 |

Data were obtained from retrospective study of neurological complications of lung cancer, performed by the authors at the Nashville Veterans Affairs Medical Center, 1988. Prevalence data are separated for patients with and without neurological complications. Specific complications are expressed as the percent of patients with complications who had each of these lesions. In adenocarcinoma and small cell, the vertical column adds up to more than 100% because some patients had more than one complication.

with adenocarcinomas, in the present series are consistent with more recent published data (4a,26).

## III. COMMON COMPLICATIONS OF LUNG CANCER

A list of potential neurological complications of lung cancer is extensive. Some, such as the paraneoplastic syndromes, have a low incidence, although they may be underdiagnosed. In our study, the most common complications were brain metastases (81% of all neurological complications), spinal cord compression (17%), neoplastic meningitis (6%), and plexopathy (5%). No cases of paraneoplastic syndromes were identified in our study. However, these syndromes may have been underdiagnosed. A large proportion of patients experienced neurological complications at the time of primary tumor diagnosis; 42% of all neurological complications were present at the time of diagnosis of the lung primary tumor. This number may be high because of the retrospective nature of the study. The high proportion of brain metastases in the present series may reflect the tendency for brain metastases to be symptomatic. Also, 20–25% of recurrences of non-small cell lung cancers are brain metastases (17,39).

SWOG Study 7415 reported 14% of extensive-stage SCLC patients had brain metastases at presentation (30a). Salvatierra et al. (56) reported a 13% incidence

**Table 3** Neurological Complications of Specific Lung Tumors

|  | Squamous | Adeno | SCLC |
| --- | --- | --- | --- |
| Survival |  |  |  |
| Median with NC | 7 mo | 10 mo | 11 mo |
| Median without NC | 6.5 mo | 7 mo | 10 mo |
| Range with NC | 1–72 mo | 1–58 mo | 1–31 mo |
| Range without NC | 1–32 mo | 1–46 mo | 1–15 mo |
| Number with mets | 29 | 35 | 19 |
| Multiple mets | 48% | 42% | 68% |
| Treatment of mets |  |  |  |
| None | 2 | 4 | 0 |
| Radiation | 27 | 29 | 18 |
| Craniotomy | 5 | 7 | 2 |
| Chemotherapy | 4 | 5 | 17 |
| Number with cord compression | 10 | 4 | 3 |

Data are from the same study described in Table 2 and in the text. NC = neurological complications; mets = metastases; mo = months; SCLC = small cell lung carcinoma.

of brain metastases at the time of diagnosis of SCLC (all stages). Others have reported brain metastases in 10% of SCLC patients at diagnosis, with another 20–25% eventually developing brain metastases (29,33). An autopsy study found brain metastases in 65% of cases (30). Sculier et al. (58) found overall that 29.5% of patients with SCLC developed a clinically evident neurological complication. Similar to the present series, the most common complications were brain metastases (76%), spinal cord compression (11%), and neoplastic meningitis (7%). Intramedullary metastases and myasthenic syndrome were rarely seen. Although short-term survival was not affected, patients with neurological complications had reduced long-term survival, in part because nervous system involvement in all forms of lung cancer usually occurs in the setting of disseminated metastases.

## A. Brain Metastases

Brain metastases may be single or multiple. The brain is the most common site of isolated relapse (39%) in patients with stage III adenocarcinoma after attempted curative resection (10,40). When lesions are multiple, their metastatic nature is obvious. However, a single lesion may be misdiagnosed as metastasis. Of patients with lung cancer and solitary brain masses, approximately 10% were not metastases. The etiology of the lesion can be abscess, other neoplasm, or, less likely, hemorrhage or infarction (49). With modern imaging techniques, the latter two possibilities are seldom confused with tumor. Abscess is especially likely in patients who have received chemotherapy or extensive bone marrow exposure to radiotherapy. Second primary neoplasms are always a concern in cancer patients. We saw at least three patients with lung cancer who were referred for resection of a presumed solitary metastasis, in whom the pathology showed malignant glioma. During the present study period, we saw two patients who received radiation for presumed brain metastasis, but did not respond. Biopsies showed *Blastomyces* abscesses.

In our retrospective study of patients with neurological complications of lung cancer, more patients with SCLC had multiple brain metastases. Of all patients with brain metastases, 68% of patients with SCLC had multiple metastases, while for squamous cell the proportion was 48% and for adenocarcinoma 42%. These figures for proportion with multiple metastases are similar to previous reports (21).

There is some controversy regarding treatment of brain metastases from lung cancer. Traditional treatment has relied on whole brain radiation. In more than half of patients, radiotherapy controls the tumor sufficiently that patients die of their systemic neoplasm (13). In our series, 89% of patients with brain metastases received radiation therapy. Chemotherapy was administered predominantly to patients with SCLC; 89% of SCLC patients received chemotherapy. Only a few patients with squamous cell and adenocarcinoma also received various investigational chemotherapies (14% for each). This low frequency of chemotherapy use in non-small cell cancer patients reflects the lack of any regimen with reliable efficacy.

Chemotherapy currently has nothing to offer in controlling brain metastases from squamous or adenocarcinomas. However, the situation is different with SCLC, which is responsive to several agents. Lee et al. (35a) reported using chemotherapy with cyclophosphamide, duxorubicin, vincristine, and etoposide as primary treatment of brain metastases of small cell carcinoma. Nine of 13 patients responded to treatment, although only one had a complete remission. Radiotherapy was given with the fourth and last cycle of chemotherapy. These and other data indicate a limited role for chemotherapy in the management of brain metastases from SCLC. Chemotherapy generally is not indicated as initial therapy for patients with brain metastases from any type of lung cancer who have stable systemic disease. We recommend considering salvage chemotherapy to control brain metastases only in SCLC patients who develop brain metastases after previous brain irradiation.

Neurosurgery was performed in 17% of our patients with brain metastases. This percentage is low by today's standards, since all of the patients received treatment prior to 1988. The distribution of surgery among the different tumor types slightly favored adenocarcinoma, with 20% having surgery. Seventeen percent of patients with squamous cell carcinoma and only 11% of patients with SCLC had craniotomy. The lower percentage for SCLC in the present series is due to the greater proportion with multiple metastases and the anticipated better response to radiation therapy and chemotherapy. Surgery should be considered in patients with single brain metastases from non-small cell lung cancer. Based on two recent studies, patients with solitary brain metastases benefit significantly from surgery followed by radiotherapy (51,64). The role of surgery in patients with multiple brain metastases is more controversial. Occasional patients with non-small cell lung cancer will do well with resection of multiple metastases. Typically, such patients have readily accessible metastases from a radioresistant primary (adenocarcinoma or squamous) and no evidence of systemic disease.

Interstitial brachytherapy and stereotactic radiosurgery have recently received attention. The latter may be beneficial for metastatic lesions (38a). Such treatment usually is tolerated well with no serious acute morbidity or mortality. One published study reported qualitatively favorable outcomes with stereotactic radiosurgery in 18 patients with metastases, not specifically selected for lung cancer (38). Seven of the 18 had lung cancer. Greater experience is needed to clarify the role of stereotactic radiosurgery in management of brain metastases from non-small cell lung cancer. At present, it is an option for single lesions that are surgically inaccessible or recurrent after initial treatment. For further discussion of brain metastases, see Chapter 1.

## B. Epidural Spinal Cord Compression (ESCC)

It is surprising that ESCC is not more common. A large percentage of patients with lung and other solid tumors will have metastases to the spine at the time of death, but the number of lung cancer patients with clinically apparent ESCC is 10% or less (53,58). Thirty-three percent of ESCC is due to lung cancer (62). Epidural spinal cord compression was observed in 17% of our patients with neurological complications of lung cancer. All tissue types were represented. Of patients with neurological complications of squamous cell carcinoma, 26% were found to develop ESCC. In 30% of patients who developed ESCC, the cord compression was not acutely symptomatic.

ESCC from lung cancer is usually due to extension of tumor that has metastasized to one or more vertebral bodies. This results in compression of the thecal sac against the posterior elements. Less commonly, there is extension of tumor from the paravertebral region through a foramen into the spinal canal (22). The most common site of ESCC is the thoracic region (70%), followed by the lumbar and cervical regions. Multiple levels of ESCC are unusual with lung cancer.

Pain occurs in 90–95% of patients with ESCC from lung cancer (20) and is often attributed to chest wall invasion, bone metastases, or port-thoracotomy pain. If a lung cancer patient with symptoms suggestive of progressive myelopathy or cauda equina compression has no pain or percussion tenderness over the spine, ESCC is unlikely. Other clinical findings are similar to those seen in patients with ESCC due to other solid tumors. ESCC should be considered in all lung cancer patients with *progressive* back pain, particularly those with new gait difficulty. Approximately 10% of the time, the cause of the lesion will not be directly related to the tumor.

Details of evaluation and treatment of ESCC are presented by Byrne in Chapter 2. The only special consideration in managing ESCC in patients with SCLC is the role of systemic chemotherapy. We recommend radiotherapy as primary treatment for ESCC from all forms of lung cancer when myelopathy is present, including SCLC. If systemic chemotherapy is indicated for treatment of the systemic disease, it is usually delayed until spinal radiotherapy is complete. If myelopathy is not present, the sequence may be reversed, with radiotherapy being administered after induction of chemotherapy. Obviously, close follow-up is mandatory in such cases. Surgery is usually not appropriate, except to establish a tissue diagnosis in patients with occult lung cancer, because ESCC in lung cancer patients rarely occurs in the absence of widespread metastases, and surgery does not improve outcome.

Intramedullary metastases, radiation myelopathy, and paraneoplastic necrotizing myelopathy must be considered in the differential diagnosis of myelopathy in cancer patients. Lung cancer is the most common cause (49%) of intramedullary spinal metastases (57) and usually presents as a progressive asymmetrical myelopathy (16). Local back pain is common, but tenderness to percussion over the spine is much less prominent compared to extradural metastases. Intramedullary metastases are highly associated with widespread systemic and intracerebral metastases (25). Radiation myelopathy occurs in lung cancer patients when the spinal cord has to be included in a thoracic radiation field. Consequently, the myelopathy is localizable to the irradiated segments of the cord, comes on after several months or several years, and is often associated with little or no pain (12a,32a,47a,b). Radiation myelopathy often begins asymmetrically but progresses to a complete transverse myelopathy. Finally, paraneoplastic myelopathy has no clear relationship to a particular type of cancer and may represent a fortuitous association (47). The diagnosis is primarily one of exclusion.

## C. Neoplastic Meningitis

Up to 10% of patients with lung cancer will develop meningeal metastases (41) although many are not diagnosed antemortem. About 25% of cases of neoplastic meningitis are due to lung cancer; most are SCLC. Squamous cell carcinomas are less likely to metastasize to the leptomeninges. Henson and Urich (28) pointed out the propensity for adenocarcinomas to metastasize to the leptomeninges. The clinical presentation of meningeal metastases is the same in lung cancer patients as in those with other solid tumors. Patients usually present with more findings than symptoms, and the findings reflect multifocal dysfunction at more than one level of the neuraxis (brain, cranial nerves, spinal cord, and spinal roots). The diagnosis and management of leptomeningeal metastases are discussed by Wasserstrom in Chapter 3.

Neoplastic meningitis was seen in 6% of our patients with neurological complications of lung cancer. Half had adenocarcinoma and half had SCLC. None had squamous cell carcinoma, even though this was the most common primary tumor. The risk of neoplastic meningitis was highest with SCLC. Among patients with neurological complications, 14% of SCLC patients had leptomeningeal involvement compared to 7% of adenocarcinoma patients. Most lung cancer patients developing meningeal involvement have widespread recurrent systemic disease. Leptomeningeal involvement by SCLC has been well documented (1,2,6,8,55,61). Radiotherapy may provide symptomatic palliation of leptomeningeal metastases from lung cancer, but intrathecal therapy is of unproven value.

## D. Paraneoplastic Syndromes

The large majority of lung cancer patients with paraneoplastic neurological syndromes have SCLC (51a). The two best-understood syndromes are "anti-HU disease," which may include any combination of central and peripheral nervous system damage, and the myasthenic syndrome of Lambert and Eaton (LEMS). Anti-HU patients most often present with peripheral nervous system signs and symptoms, typically subacute sensory neuronopathy. However, limbic encephalitis and cerebellar presentations also occur (5). Early recognition and diagnosis of these patients will often detect the underlying SCLC at an early, limited stage. The pathogenesis of these various disorders appears to be autoimmune. Most patients have detectable antibodies to the HU antigen, a basic, nonhistone nucleoprotein found in all neurons and some SCLC cells. Treatment is directed at the primary tumor. Immunosuppression, plasmapheresis, and high-dose intravenous gamma globulin are not of proven value (23). LEMS presents with proximal weakness, with or without subtle sensory signs and symptoms. Neuromuscular transmission studies reveal augmentation of compound motor potentials with repetitive stimulation. Plasmapheresis, guanidine or 4-aminopyridine, immunosuppression, and therapy of the primary tumor are all of value (44,46). The pathogenesis is an autoimmune response directed at the voltage-sensitive calcium channel that is common to neurons and some SCLC cells. A variety of other neurological syndromes have been reported rarely in patients with lung cancer. However, anti-HU and LEMS are by far the most common and best understood. Both these autoimmune paraneoplastic syndromes can produce severe disability despite successful treatment of the primary tumor. This topic is discussed in greater detail in Chapter 8.

## E. Pancoast's Syndrome and Metastatic Brachial Plexopathy

Brachial plexopathy typically develops in patients with tumors of the upper lobe. This is a rare complication, probably occurring in less than 1% of patients with cancer (32). Shoulder pain and upper extremity neurological dysfunction are common features of both Pancoast's syndrome and late-occurring brachial plexopathy in lung cancer patients. None of the patients in the present series developed brachial plexus involvement.

Pancoast's syndrome (48,52) results from invasion of the plexus by tumor extending from the chest. Patients almost always present with sensory symptoms. This syndrome usually begins as continuous, progressive pain in the shoulder and along the medial scapula. With time, the pain radiates down the arm and patients develop neurological deficits in the C8/T1 distribution, which are often confused with an ulnar neuropathy (numbness of digits IV and V, weakness of intrinsic muscles of the hand). Patients often have Horner's syndrome due to involvement of the ascending sympathetic fibers after medial spread of tumor into the paravertebral region. As many as 50% of patients with Horner's syndrome and neoplastic plexopathy from lung cancer will have extension of tumor into the epidural space.

Late-occurring metastatic brachial plexopathy is less stereotypical. Pain is present in at least 75% of patients (34). The remainder present with dysesthesias and numbness. Later, weakness develops if the tumor is untreated. Most symptoms are referable to the lower trunk and/or median cord of the plexus, since this region is nearest to the lymph nodes above the superior aspect of the lung. Clinical suspicion is raised by prominent pain radiating from the shoulder into the arm, and often by some weakness in the hand. Diagnosis may be delayed by paucity of objective findings, early in the course. Tumor in the region of the plexus is best visualized by magnetic resonance imaging (MRI). Computerized tomography is a useful alternative to MRI. With both imaging techniques, distortion or obliteration of tissue planes, with or without a mass, may be the only indication of tumor. It is important to look for intraspinal tumor extension by myelogram or MRI, making MRI the imaging procedure of choice when available. Current management involves some combination of wide-field radiotherapy and/or surgery depending on the extent of disease at diagnosis (3,41a). Occasionally surgery is necessary to distinguish between metastatic and postradiotherapy plexopathies.

In lung cancer patients with prior radiotherapy, it is important to differentiate neoplastic plexopathy from radiation plexopathy. Many patients who develop brachial plexopathy will have already received radiotherapy to the region. Table 4 presents a guide to differentiation between neoplastic and radiation plexopathy (32) in lung cancer patients. Radiation plexopathy is characterized by dysesthesias and numbness; however, pain is not as prominent as with tumor infiltration. Later in the course, pain may be more prominent. Radiation plexopathy has been reported to affect the upper plexus more frequently and more severely than metastatic invasion from the lung apex. This may be due to shielding of the lower plexus by surrounding tissues. Myokymia has been reported in patients with radiation plexopathy but not in patients with neoplastic infiltration. Myokymia is an involuntary repetitive discharge of single motor units at a frequency of 30–40/s (42). This is best detected by electromyography, although it can occasionally be seen on close examination.

An unusual but related problem is the presentation of lung cancer as unilateral face pain or headache. Patients typically develop face pain or headache ipsilateral to the lung tumor, but neurological examination reveals no deficits (9,11,15,45, 63a). The mechanism is thought to be referred pain from involvement of the vagus nerve in the chest. Indeed, 71% of cases of unilateral vocal cord paralysis (recurrent laryngeal neuropathy) are due to neoplasms, with lung cancer the cause in 34% of cases (19).

**Table 4** Differentiation of Neoplastic and Radiation Brachial Plexopathy

| Symptom/sign | Neoplastic | Radiation |
|---|---|---|
| Pain | Severe | Mild or none |
| Distribution | Lower plexus | Upper plexus |
| Lymphedema | Mild or none | Often prominent |
| Myokymia on EMG | None | Often |

Pain with radiation plexopathy is usually late in the course, dysesthesias being more prominent earlier in the course.
*Source*: Derived from Ref. 32.

**Table 5** Cause of Encephalopathy in Lung Cancer Patients

|  | Most common primary tumor type |
|---|---|
| With focal signs and symptoms | |
|   Multiple brain metastases | SCLC, adeno |
|   Leptomeningeal metastases | SCLC, adeno |
|   Anti-HU disease | SCLC only |
|   Multiple strokes (NBTE) | Adeno, any |
|   Multiple abscesses | Any |
|   Meningitis | Any |
| Without focal signs and symptoms | |
|   Hypoxia | Any |
|   Hypotension | Any |
|   Hypercalcemia | Squamous |
|   Hepatic failure | SCLC, adeno |
|   Hyponatremia | SCLC |
|   Hypercortisolemia | Carcinoid, SCLC |
|   Drug intoxication | Any |
|   Sepsis | Any |

## F. Encephalopathy

Development of encephalopathy in a lung cancer patient can be due to a variety of general and specific causes (Table 5). Aside from anti-HU disease, the spectrum of causes of encephalopathy in lung cancer patients resembles that of other patients with solid tumors. The approach to evaluating encephalopathy in a lung cancer patient must stress a careful search for focal neurological deficits indicative of metastatic invasion of the CNS. Prompt diagnosis and treatment may improve quality of survival, if not duration of life.

## REFERENCES

1. Aisner J, Aisner SC, Ostrow S, Govindan S, Mummert K, Wiernik P. Meningeal carcinomatosis from small cell carcinoma of the lung. Consequence of improved survival. Acta Cytol 1979; 23:292–296.
2. Aisner J, Ostrow S, Govindan S, Wiernik P. Leptomeningeal carcinomatosis in small cell carcinoma of the lung. Med Pediatr Oncol 1981; 9:47–59.
3. Ampil FL. Radiotherapy for carcinomatous brachial plexopathy. A clinical study of 23 cases. Cancer 1985; 56:2185–2188.
4. Anderson HA, Prakash UBS. Diagnosis of symptomatic lung cancer. In: Israel L, Chahanian P, eds. Lung cancer: natural history, prognosis and therapy. New York: Academic Press, 1976; 23–62.

4a. Anderson HA, Prakash UBS. Diagnosis of symptomatic lung cancer. Semin Respir Med 1982; 3:165–175.
5. Anderson NE, Rosenblum MK, Graus F, Wiley RG, Posner JB. Autoantibodies in paraneoplastic syndromes associated with small cell lung cancer. Neurology 1988; 38:391–398.
6. Aroney RS, Dalley DN, Chan WK, Bell DR, Levi JA. Meningeal carcinomatosis in small cell carcinoma of the lung. Am J Med 1981; 71:26–32.
7. Bach F, Larsen BH, Rohde K, Borgesen SE, Gjerris F, Boge-Rasmussed T, Agerlin N, Rasmusson B, Stjernholm P, Sorensen PS. Metastatic spinal cord compression. Occurrence, symptoms, clinical presentation, and prognosis in 398 patients with spinal cord compression. Acta Neurochir Wien 1990; 107:37–43.
8. Balducci L, Little DD, Khansur T, Steinberg MH. Carcinomatous meningitis in small cell lung cancer. Am J Med Sci 1984; 287:31–33.
9. Bindoff LA, Heseltine D. Unilateral facial pain in patients with lung cancer: a referred pain via the vagus? Lancet 1988; 1:812–815.
10. Bitran J, Golomb H, DeMeester T, et al. Combined modality therapy for stage II M0 nonsmall cell bronchogenic carcinoma. Proc Am Assoc Cancer Res Am Soc Clin Oncol 1980; 21:446.
11. Bongers KM, Willigers HMM, Koehler PJ. Referred facial pain from lung carcinoma. Neurology 1992; 42:1841–1842.
12. Bruckman JE, Bloomer WD. Management of spinal cord compression. Semin Oncol 1978; 5:135–140.
12a. Burns RJ, Jones AN, Robertson JS. Pathology of radiation myelopathy. J Neurol Neurosurg Psychiatr 1972; 35:888–898.
13. Cairncross JG, Kim JH, Posner JB. Radiation therapy for brain metastases. Ann Neurol 1982; 7:529–541.
14. Chalk CH, Murray NM, Newsom-Davis J, O'Neill JH, Spiro SG. Response of the Lambert-Eaton myasthenic syndrome to treatment of associated small-cell lung carcinoma. Neurology 1990; 40:1552–1556.
15. DesPrez RD, Freemon FR. Facial pain associated with lung cancer: a case report. Headache 1983; 23:43–44.
16. Edelson RN, Deck MDF, Posner JB. Intramedullary spinal cord metastasis. Clinical and radiographic findings in nine cases. Neurology 1972; 22:1222–1229.
17. Figlin RA, Piantadosi S, Feld R (for Lung Cancer Study Group). Intracranial recurrence of carcinoma after complete surgical resection of stage I, II and III non-small cell lung cancer. N Engl J Med 1988; 318:1300–1305.
18. Frytak S, Shaw JN, Lee Re, Eagan RT, Shaw EG, Richardson RL, Creagan ET, Coles ET, Jett JR. Treatment toxicities in long-term survivors of limited small cell lung cancer. Cancer Invest 1988; 6:669–676.
19. Gardner GM, Shaari CM, Parnes SM. Long-term morbidity and mortality in patients undergoing surgery for unilateral vocal cord paralysis. Laryngoscope 1992; 102:501–508.
20. Gilbert RW, Kim JH, Posner JB. Epidural spinal cord compression from metastatic tumor: diagnosis and treatment. Ann Neurol 1978; 3:40–51.
21. Ginsburg RJ, Kris MG, Armstrong JG. Non-small cell lung cancer. In: DeVita VT Jr,

Hellman S, Rosenberg SA, eds. Cancer: principles and practice of oncology, 4th ed. Philadelphia: JB Lippincott, 1993: 673–723.
22. Grant R, Papadopoulos SM, Greenberg HS. Metastatic epidural spinal cord compression. Neurol Clin 1991; 9:825–841.
23. Graus F, Vega F, Delattre JY. Plasmapheresis and antineoplastic treatment in CNS paraneoplastic syndromes with antineuronal autoantibodies. Neurology 1992; 42: 536–540.
24. Greenberg HS, Kim HS, Posner JB. Epidural spinal cord compression from metastatic tumor: results with a new treatment protocol. Ann Neurol 1980; 8:361–366.
25. Grem JL, Burgess J, Trump DL. Clinical features and natural history of intramedullary spinal cord metastases. Cancer 1985; 56:2305–2314.
26. Grippi MA. Clinical aspects of lung cancer. Semin Roentgenol 1990; 25:12–24.
27. Grossman SA, Moynihan TJ. Neoplastic meningitis. Neurol Clin 1991; 9:843–856.
28. Henson RA, Urich H. Cancer and the nervous system. The neurological manifestations of systemic malignant disease. Oxford: Blackwell Scientific Pub., 1982: 100–119.
29. Higgins GA, Shields TW. Experience of the Veterans Administration Surgical Adjuvant Group. In: Muggia FM, Rozencweig M, eds. Lung cancer: progress in therapeutic research. New York: Raven Press, 1979: 433–442.
30. Hirsch FR, Paulson OB, Hansen HH, et al. Intracranial metastases in small cell carcinoma of the lung: correlation of clinical and autopsy findings. Cancer 1982; 50:2433–2437.
30a. Holmes EC, Livingston R, Turrisi A. Neoplasms of the thorax. In: Holland JF, Frei E, III, Bast RC, Kufc DW, Morton DL, Weichselbaum RR, eds. Cancer Medicine, 3rd ed. Philadelphia: Lea & Febiger, 1993: 1285–1337.
31. Ihde DC, Pass HI, Glatstein EJ. Small cell lung cancer. In: DeVita VT Jr, Hellman S, Rosenberg SA, eds. Cancer: principles and practice of oncology, 4th ed. Philadelphia: JB Lippincott, 1993: 723–758.
32. Jaeckle K. Nerve plexus metastases. Neurol Clin 1991; 9:857–866.
32a. Jelling K, Sturm KW. Delayed radiation myelopathy in man. Report of 12 necropsy cases. J Neurol Sci 1971; 14:389–408.
33. Komaki R, Cox JD, Whitson W. Risk of brain metastases from small cell carcinoma of the lung related to length of survival and prophylactic irradiation. Cancer Treat Rep 1981; 65:811–814.
34. Kori SH, Foley KM, Posner JB. Brachial plexus lesions in patients with cancer: 100 cases. Neurology 1981; 31:45.
35. Lang B, Newsom-Davis J, Peers C, Prior C, Wray DW. The effect of myasthenic syndrome antibody on presynaptic calcium channels in the mouse. J Physiol (Lond) 1987; 390:257–270.
35a. Lee JS, Murphy WK, Glisson BS, Dhingra HM, Holoye PE, Hong WK. Primary chemotherapy of brain metastasis in small-cell lung cancer. J Clin Oncol 1989; 7:916.
36. Lennon VA, Lambert EH. Autoantibodies bind solubilized calcium channel-omega-conotoxin complexes from small cell lung carcinoma: a diagnostic aid for Lambert-Eaton myasthenic syndrome. Mayo Clin Proc 1989; 64:1498–1504.
37. Leys K, Lang B, Johnston I, Newsom-Davis J. Calcium channel autoantibodies in the Lambert-Eaton myasthenic syndrome. Ann Neurol 1991; 29:307–314.

38. Loeffler JS, Kooy HM, Wen PY, et al. The treatment of recurrent brain metastases with stereotactic radiosurgery. J Clin Oncol 1990; 8:576–582.
38a. Maciunas RJ, Misulis KE. Comprehensive therapy for malignant gliomas—Parts I & II. Contemp Neurosurg 1991; 13(20):1–6 and 13(21):1–5.
39. Magilligan DJ, Duvernoy C, Malik G, et al. Surgical approach to lung cancer with solitary cerebral metastasis: twenty-five years' experience. Ann Thorac Surg 1986; 42:360–364.
40. Martini N, Flehinger BJ, Nagasaki F, Hart B. Prognostic significance of N1 disease in carcinoma of the lung. J Thorac Cardiovasc Surg 1983; 86:646–653.
41. Matthews MJ. Problems in morphology and behavior of bronchopulmonary malignant disease. In: Israel L, Chahanian P, eds. Lung cancer: natural history, prognosis and therapy. New York: Academic Press 1976: 23–62.
41a. Minna JD, Pass H, Glatstein E, Ihde DC. Cancer of the lung. In: DeVita VT, Hellman S, Rosenberg SA, eds. Cancer: Principles and Practice of Oncology, 3rd ed. Philadelphia: J.B. Lippincott Co., 1989: 591–705.
42. Misulis KE. Disorders of peripheral nerve. In: Basic electronics for clinical neurophysiology. London: Butterworth-Heinemann, 1992, Chapter 24.
43. Misulis KE. Special tests of neuromuscular transmission. In: Basic electronics for clinical neurophysiology. London: Butterworth-Heinemann, 1992, Chapter 22.
44. Murray NM, Newsom-Davis JA, O'Neill JH, Spiro SG. Response of Lambert-Eaton myasthenic syndrome to treatment of associated small-cell lung carcinoma. Neurology 1990; 40:1552–1556.
45. Nestor JJ. Unilateral facial pain in lung cancer. Lancet 1991; 338:1149.
46. Newsom-Davis J, Murray NMTI. Plasma exchange and immunosuppressive drug treatment in the Lambert-Eaton myasthenic syndrome. Neurology 1984; 34: 480–485.
47. Ojeda VJ, Walters MN-I. Spinal cord disorders in patients with cancer. Pathol Annu 1984; 19:63–88.
48. Pancoast HK. Superior pulmonary sulcus tumor: tumor characterized by pain, Horner's syndrome, destruction of bone and atrophy of hand muscles. JAMA 1932; 99:1391–1396.
49. Patchell RA. Brain metastases. Neurol Clin 1991; 9:817–824.
50. Patchell RA, Cirrincione C, Thaler HT, Galicich JH, Kim JH, Posner JB. Single brain metastases: surgery plus radiation or radiation alone. Neurology 1986; 36:447–453.
51. Patchell RA, Tibbs PA, Walsh JW, et al. A randomized trial of surgery in the treatment of single metastases to the brain. N Engl J Med 1990; 322:494–500.
51a. Patel AM, Peters SG. Clinical manifestations of lung cancer. Mayo Clin Proc 1993; 68:273–277.
52. Paulson DL. Carcinomas of the superior pulmonary sulcus. J Thorac Cardiovasc Surg 1975; 70:1095–1104.
53. Pederson AG, Bach R, Melgaard B. Frequency, diagnosis and prognosis of spinal cord compression in small cell bronchogenic carcinoma: a review of 817 consecutive patients. Cancer 1985; 55:1118–1122.
54. Raichle ME, Posner JB. Treatment of epidural spinal cord compression. Neurology 1970; 20:391–396.

55. Rosen ST, Aisner J, Makuch RW, et al. Carcinomatous leptomeningitis in small cell lung cancer. Medicine 1982; 61:45–53.
56. Salvatierra A, Baamonde C, Lamos JM, Cruz F, Lopez-Pujol J. Extrathoracic staging of bronchogenic carcinoma. Chest 1990; 97:1052–1059.
57. Schwechheimer K, Lemminger JM. Intramedullary metastases: report of 4 cases and review of the literature. Clin Neuropathol 1985; 4:28–37.
58. Sculier JP, Feld R, Evans WK, et al. Neurologic disorders in patients with small cell lung cancer. Cancer 1987; 60:2275–2283.
59. Shaheen H, Abubakar A, Malik I, Altafullah I, Alam F, Khan A. Epidural spinal cord compression from metastatic cancer: clinical features and management. J Pak Med Assoc 1991; 41:60–62.
60. So NK, O'Neill BP, Eagan RT, Earnest F, Lee RE. Delayed leukoencephalopathy in survivors with small cell lung cancer. Neurology 1987; 37:1198–1201.
61. Sorenson SC, Eagan RT, Scott M. Meningeal carcinomatosis in patients with primary breast or lung cancer. Mayo Clin Proc 1984; 59:91–94.
62. Stark RJ, Henson RA, Evans SJW. Spinal metastases: a retrospective survey from a general hospital. Brain 1982; 105:189.
63. Thomas JE, Colley MY Jr. Radiation-induced or metastatic brachial plexopathy? A diagnostic dilemma. JAMA 1972; 222:1392–1395.
63a. van Moll BJ, Vecht CJ. Facial pain due to a lesion in the thorax. Ned Tijdschr Geneeskd 1992; 136:1585–1587.
64. Vecht CJ, Haaxma-Reiche H, Noordijk EM, et al. Treatment of single brain metastases: radiotherapy alone or combined with neurosurgery? Ann Neurol 1993; 33:583–590.

# 14

# Neurological Complications of Breast Cancer

### Neil E. Anderson

*Auckland Hospital, Auckland, New Zealand*

Breast cancer is the most common malignant tumor in women. The neurological complications of breast cancer are important causes of morbidity and mortality and pose difficult diagnostic and therapeutic challenges to the physician. Early diagnosis and treatment of neurological complications is important because even in patients with advanced breast cancer, prolonged survival is common.

## I. METASTASES

In autopsy studies the incidence of central nervous system (CNS) metastases (Table 1) in patients with breast cancer varies between 31 and 57% (1,2). Breast cancer is the second most common source of CNS metastases. Metastases to the nervous system usually occur in the setting of widespread metastatic disease. It is rare for metastases to be the first manifestation of breast cancer, but the CNS may be the first site of recurrent disease. Metastases in the CNS may not appear until 20 or more years after diagnosis of the primary tumor.

### A. Skull

Skull metastases are common and usually are associated with metastases in other bones. Most metastases to the calvarium are asymptomatic, but they can cause headache and localized swelling of the scalp. Rarely they produce symptoms by

**Table 1** Neurological Complications of Metastases in Breast Cancer

| Site of metastasis | Symptoms, signs | Key tests | Treatment |
|---|---|---|---|
| Skull—calvarium | None | Plain x-ray | RT |
| | Local pain | CT | |
| | Venous thrombosis | | |
| Skull—skull base (see Table 2) | Pain | CT | RT |
| | Cranial nerve palsies | Bone scan | |
| Cranial dura | None | CT | RT |
| | Pressure effects | MRI | Steroids |
| Leptomeninges | Headache | CSF | Intraventricular methotrexate |
| | Altered mentation | | |
| | Cranial nerve palsies | | RT |
| | Polyradiculopathy | | |
| Brain | Headache | CT | RT |
| | Altered mental state | MRI | Steroids |
| | Seizures | | ? Surgery |
| | Focal signs | | ? Chemotherapy |
| Optic nerve | Unilateral visual loss | MRI | RT |
| | Optic disk edema | CT | |
| Choroid | Unilateral visual loss | Fundoscopy | RT |
| Pituitary | None | MRI | Steroids |
| | Headache | CT | RT |
| | Diabetes insipidus | | Chemotherapy |
| | Ophthalmoplegia | | |
| Spinal cord—extradural | Back pain | MRI or myelogram | Steroids |
| | Progressive myelopathy | | RT |
| | | | ? Surgery |
| Spinal cord—intramedullary | Back pain | MRI | Steroids |
| | Asymmetric myelopathy | | RT |
| | Early bladder symptoms | | |
| Brachial plexus | Shoulder, arm pain | CT | RT |
| | Numbness, weakness, areflexia arm | ? Surgery | Analgesia |
| Lumbosacral plexus | Low back, buttock pain | CT | RT |
| | Unilateral leg numbness, weakness, reflex loss | | Analgesia |
| | Leg edema | | ? Chemotherapy |
| Mental nerve | Numb chin | Plain x-ray | RT |
| | Mandibular pain | CT | |

CT = Computed tomography. RT = Radiotherapy. MRI = Magnetic resonance imaging. CSF = Cerebrospinal fluid.

invading the dura and leptomeninges or compression of the superior sagittal sinus. Symptomatic lesions are treated with radiotherapy or tamoxifen.

Metastases to the skull base are less common but they often cause symptoms by compressing cranial nerves (3). Clinical manifestations depend upon the location of the metastasis (Table 2). Computed tomography (CT) and radionuclide bone scans are the most useful methods of identifying metastases in the skull base. Radiotherapy usually alleviates pain and cranial nerve palsies may improve with early treatment.

## B. Dura

Breast cancer is the most common cause of metastases to the dura (1). In autopsy studies, cranial dural metastases occur in 16–18% of patients with breast cancer (2,4). The dura is the solitary site of metastasis in the CNS in about one-half of these patients (4). Epidural lesions are associated with contiguous skull metastases, but some subdural metastases arise by hematogenous spread. Dural metastases are often asymptomatic but they can cause symptoms by compression or invasion of the brain, cranial nerves, pituitary, or venous sinuses. Care must be taken to distinguish a dural metastasis from a meningioma. Dural metastases

**Table 2** Clinical Syndromes Associated with Metastases to the Base of the Skull

| Site | Symptoms | Signs |
|---|---|---|
| Orbit | Supraorbital headache<br>Diplopia | Proptosis[a]<br>Ophthalmoplegia<br>± Facial numbness ($V_1$)<br>± Decreased vision<br>± Periorbital swelling |
| Parasellar (sella turcica, petrous apex) | Frontal headache<br>Diplopia | Ophthalmoplegia<br>Facial numbness ($V_1$)<br>Periorbital swelling |
| Gasserian ganglion (petrous ridge) | Facial numbness, paresthesias<br>Atypical facial pain | Facial numbness ($V_2$, $V_3$)<br>Abducens palsy (anterior ridge)<br>Facial palsy (posterior ridge) |
| Jugular foramen | Occipital pain<br>Hoarseness<br>Dysphagia | Cranial nerve palsies—<br>IX, X, XI |
| Occipital condyle | Occipital pain<br>Dysarthria | Cranial nerve palsy—XII |

[a]Orbital metastasis from scirrhous carcinoma of breast can present with enophthalmos, ocular immobility.

resemble meningiomas on CT scans and the incidence of meningiomas in breast cancer is higher than expected. Symptomatic lesions may respond to treatment with corticosteroids, radiotherapy, or tamoxifen.

## C. Leptomeninges

Leptomeningeal metastasis is a devastating complication which occurs in 2–5% of patients with metastatic breast cancer (2,5,6). Breast cancer is the most common cause of leptomeningeal metastases. If patients with leukemia and lymphoma are excluded, breast cancer accounts for 50% of cases. In one study there was a strong association between leptomeningeal metastases and infiltrating lobular carcinoma of the breast.

The clinical picture is characterized by the subacute onset of symptoms and signs of multiple lesions in the brain, cranial nerves, or spinal nerve roots. The signs are usually more widespread than suspected from the history. Cranial nerve palsies are present in about 80% of patients at presentation. Metastases in the spinal leptomeninges present with back or radicular pain, paresthesias, weakness, and bowel and bladder disturbances. Although these are uncommon initial symptoms, patchy weakness, impaired sensation, and loss of tendon reflexes are common signs. Headache, neck stiffness, altered mental state, nausea, vomiting, seizures, dysarthria, and gait abnormalities also occur.

The cerebrospinal fluid (CSF) may show a pleocytosis, an increased protein content, and a low glucose concentration, but any or all of these abnormalities may be absent (6). The diagnosis is confirmed by finding malignant cells in the CSF, but more than one specimen may have to be examined. If the CSF cytology is normal, other investigations may be helpful. Increased levels of beta-glucuronidase, carcinoembryonic antigen, lactic dehydrogenase isoenzyme 5, and creatine kinase BB isoenzyme in the CSF are found in many patients with breast cancer and leptomeningeal metastases (7). However, these markers may be elevated in patients with brain or epidural metastases, other primary tumors, and meningeal infections. Nodular or diffuse thickening of nerve roots may be visible on myelography or gadolinium-enhanced magnetic resonance imaging (MRI). Computed tomography or MRI scans of the brain may show ependymal enhancement, obliteration or enhancement of the sulci and cisterns, enhancing superficial cortical nodules, or hydrocephalus, but scans may be normal.

When leptomeningeal metastases are caused by breast cancer, the chance of responding to treatment is better than with other solid tumors. Most treatment regimens have employed intermittent high doses or daily small doses of intraventricular methotrexate and radiotherapy to symptomatic areas. In several studies 60–80% of patients improved or stabilized but, after a period of stabilization, about 50% of the responders progressed (8–10). The median survival with treatment was 6–8 months; 15–25% of the patients survived for 1 year or more and rarely patients lived for more than 2 years. Treated patients were more likely to die from complications of systemic metastases than from leptomeningeal disease (10). At autopsy leptomeningeal metastases were in remission in about 30% of the treated patients (9).

However, the efficacy of intrathecal methotrexate is not clearly established. Boogerd and colleagues treated 44 patients with breast cancer and leptomeningeal metastases with daily small doses of intraventricular methotrexate (6). Although 50% of the patients had improved or stabilized after 6 weeks, the median survival was only 12 weeks. About one-third of the patients died within 6 weeks. The overall survival of these patients did not differ significantly from the survival of 14 patients who did not receive intrathecal chemotherapy. Inclusion of patients with widespread and progressive systemic disease may explain the disappointing outcome of treatment with intraventricular methotrexate in this study.

## D. Brain

In autopsy studies brain metastases are found in 18–22% of patients with breast cancer (2,4). Breast cancer accounts for 15–20% of symptomatic brain metastases (11) and it is the most common cause of brain metastases in women. Single brain metastases occur in 56–58% of patients and multiple lesions are found in 42–44% (11). Brain metastases develop more frequently and earlier in the course of the disease in premenopausal patients with breast cancer than in postmenopausal patients (12). However, menopausal status does not affect survival after diagnosis of brain metastases (12,13).

Symptoms usually develop over 1 to 3 months. Headache, altered mental state and behavior, seizures, and an abnormal gait are the most frequent presenting symptoms. The neurological signs depend upon the number, size, and site of the lesions and the severity of the cerebral edema. Focal neurological signs, impairment of cognitive function and consciousness, and papilledema may appear alone or in varying combinations.

Brain metastases are usually visible on CT scans (Fig. 1) but occasionally the scan is normal. CT scans after a double dose of contrast, $T_2$-weighted MRI, and gadolinium-enhanced MRI are more sensitive methods of detecting metastases. If a solitary metastasis cannot be distinguished from a primary brain tumor, infarct, or abscess, the scan should be repeated after a few weeks, or the lesion can be excised.

Although brain metastases usually occur with disseminated disease, treatment often controls the neurological symptoms. After treatment with whole-brain radiotherapy and dexamethasone, about 70% of patients with breast cancer and brain metastases improve, 25% stabilize, and 5% continue to deteriorate (11). Long-term improvement is maintained in 75% of the responders. Follow-up CT scans show disappearance of the lesions in 35% of the patients and a major

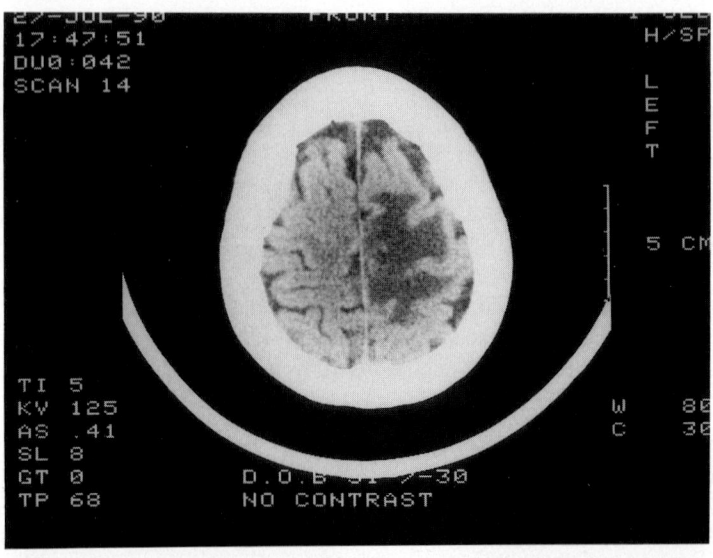

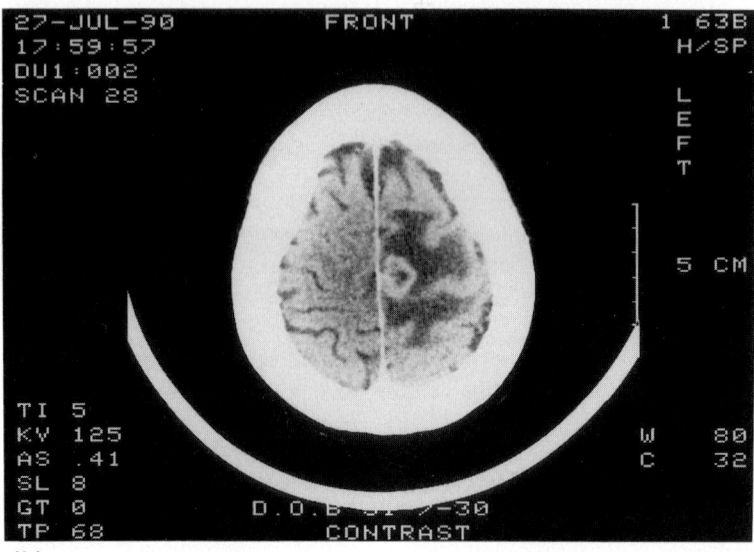

**Figure 1(a,b)** Computed tomography scans of the brain (a) before and (b) after intravenous contrast. Single metastasis and surrounding edema in left parietal lobe.

improvement in 40% (11). Patients who are treated with radiotherapy probably live longer than those who are untreated. Forty-one percent survive for more than 6 months, and 22% live for more than 1 year (11). The median survival with radiotherapy is 3–4 months. Most patients die from complications of systemic metastases.

Surgical resection of an accessible single brain metastasis followed by radiotherapy may be preferable to radiotherapy alone if there are no systemic metastases, if systemic disease can be controlled, or if the metastasis recurs after maximal doses of radiotherapy. A solitary brain metastasis that recurs or persists after whole-brain radiotherapy can be controlled with stereotactic radiosurgery or interstitial brachytherapy.

Breakdown of the blood-brain barrier in tumors permits systemically administered drugs to reach brain metastases. The main potential advantage of systemic chemotherapy is that it may control both extracranial and cerebral metastases. Rosner treated 100 patients with breast cancer and brain metastases with different combinations of cyclophosphamide, 5-fluorouracil, methotrexate, vincristine, adriamycin, and prednisone (14). Ten percent had a complete clinical and CT response, 40% had a partial response, 9% were stable, and 41% did not respond. The median survival for the whole group was 5.5 months and 31% of the patients lived for 1 year or longer. Chemotherapy has not been compared with radiotherapy in a prospective randomized trial, but it may have a role in patients with multiple brain metastases who already have received radiotherapy or in patients with brain metastases and widespread systemic disease. Brain metastases also can regress during treatment with tamoxifen, megestrol acetate, fluoxymesterone, and bromocriptine.

## E. Optic Nerve and Choroid (15)

Optic nerve metastases are rare but breast cancer is the most common cause of these lesions. The patient experiences an acute or slowly progressive painless loss of vision in one eye with optic disk edema. The clinical picture can be confused with optic neuritis or ischemic optic neuropathy.

Metastases in the choroid are relatively common, but they often are asymptomatic. They can be found in about 10% of patients who have advanced breast cancer but no ocular symptoms. The most common presenting symptoms are decreased visual acuity or a scotoma. Radiotherapy is required if the metastasis is affecting vision or if it is associated with a serous retinal detachment.

## F. Pituitary

Pituitary metastases have been discovered at autopsy in 9% of patients with breast cancer and in 25% of patients who have had a hypophysectomy as treatment for bony metastases. The pituitary gland may be invaded by hematogenous spread, direct extension from a metastasis in the sella turcica, or leptomeningeal metastases in the suprasellar cistern (16). Most pituitary metastases are asymptomatic. When symptoms occur, headache, diabetes insipidus, and external ophthalmoplegia are the usual manifestations; visual loss and hypopituitarism are uncommon. A pituitary adenoma should be suspected if there is hypopituitarism or visual loss and there are no other metastases. Bony erosion and soft tissue invasion on CT or MRI can occur with either invasive adenomas or metastases. If the clinical features suggest there is a metastasis, corticosteroids and radiotherapy should be used. Symptoms also may improve with systemic chemotherapy (16). Resection of a metastasis is usually difficult because cavernous sinus infiltration is common and the tumor can bleed profusely. An operation is indicated if the clinical features suggest an adenoma, there are no other metastases, and expected survival is greater than 6 months.

## G. Spinal Cord (see also Chap. 2)

Compression of the spinal cord or cauda equina by an epidural metastasis is a common complication of breast cancer. Without correct diagnosis and treatment it causes progressive pain and paralysis, yet patients often survive for 1 year or longer. In cancer hospitals, breast cancer is the most common cause of epidural spinal cord compression (ESCC) and accounts for 22% of cases. In general hospitals, lung cancer is more common because ESCC is rarely the first manifestation of breast cancer.

In breast cancer patients, ESCC is caused by metastases in the vertebral body or, less commonly, in the posterior elements of the spine. Vertebral metastases occur in 60% of patients with metastatic breast cancer. The high incidence of vertebral metastases may be related to spread of tumor cells through the vertebral venous plexus which can be filled by the mammary veins. Nerve roots and the spinal cord are compressed either by expansion of the tumor into the epidural tissues or intervertebral foramina or by collapse of the vertebral body and encroachment of tumor and bone upon the epidural space. In some patients the neurological deficit is caused by ischemia of the spinal cord. In breast cancer patients, ESCC occurs in the thoracic spine in 75–80%, the cervical spine in about 15%, and the lumbosacral spine in 6–7% (17,18). *Spinal cord or cauda equina compression at more than one level is common.*

Pain is the initial complaint in most patients, but ataxia, weakness, or sensory loss may be the first symptom. Pain usually begins as a constant ache in the middle of the back, but later it is accompanied by radicular pain. The affected vertebrae are usually tender to percussion. Without treatment other symptoms and signs appear weeks or months later. Weakness and ataxia leading to paraplegia or quadriplegia develop over several days but a sudden deterioration occurs in about

20% of patients (18). Sensory loss parallels the degree of weakness. Urinary retention and constipation typically occur after weakness appears, but may precede weakness and sensory loss if the lesion is between the T10 and L1 vertebrae. The location of the pain is usually a reliable indicator of the site of the spinal cord compression.

Urgent investigation is required if ESCC is suspected. Plain radiographs of the spine are abnormal at the symptomatic level in 94% of patients with breast cancer and ESCC (18). Eighty-two percent of these patients have metastases in other vertebrae. Computed tomography and radionuclide bone scans may identify a vertebral metastasis that is not visible on plain films. Epidural spinal cord compression is unlikely if the neurological examination, spine radiographs, radionuclide scan, and CT are normal or if the metastasis is restricted to the vertebral body without major collapse or pedicle erosion. In patients with a normal neurological examination, the likelihood of ESCC is higher if the spine radiographs or CT show vertebral body collapse or pedicle erosion. In these patients and those with neurological signs, urgent myelography or MRI is required to determine if there is compression of the spinal cord or nerve roots, to assess the severity of the compression, and to identify asymptomatic lesions (Figs. 2,3).

The aims of treatment for breast cancer patients with ESCC are to relieve pain and retain ambulation. Corticosteroids and radiotherapy should be given immediately. Dexamethasone should be started before the myelogram if there are symptoms or signs of a progressive myelopathy. Dexamethasone reduces pain and may stabilize the neurological signs for a short time. The optimal dose of dexamethasone is controversial. Ambulation is usually maintained if radiotherapy is commenced while the patient is still able to walk (17). If treatment is delayed until the patient cannot walk, independent ambulation is usually not achieved, although exceptions occur.

The role of surgery in the management of ESCC from breast cancer is controversial (see Chap. 2). It is uncommon for ESCC to be the first manifestation of breast cancer and therefore surgery is usually not needed for a tissue diagnosis. The response to chemotherapy and hormonal therapy is delayed and uncertain and these treatments should not be used alone.

Intramedullary spinal metastases are rare, but breast cancer accounts for about 15% of the cases. Many patients also have brain metastases. Patients typically present with back pain and a progressive myelopathy. Clues to the diagnosis include a Brown-Séquard's syndrome; asymmetric motor findings; atrophy, fasciculations, or dissociated sensory loss at the level of the lesion; early involvement of bladder and bowel function; and the absence of metastases in adjacent vertebral bodies in spine radiographs. Magnetic resonance imaging is the best method of demonstrating an intramedullary metastasis. Symptoms may improve or stabilize if dexamethasone and radiotherapy are commenced promptly.

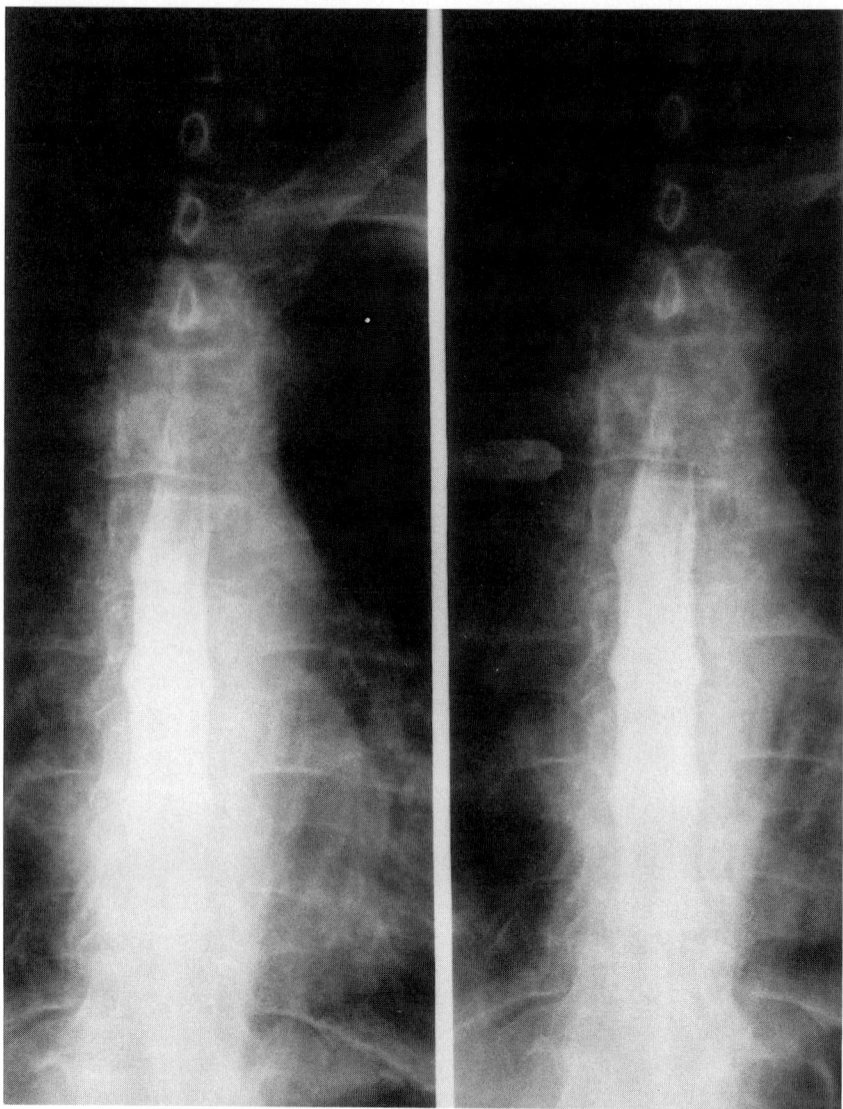

**Figure 2** Myelogram showing lower end of complete block at level of T4 vertebra. Note loss of pedicles in T4 and collapse of T3 vertebral body.

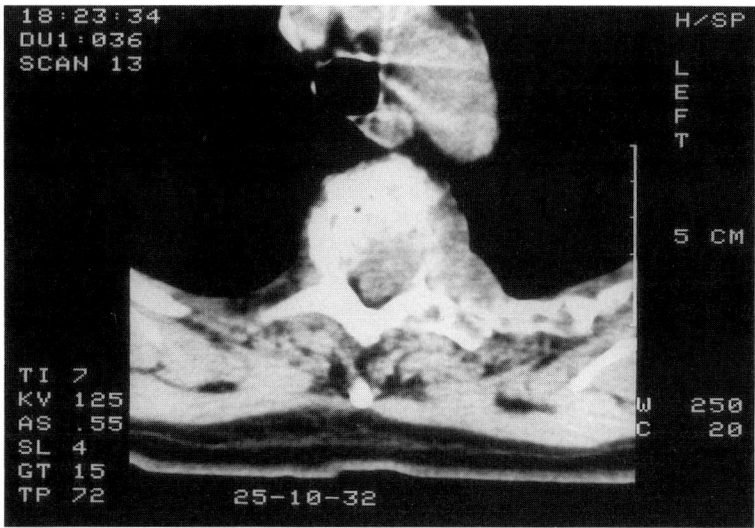

(a)

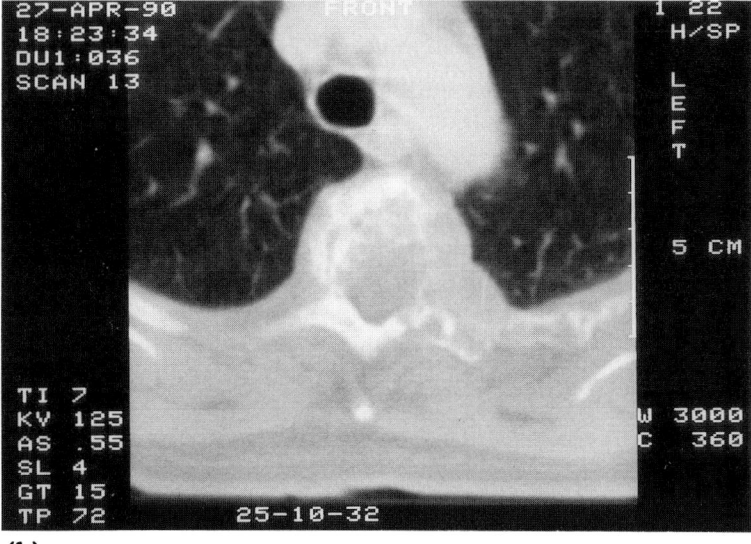

(b)

**Figure 3(a,b)** Computed tomography scans of thoracic spine in patient with breast cancer and epidural spinal cord compression. Tumor in vertebral body, pedicle, paravertebral tissues, and spinal canal.

## H. Peripheral Nerve (see also Chap. 4)

### 1. Brachial Plexus (19, 20)

Malignant infiltration of the brachial plexus is caused by breast cancer in 32–56% of the cases. Malignant brachial plexopathy occurs in 2.5% of patients with breast cancer. The whole plexus, the lower trunk, or, uncommonly, the upper trunk can be involved and the tumor can spread into paraspinal and epidural tissues. Unremitting severe pain in the shoulder and arm usually precedes other symptoms by several weeks or months. Sensory symptoms, wasting, and weakness appear later on. The motor and sensory signs depend on the location of the lesion in the brachial plexus. A Horner's syndrome is common when metastases in the lower trunk extend into paraspinal or epidural tissues. Other signs of malignant infiltration of the brachial plexus may include induration and tenderness in the supraclavicular fossa, lymphedema, and trophic changes in the skin and nails.

Nerve conduction studies may show prolonged or absent F waves and low-amplitude sensory and compound muscle action potentials. Electromyography (EMG) shows fibrillations and neurogenic changes in motor unit potentials. Paraspinal muscles are normal, unless the tumor extends into the epidural space. Myokymia is uncommon but can occur in patients who have received radiotherapy (20).

The most common finding on the CT scan is a mass in the brachial plexus (Fig. 4), but in some patients the CT is normal or only shows a loss of normal tissue planes. Paravertebral extension and erosion of the vertebral bodies can be seen on CT but epidural infiltration may not be obvious. Myelography or MRI is required if epidural disease is suspected. If the diagnosis is uncertain, surgical exploration of the plexus is required, but even then, microscopic infiltration of the nerves may be missed (19). If the patient has a progressive brachial plexopathy and surgical exploration is negative, the CT and exploration should be repeated after 3–6 months.

Radiotherapy may partly relieve pain but narcotic analgesics, nerve blocks, and cordotomy are often required. The other symptoms usually worsen despite treatment.

Malignant infiltration of the brachial plexus must be distinguished from the effects of radiation on the brachial plexus, trauma to the plexus during surgery, the postmastectomy pain syndrome, and brachial neuritis.

### 2. Lumbosacral Plexus

Malignant infiltration of the lumbosacral plexus is a relatively uncommon complication of breast cancer. The lumbosacral plexus is invaded by bone metastases in the pelvis and sacrum. There is an insidious onset of pain in the low back, buttock, or thigh. Unilateral or asymmetric weakness, sensory loss, reflex loss, and leg edema appear weeks to months later. Bowel and bladder symptoms are uncommon unless there is epidural extension of the tumor. A mass may be palpable on rectal

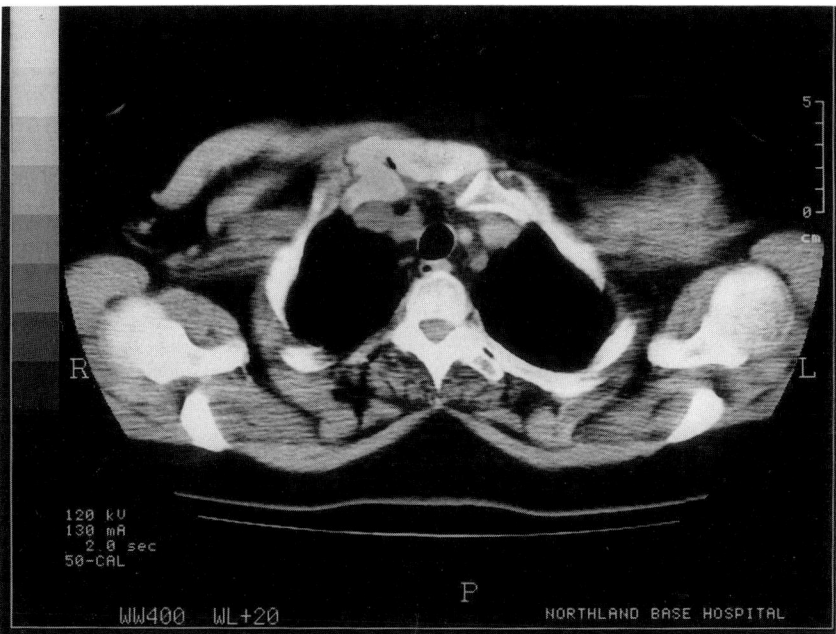

**Figure 4** Computed tomography scan of brachial plexus. Mass in left brachial plexus in a patient with breast cancer and malignant brachial plexopathy.

examination. Nerve conduction velocities are normal, but the compound muscle and sensory action potentials are reduced. Fibrillations and chronic neurogenic motor unit changes are seen in the EMG. CT shows a tumor mass, lymphadenopathy, or bone erosion. Other causes of a lumbosacral plexopathy, such as a retroperitoneal hemorrhage, vasculitis, and diabetes, need to be excluded. Malignant lumbosacral plexopathy can be confused with leptomeningeal metastases or compression of the cauda equina by an epidural metastasis. Leptomeningeal and epidural metastases usually affect bladder and bowel function, although a rectal mass and leg edema are absent.

Radiotherapy and chemotherapy may stabilize the symptoms but eventually the symptoms progress until the patient succumbs to progressive metastatic disease. Narcotic analgesics, epidural or intrathecal morphine, and cordotomy assist in pain relief.

## 3. *Mental Nerve*

Metastases in the mandible may affect the mental nerve (3). Patients experience unilateral numbness of the lower lip, chin, and the mucous membrane on the inside of the lip. There may be swelling and pain in the mandible. Mandibular metastases are visible on plain radiographs or CT. The facial numbness caused by dural or leptomeningeal metastases is usually more extensive. Radiotherapy is the treatment of choice.

## II. NONMETASTATIC COMPLICATIONS

### A. Metabolic Disorders

A metabolic encephalopathy is one of the most common neurological complications of breast cancer and often occurs as part of the terminal events. Symptoms begin acutely or subacutely and often fluctuate. The clinical picture is characterized by mental and behavioral changes, disorders of consciousness, tremor, asterixis, and myoclonus. There are many causes of a metabolic encephalopathy but hypercalcemia is probably the most common in breast cancer. Other neurological manifestations of hypercalcemia are proximal muscle weakness and paresthesias. The encephalopathy is reversible if the underlying metabolic abnormality can be treated successfully.

### B. Complications of Treatment

#### 1. Chemotherapy (see also Chap. 11)

Several of the drugs used to treat breast cancer have adverse effects on the nervous system (Table 3), but adrenocorticosteroids, vincristine, and methotrexate are the most common causes of complications. An acute meningoencephalopathy presenting with headache, fever, neck stiffness, vomiting, and confusion can develop 2–4 h after an intrathecal injection of methotrexate (8). The CSF may show an increase in the white cell count and protein content above the pretreatment values, but cultures are sterile. The symptoms resolve after 12–72 h and they do not recur with subsequent methotrexate treatments. Sudden death or a myelopathy are rare, early complications of intrathecal methotrexate.

A mild fever and encephalopathy can appear after the second or third intrathecal treatment. This syndrome is not associated with neck stiffness or changes in the CSF (21). The symptoms resolve after 1 or 2 weeks but there is a possible relationship between this syndrome and later development of a necrotizing leukoencephalopathy (21).

Leukoencephalopathy develops in more than 50% of breast cancer patients who survive for 1 year or longer after receiving repeated intrathecal injections of methotrexate for leptomeningeal metastases (6). This complication usually occurs when intrathecal methotrexate is combined with whole-brain radiotherapy or intravenous methotrexate and, if possible, these combinations of treatment should be avoided. Behavioral changes, confusion, dementia, somnolence, ataxia, seizures, hemiparesis or quadriparesis begin insidiously or abruptly 3 months or

**Table 3** Neurological Complications of Chemotherapy in Breast Cancer

| Agent | Drug | Neurotoxicity |
|---|---|---|
| Adrenocorticosteroids | Prednisone, prednisolone, dexamethasone | Myopathy,[a] psychiatric,[a] epidural lipomatosis, withdrawal syndrome, hiccups, tremor, abnormal taste and olfaction |
| Hormonal | Tamoxifen | Encephalopathy, cerebellar disorders, retinopathy, optic neuropathy |
|  | Aminoglutethimide | Lethargy, drowsiness, ataxia |
| Plant alkaloids | Vincristine, vinblastine, vindesine | Sensorimotor neuropathy,[a] autonomic neuropathy, cranial neuropathy, seizures secondary to inappropriate ADH secretion |
| Antimetabolites | Methotrexate (IT) | Acute meningoencephalopathy,[a] subacute optic neuropathy, delayed leukoencephalopathy,[a] necrotizing myelopathy |
|  | 5-Fluorouracil (high dose) | Acute reversible cerebellar disorder, encephalopathy, parkinsonian syndrome, optic neuropathy |
|  | Arabinosylcytosine (only IT) | Acute meningoencephalopathy, necrotizing myelopathy |
| Alkylating agents | Thio-TEPA (IT only) | Myelopathy, radiculopathy |

[a]Common complications
IT = Intrathecal. ADH = Antidiuretic hormone

more after treatment is commenced. Computed tomography and MRI show periventricular white matter abnormalities. The symptoms can stabilize or improve when methotrexate is stopped, or there may be progression to coma and death.

A retinopathy characterized by refractile deposits in the inner retinal layers of the macula and paramacular area may develop during treatment with tamoxifen (22). It is often associated with subepithelial corneal opacities, macular edema, and impaired vision. Retinopathy usually develops after high doses of tamoxifen but it can occur with conventional doses. Vision may improve after treatment is withdrawn. Optic neuropathy has been attributed to tamoxifen therapy in a few patients. Other rare complications of tamoxifen include depression, headache, encephalopathy, syncope, and cerebellar symptoms (23). Lethargy, drowsiness, depression, ataxia, and dizziness are common reversible side effects of aminoglutethimide.

## 2. Radiation Therapy (see also Chap. 10)

Brain, spinal cord, and optic nerve complications of radiotherapy are rare among patients with breast cancer (Table 4), but peripheral nerve effects are common.

Radiotherapy can affect the brachial plexus in several ways. A reversible brachial plexopathy may develop 1.5–14 months after radiotherapy is completed. This disorder was observed in 8 of 565 (1.4%) patients with breast cancer after irradiation of the axilla with 46–56 Gy (24). The initial symptoms are numbness and paresthesias in the hand and forearm. Shoulder and axillary pain may appear but it is not severe. In some patients there is weakness and wasting but the scapular and rhomboid muscles are spared. The symptoms and signs usually resolve over a few months, but there may be mild residual sensory symptoms. The pathogenesis of this disorder is unknown.

A delayed, irreversible, radiation-induced brachial plexopathy is caused by perineural fibrosis. In most series, 2–4% of patients with breast cancer develop a brachial plexopathy after radiotherapy but incidences as high as 15% have been reported. A brachial plexopathy is more likely to develop after total doses of 60 Gy or more but it can occur with smaller doses, especially if they are administered in fractions of more than 2 Gy (25). Concomitant chemotherapy may be a contributing factor. The disorder usually occurs 6 months or more after radiotherapy but shorter latent intervals have been reported. Initially the upper trunk of the plexus is usually affected, but the lower trunk or whole plexus may become involved. Paresthesias and numbness are the dominant presenting symptoms; lymphedema, induration of the supraclavicular fossa, and weakness of the arm develop later (19). Pain is usually less severe than in malignant brachial plexus infiltration, and Horner's syndrome is uncommon. The weakness either deteriorates slowly or stabilizes after a few months, and extended survival is usual. Myokymia is usually seen in the EMG but may be absent (20). Fibrillations in paraspinal muscles and fasciculations are common but the other neurophysiological findings are similar to malignant brachial plexopathy. Computed tomography results either are normal or show a loss of normal tissue planes without a discrete mass.

Radiation fibrosis must be distinguished from malignant infiltration of the plexus. Radiation plexopathy is the more likely diagnosis if there is little or no pain at the outset, the EMG shows myokymia, and the CT is normal or shows an ill-defined loss of tissue planes.

Peripheral nerve sheath tumors are rare, late complications of radiotherapy to the supraclavicular fossa. These lesions develop after many years when patients are cured of their original tumors. They present with a painful mass and a progressive brachial plexopathy.

## 3. Surgery

Phantom sensations in the breast occur in about one-third of patients after a mastectomy. Pain and altered sensation around the mastectomy scar also are

**Table 4** Brain, Spinal Cord, and Optic Nerve Complications of Radiotherapy in Breast Cancer

| Syndrome | Onset | Symptoms | Course | Pathogenesis |
|---|---|---|---|---|
| *Brain* | | | | |
| Acute encephalopathy | Minutes–days | Headache, nausea, somnolence, focal signs | Reversible | Vasogenic edema |
| Early delayed encephalopathy | 4–8 weeks | Simulates tumor progression | Reversible | ? Demyelination |
| Necrosis | Months–years | Focal signs Raised ICP | Improves with resection, steroids | ? Vascular |
| Cerebral atrophy | Months–years | Dementia, ataxia, urinary incontinence | Irreversible | ? |
| Hydrocephalus | Months–years | Ataxia, dementia | Improves with shunt | Radiation induced arachnoiditis |
| *Optic Nerve* | | | | |
| Optic neuropathy | 6–24 months | Visual loss, optic disk edema | Irreversible or partial improvement | ? Vascular |
| *Spinal Cord* | | | | |
| Early delayed | Weeks | Lhermitte's sign | Reversible | Demyelination |
| Delayed (necrosis) | Months–years | Brown-Séquard's syndrome, partial transverse myelopathy | Progressive or stabilizes | Glial, vascular destruction |

ICP = Intracranial pressure

common symptoms. Carpal tunnel syndrome and brachial plexopathy have been attributed to lymphedema following radical mastectomy, but the evidence for a causative link is not convincing.

A postmastectomy pain syndrome occurs after 4–6% of breast operations, particularly those involving an axillary lymph node dissection (26). It is caused by interruption of the intercostobrachial nerve and, in some patients, cutaneous branches of other intercostal nerves. This syndrome is more common when the early postoperative course is complicated by local swelling and infection. Pain can begin immediately after the operation or as late as 6 months. There is a constricting, burning sensation and sensory loss in the axilla, posteromedial upper arm, and anterior chest wall. The pain is exacerbated by shoulder movement and a frozen shoulder can develop. Typically there is a trigger point in the axilla or anterior chest wall. Treatment with analgesics, amitriptyline, carbamazepine, and nerve blocks has had limited success but topical capsaicin may be more effective.

## C. Cerebrovascular Disease (see also Chap. 8)

### 1. Intracerebral Hemorrhage

In breast cancer patients, less than 1% of brain metastases are hemorrhagic. Intracerebral hemorrhage also may occur with thrombocytopenia caused by bone marrow invasion, radiotherapy, or chemotherapy. The clinical picture resembles a stroke.

### 2. Subdural Hematoma

Subdural hematoma is an uncommon complication of breast cancer which can be caused by dural metastases, head injury, anticoagulant therapy, or a coagulopathy. Neoplastic invasion of veins in the outer layer of the dura causes obstruction of venous flow from the vascular inner layer, leading to rupture of the capillaries in the subdural space. Subdural hematoma also may be caused by hemorrhage into an effusion produced by the tumor, or bleeding into a dural metastasis. The clinical manifestations are similar to those of a subdural hematoma in the general population. If a subdural hematoma is associated with a metastasis, surgery should be followed by radiotherapy.

### 3. Disseminated Intravascular Coagulation (DIC)

Breast cancer is one of the most common causes of DIC in malignancy. In an autopsy study, 1% of the patients with breast cancer had DIC with CNS involvement. Patients present with an acute encephalopathy, which may be associated with focal seizures, focal neurological signs, and systemic bleeding. Symptoms can fluctuate but death usually occurs within 3 weeks of the onset. The neurological complications of DIC must be distinguished from other causes of a diffuse or multifocal encephalopathy, especially a metabolic encephalopathy, infection, and metastases. Coagulation studies usually are abnormal, but CT scans and cerebral angiography are normal. Heparin is usually not beneficial. At autopsy there are multiple small cerebral infarcts and fibrin thrombi in small penetrating vessels and capillaries in the brain and other organs.

### 4. *Nonbacterial Thrombotic Endocarditis (NBTE)*

Neurological signs in NBTE may be caused by cardiogenic emboli or DIC, which commonly accompanies this disorder. Five to ten percent of patients with NBTE have breast cancer. Most patients have disseminated metastases but occasionally the systemic disease is stable. Patients present with acute focal neurological symptoms and signs (transient ischemic attacks or a stroke), a diffuse encephalopathy, or both. There may be systemic emboli, venous thrombophlebitis, and a heart murmur, but neurological signs may be the only evidence of NBTE. Single or multiple cerebral infarcts are visible on CT scans, and arteriograms show multiple embolic occlusions of cerebral arteries. Valvular vegetations are usually not seen on echocardiograms. Occasionally intravenous heparin is beneficial but most patients die without recovery. The pathological findings include multiple infarcts in the brain and other organs, and sterile platelet-fibrin vegetations on one or more heart valves.

### 5. *Tumor Embolism*

This is a rare cause of a cerebral infarct in patients with breast cancer. Occlusion of a large cerebral artery by a tumor embolus causes abrupt development of focal signs which worsen later on. The source of the embolus is usually a metastatic tumor in the lung.

### 6. *Cerebral Venous Thrombosis*

Superior sagittal sinus thrombosis is a rare complication of breast cancer that can be caused by a coagulopathy, meningitis, or compression of the superior sagittal sinus by a metastasis. Headache, papilledema, seizures, focal neurological signs, or a diffuse encephalopathy develop over a few days. Venous thrombosis can be demonstrated by MRI, angiography, or CT. The treatment is controversial because anticoagulation may increase the risk of hemorrhagic infarction. Radiotherapy is usually unhelpful in patients with metastatic superior sagittal sinus thrombosis.

### 7. *Intravascular Mucin*

Embolization of mucin and fat to capillaries and small arteries in the CNS is a rare complication of disseminated breast cancer (27). The clinical picture consists of an encephalopathy and multiple acute strokes. The course is rapidly progressive and death occurs within 3 weeks. At autopsy examination there are multiple hemorrhagic cerebral infarcts.

## D. Infections

CNS infections are uncommon in patients with breast cancer. Defects in the immune system which increase susceptibility to infections can develop after chemotherapy or corticosteroid treatment. These disorders are reviewed in Chapter 7.

## E. Paraneoplastic Syndromes (see also Chap. 8)

The neurological paraneoplastic syndromes are rare complications of breast cancer which often precede diagnosis of the tumor. Recognition of these syndromes may lead to early diagnosis of the breast cancer. Breast cancer only occasionally causes most of these disorders, but it does have a striking association with subacute cerebellar degeneration and opsoclonus with ataxia.

Breast cancer is one of the most common causes of paraneoplastic cerebellar degeneration (PCD) (28). Truncal and appendicular ataxia, dysarthria, and nystagmus develop progressively over a few days or weeks. The symptoms eventually stabilize but by then the patient is severely incapacitated. The CSF often shows a mild pleocytosis, oligoclonal bands, and increased protein and IgG concentrations. Initially the CT and MRI are normal but later they show cerebellar atrophy. The main pathological abnormality is a severe, diffuse loss of cerebellar Purkinje cells. An anti–Purkinje cell antibody (anti-Yo) is present in serum and CSF of most patients with breast cancer and PCD (28). The same antibody is found in women with PCD and gynecological tumors, but it does not occur in breast cancer patients who do not have neurological symptoms. Treatment of the tumor, steroids, cyclophosphamide, and plasmapheresis do not improve the neurological symptoms, although prolonged survival is usual (28).

Another antineuronal antibody (anti-Ri) is harbored by women with breast cancer and a syndrome characterized by the subacute onset of ataxia and abnormal eye movements, usually opsoclonus (29). The ataxia varies from a mild unsteadiness of gait to a severe truncal and appendicular ataxia. The symptoms usually stabilize and partial remissions can occur. The CSF may show a mild pleocytosis and increased protein content, while CT and MRI are usually normal. The pathological lesion is unknown.

## REFERENCES

1. Posner JB, Chernik NL. Intracranial metastases from systemic cancer. In: Schoenberg BS, ed. Advances in neurology, Vol. 19. New York: Raven Press, 1978:579–591.
2. Cifuentes N, Pickren JW. Metastases from carcinoma of mammary gland: an autopsy study. J Surg Oncol 1979; 11:193–205.
3. Hall SM, Buzdar AU, Blumenschein GR. Cranial nerve palsies in metastatic breast

cancer due to osseous metastasis without intracranial involvement. Cancer 1983; 52:180–184.
4. Tsukada Y, Fouad A, Pickren JW, Lane WW. Central nervous system metastasis from breast carcinoma: autopsy study. Cancer 1983; 52:2349–2354.
5. Yap H-Y, Yap B-S, Tashima CK, DiStefano A, Blumenschein GR. Meningeal carcinomatosis in breast cancer. Cancer 1978; 42:283–286.
6. Boogerd W, Hart AAM, van der Sande JJ, Engelsman E. Meningeal carcinomatosis in breast cancer. Prognostic factors and influence of treatment. Cancer 1991; 67: 1685–1695.
7. Twijnstra A, van Zanten AP, Nooyen WJ, Ongerboer de Visser BW. Sensitivity and specificity of single and combined tumour markers in the diagnosis of leptomeningeal metastasis from breast cancer. J Neurol Neurosurg Psychiatry 1986; 49:1246–1250.
8. Wasserstrom WR, Glass JP, Posner JB. Diagnosis and treatment of leptomeningeal metastases from solid tumors: experience with 90 patients. Cancer 1982; 49: 759–772.
9. Yap H-Y, Yap B-S, Rasmussen S, Levens ME, Hortobagyi GN, Blumenschein GR. Treatment for meningeal carcinomatosis in breast cancer. Cancer 1982; 49:219–222.
10. Ongerboer de Visser BW, Somers R, Nooyen WH, van Heerde P, Hart AAM, McVie JG. Intraventricular methotrexate therapy of leptomeningeal metastasis from breast carcinoma. Neurology 1983; 33:1565–1572.
11. Cairncross JG, Kim J-H, Posner JB. Radiation therapy for brain metastases. Ann Neurol 1980; 7:529–541.
12. DiStefano A, Yap HY, Hortobagyi GN, Blumenschein GR. The natural history of breast cancer patients with brain metastases. Cancer 1979; 44:1913–1918.
13. Kamby C, Soerensen PS. Characteristics of patients with short and long survivals after detection of intracranial metastases from breast cancer. J Neurooncol 1988; 6:37–45.
14. Rosner D, Nemoto T, Lane WW. Chemotherapy induces regression of brain metastases in breast carcinoma. Cancer 1986; 58:832–839.
15. Bullock JD, Yanes B. Ophthalmic manifestations of metastatic breast cancer. Ophthalmology 1980; 87:961–973.
16. Yap H-Y, Tashima CK, Blumenschein GR, Eckles N. Diabetes insipidus and breast cancer. Arch Intern Med 1979; 139:1009–1011.
17. Gilbert RW, Kim J-H, Posner JB. Epidural spinal cord compression from metastatic tumor: diagnosis and treatment. Ann Neurol 1978; 3:40–51.
18. Stark RJ, Henson RA, Evans SJW. Spinal metastases: a retrospective survey from a general hospital. Brain 1982; 105:189–213.
19. Kori SH, Foley KM, Posner JB. Brachial plexus lesions in patients with cancer: 100 cases. Neurology 1981; 31:45–50.
20. Harper CM, Thomas JE, Cascino TL, Litchy WJ. Distinction between neoplastic and radiation-induced brachial plexopathy, with emphasis on the role of EMG. Neurology 1989; 39:502–506.
21. Boogerd W, vd Sande JJ, Moffie D. Acute fever and delayed leukoencephalopathy following low dose intraventricular methotrexate. J Neurol Neurosurg Psychiatry 1988; 51:1277–1283.

22. Kaiser-Kupfer MI, Kupfer C, Rodrigues MM. Tamoxifen retinopathy: a clinicopathologic report. Ophthalmology 1981; 88:89–93.
23. Pluss JL, DiBella NJ. Reversible central nervous system dysfunction due to tamoxifen in a patient with breast cancer. Ann Intern Med 1984; 101:652.
24. Salner AL, Botnick LE, Herzog AG, Goldstein MA, Harris JR, Levene MB, Hellman S. Reversible brachial plexopathy following primary radiation therapy for breast cancer. Cancer Treat Rep 1981; 65:797–802.
25. Barr LC, Kissin MW. Radiation-induced brachial plexus neuropathy following breast conservation and radical radiotherapy. Br J Surg 1987; 74:855–856.
26. Vecht CJ, Van de Brand HJ, Wajer OJM. Post-axillary dissection pain in breast cancer due to a lesion of the intercostobrachial nerve. Pain 1989; 38:171–176.
27. Deck JHN, Lee MA. Mucin embolism to cerebral arteries: a fatal complication of carcinoma of the breast. Can J Neurol Sci 1978; 5:327–330.
28. Anderson NE, Rosenblum MK, Posner JB. Paraneoplastic cerebellar degeneration: clinical-immunological correlations. Ann Neurol 1988; 24:559–567.
29. Luque FA, Furneaux HM, Ferziger R, et al. Anti-Ri: an antibody associated with paraneoplastic opsoclonus and breast cancer. Ann Neurol 1991; 29:241–251.

# 15
# Neurological Complications of Malignant Melanoma and Other Cutaneous Malignancies

### John W. Henson
*Massachusetts General Hospital and Harvard Medical School, Boston, Massachusetts*

## I. INTRODUCTION

Skin cancer is often detected early in its development, at a time when therapy is curative. As a result, patients with cutaneous malignancies usually have a better outcome than those with malignancies of other organs. When initial therapy is not curative, however, certain cutaneous malignancies commonly produce neurological complications. For example, malignant melanoma is the third most common cause of brain metastases, after lung and breast cancer, even though melanoma accounts for only 1% of all cancers (1). Less frequently, cutaneous cancers in the head and neck region and cutaneous lymphomas may produce neurological symptoms and signs. Skin cancers produce neurological complications by a variety of mechanisms, including direct invasion, compression from metastases to adjacent structures, vascular compromise, and systemic metabolic disturbances secondary to visceral metastases. This chapter addresses the clinical features and therapeutic issues of these complications.

## II. MALIGNANT MELANOMA

### A. Introduction

Cutaneous malignant melanoma is an increasingly common form of cancer, almost doubling in incidence every decade (2). The cause of the rising incidence is unknown, but higher levels of exposure to ultraviolet light have been suggested as one possible factor. As a result of the rising incidence, the mortality rate from malignant melanoma is also increasing.

Neurological complications are common and grave events in the progression of malignant melanoma. Fifty percent of patients with metastatic melanoma develop clinically apparent neurological complications, and 90% have central nervous system (CNS) involvement at autopsy (3). In the majority of patients these complications arise in the setting of disseminated, progressive systemic disease, thereby confirming an already grim prognosis.

While metastatic melanoma is notorious for its aggressive biological nature, there are occasional patients in whom the disease does not progress relentlessly. Melanoma can act in an unpredictable manner, with metastatic disease becoming indolent or, on rare occasions, spontaneously regressing. Spontaneous tumor regression occurs in 0.2% of patients with metastatic melanoma, making it one of the most common tumors to exhibit this phenomenon (4). Long-term survivals occasionally follow surgical resection of brain metastases.

Melanomas arise from melanocytes, which are neural crest–derived cells found in the skin, hair follicles, mesentery, iris and choroid, leptomeninges, and occasionally other sites in the body. Melanin, the pigment of melanocytes, is produced from tyrosine by the enzyme tyrosinase. Conversion of tyrosine to catecholamines occurs through a separate enzymatic pathway. Melanin is bound to proteins within intracellular organelles called melanosomes. Melanin absorbs ultraviolet light, partially protecting the skin from this form of irradiation. This may explain the lower incidence of melanoma in blacks (about 7.5 times lower) compared with whites.

Cutaneous melanomas are clinically and pathologically classified into four groups: lentigo maligna, superficial spreading melanoma, nodular melanoma, or acral-lentiginous melanoma. Initially, tumor cells extend in a radial (horizontal) plane. The development of vertical growth heralds an invasive phase in the progression of the tumor. The depth of invasion (Clark's or Breslow's levels) at the time of resection is highly correlated with the likelihood of metastatic disease and survival. Other characteristics associated with a poor prognosis include nodular melanoma subtype (reflects vertical growth), lesions located on the scalp, hands, or feet, and older age at diagnosis (2). When metastases occur, the organs most likely to be involved are the skin, lymph nodes, lung, and brain.

## B. Neurological Complications of Cutaneous Melanoma

Most of the neurological complications from malignant melanoma result from metastases directly to the nervous system or to adjacent structures with secondary neural compromise. Nonmetastatic complications, such as vascular disorders (e.g., nonbacterial thrombotic endocarditis and disseminated intravascular coagulation (DIC) and paraneoplastic disorders, are uncommon.

Although there are numerous studies describing the incidence and clinical course of melanoma brain metastases, there is little data about the overall pattern of involvement of the nervous system. To assess the spectrum of neurological disorders in patients with metastatic melanoma, a retrospective study of all neurological complications from malignant melanoma was performed by reviewing the records of 208 patients referred to the medical Oncology Clinic at Vanderbilt University Medical Center. Study methods are presented in the Appendix at the end of this chapter.

## 1. Incidence

Of the 208 melanoma patients seen at Vanderbilt, 174 (84%) developed systemic metastases. This high percentage most likely reflects the bias in the types of patients referred to university hospitals. Clinically recognized neurological complications occurred in 47% (82/174) of patients with metastases. The nervous system was the initial site of metastasis in 5% of these 82 patients and two patients (1%) had nervous system metastases at the time of diagnosis of their melanoma. Other studies have reported symptomatic metastases to the nervous system in a similar percentage of patients (5). Postmortem studies have found neural metastases in 75% to 90% of patients with metastatic melanoma, suggesting that many patients harbor clinically undetected disease (3,6). The median interval from initial diagnosis of melanoma to the diagnosis of nervous system complications was 37 months, but 21 patients (25%) were more than 5 years from diagnosis and 9 patients (11%) were more than 10 years from initial diagnosis.

The nervous system was not the sole site of metastatic disease in any patient in our series. Similarly, Byrne et al. found that only 4% of 80 patients with brain metastases had no other systemic metastases (7). However, these figures may also result from referral bias, because isolated brain metastases are more common in population-based series of melanoma patients. Bullard et al. found isolated disease in 22% of 107 patients with brain metastases (8), and Choi et al. reported that 22% of 194 patients had no identifiable second site of disease at the time brain metastases were diagnosed (9). Therefore, as many as one in five patients with brain metastases have isolated CNS disease.

Lung metastases are the most common site of extracranial disease in patients with brain metastases, occurring twice as often as any other systemic site. This pattern has been noted with brain metastases from many types of cancer and suggests that the lungs are a common source for hematogenous spread to the brain.

In the Vanderbilt series, melanoma primaries located on the head, neck, and trunk were more likely to cause nervous system and systemic metastases than were primaries on the lower extremities. Other authors have also reported a predisposition for metastatic spread of lesions of the upper body (8).

**Table 1** Site of Nervous System Involvement in 78 Patients from a Total Sample of 208 Patients with Malignant Melanoma[a]

| Location | Number (%) | Location | Number (%) |
|---|---|---|---|
| Brain | 61 (82%)[b] | Spinal cord | |
| Supratentorial | 56 | Epidural | 2 (3%) |
| Infratentorial | 10 | Intramedullary | 0 |
| Number of lesions | | Meningeal | |
| 1 | 26 (46%)[c] | Total | 9 (12%) |
| 2 | 10 (18%) | Meningeal + brain | 3 |
| 3 or more | 20 (36%) | Cranial and Peripheral nerve | 13 (17%) |

[a]12 patients had involvement of two nervous system sites.
[b]5 patients had metastases above and below the tentorium.
[c]46% of the 56 patients for whom lesion number is known.

The specific sites of metastasis could be ascertained in 78 of the 82 patients with neurological complications in the Vanderbilt series (Table 1). Brain metastases were the most common neurological complication, but spinal metastases, meningeal metastases, and cranial and peripheral nerve lesions also occurred.

## 2. Brain Metastases from Malignant Melanoma

The majority of the neurological complications from malignant melanoma result from metastases directly to nervous system structures. The most frequent site of metastasis is the brain (see Table 1). In our series, brain metastases occurred in 61 of 174 (35%) patients with metastatic melanoma. The distribution of lesions between supratentorial and infratentorial compartments (see Table 1) is similar to that of brain metastases in general (1). Of 56 patients for whom the number of lesions was estimated by computed tomography (CT) scan, 26 (46%) had a single lesion, and 30 (54%) had two or more lesions. These figures are similar to those for brain metastases from all cancers (1) and to other reports of patients with metastatic melanoma (7). Postmortem studies have found a higher percentage (91%) of patients with multiple lesions than have CT-based studies (3).

*Symptoms and Signs.* Headache, focal neurological deficits, cognitive changes, and seizures are the most common presenting features of brain metastases. In our series, 15 of 56 (27%) patients with supratentorial brain metastases developed seizures at some time during their course. Five of these patients had seizures as the presenting sign of their brain metastasis. Reports of the percentage of patients with seizures from brain metastases originating from other cancers (10) and from metastatic melanoma (5,9) have described similar figures. However, Hagen et al. found seizures at presentation in 37% (13/35) of their patients with melanoma (11), and Byrne et al. reported a still higher figure of 48% of 80 patients

(7). Therefore, the available data suggest but do not clearly demonstrate a higher risk for seizures among patients with brain metastases from melanoma.

The risk of developing seizures after diagnosis of brain metastases determines whether patients should receive prophylactic anticonvulsants. In the Vanderbilt series, 10 of 51 patients (20%) developed seizures after the diagnosis of brain metastases. Byrne et al. found late-onset seizures in 21 of 63 (37%) melanoma patients (7). Cohen et al. observed late-onset seizures in only 16 of 195 (8%) patients with brain metastases from a variety of solid tumors (10). In the latter study, multiple cerebral metastases correlated positively with the development of late-onset seizures.

Patients with multiple brain metastases from melanoma may develop a diffuse (nonfocal) encephalopathy that suggests a metabolic etiology. While there are usually other clues to the presence of structural disease such as visual field loss, subtle focal weakness, or headache, these may be absent early. Also, patients with brain metastases have a lower threshold for the development of encephalopathy secondary to metabolic derangements or CNS-depressant drugs than do those without such underlying brain abnormalities. Leptomeningeal metastases should be considered in melanoma patients with encephalopathy of unknown cause. Other unusual presentations of brain metastases from melanoma may mimic subarachnoid hemorrhage (12) or subdural hematoma (13).

*Diagnosis.* The diagnosis of brain metastasis is confirmed by magnetic resonance imaging (MRI) or CT scanning. Because of the high frequency of brain metastases in patients with metastatic melanoma and because at autopsy patients have previously undetected brain metastases, a CT or MRI scan is appropriate for melanoma patients with only headache, personality changes, or encephalopathy. MRI with gadolinium is more sensitive in the detection of metastatic deposits than CT, even when double-dose contrast CT is used (14). Gadolinium-enhanced MRI is the study of choice when resection of a presumed solitary metastasis is contemplated.

The typical radiographic finding is single or multifocal parenchymal brain lesions that enhance following contrast administration. Extra-axial (subarachnoid or dural) lesions are also seen (15). Approximately 25% of pre–contrast CT scans demonstrate lesions with increased density, which reflects the presence of melanin or hemorrhage. Magnetic resonance imaging may be able to differentiate between melanotic melanoma, amelanotic melanoma, and hemorrhagic melanoma metastasis (16). Melanotic melanomas can give increased intensity on $T_1$-weighted sequences and mildly hypo- or isointense $T_2$-weighted signals, which is the reverse of the findings with most metastases (Fig. 1). This MRI finding is suggestive, although not diagnostic, of metastatic melanoma. Hemorrhagic lesions may be distinguished from melanotic metastases because of the marked decreased intensity on $T_2$-weighted sequences typically seen with hemorrhagic metastases. Amelanotic melanoma metastases give MRI signal intensities that are

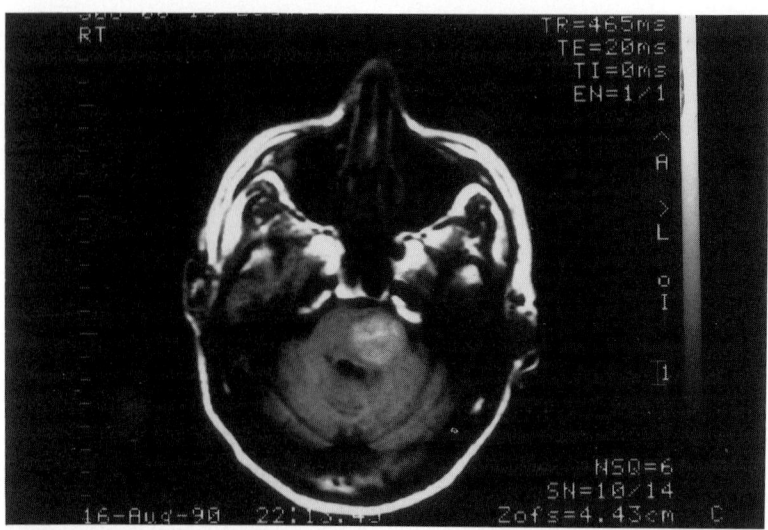

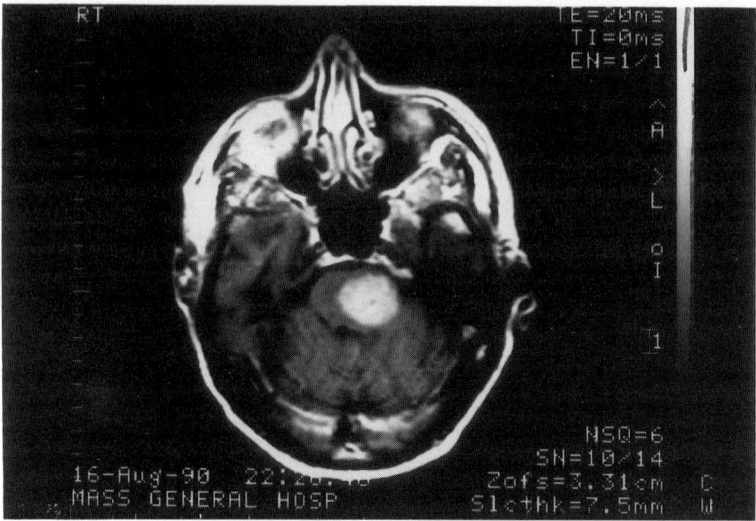

**Figure 1** Magnetic resonance and computed tomography images of a brain metastasis from malignant melanoma. The radiographic findings suggest a melanotic metastasis (see text). The $T_1$-weighted image (a, TE = 20 ms, TR = 264 ms) shows mildly hyperintense signal within the lesion, with marked enhancement following the administration of gad-

## Malignant Melanoma

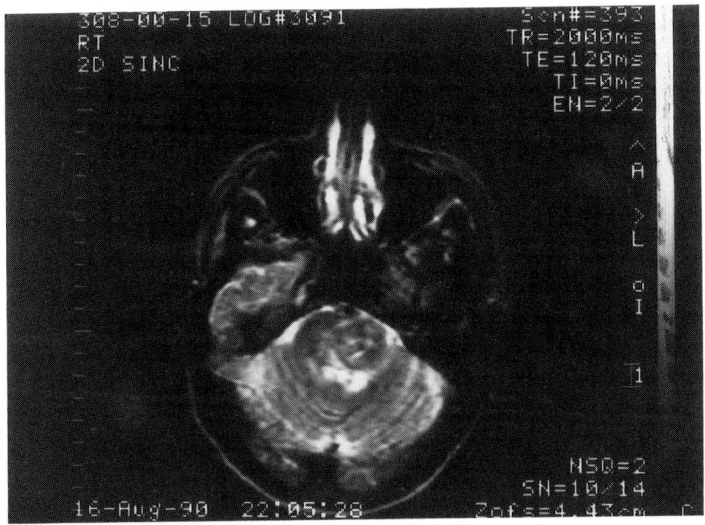

(c)

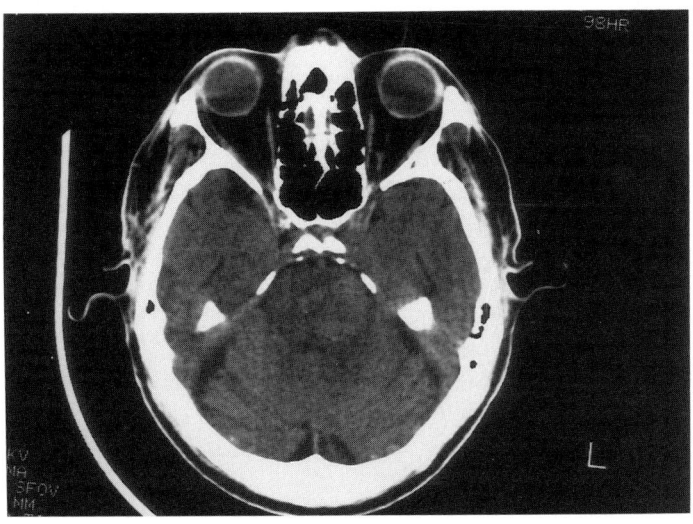

(d)

olinium (b). The $T_2$-weighted image (c, TE = 120 ms, TR = 2000 ms) reveals isointense to slightly hypointense signal characteristics. Hemorrhagic brain metastases typically are markedly hypointense on $T_2$-weighted sequences. Computed tomography scan shows homogeneous, mild hyperdensity in the lesion (d). (Courtesy of Bradley R. Buchbinder, M.D., Division of Neuroradiology, Massachusetts General Hospital.)

indistinguishable from those seen with metastases from other primaries (decreased intensity on $T_1$, increased intensity on $T_2$ sequences).

Magnetic resonance imaging with gadolinium is more sensitive in the detection of small metastatic deposits than CT. Gadolinium-enhanced MRI is the study of choice in patients with suspected brain metastases, particularly when resection of a suspected solitary metastasis is contemplated.

When radiological abnormalities consistent with brain metastases are seen, the diagnosis can be accepted with a high degree of confidence. However, the possibility of nonmetastatic diseases must always be kept in mind. In a recent prospective surgical series of cancer patients with a single brain lesion thought to represent a metastasis, 6 of 54 (11%) patients were found to have other diseases at biopsy (17). Second malignancies occur in 5% of patients with metastatic melanoma. For these reasons, surgical biopsy should be considered for patients with a history of melanoma and solitary brain lesion in the absence of progressive systemic disease.

In patients with neurological complaints but whose CT or MRI scan does not reveal a parenchymal abnormality, metastases to the leptomeninges and skull base must be considered. Hydrocephalus, leptomeningeal enhancement, and brain parenchymal lesions that abut the ventricles or the subarachnoid space suggest the possibility of leptomeningeal metastases. Computed tomography with bone window settings can be useful in the detection of metastases to the skull base.

*Therapy of Brain Metastases (see also Chaps. 1 and 5). Glucocorticoids.* Symptoms and signs from melanoma brain metastases, usually respond dramatically to dexamethasone 4 mg given orally (p.o.) four times daily (q.i.d.). Dexamethasone should be tapered in patients whose neurological deficits are stable or improving during radiation therapy (RT). However, many patients will not be able to tolerate completely stopping glucocorticoids. Byrne et al. found that 86% of 80 patients with brain metastases from melanoma were steroid dependent until death (7).

*Anticonvulsants.* Because of its efficacy, ease of management, and low cost, phenytoin is the first-choice anticonvulsant for melanoma patients with seizures from brain metastases. The risk of Stevens-Johnson syndrome may be increased in patients on phenytoin during radiation therapy so that special caution should be used when a rash occurs in this setting. Determination of free phenytoin levels may be useful in patients with hypoalbuminemia (phenytoin is extensively bound by serum proteins), in those taking numerous medications, and in those who develop signs of nervous system toxicity in the presence of a normal total phenytoin level. Second-line agents include phenobarbital and valproic acid. The addition of valproic acid to phenobarbital results in a decrease in phenobarbital elimination so that serum levels may rise rapidly, leading to sedation. Carbamazepine is usually avoided because of the potential to worsen the leukopenia resulting from chemotherapy and radiation therapy. If carbamazepine must be used, blood counts should be monitored.

Some authors have recommended prophylactic anticonvulsants for patients with brain metastases form melanoma (7). This recommendation is based on reports of a high risk for seizures in these patients (see above). Three conclusions are justified: (1) seizures occur in at least 20% to 30% of melanoma patients with brain metastases, of which some are late in onset; (2) patients with multiple cerebral metastases may be at a higher risk for seizures than those with solitary or posterior fossa lesions; and (3) prophylactic anticonvulsants at therapeutic levels likely reduce the risk of late-onset seizures. One approach is to administer prophylactic anticonvulsants to patients with multiple cerebral metastases and to withhold anticonvulsants until a first seizure in the remainder of patients. Patients with newly diagnosed brain metastases should be advised not to engage in potentially hazardous activities.

*Radiation therapy (see also Chap. 10).* Melanoma is a radioresistant cancer, and there is no convincing evidence that conventional, external-beam RT is beneficial to patients with brain metastases from melanoma. Metastases are treated with very high doses in a single fraction (equivalent to approximately 6000 cGy). Stable disease or partial responses are routinely obtained at the treatment site, and symptomatic radionecrosis has not been common. Stereotactic external-beam RT is of limited usefulness in patients with multiple (3 or more) or large (>3 cm) lesions, and is not widely available. However, it may become the treatment of choice for patients who develop one or two brain metastases 3 cm or less in diameter, particularly when the lesion is not surgically accessible (18,19).

Many studies of radiation therapy for brain metastases from melanoma have been published. The majority of these studies are difficult to interpret because they are not prospective or controlled, and because there is no direct measurement of the response of the brain metastases to radiation therapy. When neurological symptoms and signs are used to measure response, glucocorticoid therapy may be responsible for apparent responses. Also, rapidly progressive systemic disease can obscure any benefit of cranial irradiation on survival. Hagen et al. reported 35 patients with a single metastasis that was surgically removed (11). Nineteen patients received postoperative RT and 16 did not. Relapse was measured by CT or MRI appearance of progressive disease. The irradiated group had a significantly longer interval to progression than did the nonirradiated group (26 months versus 5.7 months, respectively). However, median survival times were the same for the two groups. Byrne et al. used discontinuation of glucocorticoids and CT scans to indicate responses to irradiation in 66 melanoma patients (7). Using these criteria, approximately 10% to 15% of patients showed a response to irradiation. Accelerated fractionation schedules have been tested because of their beneficial effect on other systemic sites of disease. No convincing evidence has emerged to show benefit over conventional fractionation in patients with brain metastases from melanoma (9). However, several authors have reported short-term toxicity (headache and increase in focal neurological deficits) in patients receiving high-dose fractions (20,21). In conclusion, conventional external-beam RT may have limited palliative benefit for melanoma brain metastases in some patients, with or without surgical resection.

Recent experience with stereotactic external-beam RT suggests that this approach is more effective than conventional RT in the treatment of melanoma brain metastases. Metastases are treated with very high radiation doses (equivalent to approximately 6000 cGy) in a single fraction. Since 1986, 45 patients with recurrent, solitary melanoma brain metastases 3 cm or less in diameter have been treated with this technique at one center (J. Loeffler, personal communication). This treatment has produced stable disease or partial responses at the treatment site, without subsequent progression. Symptomatic radionecrosis has not occurred in any patient. Stereotactic external-beam RT is of limited usefulness in patients with multiple (three or more) or large lesions; it is very expensive and not widely available. However, stereotactic RT may become the treatment of choice for patients with limited systemic disease who develop one or two brain metastases 3 cm or less in diameter, particularly when the lesion is not surgically accessible.

*Surgery.* Resection of brain metastases is an increasingly common practice. In a prospective, randomized study comparing surgery plus conventional RT to RT alone in the treatment of solitary brain metastases from a variety of cancers, those patients undergoing surgery had a longer duration of survival, maintained functional independence for a longer period of time, and had a lower rate of local recurrence compared with the RT-only group (17).

Most retrospective surgical series report longer survivals after surgery plus RT compared with RT alone in patients with metastatic melanoma, but selection bias may account for most of the reported differences. Patient age, performance status, extent of systemic disease, and rate of disease progression all affect the clinical decision to operate. Nonetheless, postoperative survivals are usually longer than would be expected when brain metastases are treated with RT alone. In addition, the only long-term survivals in patients with melanoma metastases to brain are in those undergoing surgery plus RT. This suggests that in selected patients, surgical excision of brain metastases is beneficial.

Median survivals for patients undergoing surgical resection of a melanoma brain metastasis range from 5 to 10 months, with the longer durations appearing in series from recent years (23,24). The extent of systemic disease is the key factor determining the duration of survival following surgery. Hagen et al. found a median survival of 19.2 months in those patients undergoing surgery with systemic disease that was undetectable or limited to the primary site (11). In those with disseminated disease, the median postoperative survival was 3.7 months.

Survivals of 24 months or more have been reported in several series of patients undergoing resection of cerebral metastases from melanoma. Of 133 patients pooled from six surgical series, 16 (12%) survived 24 or more months. At least three (2%) of these patients survived for more than 5 years.

Several factors must be considered when surgical resection of brain metastasis from melanoma is contemplated. These factors include lesion number and surgical accessibility, status of systemic disease, and the physical condition of the patient. Gadolinium-enhanced MRI is the most sensitive way to assess the number of brain metastases (14). Patients with one or two lesions that are surgically accessible should be considered for surgery. Some patients with brain metastases (10%, see below) will have clinically detectable, coexistent leptomeningeal metastases (LM). Lumbar puncture should be performed prior to surgery, if not contraindicated by mass effect, to rule out LM. The presence of leptomeningeal enhancement, hydrocephalus, and lesions abutting CSF spaces is suggestive of LM. Surgical candidates should undergo a thorough staging evaluation. Only 5% to 20% of patients with brain metastases from melanoma will not have identifiable systemic metastases (7,9). However, in patients with limited systemic disease, brain metastases may herald a more aggressive phase of tumor growth which has yet to become clinically apparent.

*Chemotherapy.* Chemotherapy for brain metastases has a limited role as salvage therapy. Chemotherapy can be considered when the brain is the major symptomatic site of disease in patients whose lesions have not responded to RT. The only presently available drug reported active against brain metastases from melanoma is cisplatin, administered intra-arterially (25,26). Systemic disease may progress during an intracranial response to intra-arterial cisplatin. The currently available nitrosoureas (e.g., BCNU, CCNU) and DTIC have limited activity in extracranial disease (25% response rate) but are not active against brain metastases (27–29).

Fotemustine (an aminophosphonic acid–linked nitrosourea) has shown activity against brain and systemic metastases from melanoma in European trials (30,31). In 39 patients treated with fotemustine prior to RT for brain metastases from melanoma, intracranial responses were measured in 11 (28%; two complete responses, nine partial responses). Fotemustine should soon be commercially available in the United States.

## 3. Spinal Cord Compression from Metastatic Melanoma

In the Vanderbilt series, epidural spinal cord compression (SCC) occurred in 2 of 78 (3%) patients with neurological complications. In both patients SCC occurred as a result of extension of a vertebral body metastasis into the spinal canal. This percentage is in the range reported by Amer et al. (5), who found SCC in 4 of 56 (7%) and by Bullard et al. (8), who found SCC in 9.3% of 86 patients with neural metastases from melanoma. These figures are also close to the 5% reported for SCC from all cancers (32). The signs, symptoms, and diagnosis of metastases SCC are similar to those occurring in patients with other types of cancer and are discussed in Chapter 16. Spinal cord compression from intradural masses secondary to leptomeningeal metastases may be more common in patients with melanoma than in patients with other types of cancer.

Two recent studies have reported responses to radiation therapy in 75% of patients with spinal cord or cauda equina compression from metastatic melanoma, as determined by clinical evaluation 1 month following completion of RT (33,34). Therefore, radiation therapy is the first line of treatment for most patients with SCC from metastatic melanoma. High-dose corticosteroids are useful at the time of diagnosis of SCC. Surgical treatment (anterior decompression) may be considered in patients with spinal instability or cord compression from displaced bone and disk fragments or, rarely, in those with disease progression following maximal RT.

### 4. Leptomeningeal Metastases from Metastatic Melanoma

Leptomeningeal metastases (LM) were clinically diagnosed in 9 of 78 (12%) patients with neurological complications in our series. This is similar to the frequency reported in other series of patients with metastatic melanoma (5) and is higher than the frequency in most other cancers. Autopsy series report LM in 24% to 63% of melanoma patients (6,35).

Leptomeningeal metastases and brain metastases commonly coexist. Parenchymal brain lesions were noted in 4 of 9 patients with LM in the Vanderbilt patients. Similar findings were noted by Amer et al. (5). Approximately 10% of patients with brain metastases from malignant melanoma will have clinically evident LM. Autopsy studies have reported that 50% of patients with brain metastases also have LM. This may reflect more disseminated disease by the time of death or the detection of clinically inapparent cases at autopsy. The signs, symptoms, and diagnosis of LM are discussed in Chapter 3. Immunocytology may be useful in the diagnosis of suspected LM from melanoma (36).

There is little information available about the efficacy of treatments for LM from melanoma. Radiation therapy may be helpful when administered to clinically symptomatic areas. Two of 11 (18%) patients with LM from melanoma responded to RT plus intrathecal methotrexate in the study of Wasserstrom and coworkers (37). In melanomatous meningitis, it is not known whether the addition of methotrexate to RT is beneficial. Experience with intrathecal injections of interferon alpha and dacarbazine are anecdotal and these therapies should be considered experimental (38,39).

### 5. Peripheral Nerve Complications

A total of 10 of 78 (13%) of patients with neurological complications from metastatic melanoma had cranial nerve or peripheral nerve complications. Each appeared to be secondary to metastases to nonneural sites (e.g., lymph nodes, bone) with compression of adjacent nerves. In the Vanderbilt patients, there was clinical evidence of brachial plexopathy in four cases. In each case, cervical or axillary nodes were enlarged. Leg pain, reflex loss, and weakness occurred in two patients. One had enlarged inguinal nodes and the second had a pelvic mass. A seventh patient developed incontinence from a destructive sacral lesion. There are a modest number of reports describing a rare and somewhat indistinct clinicopathological entity known as "neurotropic melanoma," which is described under Perineural Spread of Cutaneous Carcinoma in the following section (40). Cranial nerve complications included one superior orbital fissure syndrome associated with a mass at the cavernous sinus, one jugular foramen syndrome associated with a skull base metastasis, and one orbital mass with vision loss and pupillary paralysis.

## 6. Survival

Median survival form diagnosis of melanoma for the Vanderbilt patients with neurological complications was 45 months. Patients with systemic metastases, but not nervous system metastases, had the same duration of survival. Eighty-one patients with nervous system metastases are known to have died, with a median survival of 4 months from the diagnosis of their nervous system metastases. Of 39 patients for whom the cause of death could be determined, 23 (60%) died as a direct result of their neurological disease.

## 7. L-Dopa Therapy and Malignant Melanoma

A temporal link has been reported between L-dopa therapy of Parkinson's disease and development or progression of malignant melanoma (41). However, melanoma is not overrepresented as a co-morbid condition in patients with Parkinson's disease. There is no evidence to suggest that L-dopa or melanin stimulates the growth of melanocytes. Wick et al. found L-dopa without activity as a chemotherapy agent against melanoma (42). Thus, there is no convincing evidence that L-dopa has any effect on melanoma.

## C. Metastatic Complications of Noncutaneous Melanomas

### 1. Primary Nervous System Melanoma

Two types of cutaneous melanotic lesions are associated with primary central nervous system melanoma: neurocutaneous melanosis and oculodermal melanosis. In the former, congenital, giant cutaneous pigmented nevi are associated with meningeal melanosis. Malignant melanoma may arise in the skin or the meningeal lesion (43). In oculodermal melanosis, pigmentation of the conjunctiva and periorbital skin, usually unilaterally (Ota's nevus), may be associated with primary central nervous system melanoma (44).

Melanoma can also arise in the brain without a predisposing neurocutaneous syndrome. Primary melanoma of the nervous system more commonly arises from the leptomeninges, sometimes with associated brain infiltration, but without a detectable systemic primary site (45).

## 2. Metastatic Ocular Melanoma

Ocular melanomas occur with one-eighth the incidence of cutaneous melanomas and may metastasize throughout the body, including the nervous system. The organs most often involved are liver, lung, and bone. An autopsy study of 92 patients who died from metastatic melanoma revealed a significantly lower frequency of brain metastases in patients with ocular melanoma (2 of 9 or 22%) compared to nonocular melanoma (48/73, or 66%) (46). In a retrospective study of 41 patients with metastatic ocular melanoma, three (7%) had clinically detectable neurological metastases at first diagnosis of metastases (47). However, an autopsy study which included four patients with ocular melanoma found brain metastases in three (6). Skeletal metastases from metastatic ocular melanoma can lead to epidural spinal cord compression. Rarely, ocular melanoma extends intracranially along an optic nerve (48). Metastatic ocular melanoma, like cutaneous melanoma, responds poorly to available therapy.

## D. Summary

The incidence of melanoma is rising rapidly; therefore, physicians will be called upon more often than before to manage the complications of this malignancy. Metastatic complications may appear 10 years or more after the initial diagnosis of melanoma; therefore, clinical suspicion of recurrent disease must remain permanently high in patients with a history of melanoma. Three advances in the management of melanoma brain metastases have been achieved recently. Surgical resection can lead to long-term survivals in selected patients, and to significant palliation in others. Stereotactic exernal RT is an effective approach in the control of brain metastases 3 cm or less in size. Results with the chemotherapeutic agent fotemustine give cause for cautious optimisim for a useful medical approach to brain metastases. Prevention and early detection and treatment represent the optimal management of melanoma patients.

## III. NEUROLOGICAL COMPLICATIONS OF OTHER CUTANEOUS MALIGNANCIES

### A. Introduction

At least two other malignancies arising in the skin can cause neurological complications. Perineural spread of cutaneous carcinoma of the head and neck region can cause diagnostic difficulty because of progressive, focal cranial nerve deficits. Cutaneous T-cell lymphomas (CTCL) cause complications that are similar to those arising from other lymphomas. This section discusses the presentation and diagnosis of neurological complications from these malignancies.

## B. Perineural Spread of Cutaneous Carcinoma

Migration of tumor cells along peripheral nerves is a common event in the spread of cancer. Such spread rarely causes clinical symptoms. However, when perineural spread of tumor cells occurs along cranial nerves, significant neurological morbidity may result. Cutaneous neoplasms of the head and neck, particularly squamous cell carcinoma and less commonly basal cell carcinoma, can cause multiple cranial nerve deficits by this mechanism (49). Carcinomas of oro- and nasopharynx or sinuses may also cause this syndrome.

Patients develop slowly progressive (weeks to months) cranial nerve deficits in proximity to the site of the primary tumor. The most commonly reported deficits are (1) facial sensory loss, often focal at first followed by gradual spread; (2) facial weakness, also often focal at first; and (3) extraocular muscle palsies. The abnormalities are unilateral. Pain may be absent or occurs concurrently with motor and sensory deficits. Exposure keratitis may require tarsorrhaphy. The history of skin cancer may be recent or distant.

Once the diagnosis is suspected, evaluation should include CT or MRI through the orbits, facial bones, and base of the skull. Nerves enlarged by infiltrating tumor or enlarged neural foramina can sometimes be detected. Tumor cell infiltration may extend along cranial nerves all the way to the brain stem. Soft tissue masses may yield a clue to the correct diagnosis. Lumbar puncture may be necessary to rule out meningeal diseases causing multiple cranial nerve palsies. Histological confirmation of the diagnosis can be obtained by nerve biopsy (e.g., inferior orbital nerve biopsy in a patient with complete sensory loss, see Fig. 2). Histological examination of tumor-infiltrated nerve tissue in "neurotropic melanoma" is said to reveal tumor cells with the appearance of Schwann cells that do not synthesize melanin, intermixed with normal appearing Schwann cells (40). Direct infiltration of cutaneous nerves from the adjacent melanocytic lesion can sometimes be seen.

Treatment consists of palliative radiation therapy to the affected nerve. Deficits, especially if severe, are unlikely to improve with therapy, but further deterioration may be halted.

## C. Neurological Complications of Cutaneous T-Cell Lymphomas

Approximately 25% of non-Hodgkin's lymphomas present at extranodal sites. Cutaneous T-cell lymphomas, including mycosis fungoides and Sézary syndrome, are among these extranodal lymphomas. In CTCL, malignant T cells infiltrate the epidermis, and to a lesser extent the dermis, resulting in characteristic skin lesions.

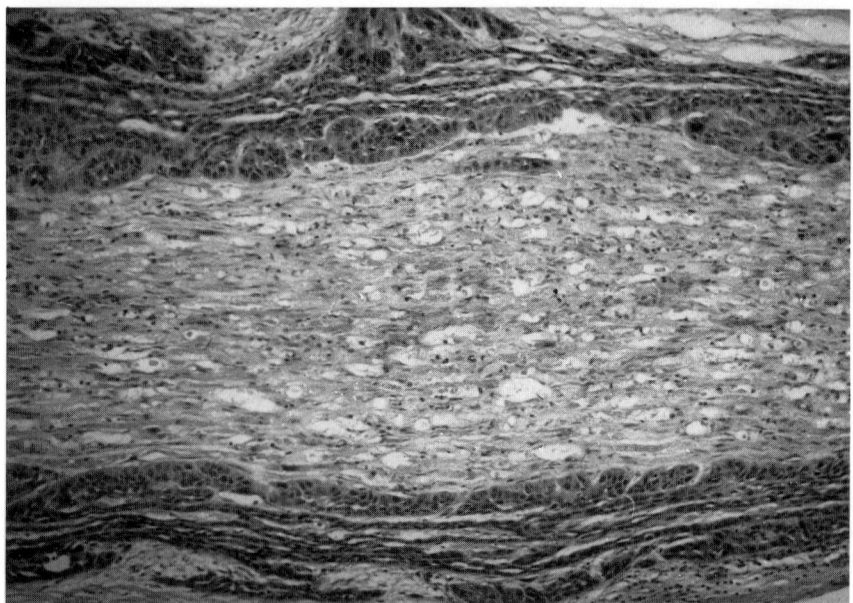

**Figure 2** Longitudinal section of facial nerve showing epineurial infiltration by cutaneous squamous carcinoma. (Hematoxylin and eosin, ×100. Courtesy of Paul Clouston, M.D., Neurology Department, Repatriation General Hospital, Sydney, Australia.)

Initially these cutaneous lesions are discrete but later become diffuse and tumor nodules appear in the skin.

Cutaneous T-cell lymphoma is usually disseminated at onset, with extracutaneous involvement becoming more prominent in the later stages of the illness. An autopsy study of 86 patients who died of mycosis fungoides revealed parenchymal brain involvement in 11 (13%), meningeal involvement in eight (9%), and peripheral nerve infiltration in four (5%) (50). While these lesions are often clinically silent, patients may present with intracerebral hemorrhage, mass lesions, white matter lesions, or meningeal involvement. Chapter 23 discusses the neurological complications of lymphoma in greater detail.

## D. Summary

Although these cutaneous malignancies cause neurological complications less commonly than does melanoma, they can result in diagnostic confusion and disabling neurological morbidity. Early diagnosis and local therapy may be beneficial.

## ACKNOWLEDGMENTS

I wish to thank Ronald G. Wiley for the idea of reviewing the neurological complications of melanoma patients at Vanderbilt, and David N. Louis (Division of Neuropathology, Massachusetts General Hospital) for helpful comments on the manuscript.

## APPENDIX

The charts of 233 patients referred to the Medical Oncology department at Vanderbilt University Medical Center between 1976 and 1986 were reviewed. Clinical and laboratory data for each patient was collected in chronological form and then entered into a computerized data base for analysis. Only clinically diagnosed neurological complications were recorded. Since computed tomography (CT) was in routine use by 1976, this source was used to collect data regarding such information as site, number, and presence of hemorrhage in brain metastases. Outcome was defined as the clinical state (alive or deceased) at the time of data acquisition. Telephone interviews were used to follow up any living patient not seen at Vanderbilt within 1 month prior to data acquisition. Of 233 patients, outcome was known for 225; adequate follow-up to determine the presence of a neurological complication was available for 208 (89%). Demographic information for these 208 included 115 men, 93 women; average age at diagnosis 45.2 years.

## REFERENCES

1. Delattre J-Y, Krol G, Thaler HT, Posner JB. Distribution of brain metastases. Arch Neurol 1988; 45:741–744.
2. Koh HK. Cutaneous melanoma. N Engl J Med 1991; 325:171–182.
3. Chason JL, Walker FB, Landers JW. Metastatic carcinoma of the central nervous system and dorsal root ganglia. Cancer 1963; 16:781–787.
4. Nathanson L. Spontaneous regression of malignant melanoma: a review of the literature on incidence, clinical features and possible mechanisms. Natl Cancer Inst Monogr 1976; 44:67–76.
5. Amer MH, Al-Sarraf M, Baker LH, Vaitkevicius VK. Malignant melanoma and central nervous system metastases. Cancer 1978; 42:660–668.
6. de la Monte SM, Moore GW, Hutchins GM. Patterned distribution of metastases from malignant melanoma in humans. Cancer Res 1983; 43:3427–3433.
7. Byrne TN, Cascino TL, Posner JB. Brain metastases from melanoma. J Neurooncol 1983; 1:313–317.
8. Bullard DE, Cox EB, Seigler HF. Central nervous system metastases in malignant melanoma. Neurosurgery 1981; 8:26–30.
9. Choi KN, Withers R, Rotman M. Intracranial masses from melanoma. Cancer 1985; 56:1–9.

10. Cohen N, Strauss G, Lew R, Silver D, Recht L. Should prophylactic anticonvulsants be administered to patients with newly-diagnosed cerebral metastases? A retrospective analysis. J Clin Oncol 1988; 6:1621–1624.
11. Hagan NA, Cirrincione C, Thaler HT, DeAngelis LM. The role of radiation therapy following resection of single brain metastasis from melanoma. Neurology 1990; 40: 158–160.
12. Clifford JR, Kirgis HD, Connolly ES. Metastatic melanoma of the brain presenting as subarachnoid hemorrhage. South Med J 1975; 68:206–208.
13. Palmer FJ, Poulgrain AP. Metastatic melanoma simulating subdural hematoma. J Neurosurg 1978; 49:301–302.
14. Davis PC, Hudgins PA, Petermin SB, Hoffman JC. Diagnoses of cerebral metastases: double-dosed delayed CT vs contrast-enhanced MR imaging. Am J Neuroradiol 1991; 12:293–300.
15. McGann GM, Platts A. Computed tomography of cranial metastatic malignant melanoma: features, early detection and unusual cases. Br J Radiol 1991; 64:310–313.
16. Atlas SW, Grossman RI, Gomori JM, Guerry D, Hackney DB, Goldberg HI, Zimmerman RA, Bilaniuk LT. MR imaging of intracranial metastatic melanoma. J Comput Assist Tomogr 1987; 11:577–582.
17. Patchell RA, Tibbs PA, Walsh JW, Dempsey RJ, Maruyama Y, Kryscio RJ, Markesbery WR, MacDonald JS, Young B. A randomized trial of surgery in the treatment of single metastases to the brain. N Engl J Med 1990; 322:494–500.
18. Somaza S, Kondziolka D, Lunsford LD, Kirkwood JM, Flickinger JC. Stereotactic radiosurgery for cerebral metastatic melanoma. J Neurosurg 1993; 79:661–666.
19. Loeffler JS, Kooy HM, Wen PK, Fine HA, Cheng CW, Mannarino EG, Tsai JS, Alexander E. The treatment of recurrent brain metastases with stereotactic radiosurgery. J Clin Oncol 1990; 8:576–582.
20. Vlock DR, Kirkwood JM, Leutzinger C, Kapp DS, Fischer JJ. High-dose fraction radiation therapy for intracranial metastases of malignant melanoma. Cancer 1982; 49:2289–2294.
21. Ziegler, JC, Cooper JS. Brain metastases from malignant melanoma: conventional vs. high-dose-per-fraction radiotherapy. Int J Radiat Oncol Biol Phys 1986; 12:1839–1842.
22. Stevens G, Firth I, Coates A. Cerebral metastases from malignant melanoma. Radiotherapy Oncol 1992; 23:185–191.
23. Fell DA, Leavens ME, McBride CM. Surgical versus nonsurgical management of metastatic melanoma of the brain. Neurosurgery 1980; 7:238–242.
24. Brega K, Robinson WA, Winston K, Wittenberg W. Surgical treatment of brain metastases in malignant melanoma. Cancer 1990; 66:2105–2110.
25. Weiden PL. Intracarotid cisplatin as therapy for melanoma metastatic to brain: ipsilateral response and contralateral progression. Am J Med 1988; 85:439–440.
26. Feun LG, Lee YY, Plager C, Papadopoulos N, Savaraj N, Charnsangavej C, Benjamin RS, Wallace S. Intracarotid cisplatin-based chemotherapy in patients with malignant melanoma and central nervous system metastases. Am J Clin Oncol 1990; 13:448–451.
27. Moon JH, Gailani S, Cooper MR, Hayes DM, Rege VB, Blom J, Falkson G, Maurice

P, Brunner K, Glidewell O, Holland JF. Comparison of the combination of 1,3-bis(2-chloroethyl)-1-nitrosourea (BCNU) and vincristine with two dose schedules of 5-(3,3-dimethyl-1-triazino)imidazole 4-carboxamide (DTIC) in the treatment of disseminated malignant melanoma. Cancer 1975; 35:368–3671.
28. Costanzi JJ. DTIC (NSC-45388) studies in the Southwest Oncology Group. Cancer Treat Rep 1976; 60:189–192.
29. Merimsky O, Inbar M, Reider I, Chaitchik S. Brain metastases of malignant melanoma in interferon complete responders: clinical and radiological observations. J Neuro-Oncol 1992; 12:137–140.
30. Jacquillat C, Khayat D, Banzet P, Weil M, Avril MF, Fumoleau P, Namer M, Bonneterre J, Kerbrat P, Bonerandi JJ, Bugat R, Montcuquet P, Audhuy B, Cupissol D, Lauvin R, Grosshans E, Vilmer C, Prache C, Bizzari JP. Chemotherapy by fotemustine in cerebral metastases of disseminated malignant melanoma. Cancer Chemother Pharmacol 1990; 25:263–266.
31. Khayat D, Avril MF, Gerard B, Bertrand B, Bizzari JP, Cour V. Fotemustine: an overview of its clinical activity in disseminated malignant melanoma. Melanoma Res 1992; 2:147–151.
32. Barron KD, Hirano A, Araki S, Terry RD. Experiences with metastatic neoplasm involving the spinal cord. Neurology 1959; 9:91–106.
33. Rate WR, Solin LJ, Turrisi AT. Palliative radiotherapy for metastatic malignant melanoma: brain metastases, bone metastases, and spinal cord compression. Int J Radiat Oncol Biol Phys 1988; 15:859–864.
34. Herbert SH, Solin LJ, Rate WR, Schultz DJ, Hanks GE. The effect of palliative radiation therapy on epidural compression due to metastatic malignant melanoma. Cancer 1991; 67:2472–2476.
35. Patel JK, Didolkar MS, Pickren JW, Moore RH. Metastatic pattern of malignant melanoma. Am J Surg 1978; 135:807–810.
36. Moseley RP, Davies AG, Bourne SP, Popham C, Carrel S, Monro P, Coakham HB. Neoplastic meningitis in malignant melanoma: diagnosis with monoclonal antibodies. J Neurol Neurosurg Psychiatry 1989; 52:881–886.
37. Wasserstrom WR, Glass JP, Posner JB. Diagnosis and treatment of leptomeningeal metastases from solid tumors. Cancer 1982; 49:759–772.
38. Dorval T, Beuzeboc P, Garcia E, Jouve M, Palangie T, Pouillart P. Malignant melanoma: treatment of metastatic meningitis with interferon alpha-2b. Eur J Cancer 1992; 28:244–245.
39. Champagne MA, Silver HKB. Intrathecal dacarbazine treatment of leptomeningeal melanoma. J Natl Cancer Inst 1992; 84:1203–1204.
40. Mack EE, Gomez EC. Neurotropic melanoma. J Neuro-Oncol 1992; 13:165–171.
41. Rampen FHJ. Levodopa and melanoma: three cases and review of literature. J Neurol Neurosurg Psychiatry 1985; 48:585–588.
42. Wick MM. The chemotherapy of malignant melanoma. J Invest Derm 1983; 80: 61s–62s.
43. Reyes-Mugica M, Chou P, Byrd S, Ray V, Castelli M, Gattuso P, Gonzalez-Crussi F. Nevomelanocytic proliferations in the central nervous system of children. Cancer 1993; 72:2277–2285.

44. Sang DN, Albert DM, Sober AJ, McMeekin TO. Nevus of Ota with contralateral cerebral melanoma. Arch Ophthalmol 1977; 95:1820–1824.
45. Rodreiquez y Baena R, Paolo Gaetani P, Danova M, Bosi F, Zappoli F. Primary solitary intracranial melanoma: case report and review of the literature. Surg Neurol 1992; 38:26–37.
46. Zakka KA, Foos RY, Omphroy CA, Straatsma BR. Malignant melanoma: analysis of an autopsy population. Ophthalmology 1980; 87:549–556.
47. Lorigan JG, Wallace S, Mavligit GM. The prevalence and location of metastases from ocular melanoma: imaging study in 110 patients. Am J Radiol 1991; 157:1279–1281.
48. Jones DR, Scobie IN, Sarkies NJC. Intracerebral metastases from ocular melanoma. Br J Ophthalmol 1988; 72:246–247.
49. Clouston PD, Sharpe DM, Corbett AJ, Kos S, Kennedy PJ. Perineural spread of cutaneous head and neck cancer. Arch Neurol 1990; 47:73–77.
50. Epstein EH, Levin DL, Croft JD, Lutzner MA. Mycosis fungoides. Medicine 1972; 15:61–72.

# 16

# Neurological Disorders in Head and Neck Cancers

**Paul L. Moots**

*Vanderbilt University Medical Center, Nashville, Tennessee*

**Ronald G. Wiley**

*Vanderbilt University Medical Center and Veterans Affairs Medical Center, Nashville, Tennessee*

## I. INTRODUCTION

Head and neck cancers are typically squamous carcinomas and present as masses or bleeding with local or referred pain (1,2). Adenocarcinomas occur in the paranasal sinuses or upper nasal cavity, ethesioneuroblastomas also occur in the upper nasal cavity, and adenocarcinomas are the typical salivary gland tumors. Involvement of the nervous system varies depending on the location of the primary tumor, the extent of local invasiveness, metastases, and complications of therapy. The spectrum of neurological complications seen with squamous carcinomas is described in detail later. The rest of the Introduction will focus on neurological presentations (Table 1).

*Diplopia* may result from invasion of the orbit or involvement of the cavernous sinus. Cavernous sinus invasion produces some combination of dysfunction of cranial nerves III, IV, VI, and the ophthalmic division of V. If occlusion of the sinus occurs, headache, papilledema, chemosis, and proptosis ensue (3,4). Frontal, maxillary, or ethmoid sinus tumors may invade the orbit, while sphenoid sinus tumors may spread to involve the cavernous sinus.

*Ear pain* is common with head and neck carcinomas at a variety of primary sites. Since several cranial nerves (V, VII, IX, and X) provide sensory innervation to the ear, referred pain can occur with involvement of branches of any of these four cranial nerves. Chronic ear pain with a sense of fullness in the ear and serous

353

**Table 1** Neurological Symptoms of Head and Neck Cancers

| Symptom/sign | Tumor location |
| --- | --- |
| Anosmia | Frontal sinus, olfactory epithelium (esthesioneuroblastoma) |
| Diplopia | Frontal, maxillary, or ethmoid sinus, cavernous sinus invasion (sphenoid sinus) |
| Otalgia | Any tumor involving nerve V, VII, IX, or X, occlusion of eustachian tube (nasopharyngeal or nasal) |
| Trismus | Metastatic spread to pterygoid fossa and muscles of mastication |
| Headache | Any sinus occlusion, base of skull invasion (usually nasopharyngeal), increased intracranial pressure with venous occlusion or intracranial mass |
| Hoarseness | Laryngeal, pharyngeal, vagal involvement from any other primary |
| Facial pain/ paresthesia/ numbness | Perineural spread into branches of nerve V from variety of primaries (nasal, maxillary sinus, etc.) |
| Facial weakness | Parotid, nasopharyngeal (spread to base of skull) |
| Dysarthria | Parotid, oropharyngeal, tongue, lip, palatal |
| Dysphagia/ odynophagia | Pharyngeal, base of tongue, tonsillar, invasion of pharyngeal muscles |

otitis media can result from obstruction of the eustachian tubes by tumor (nasopharyngeal, nasal). Spread of nasopharyngeal, oropharyngeal, buccal, or parotid tumors to the pterygoid fossa can produce local (periauricular) pain or trismus (5).

*Hoarseness* obviously can occur with laryngeal tumors, but in published series, the most common tumors to cause hoarseness with vocal paralysis are lung carcinomas and thyroid carcinomas (6–8). Interestingly, some lung cancer patients also may develop ipsilateral face/head pain that is thought to be referred pain from vagus nerve involvement in the chest by the lung tumor (9–11).

*Progressive facial pain, numbness, and paresthesias* can result from trigeminal involvement with a variety of primary head and neck squamous carcinomas (3), often due to perineural infiltration. Perineural spread of squamous carcinomas is well documented as a cause of pain and neurological deficits (12–14) and is considered a poor prognosticator indicative of a biologically aggressive tumor. Progressive facial numbness, particularly mental neuropathies ("numb chin syndrome"), often result from other processes including vascular anomalies, benign tumors, metastases, carcinomatous meningitis, and intrinsic lesions of the brainstem (3,15–18). However, invasive nasopharyngeal tumors have a tendency to involve the trigeminal nerve at the base of the skull causing midface pain and numbness.

*Weakness* can involve the face with parotid tumors, in which case the weakness is most prominent at the ipsilateral corner of the mouth with or without pain (local or ear) or trismus (1). Weakness or mechanical distortion also can occur with carcinoma of the tongue or spread of tumor into the pharyngeal muscles leading to dysphagia and dysarthria. Often pathological analysis of the surgical specimen is necessary to determine the extent of nerve involvement in such cases.

*Nasal tumors* typically present as nonhealing ulcers, occasional bleeding, and unilateral obstruction. Neurological symptoms are not common initially with limited stage disease but metastatic spread into the orbit can produce diplopia with or without pain and proptosis. Occlusion of the ostia of paranasal sinuses can produce persistent headache or face pain appropriate to the involved sinus (1,2). Rarely, squamous carcinoma or esthesioneuroblastoma will extend superiorly into the frontal fossa producing headache, anosmia, and personality change due to frontal lobe involvement.

*Paranasal sinus tumors* have varying presentations depending on which site is initially involved, but a mass or swelling and local pain dominate the early phases. As mentioned above, diplopia or cavernous sinus involvement may develop by local extension. Maxillary sinus tumors may spread perineurially along the trigeminal nerve and even into the middle cranial fossa producing ipsilateral facial pain and numbness followed by symptoms of intracranial involvement such as focal cerebral deficits.

*Nasopharyngeal tumors* most often (90%) present with a mass in the neck (1,2). However, altered hearing, chronic serous otitis media, tinnitus, nasal obstruction, and ear pain also occur. Extension along the base of the skull or into the cervical lymph nodes can produce deficits affecting almost any combination of cranial nerves, although evolution of cranial nerve deficits usually occurs by contiguous spread.

*Oral and oropharyngeal tumors* typically present with local pain and mass effects. Bleeding and dysphagia are common with some primary tumor locations. Neurological symptoms most often reflect advanced or recurrent disease. Base of the tongue tumors may produce referred ear pain due to perineural spread along branches of the ninth nerve. Tumors of the pharyngeal walls or hypopharynx may produce referred ear pain by involvement of tenth nerve branches. Odynophagia, dysphagia, and dysarthria may reflect mechanical mass effects more often than neurological deficits in patients with these tumors. Laryngeal tumors rarely produce neurological signs or symptoms until far advanced or metastatic.

## II. SQUAMOUS CELL CARCINOMA

### A. Clinical Features

#### 1. Presentation, Natural History, Staging

Squamous cell carcinoma is the principal neoplasm included under the general category of head and neck cancers. This includes the vast majority of carcinomas arising in the oral cavity, the naso- and oropharynx, the larynx, and less commonly the nasal cavity. These neoplasms occur with a marked preponderance in males (4:1 male-to-female ratio) and are strongly associated with tobacco and alcohol abuse. Chronic pulmonary, hepatic, and nutritional disorders are common among these patients. Most patients are greater than 40 years of age at diagnosis.

The natural history of squamous cell carcinomas of the head and neck is notable for relatively predictable patterns of locoregional involvement (19). Increasing size of the primary tumor is associated with a poorer prognosis. Regional lymph node involvement at diagnosis varies from 10 to 75% depending on the site of the primary tumor. The frequency of lymph node involvement increases with the size of the primary. Distant metastases occur in 10–30% of patients (20,21). From these patterns derives a T,N,M staging system that is valuable in treatment planning and assessment of prognosis (see Table 2).

Carcinomas arising in the oral cavity tend to be diagnosed relatively early (i.e., T1 or T2). This is particularly true of neoplasms arising on the lip or anterior tongue. Lymph node involvement at diagnosis varies greatly, but in general is somewhat less common than with neoplasms of the oropharynx or larynx. The incidence ranges from 5–20% for neoplasms of the lip to 30–35% for anterior tongue, buccal mucosa, and floor of the mouth primaries. The last of these has a high frequency of bilateral node involvement.

Carcinomas of the oropharynx include neoplasms arising from the base of tongue, tonsils, soft palate, and pharynx. The interdigitating muscular and fascial barriers at the base of the tongue and lateral pharyngeal walls often fail to provide an effective barrier to local extension. Lateral extension into the parapharyngeal space is an important antecedent to cranial nerve and base of skull involvement. In addition to incomplete local barriers, the early symptoms tend to be minor and insidious. Thus primaries in this region are often relatively large (i.e., T3 or T4) at

**Table 2** T, N, M Staging for Squamous Cell Carcinoma of the Head and Neck

| Stage | T[a] | N[b] | M | Stage | T[a] | N[b] | M |
|---|---|---|---|---|---|---|---|
| I | T1 | N0 | — | IV | T1-3 | N2-3 | — |
| II | T2 | N0 | — |  | T4 | N0-3 | — |
| III | T1-2 | N1 | — |  | T1-4 | N0-3 | + |
|  | T3 | N0 | — |  |  |  |  |

[a]T dimension varies with site.
[b]N staging system is the same for all sites: N0, clinically negative; N1, single homolateral node <3 cm; N2, single homolateral node 3–6 cm or multiple homolateral nodes <6 cm; N3, massive homolateral nodes, bilateral or contralateral nodes.

diagnosis. The size and extent are frequently underestimated clinically. There is a high incidence of lymph node involvement. For example, neoplasms of the base of the tongue are noted for late presentation with large (i.e., T3 and T4) primary tumors and a 75% incidence of clinically positive neck nodes. In 30% the nodes are bilateral.

Insidious growth, late presentation, and a tendency for local extension into the parapharyngeal and retropharyngeal spaces are also characteristic of primaries in the hypopharynx. These primaries characteristically have a poor prognosis.

Carcinomas of the larynx include predominantly supraglottic and glottic primaries, subglottic tumors being rare. Supraglottic tumors tend to present as relatively small exophytic lesions causing pain with little involvement of adjacent structures (i.e., T1 or T2). However, early lymph node involvement is common (55%) and frequently bilateral. Carcinomas of the glottis, including the vocal cords, also present early. The presenting symptom is generally hoarseness, while pain is a late symptom. Lymph node involvement is rare given the absence of lymphatics draining the true vocal cords.

## 2. Associated Diseases

Second primary neoplasms are found in 10–25% of patients with head and neck cancers. The most commonly reported sites are the lungs, the head and neck region, and the esophagus (20,22,23). The incidence of second primaries increases with duration of survival, being 10% at 3 years, 15% at 5 years, and 23% at 8 years. This frequency is sufficient to warrant detailed evaluation including tissue diagnosis for unexpected patterns of cervical lymph node involvement, and for apparent late relapses at distant sites.

Nutritional deficiencies associated with chronic ethanol abuse or consequent to tumor-related trismus or dysphagia add to the list of associated disorders that may produce neurological symptoms.

## B. Therapy

## 1. Stages I and II

Stage I and most stage II neoplasms can be treated with excellent long-term results by either surgery or radiation. Factors favoring a surgical approach include: tumors located in sites where resection can be performed without significant functional impairment, and a medical status that does not suggest an increased risk of postoperative complications. The lack of late delayed complications also favors the surgical approach. Conversely, radiation may provide better end-organ functional preservation. Therefore, stage I and II patients who are poor surgical candidates or who have primaries in the pharynx or larynx where surgical morbidity is often high and functional disability great are more often treated with radiotherapy. The long-term disease-free survival for stage I and II patients treated by either modality should be greater than 85%.

## 2. Stages III and IV

Treatment of the primary site in patients with advanced-stage (III and IV) head and neck carcinomas generally requires combined modality therapy to achieve long-term survival. Patients with resectable primaries who receive postoperative radiation have a 40% 5-year survival. Patients with unresectable primaries or in whom poor medical condition precludes surgery achieve local control by radiation alone in about 20% of cases.

Adjuvant and neo-adjuvant chemotherapy have demonstrated significant response rates in patients with advanced disease (24). Active single agents include cisplatin, methotrexate, 5-fluorouracil (5-FU), and bleomycin. The highest single-agent response rates are observed with cisplatin (40%) and methotrexate (35%). Combination chemotherapy, for example using cisplatin and 5-FU, has a somewhat higher response rate. The use of combination chemotherapy in the neo-adjuvant setting has demonstrated response rates of 50–70%, with complete responses in 20%. In conjunction with organ-preserving surgical procedures, or as an alternative to surgery prior to radiation, chemotherapy adds an important option for patients with advanced-stage disease. However, randomized trials of neo-adjuvant chemotherapy have not demonstrated an increase in survival.

## 3. Management of the Neck

In addition to treatment of the primary site, the high likelihood of cervical lymph node involvement necessitates a strategy for assessment and treatment of the neck. Radiation can provide adequate control of node involvement in the neck, particularly if involvement is subclinical (e.g., clinical stage N0). Surgical treatment of the clinically uninvolved neck has some distinct advantages including: pathological staging, specific tailoring of the surgical approach to the site of the primary, and fewer delayed sequelae than radiation when "functional" dissections are employed (see below). However, even with the standard radical neck dissection certain groups of cervical lymph nodes routinely escape removal (i.e., retro- and parapharyngeal nodes), and despite treatment the neck remains the most common site of recurrence. The presence of multiple nodes, multiple levels of nodal involvement, or extension through the capsule indicates the need for postoperative radiation. Fixed nodes have generally been treated by radiation prior to surgery, but the use of chemotherapy in this situation is increasing.

## C. Neurological Sequelae of Metastatic Disease

### 1. Direct Extension

Direct extension and spread via lymphatics are the principal means of metastasis for carcinomas of the head and neck. The pattern of progression of locoregional disease is outlined above. Direct invasion of peripheral nerves, while uncommon, is associated with a poor prognosis. These patients have a higher than expected rate of cervical node involvement. In addition, the long-term survival in this group is poor, with a 2-year survival of only 46% (12).

Histologically documented nerve invasion was found in 25 of 1308 (2%) patients with squamous cell carcinoma of the lower lip (12). In a report of 80 cases of nerve invasion from head and neck cancers by Ballantyne et al., 43 arose from the skin or lip (13). Mental nerve involvement by primary lip cancers produced the most characteristic syndrome (i.e., "numb chin" syndrome), but multiple distal ramifications of the trigeminal nerve were frequently affected. Conversely reports describing cranial neuropathies and base of skull involvement in cancer patients indicate that about 15% of these cases are due to head and neck primaries (3,15).

Although some patients are asymptomatic, many complain of burning or lancinating pain often for months before the tumor becomes apparent. The pace of growth is often sufficiently slow that enlargement of the mandibular canal, foramen ovale, or other bony foramen is an important radiographic clue to neural extension. Intracranial extension may lead to the development of a tumor mass in the cerebellopontine angle or to meningeal dissemination (see below).

Paroxysmal hypotension is another consequence of nerve invasion, usually in patients with disease recurrent after neck dissection (25–27). Some patients have pain attacks resembling glossopharyngeal neuralgia in association with the syncopal episodes that occur even when supine (27–30). Frequently, atropine and cardiac pacemakers are ineffective in preventing the life-threatening syncopal attacks. Some success has been reported with anticonvulsants such as phenytoin and carbamazepine (27,28). Pathophysiologically, the patients experience vasodepressor syncope. Presumably, infiltration of the ninth and/or tenth cranial nerves results in barrages of inappropriate nerve discharges involving pain and baroreceptor fibers. During hypotensive episodes, patients may have inappropriately low plasma catecholamine levels consistent with failure of sympathetic function (30). Autopsy findings include the expected extracranial nerve infiltration, usually without intracranial extension. Thus, intractable cases can be managed by intracranial transection of the ninth and rostral half of the tenth nerves. Since the new onset of syncope invariably means recurrent tumor in patients previously treated for head and neck squamous carcinoma, other forms of salvage antitumor therapy also should be considered.

## 2. Meningeal Carcinomatosis

The incidence of carcinomatous meningitis in carcinomas of the head and neck is about 1–2%, or somewhat less than the 5% incidence that is generally stated as the overall incidence of meningeal metastases in cancer patients (31–33). Perineural invasion appears to be the predominant route of spread to the meninges (31,34,35). In comparison with meningeal dissemination by other solid tumors, spinal cord and spinal nerve root involvement are uncommon. Since methotrexate is an active agent against squamous cell carcinomas of the head and neck, it is not surprising that intrathecal methotrexate may produce a response in patients with meningeal involvement by this neoplasm. Two of four patients treated by Redman et al. had significant responses and two had stable disease with a median survival of 10 months (31). This exceeds the median survival of patients treated for meningeal involvement by breast cancer.

## 3. Brachial Plexopathy

Involvement of the brachial plexus is occasionally observed in patients with advanced head and neck cancers, usually in the setting of cervical lymph node involvement with capsular extension and involvement of adjacent tissues. Capsular extension producing truly fixed lymph nodes is rare in nodes smaller than 6 cm (36). In large series about 7% of patients have truly fixed nodes at diagnosis. The incidence is higher for cancers of the oropharynx and hypopharynx than for other primary sites. However, in a series of 23 surgically treated patients with fixed nodes reported by Stell et al., none had involvement of the brachial plexus (36). Conversely, in two series reported from the Memorial Sloan-Kettering Cancer Center including more than 75 patients with brachial plexopathy due to neoplastic infiltration, four patients had head and neck cancers (37,38).

## 4. Spinal Epidural Metastases

Given the infrequency of metastatic dissemination of head and neck cancers beyond the cervical lymph nodes (10% or less at diagnosis and 30% in patients with advanced disease), involvement of the spinal epidural space would likely be uncommon (35,36). The most common sites of distant metastasis by head and neck cancers are lung and bone, accounting for 50 and 20% of distant sites, respectively (35,36). Approximately 80% of distant metastases are detected within 2 years of diagnosis of the primary cancer. As spinal epidural metastasis is the sequela of vertebral bone involvement in 80–85% of cases, most studies of epidural metastases include a small percentage of patients with head and neck primaries. In two large studies from the Memorial Sloan-Kettering Cancer Center, including a total of 318 patients, 19 patients (6%) had head and neck primaries (39,40). Epidural involvement was observed in the cervical, thoracic, and lumbosacral regions with equal frequency in the few patients ($n = 5$) for whom the level was reported. Treatment outcome with high-dose dexamethasone and radiotherapy was similar to that observed with other carcinomas (40). Given the relative rarity of these metastases, epidural involvement in a head and neck cancer patient without any other evidence of active disease, particularly if more than 2 years from the initial diagnosis, should raise the suspicion of a second primary neoplasm. Surgery or needle biopsy for tissue diagnosis is usually needed in such cases.

## 5. Parenchymal Metastases

Parenchymal brain metastases are generally hematogenous in origin, and for many cancers are strongly associated with lung involvement (41,42). As mentioned previously, the lungs are the most frequent site of distant metastases from head and neck cancers. Thus, it is not surprising that the brain is occasionally the site of distant metastasis by head and neck cancers. In an autopsy study of 2452 patients performed at the Memorial Sloan-Kettering Cancer Center, 3% of all intracranial metastases were observed in head and neck cancer patients. In that report seven of 118 (6%) head and neck cancer patients had intracerebral metastases (41). In another postmortem series, brain lesions accounted for five of 71 metastatic sites documented in 63 head and neck cancer patients (20). Clinical series have indicated a slightly lower percentage of patients with brain metastases from head and neck cancer (20,43,44). Treatment approaches rely on extrapolation of results obtained with the solid tumors most commonly associated with brain metastases (i.e., lung and breast cancer), and probably have a similar efficacy. As noted in regard to epidural metastases, brain metastases appearing in a head and neck cancer patient with a long disease-free interval should raise suspicion regarding a second primary neoplasm. Thus, a search for systemic tumor and tissue diagnosis would be appropriate.

## D. Nonmetastatic Sequelae
### 1. Paraneoplastic Disorders
Paraneoplastic neurological syndromes are rare degenerative disorders that may involve any level of the central or peripheral nervous system. The most common are cerebellar degeneration and/or diffuse encephalomyelitis, sensory neuropathy, and Lambert-Eaton myasthenic syndrome. These disorders are most commonly associated with lung cancers, particularly small cell carcinomas, breast cancer, and ovarian cancer. Approximately half these patients have antineuronal or other antibodies, supporting the thesis that the pathogenesis is immunological (45). Although a number of relatively large series have been reported, none include any patients with head and neck carcinomas (46,47).

One of the authors (PLM) has personally followed a 66-year-old man who developed slowly progressive, moderately severe limb and gait ataxia and dysarthria 2 years after resection of a small supraglottic adenocarcinoma. Magnetic resonance imaging demonstrated severe atrophy of the cerebellar hemispheres. Studies of serum and cerebrospinal fluid did not demonstrate antineuronal antibodies. There was no significant history of alcohol or other toxin exposure and no family history of neurological degeneration. Two years following the onset of the neurological symptoms no evidence of recurrent tumor or second primary has been found, and the patient remains ambulatory with the assistance of a cane.

## E. Neurological Sequelae of Treatment
### 1. Surgery
Resection of primary head and neck cancers often requires severing of terminal branches of sensory nerves to the face, oral, and nasal cavity (trigeminal nerve),

the oropharynx and hypopharynx (glossopharyngeal nerve), or dermatomal branches of the upper cervical nerve roots. The subsequent development of neuropathic pain syndromes can be a major clinical problem. Referred pain involving the ear is another common sequela. Such pain syndromes require careful reexamination and repeated imaging to exclude recurrent tumor, particularly with perineural extension, which is often difficult to demonstrate. Pain syndromes with burning dysesthetic sensations or lancinating pains that appear confined to the territory of a peripheral nerve may be treated with amitriptyline or anticonvulsants such as carbamazepine or phenytoin.

The most characteristic postoperative neurological complications seen in patients with head and neck cancer are those related to neck dissection. The standard radical neck dissection involves removal of the sternocleidomastoid, digastric, and stylohyoid muscles, the internal and external jugular veins, the submaxillary gland, and the spinal accessory nerve. The procedure can be followed by significant morbidity due to trapezius weakness and neck instability. Less frequently other cranial nerves, particularly the facial, vagus, and hypoglossal nerves, may be injured. Horner's syndrome due to injury to the sympathetic fibers accompanying the carotid artery is not uncommon. Burning dysesthetic pain occurs due to the interruption of the anterior cervical nerve roots with subsequent neuroma formation. This is the most common posttreatment complaint in patients who have undergone radical neck dissection. In conjunction with muscle instability, this can produce a disabling and difficult to manage pain syndrome.

Carotid exposure and rupture can be another means of neurological complication from the neck dissection (48). Invasion of the carotid artery by neoplasm is more often seen at the time of recurrence than at initial diagnosis. Many surgeons favor resection of the tumor along with the involved carotid artery. This is accompanied by reconstruction of the vessel. Ligation of the carotid appears to have a higher incidence of cerebrovascular events and a higher mortality than reconstruction. Occasionally, unilateral removal of the jugular veins is followed by intracranial hypertension. When bilateral neck dissections are required, one internal jugular vein must be preserved.

Functional or "conservative" neck dissections in which the sternocleidomastoid muscle, internal jugular vein, and spinal accessory are left intact have gained wide acceptance as the surgical approach to the patient with clinically negative or very limited cervical lymph node involvement (49).

## 2. Radiation Therapy

Radiotherapy for head and neck cancers typically involves the administration of doses between 55 and 70 Gy in daily fractions of 180–225 cGy to ports that include the primary site and all tissues at risk of involvement. In selected primary sites interstitial implantation may be used. Patients with hypopharyngeal and laryngeal primaries and those with advanced nodal disease (i.e., N2 or N3) receive substantial radiation doses to the cervical spine. Bilateral parallel opposed fields are frequently used. They generally include 5–15 cm (e.g., two to eight vertebral bodies) of the cervical spine. With limited neck disease a single anterior posterior field with a midline block is sometimes used. Field reductions at 45–50 Gy can also be used to limit the dose to the spinal cord depending on the location of the primary neoplasm. Primaries in the nasopharynx necessitate inclusion of the base of the skull, and not infrequently portions of the anterior and middle cranial fossae.

Acute neurological complications associated with radiotherapy are rare. The major neurotoxicities are categorized temporally as early- and late-delayed radiation toxicities. The most common early-delayed effect is Lhermitte's sign. The incidence of Lhermitte's sign in head and neck cancer patients is about 4% (50). In most patients this is transient, lasting a few weeks. In the absence of pain or other signs of myelopathy, close follow-up is all that is needed. However, occasionally these patients will go on to develop more serious late-delayed sequelae or radiation myelopathy (50).

Late-delayed radiation myelopathy is characterized by small-vessel thrombosis with parenchymal necrosis, inflammation, and eventual atrophy of the affected segment. There is subsequent degeneration of the involved nerve fiber tracts. The latent period following irradiation is usually 6 months and often more than 1 year. There is not an absolute relation between total dose and the likelihood of myelopathy; however, the incidence increases progressively with doses above 5500 cGy. In addition, high-dose fractions (e.g., 300 cGy/fraction) and longer lengths of irradiated spinal cord are associated with an increased risk of radiation myelopathy (55). The incidence in head and neck cancer patients is probably 0.5–1%, although some series report an incidence as high as 5% (54,55).

The clinical syndrome of radiation myelopathy evolves with subacute progressive symptoms over weeks or months. Pain in a dermatomal pattern followed by sensory loss, weakness and corticospinal tract signs that are often asymmetrical, and bladder or bowel dysfunction are typical. Brown-Séquard syndrome is relatively common, and often the motor deficits are partial (36).

Delayed cerebral radionecrosis has been reported following treatment of a variety of neoplasms originating in the head and neck region (53). Frontal and temporal masses with evidence of microvascular injury are seen. These lesions behave as progressive space-occupying masses and must be distinguished from malignant gliomas or metastatic tumors.

Cranial neuropathy is a relatively rare complication of radiation therapy. The latent period to the development of cranial neuropathies is generally greater than 2 years. This interval is inversely related to the dose of radiation. For patients with head and neck cancers the twelfth nerve is most commonly affected, followed by the tenth (54). The distinction from recurrent tumor is often difficult and requires serial observations to be established with certainty. Brachial plexopathy may also

Table 3  Neurotoxicity in Selected Chemotherapy Trials for Head and Neck Cancer

| Study | Design | Treatment plan | Number of patients | | Neurotoxicity | | |
|---|---|---|---|---|---|---|---|
| | | | | | Ototoxicty | Neuropathy | Other |
| Forastiere et al. J. Clin. Oncol. 1992 (42) | Randomized trial for recurrent and metastatic S.C.C. | Cisplatin (100 mg/m²) + 5-FU (1000 mg/m² per day × 4 days) every 3 weeks | 87 (60% rec'd 3 or more courses) | Mild Severe | 8% 4% | 5% 1% | NR |
| | | Carboplatin (300 mg/m² + 5-FU (1000 mg/m²/d × 4) every 4 weeks | 86 (46% rec'd 3 or more courses) | Mild Severe | 0 0 | 2% 0 | NR |
| | | Methotrexate (40 mg/m² wk) (3 weeks = 1 course) | 88 (49% rec'd 3 or more courses) | Mild Severe | 0 0 | 0 0 | NR |
| Jacobs et al. J. Clin. Oncol. 1992 (45) | Randomized trial for recurrent and metastatic S.C.C. | Cisplatin (100 mg/m²) + 5-FU (1000 mg/m²/d × 4) every 3 weeks | 78 | Mild Severe | 10% 3% | NR[a] | NR[a] |
| | | Cisplatin (100 mg/m²) every 3 weeks | 83 | Mild Severe | 3% 1% | NR[a] | NR[a] |
| | | 5-FU (1000 mg/m²/d × 4) every 3 weeks) | 82 | Mild Severe | 2% 2% | NR[a] | NR[a] |
| H & N Contracts Program Cancer 1987 (43) | Randomized trial of surgery + RT vs | Surgery and radiation | | | NR | NR | NR |
| | | Cisplatin (100 mg/m²) + bleomycin followed by surgery & RT | 140 | | 1% | NR | |

| Study | Treatment | Regimen | N | | | |
|---|---|---|---|---|---|---|
| | S, RT, neoadjuvant chemo *vs* S, RT, neoadjuvant and maintenance chemo for H & N Ca | CDDP + bleomycin → surgery → RT → CDDP (80 mg/m²/month × 6) | 151 (only 27% completed 3 cycles of maintenance chemotherapy) | 2% (7 of 245 cycles) | NR | NR |
| Ensley et al. J Clin Oncol 1988 (44) | Intensive neoadjuvant chemotherapy for advanced S.C.C. | Course 1, 3, 5: CDDP (100 mg/m²) + 5-FU (1000 mg/m²/d × 5) Course 2, 4: MTX (250 mg/m²/wk × 3) + 5-FU (600 mg/m²/wk × 3) (Each course 28 days) Prior to surgery and RT (66 Gy) | 46 (31 completed chemotherapy) | 0 | 0 | 0 |
| Denham and Abbott J Clin Oncol 1991 (46) | Concurrent radiation and chemotherapy for advanced S.C.C. | CDDP (50 mg/m²) + 5-FU (350 mg/m²/d × 5) (2 courses during RT) And 60–64 Gy | 23 | 0 Note: No myelopathy reported with minimum follow-up of 38 months. | 0 | 0 |

NR, not reported.

[a] <5% of patients in any arms had greater than WHO grade 1 neurotoxicity.

occur following radiation. However, in a series of 27 patients with well-documented radiation plexopathy reported from the Memorial Sloan-Kettering Cancer Center none had head and neck cancers (36,37).

Vasculopathy is another important delayed complication of radiation therapy for head and neck cancers that can result in neurological symptoms. Cerebral radionecrosis largely results from endothelial and small-vessel damage. Large-vessel injury has also been associated with radiation (55). Rarely, intimal necrosis, inflammation, sinus formation, or infection leads to lethal carotid rupture, usually within weeks after treatment. This is more clearly related to local factors than to radiation (56). Carotid stenosis and carotid occlusion have both been reported following radiation, often in the absence of coronary or peripheral vascular disease (57,58). Atherosclerosis following radiation occurs with a long latent period and thus is not a complication seen with high incidence in the head and neck cancer patients. The frequency of atherosclerotic changes appears to be inversely related to vessel size based on comparisons of intracranial versus extracranial carotid artery disease (57). These changes evolve slowly. The latency to onset of symptoms is up to 4 years for intracranial carotid disease as compared to 19 years for extracranial carotid disease (57). Distal carotid stenosis or occlusion following radiation is often associated with the development of a moyamoya-like abnormality.

Despite compelling laboratory and clinical evidence that radiation produces vascular injury, the significance for head and neck cancer patients is unclear. This population has multiple risk factors for atherosclerosis and stroke. Among 52 patients surviving an average of 5.5 years after treatment for a head and neck cancer reported by Lopez et al., stroke risk factors included: male gender—84%, smoking—92%, hypertension—17%, diabetes—8%, and coronary artery disease 23% (59). Of those 52 patients, 28 who had received radiation underwent carotid duplex scanning. Five carotid stenoses of 50–75% and three of greater than 75% were detected. In six nonirradiated patients, two asymptomatic carotid stenoses of 50–75% were detected. Two of 34 patients studied had symptomatic cerebral ischemia, both of whom had received radiation and had 50–75% stenosis (59). Although this study demonstrates the multiplicity of stroke risk factors common to head and neck cancer patients, the size of the study is too small to assess the significance of radiation as an added risk factor. These authors do not recommend carotid Doppler studies as part of the routine long-term follow-up evaluation of head and neck cancer patients (59).

## 3. Chemotherapy

Current chemotherapeutic approaches to the treatment of head and neck cancers frequently include agents with significant neurotoxicities, particularly methotrexate, cisplatin, and 5-FU (24). However, the doses and schedules used in most head and neck cancer chemotherapy protocols tend to be less intensive than those likely to produce central or peripheral neurotoxicity.

The principal form of neurotoxicity associated with intravenous administration of methotrexate is leukoencephalopathy (60). This is generally associated with high-dose methotrexate therapy (e.g., repeated doses of $>1-3$ g/m$^2$) and would be very unusual in the dose ranges commonly utilized in the treatment of head and neck cancers (see Table 3).

Cisplatin produces dose-related ototoxicity and peripheral neuropathy. It occasionally causes Lhermitte's sign (61). Chemotherapy protocols for head and neck cancers using cisplatin rarely achieve the cumulative dose of cisplatin sufficient to produce a high incidence of peripheral neuropathy (e.g., cumulative dose $>400$ mg/m$^2$) (58–64; see also Table 2). The incidence of severe ototoxicity is generally less than 5%. Severe neuropathy is reported as 1% or less. Central nervous system complications such as radiation myelopathy and cerebral radionecrosis are reported even less commonly in the large randomized trials despite the evidence that cisplatin and radiation may have synergistic effects in the production of neurotoxicity (67,68). Notably, the concurrent use of cisplatin/5-FU in moderate doses with radiation resulted in no instances of myelopathy or other central nervous system complications (66).

The principal neurotoxicity associated with high-dose 5-FU is an acute, transient cerebellar syndrome, which is seen in 2–7% of patients (69). Less commonly encephalopathy, parkinsonism, and other neurological syndromes are observed. These problems are most frequent with doses $>1$ g/m$^2$ given by intravenous bolus. Neurotoxicity is rarely associated with continuous infusion of 5-FU, the method of administration used in essentially all the head and neck cancer protocols for 5-FU (62,63,65,66; see also Table 2).

## REFERENCES

1. Lane M, Donovan DT. Neoplasms of the head and neck. In: Calabresi P, Schein PS, eds. Medical oncology. Basic principles and clinical management of cancer, 2nd ed. New York: McGraw-Hill, 1992:568–92.
2. Schantz SP, Harrison LB, Hong WK. Tumors of the nasal cavity and paranasal sinuses, nasopharynx, oral cavity and oropharynx. In: Devita VT, Hellman S, Rosenberg SA, eds. Cancer. Principles and practice of oncology, 4th ed. Philadelphia: JB Lippincott, 1993:574–630.
3. Greenberg HS, Deck MDF, Vikram B, Chu FCH, Posner JB. Metastasis to the base of the skull: clinical findings in 43 patients. Neurology 1981; 31(5):530–7.
4. Dalmau J, Graus F. Neuropatia craneal y cancer. Neurologia (Esp), 1986; 1:202–11.
5. Tveteras K, Kristensen S. The aetiology and pathogenesis of trismus. Clin Otolaryngol 1986; 11:383–7.
6. Titche LI. Causes of recurrent laryngeal nerve paralysis. Arch Otolaryngol 1976; 102:259–61.
7. Kearsley JH. Vocal cord paralysis (VCP)—an aetiologic review of 100 cases over 20 years. Aust NZ J Med 1981; 11:663–6.

8. Gardner GM, Shaari CM, Parnes SM. Long-term morbidity and mortality in patients undergoing surgery for unilateral vocal cord paralysis. Laryngoscope 1992; 102: 501–8.
9. Des Prez RD, Reemon FR. Facial pain associated with lung cancer: a case report. Headache 1983; 23:43–4.
10. Bindoff LA, Heseltine D. Unilateral facial pain in patients with lung cancer: a referred pain via the vagus? Lancet 1988; 1:812–5.
11. Bongers KM, Willigers HMM, Koehler PJ. Referred facial pain from lung carcinoma. Neurology 1992; 42:1841–2.
12. Byers RM, O'Brien J, Waxler J. The therapeutic and prognostic implications of nerve invasion in cancer of the lower lip. Int J Radiat Oncol Biol Phys 1978; 4:215–7.
13. Ballantyne AJ, McCarten AB, Ibanez ML. The extension of cancer of the head and neck through peripheral nerves. Am J Surg 1963; 106:651–67.
14. Carter RL, Pittam MR, Tanner NSB. Pain and dysphagia in patients with squamous carcinomas of the head and neck: the role of perineural spread. J Roy Soc Med 1982; 75:598–606.
15. Gupta SR, Zdonczyk DE, Rubino FA. Cranial neuropathy in systemic malignancy in a VA population. Neurology 1990; 40:997–9.
16. Yuh WTC, Wright DC, Barloon TJ, Schultz DH, Sato Y, Cervantes CA. MR imaging of primary tumors of trigeminal nerve and Meckel's cave. Am J Neuroradiol 1988; 9:665–70.
17. Kuntzer T, Bogousslavsky J, Rilliet B, Uldry P-A, de Tribolet N, Regli F. Herald facial numbness. Eur Neurol, 1992; 32:297–301.
18. Delaney P, Khoa N, Saini N. Isolated trigeminal neuropathy. An unusual complication of carcinoma of the lung. JAMA 1977; 237:2522–3.
19. Million RR, Cassisi NJ, Wittes RE. Cancer of the head and neck. In: DeVita VT, Hellman SH, Rosenberg SA, eds. Cancer: principles and practice of oncology, 2nd ed. Philadelphia: JB Lippincott, 1985:407–506.
20. Papac RJ. Distant metastases from head and neck cancer. Cancer 1984; 53:342–5.
21. Merino OR, Lindberg RD, Fletcher GH. An analysis of distant metastases from squamous cell carcinoma of the upper respiratory and digestive tracts. Cancer 1977; 40:145–51.
22. Kotwall C, Razack MS, Sako K, Rao U. Multiple primary cancers in squamous cell cancer of the head and neck. J Surg Oncol 1989; 40:97–9.
23. Cooper JS, Pajak TF, Rubin P, et al. Second malignancies in patients who have head and neck cancer: incidence, effect on survival and implications based on the RTOG experience. Int J Radiat Oncol Biol Phys 1989; 17:449–56.
24. Jacobs C. Adjuvant and neoadjuvant treatment of head and neck cancers. Semin Oncol 1991; 18(6):504–14.
25. MacDonald DR, Strong E, Nielsen S, Posner JB. Syncope from head and neck cancer. J Neuro-oncol 1983; 1:257–68.
26. Patel AK, Yap VU, Fields J, Thomsen JH. Carotid sinus syncope induced by malignant tumors in the neck. Arch Intern Med 1979; 139:1281–4.
27. Papay FA, Roberts JK, Wegryn TL. Evaluation of syncope from head and neck cancer. Laryngoscope 1989; 99:382–8.

28. Metheetrairut C, Brown DH. Glossopharyngeal neuralgia and syncope secondary to neck malignancy. J Otolaryngol 1993; 22:18–20.
29. Weinstein RE, Herec D, Friedman JH. Hypotension due to glossopharyngeal neuralgia. Arch Neurol 1986; 43:90–2.
30. Onrot J, Wiley RG, Fogo A, Biaggioni I, Robertson D, Hollister AS. Neck tumour with syncope due to paroxysmal sympathetic withdrawal. J Neurol Neurosurg Psychiatry 1987; 50:1063–6.
31. Redman BG, Tapazoglou E, Al-Sarraf M. Meningeal carcinomatosis in head and neck cancer. Cancer 1986; 58:2656–61.
32. Olson ME, Chernik NL, Posner JB. Infiltration of the leptomeninges by systemic cancer. Arch Neurol 1974; 30:122–37.
33. Wasserstrom WR, Glass JP, Posner JB. Diagnosis and treatment of leptomeningeal metastases from solid tumors: experience with 90 patients. Cancer 1982; 49:759–72.
34. Kokkoris CP. Leptomeningeal carcinomatosis: how does cancer reach the pia-arachnoid? Cancer 1983; 51:154–60.
35. Banerjee TK, Gottschalk PG. Unusual manifestations of multiple cranial nerve palsies and mandibular metastasis in a patient with squamous cell carcinoma of the lip. Cancer 1984; 53:346–8.
36. Stell PM, Dalby JE, Singh SD, Taylor W. The fixed cervical lymph node. Cancer 1984; 53:336–41.
37. Kori SH, Foley KM, Posner JB. Brachial plexus lesions in patients with cancer: 100 cases. Neurology 1981; 31:45–50.
38. Cascino TL, Kori S, Krol G, Foley KM. CT of the brachial plexus in patients with cancer. Neurology 1983; 33:1553–7.
39. Gilbert RW, Kim J-H, Posner JB. Epidural spinal cord compression from metastatic tumor: diagnosis and treatment. Ann Neurol 1978; 3:40–51.
40. Greenberg HS, Kim J-H, Posner JB. Epidural spinal cord compression from metastatic tumor: results with a new treatment protocol. Ann Neurol 1980; 8:361–6.
41. Posner JB, Chernik NL. Intracranial metastases from systemic cancer. Adv Neurol 1978; 19:579–92.
42. Zimm S, Wampler GL, Stablein D, Hazra T, Young HF. Intracerebral metastases in solid-tumor patients: natural history and results of treatment. Cancer 1981; 48:384–94.
43. Cairncross JG, Kim J-H, Posner JB. Radiation therapy for brain metastases. Ann Neurol 1980; 7:529–41.
44. Patchell RA, Tibbs PA, Walsh JW, et al. A randomized trial of surgery in the treatment of single metastases to the brain. N Engl J Med 1990; 332:494–500.
45. Anderson NE, Cunningham JM, Posner JB. Autoimmune pathogenesis of paraneoplastic neurological syndromes. CRC Crit Rev Neurobiol 1987; 3:245–99.
46. Dalmau J, Graus F, Rosenblum MK, Posner JB. Anti-HU-associated paraneoplastic encephalomyelitis/sensory neuronopathy: a clinical study of 71 patients. Medicine 1992; 71(2):59–72.
47. Hammack JE, Kimmel DW, O'Neill BP, Lennon VA. Paraneoplastic cerebellar degeneration: a clinical comparison of patients with and without Purkinje cell cytoplasmic antibodies. Mayo Clin Proc 1990; 65:1423–31.

48. Karam F, Schaefer S, Cherryholmes D, Dagher FJ. Carotid artery resection and replacement in patients with head and neck malignant tumors. J Cardiovasc Surg 1990; 31:697–701.
49. Bocca E, Pignataro O. A conservation technique in radical neck dissection. Ann Otol Rhinol Laryngol 1967; 76:975–87.
50. Jeremic B, Djuric L, Mijatovic L. Incidence of radiation myelitis of the cervical spinal cord at doses of 5500 cGy or greater. Cancer 1991; 68:2138–41.
51. Abbatucci JS, Delozier T, Quint R., Roussel A, Brune D. Radiation myelopathy of the cervical spinal cord: time, dose and volume factors. Int J Radiat Oncol Biol Phys 1978; 4:239–48.
52. Cascino TL. Radiation myelopathy. In: Rottenberg DA, ed. Neurological complications of cancer treatments. Boston: Butterworth-Heinemann, 1991:69–78.
53. Rottenberg DA, Chernik NL, Deck MDF, Ellis F, Posner JB. Cerebral necrosis following radiotherapy of extracranial neoplasms. Ann Neurol 1977; 1:339–57.
54. Berger PS, Bataini JP. Radiation-induced cranial nerve palsy. Cancer 1977; 40:152–5.
55. Conomy JP, Kellermeyer RW. Delayed cerebrovascular consequences of therapeutic radiation. Cancer 1975; 36:1702–8.
56. Fajardo LF, Lee A. Rupture of major vessels after radiation. Cancer 1978; 36:904–13.
57. Silverberg GD, Britt RH, Goffinet DR. Radiation-induced carotid artery disease. Cancer 1978; 41:130–7.
58. Murros KE, Toole JF. The effect of radiation on carotid arteries. Arch Neurol 1989; 46:449–55.
59. Lopez M, El-Bayer H, Hye RJ, Freischlag J. Carotid artery disease in patients with head and neck carcinoma. Am Surg 1990; 56:778–81.
60. Bleyer WA. Neurologic sequelae of methotrexate and ionizing radiation: a new classification. Cancer Treat Rep 1981; 65(Suppl 1):89–98.
61. Hamers FPT, Gispen WH, Neijt JP. Neurotoxic side-effects of cisplatin. Eur J Cancer 1991; 27:372–6.
62. Forastiere AA, Metch B, Schuller DE, Ensley JF, Hutchins LF, Triozzi P, Kish JA, McClure S, VonFeldt E, Williamson SK, Von Hoff DD. Randomized comparison of cisplatin plus fluorouracil and carboplatin plus fluorouracil versus methotrexate in advanced squamous cell carcinoma of the head and neck: a Southwest Oncology Group Study. J Clin Oncol 1992; 10:1245–51.
63. Final Report of the Head and Neck Contracts Program: Adjuvant chemotherapy for advanced head and neck squamous carcinoma. Cancer 1987; 60:301–11.
64. Ensley J, Kish J, Tapazoglou E, Jacobs J, Weaver A, Atkinson D, Ahmed K, Mathog R, Al-Sarraf M. An intensive, five course, alternating combination chemotherapy induction regimen used in patients with advanced, unresectable head and neck cancer. J Clin Oncol 1988; 6:1147–53.
65. Jacobs C, Lyman G, Velez-Garcia E, Sridhar K, Knight W, Hochster H, Goodnough L, Mortimer J, Einhorn L, Schacter L, Cherng N, Dalton T, Burroughs J, Rosencweig M. A phase III randomized study comparing cisplatin and fluorouracil as single agents and in combination for advanced squamous cell carcinoma of the head and neck. J Clin Oncol 1992; 10:257–63.
66. Denham JW, Abbot RL. Concurrent cisplatin, infusional fluorouracil, and conven-

tional fractionated radiation therapy in head and neck cancer: dose-limiting mucosal toxicity. J Clin Oncol 1991; 9:458–63.
67. Bertolone SJ, Baum ES, Krivit W, Hammond GD. A phase II study of cisplatin therapy in recurrent childhood brain tumors. J Neuro-Oncol 1989; 7:5–11.
68. Bloss JD, DiSaia PJ, Mannel RS, Hyden EC, Manetta A, Walker JL, Berman ML. Radiation myelitis: a complication of concurrent cisplatin and 5-fluorouracil chemotherapy with extended field radiotherapy for carcinoma of the uterine cervix. Gynecol Oncol 1991; 43:305–8.
69. Phillips PC, Reinhard CS. Antipyrimidine neurotoxocity: cytosine arabinoside and 5-fluorouracil. In: Rottenberg DA, ed. Neurological complications of cancer treatment. Boston: Butterworth-Heinemann, 1991: 97–114.

# 17

# Neurological Complications of Genitourinary Cancer

**Camilo E. Fadul**

*Dartmouth-Hitchcock Medical Center, Lebanon, New Hampshire*

## I. GENERAL PRINCIPLES

### A. Incidence

Neurological complications are not common among genitourinary (GU) cancer patients compared with other malignancies. The frequency and type of complications vary depending on the primary cancer, its biological characteristics, and the stage of the disease. Metastatic neurological complications are more common than nonmetastatic. At the National Cancer Institute of Colombia (NCIC), a tertiary referral cancer center, lumbosacral plexopathy is the most usual complication of GU neoplasms, followed by metastatic epidural spinal cord compression.

### 1. Metastatic

Lumbosacral plexopathy develops in 4% of cervical cancer patients, when most of them have stage II or less disease (1). However, in countries where advanced cervical cancer is the most frequent neoplasm, tumor involvement of the lumbosacral plexus occurs in approximately 12% of the patients. The most frequent GU neoplasm causing epidural spinal cord compression is prostate carcinoma, which combined with renal and cervix tumors, is responsible for 24% of all patients with metastatic cord compression diagnosed at our center.

Distant metastases to the brain or leptomeningeal carcinomatosis are rare events, although their incidence may be increasing because of prolonged survivals resulting from more effective treatment for systemic disease. In a Radiation Therapy Oncology Group (RTOG) study, 3.6% of all patients with brain metastases had GU primaries; most were renal cell carcinomas (2). In our center, a review of 100 consecutive patients diagnosed with brain metastases showed that 14% had a GU primary neoplasm (Table 1).

## 2. Nonmetastatic

Cancer treatment neurotoxicity is common among patients with GU cancer. New chemotherapeutic agents effective for advanced gynecological cancer and germ cell tumors are particularly neurotoxic. Subacute cerebellar degeneration, with high titer of typical anti–Purkinje cell antibody, is the paraneoplastic syndrome most frequently associated with gynecological, specifically ovarian, cancer.

Metabolic encephalopathy occurs in patients with bilateral ureteral obstruction from pelvic tumors and in patients with hepatic metastases. Occasionally, hypoglycemia has been described in patients with large retroperitoneal metastases of GU tumors. Despite severe bone involvement, metastatic prostate cancer rarely produces hypercalcemia. The most frequent neurological complications according to the primary GU tumor are shown in Table 2.

## B. Pathogenesis

The lumbosacral plexus, because of its pelvic and retroperitoneal location, is frequently involved by direct extension of GU neoplasms or by metastases to lymph nodes. Extension of retroperitoneal metastases into the spinal canal or encroachment of vertebral bone metastases can produce epidural spinal cord

**Table 1** Frequencies of Brain Metastases with Genitourinary Neoplasms: Comparison of Series from RTOG and NCIC

| Primary neoplasm | RTOG[a] 1865 patients | NCIC[b] 100 patients | Combined 1965 patients |
|---|---|---|---|
| Kidney | 43 | — | 43 (2.2%) |
| Uterus | — | 9 | 9 (0.5%) |
| Testicle | 11 | 1 | 12 (0.6%) |
| Prostate | 7 | 1 | 8 (0.4%) |
| Bladder | 7 | 1 | 8 (0.4%) |
| Ovary | — | 2 | 2 (0.1%) |
| Total | 68 (3.6%) | 14 (14%) | 82 (4%) |

[a]Radiation Therapy Oncology Group (2)
[b]National Cancer Institute of Colombia

**Table 2** Most Frequent Neurological Complications of Genitourinary Cancer

| Primary cancer | Neurological complications | |
|---|---|---|
| | Metastatic | Nonmetastatic |
| Prostate | Spinal cord compression | |
| | Intracranial metastases | |
| Uterus | Lumbosacral plexopathy | Metabolic encephalopathy |
| | Brain metastases | |
| Ovary | Brain metastases | Paraneoplastic cerebellar syndrome |
| | Neoplastic meningitis | Chemotherapy toxicity |
| Kidney | Brain metastases | Postnephrectomy pain |
| | Spinal cord compression | |
| Testicle | Brain metastases | Radiation plexopathy |
| | Spinal cord compression | Chemotherapy toxicity |
| Bladder | Brain metastases | Chemotherapy toxicity |
| | Neoplastic meningitis | |

compression. Vertebral metastases may develop either by hematogenous spread to marrow or by epidural venous emboli.

Genitourinary cancer may metastasize to the brain by hematogenous spread, but in many patients, there is no evidence of lung involvement. Retrograde migration of neoplastic cells through the valveless vertebral epidural venous system, when abdominal pressure increases, may be an alternative metastatic pathway. Although this mechanism of dissemination has not been confirmed in experimental models, it may explain why brain metastases from pelvic neoplasms have a tendency to localize in the posterior fossa (3).

## C. Clinical Presentation

Pain is usually the first and sole manifestation of a neurological complication from GU cancer. Seventy-five percent of men and 70% of women with advanced neoplasms experience moderate to severe pain. Even patients without metastases may have significant pain (4). Therefore, the clinician must be alert for any associated symptoms and physical findings which may indicate the cause of the pain syndrome. A high level of suspicion is necessary to make the diagnosis, especially in the rare situation when the neurological symptoms are the first manifestation of GU cancer. A useful clinical indicator of neoplasm is progressively increasing pain severity. Other neurological manifestations are related to retroperitoneal lymph node and osseous metastases.

**Table 3** Neurological Complications of Genitourinary Cancer Treatment

| Treatment | Type | Cancer | Complication |
|---|---|---|---|
| Surgery | Radical pelvic | Gynecological | Mononeuropathy |
|  |  |  | Plexopathy |
|  | Nephrectomy | Kidney | Pain L1 |
| Radiation therapy | Pelvic | Uterine | Lumbosacral |
|  |  | Prostate | plexopathy |
|  | Para-aortic lymph nodes | Testicle | Motor caudal radiculopathy |
| Chemotherapy | Cisplatin | Germ cell | Neuropathy |
|  |  | Ovary | Hearing loss |
|  |  | Bladder | Seizures |
|  |  |  | Lhermitte's sign |
|  | Taxol | Ovary | Neuropathy |
|  |  |  | Myalgias |
|  | Pelvic chemoembolization | Advanced pelvic | Mononeuropathy |
|  |  |  | Plexopathy |
|  | Ketoconazole | Prostate | Confusion |

## D. Treatment and Prognosis

Treatment of most neurological complications from GU neoplasm is palliative, trying to improve the quality of life and prolong survival.

### 1. Surgery

Surgical excision of solitary GU metastases in brain or vertebral body has been recommended, although the absence of controlled clinical trials in GU neoplasms to support efficacy and define the best indications precludes any general conclusion.

### 2. Radiation Therapy

Metastatic deposits of GU cancer have been considered less responsive to radiation therapy than those of other primaries. However, radiation therapy for brain and bone metastases from GU primary neoplasms provides comparable and sometimes better symptomatic relief than for metastases from other types of neoplasms (2).

### 3. Chemotherapy

Chemotherapy plays an important role, alone or in combination with other treatment, in the management of neurological complications produced by metastatic germ cell tumors. The efficacy of systemic chemotherapy that crosses the blood-brain barrier as adjuvant treatment for brain metastases of chemoresponsive GU neoplasms remains to be proven.

Neurological complications usually occur in patients with advanced GU neoplastic disease; the approximate median survival for those patients after treatment is 30 weeks (5). However, the majority of treated patients die of complications from systemic neoplastic disease, unrelated to the neurological involvement.

## E. Cancer Treatment Complications

Neurological complications of GU cancer treatment may be the result of a surgical procedure or radiation therapy or an adverse effect of chemotherapy, as shown in Table 2.

### 1. Surgery

Postsurgical neurological complications have been described after radical pelvic surgery for gynecological cancer and after nephrectomy for renal carcinoma. Nerve injuries occur in 1% of all radical pelvic surgical procedures for gynecological cancer. The neuropathy is usually caused by direct pressure due to positioning of the patient or injury from a retractor or as a complication of intraoperative hemorrhage from the hypogastric venous plexus.

The femoral and sciatic nerves are the most frequently injured during surgery for genital cancer (6). Obturator nerve damage has been associated with surgery for uterine cancer and pelvic lymphadenectomy (1). A careful surgical technique and proper positioning of the patient prevents these complications. Treatment includes physical therapy and braces. Recovery depends on the degree of injury.

The nerve arising from the L1 spinal segment may be injured by the surgical exposure during nephrectomy for renal carcinoma. The clinical manifestation is a pain syndrome with numbness in the distribution of the involved dermatome. A careful history, examination, and diagnostic imaging studies are needed to rule out paraspinal tumor. Treatment includes a corset for abdominal wall support, physical therapy, and amitriptyline (7).

### 2. Radiation Therapy

Although high doses of external radiation therapy plus intracavitary brachytherapy are used to treat cervix carcinoma, the incidence of clinically evident radiation-induced plexus injury is low. Lumbosacral plexus injury caused by radiation for uterine cancer may be rare because of shielding by pelvic bone structures. Modifications of the treatment technique, such as protection of the plexus when lateral fields are used and delivery of lower doses to the whole pelvis, may prevent this complication (8).

A lesion of the caudal roots has been described after irradiation of para-aortic lymph nodes for testicular cancer (9). Clinically, a flaccid paraparesis appears several years after therapy, without sensory or sphincter disturbances. Neurophysiological examination reveals myokymic discharges with normal nerve conduction velocities and prolonged latencies on somatosensory evoked potentials of tibial nerve. The etiology and risk factors for developing this complication are unknown. Even patients who received below the suggested tolerance limit for radiation of para-aortic lymph nodes (40 Gy in 20 fractions) can develop this neurological complication.

## 3. Chemotherapy

Cisplatin and taxol are the two agents most frequently responsible for neurological complications from GU cancer chemotherapy.

Cisplatin is a potent antineoplastic drug efficacious against most gynecological cancers and germ cell tumors. A sensory peripheral neuronopathy, primarily affecting large myelinated fibers, is the most common neurological complication. The nerve injury occurs in almost all patients after a cumulative dose of 300 mg/m$^2$, but causes symptoms only in approximately 50% (10). The initial symptom of neurotoxicity is paresthesia in the feet. Early findings on examination include a decrease of vibratory sensation in the feet and loss of ankle jerks (11). Severe neuropathy with inability to walk is rare. In some instances, delayed symptoms of neuropathy may occur 3 to 8 weeks after cisplatin is discontinued. The neuropathy may progress several weeks before stabilizing (12).

No risk factors for developing cisplatin-related neuropathy have been identified (10). In a considerable number of patients the neuropathy is irreversible, and in those who recover, the process is slow. Neuroprotective agents administered in combination with cisplatin are under investigation to prevent this complication, including nerve growth factor.

After therapy with cisplatin, some patients may experience Lhermitte's sign and have slow central conduction velocity, as measured by somatosensory evoked response, indicating involvement of the spinal cord dorsal columns. Seizures and autonomic neuropathy also have been described after administration of this agent.

Ototoxicity (hearing loss and tinnitus) is bilateral and symmetric and predominantly affects high frequencies. The likelihood of developing this complication after treatment with cisplatin is greater in older patients and in those with a preexisting hearing loss (13).

Taxol is a promising new agent active against refractory ovarian cancer. Peripheral nerve toxicity is frequently the dose-limiting adverse effect. The drug affects predominantly sensory fibers at cumulative doses above 200 mg/m$^2$ (14). The symptoms appear rapidly after taxol administration, involving hands and feet in a simultaneous, symmetric pattern. Neurotoxicity is reversible after treatment is suspended.

Chemoembolization is an effective approach for treatment and palliation of symptoms related to pelvic malignancies; it includes local intra-arterial cisplatin infusion and collagen embolization of the internal iliac artery. The procedure may result in an acute nonprogressive neurological complication within 48 h of the procedure, characterized by painful motor and sensory deficit of a lower limb. Presumably, the nerves suffer a vascular insult due to ischemia, although direct toxicity of the chemotherapeutic agent also may contribute (15). In most patients, no predisposing factor exists. However, the procedure is not recommended for patients at high risk for vascular injury. The neurological dysfunction has a poor prognosis, with partial recovery occurring only in a few patients.

Ketoconazole has an inhibitory effect on testosterone synthesis in the testes and adrenal glands. Therefore, it is an alternative for the treatment of metastatic prostate cancer. A neurological disorder consisting of confabulation, disorientation, apathy, and asthenia has been related to its administration in cancer patients. The pathogenesis of this neurological complication is unknown, but the symptoms improve after withdrawal of the medication (16).

## F. Associated Primary Neoplasms of the GU and Central Nervous Systems

An interesting aspect of GU tumors is their association with certain intracranial primary neoplasms. The following associations have been described: meningioma and genital cancer, hemangioblastoma and renal cancer, and primary primitive tumors of the kidney and brain.

### 1. Sphenoid Ridge Meningioma and Genital Cancer

Women with sphenoid ridge meningiomas seem to be at higher risk of developing two additional tumors, usually breast or genital (endometrial or cervical) cancer (17). The associated tumor can precede or follow the diagnosis of meningioma by several years. Therefore, a sphenoid ridge lesion in a woman with these GU neoplasms may be a meningioma rather than metastases of her primary cancer. Patients with a sphenoid ridge meningioma and other cancer should be followed carefully for the appearance of a third tumor. The etiology of this combination of neoplastic lesions in a single patient is unknown.

### 2. Cerebellar Hemangioblastoma and Renal Carcinoma

The association between cerebellar hemangioblastoma and renal carcinoma has been described in patients with von Hippel–Lindau disease, a low-penetrance dominantly inherited disorder. The most relevant clinical manifestations are retinal angiomatosis and a cerebellar syndrome caused by posterior fossa hemangioblastomas. Renal tumors associated with hemangioblastoma are carcinomas with a malignant behavior. The likelihood of developing the kidney neoplasm is higher if there is a positive family history (18). Also, renal hamartomas have been described in patients with tuberous sclerosis; however, malignant transformation is rare.

## 3. Embryonal Renal and Brain Tumors

In infants younger than 2 years of age, an embryonal renal tumor may coexist with an embryonal primary central nervous system tumor. A malignant rhabdoid tumor is the most common histological type in the kidney, as medulloblastoma is in the brain (19). However, primary malignant rhabdoid tumor has also been described in the brain and associated with kidney tumors of the same histology (20). The precursor cell of these primitive neoplasms may be related.

## II. PROSTATE CARCINOMA

Nearly 80% of patients with prostate carcinoma have bone metastases at autopsy, usually involving the pelvis and vertebrae (5). Most neurological complications associated with prostate cancer are secondary to compression of neural structures from bone metastases. Vertebrae eroded by metastatic spread may collapse. Extraosseous extension can cause cord compression or nerve entrapment. Likewise, metastatic involvement of the pelvis can cause lumbosacral plexus injury, or metastases to the base of the skull may involve cranial nerves.

Intracranial metastases occur by epidural extension of calvarial metastases or by direct hematogenous spread to the dura, sometimes causing subdural collections. Intraparenchymal brain metastases from prostate carcinoma are rare. They can be identified by immunoperoxidase staining for prostatic acid phosphatase and prostate-specific antigen.

Neurological complications from prostate cancer occur usually in patients with advanced disease. Treatment is palliative. The therapeutic response varies depending on whether the patient received previous hormonal treatment. Prostate cancer patients who develop a neurological complication, including brain metastasis, without prior hormonal manipulation may have a dramatic regression with this endocrine treatment (21).

### A. Epidural Spinal Cord Compression

In our cancer center, adenocarcinoma of the prostate is the most common primary malignancy responsible for spinal cord compression in the male population. Many patients with back pain and vertebral bone metastases never develop cord compression. Approximately 7% of all prostate cancer patients develop symptomatic spinal cord compression. Outcomes depend on early diagnosis and treatment, degree of tumor differentiation, and stage of the disease at presentation.

In patients with poorly differentiated tumor, cord compression develops in 12.2%; in those with well-differentiated tumors, it occurs only in 2.9% (5). Patients with stage D2 disease at presentation have a higher risk of developing cord compression, compared with patients without bone metastases. Therefore, patients with poorly differentiated prostate cancer and bone metastases at diagnosis should be carefully followed for early detection of spinal metastases.

Most lesions are extradural and the lower thoracic spine is the region most frequently involved. The median time interval between primary cancer diagnosis and cord compression is 24 months, with stage D2 patients at diagnosis having a shorter interval. In 30% of patients with spinal cord compression from prostate cancer, the neurological complication is the initial manifestation of systemic malignancy (22). These patients usually have an abnormal prostate gland on rectal examination, with an elevated serum acid phosphatase.

Patients with metastatic prostate carcinoma should be alerted about the risk of cord compression and instructed to seek medical help promptly should symptoms appear. Like any metastatic cord compression, new back pain is the cardinal symptom of cord compression and precedes other neurological deficits.

Bony abnormalities on plain spine films highly correlate with the myelographic level of cord compression (5). Radionuclide bone scans are very sensitive for detection of prostate bone metastases but correlate less well with the site of compression than plain films (22). The investigation of choice, magnetic resonance imaging (MRI) or myelography, for confirming the diagnosis of epidural spinal cord compression is controversial. Specifically, in patients with prostate metastases who have two separate sites of compression, MRI restricted to a small region of the spine may fail to detect both lesions (22).

The objectives of treatment are maintenance or restoration of ambulation, pain relief, and improvement of survival. No randomized controlled studies have defined what is the most efficacious and least deleterious treatment for patients with cord compression from prostate cancer.

Steroids and radiotherapy are recommended for ambulatory and moderately paraparetic patients. The indications for surgery are controversial. Surgical decompression has been reserved for patients who (1) do not have a tissue diagnosis of malignancy; (2) have an acceptable expected lifespan; (3) have a low anesthetic risk; (4) are paraplegic at diagnosis; (5) deteriorated during radiation; (6) failed previous radiation; or (7) have an unstable spine from a pathological fracture or dislocation. In patients without the diagnosis of cancer, who are not suitable for surgery, a percutaneous biopsy prior to radiotherapy will identify the histology of the primary neoplasm. Whether to do an anterior decompression with vertebral body resection or a laminectomy for posterior decompression depends on the tumor location and condition of the patient.

Androgen deprivation plays an important role in the treatment of spinal cord compression patients without previous endocrine therapy. The survival of patients who respond to hormonal manipulation is better, compared with survival of patients in relapse after hormone therapy (22).

Although vital organs are not usually affected by prostate metastases, the prognosis of patients with spinal cord compression depends on the progression of systemic disease. The median survival after the diagnosis of cord compression from prostate cancer is 6 months, with 34% surviving at least 1 year (3). Patients who are ambulatory after treatment have a greater likelihood of more prolonged and better quality survival than nonambulatory patients.

## B. Intracranial Metastases

### 1. Metastases to the Base of the Skull

Among males, prostate carcinoma, because of its predilection for bone, is the most common malignancy causing cranial neuropathy from metastases to the base of the skull (23). This phenomenon appears late in the course of the disease and carries a bad prognosis, with a median survival time of 5 months after initial cranial nerve symptoms (24).

The clinical characteristics vary according to the site of metastases; prostate carcinoma may cause any of the neurological syndromes described with metastases to the base of the skull (25). The appearance of craniofacial pain is the clue to alert the clinician about this neurological complication. Nearly 50% of patients with cranial nerve palsies due to prostate metastasis experience other neurological complications, such as cord compression or radiculopathy (26).

Normal imaging studies do not rule out the diagnosis of metastases to the base of the skull. Plain films, bone scan, and CT scan with bone windows are in ascending order the most sensitive ways to confirm the diagnosis of skull metastases.

Symptomatic relief of pain after palliative treatment with radiation therapy and glucocorticoid occurs in most patients. Improvement of cranial nerve function is less common. Cranial neuropathies from prostate cancer do not respond well to treatment (23,24). Early treatment after onset of symptoms (less than 1 month) and high doses of radiation therapy (36 Gy) improve the prognosis of the neurological deficit (23).

### 2. Subdural Hematoma

Another neurological complication that may develop in patients with prostate cancer is an intracranial subdural hematoma. Although skull or dural metastasis may be the cause of the subdural collection, other factors, like trauma, anticoagulant use, and coagulopathy are frequently associated with this complication. Among patients with solid tumors, those with prostate or breast cancer have been most commonly associated with subdural hematoma. The clinical manifestations are the same as subdural hematoma in a patient without cancer, but a history of predisposing risk factors may point to the diagnosis.

During surgery, adequate specimens of the bone, dura, and membrane of the hematoma should be obtained for histological examination looking for metastatic deposits. If dural involvement is confirmed, adjuvant radiation therapy is recommended. Cancer patients with subdural hematoma and an abnormal coagulation profile have a poor prognosis (27).

### 3. Intraparenchymal Brain Metastases

Approximately 1% of patients who die with prostate cancer have intraparenchymal cerebral metastases at autopsy (28). This neurological complication is a late event in the course of the disease and is most commonly associated with stage C and D cancer. The histological examination of brain metastases denotes that most are moderately or poorly differentiated adenocarcinomas (29). Patients with cerebral metastases seem to be younger than the overall population of patients with this neoplasm. The median interval between the diagnosis of the primary cancer and brain metastases is 4 years, whereas the median duration of survival after neurological symptoms appear is less than a year.

Immunostaining for prostatic acid phosphatase and prostate-specific antigen will confirm the origin of the metastasis. This technique is especially useful for the exceptional patient whose first manifestation of adenocarcinoma of the prostate is a brain metastasis.

Craniotomy and resection of a solitary metastasis in good surgical candidates, combined with radiation therapy, can result in long-term survival. Whole-brain external radiation or stereotactic radiosurgery provide palliation for patients not suitable for resection. In a patient without previous treatment, regression of brain metastasis from prostate cancer has been reported with only androgen deprivation and hormonal therapy (21). However, most patients relapse after hormonal manipulation and the efficacy of this approach has yet to be established.

## C. Paraneoplastic Syndromes

The Lambert-Eaton myasthenic syndrome, an autoimmune paraneoplastic disorder frequently associated with small-cell carcinoma of the lung, has been described in a patient with prostate cancer (30). The histological examination of prostatic tissue demonstrated an adenocarcinoma mixed with areas of small-cell carcinoma, staining for neuron-specific enolase and serotonin. Therefore, regardless of its site of origin, small-cell carcinoma sometimes associates with the Lambert-Eaton syndrome. Other paraneoplastic syndromes have not been associated with prostate cancer.

## III. UTERUS

### A. Uterine Cervix

Cancer of the uterine cervix affects the nervous system more frequently than cancer of the uterine body. Neurological complications occur in 8% of patients presenting with stage I or greater cervical cancer. Half have lumbosacral plexus metastatic disease (1). The percentage of patients with associated neurological disorders increases with more advanced disease stages.

## 1. Lumbosacral Plexopathy

Metastatic lumbosacral plexopathy is the most frequent neurological complication of established cervical squamous cell carcinoma and the first manifestation of malignancy in many patients with advanced disease. Only half of the patients with retroperitoneal metastases develop neurological symptoms of plexopathy. The median interval between diagnosis of cervical cancer and diagnosis of lumbosacral plexopathy is 20 months (range: 0–86 months) (1).

Although most GU neoplasms cause an asymmetric panplexopathy, cervical cancer usually involves the lower plexus (L4-S1). The neurological manifestations include pain in these dermatomes, focal distal lower extremity weakness, loss of ankle jerks, and sensory deficit. Ipsilateral leg lymphedema occurs in 46% of the patients secondary to lymph node metastatic spread. Only 4% of patients have bilateral involvement of the plexus. The differential diagnosis may include surgical trauma, spinal metastases, or radiation-induced plexus injury, a rare complication with the standard radiation fields and dose fractionation.

Plain x-ray films play an important role in diagnosis of lumbosacral plexopathy, because more than half of patients have associated vertebral bone destruction. Ipsilateral hydronephrosis is detected in 70% of patients. Computed tomography scan of the lumbosacral plexus, including visualization from the upper lumbar segments all the way down to the sciatic notch, confirms the diagnosis.

Additional radiation treatment has been attempted, usually with poor results; pain and neurological deficits often respond poorly. The median survival after diagnosis of lumbosacral plexopathy from cervical cancer is 5 months.

## 2. Brain Metastases

Brain metastases from uterine cervix cancer are uncommon. However, because of the high incidence of cervical cancer in our population, 7% of all our patients with cerebral metastases have a primary tumor in this location (1). Review of histological types show that although most are squamous cell carcinoma, approximately one-third are adenocarcinoma alone or mixed with areas of squamous cell carcinoma. Lung metastases are documented by chest x-ray in most patients with brain metastases, suggesting hematogenous spread to the brain. Patients usually have advanced neoplastic disease. In no patient was a brain metastasis the initial manifestation of cancer.

## 3. Neoplastic Meningitis

Leptomeningeal carcinomatosis is a rare complication of cervical cancer. One of our patients had concomitant brain metastases. The clinical manifestations are similar to those seen with meningeal carcinomatosis arising from solid tumors in other locations.

### 4. Metabolic Encephalopathy

Seizures and metabolic encephalopathy may develop in patients with renal failure secondary to bilateral ureteral obstruction in advanced-stage cervical cancer. Renal failure is frequently the cause of death in these patients, and the focus of treatment is symptomatic relief.

## B. Uterine Body

Adenocarcinoma of the endometrium may produce any neurological complication, including lumbosacral plexopathy, spinal cord compression, or brain metastases, but in our experience, they are even more uncommon than those caused by cervix cancer. Brain metastasis usually occurs associated with widespread disease. However, it may be the initial manifestation of malignancy when the endometrial carcinoma is undifferentiated and deeply invades myometrium and blood vessels (31). There are case reports of dural metastases, nontraumatic subdural hematomas, and atrial metastases producing recurrent embolic strokes, associated with cancer of the uterine body.

## IV. OVARY

Epithelial ovarian carcinoma rarely involves the nervous system. However, recent therapeutic advances for widespread disease, resulting in improved survival, will increase the incidence of these complications.

## A. Brain Metastases

Ovarian cancer is rarely the origin of brain metastases, but the incidence may be increasing as a result of more effective chemotherapeutic regimens for systemic disease. The median interval between diagnosis of the primary neoplasm and diagnosis of cerebral metastases is 14.5 months (range: 0–72 months). The interval is shorter with advanced clinical stage at diagnosis. Characteristically, these patients are younger, have a longer survival after diagnosis of the primary cancer, and have extraperitoneal metastases, when compared with other ovarian cancer patients (32).

The brain metastases may develop even following negative "second look" procedures. Serous cystadenocarcinoma is the most common histological subtype of ovarian cancer and the one most frequently associated with central nervous system involvement. Infrequently, an adenocarcinoma from another origin, like breast, may metastasize to the ovary and the brain, giving the erroneous impression of a primary ovarian cancer spreading to the brain.

On CT scan, most brain metastases from ovarian cancer are single lesions; some may be calcified or have a cystic appearance. Spread to the lung parenchyma is frequently detected at diagnosis of brain metastases, although in some patients the chest x-ray may be normal.

In patients without evidence of active ovarian carcinoma and suspicion of central nervous system involvement, elevated serum CA 125 may be a useful tumor marker to confirm the clinical impression. Repeated CA 125 determinations may correlate with response of the lesions to treatment (33).

Clinical stage at diagnosis of primary ovarian cancer, number of cerebral metastases (single versus multiple), and the presence of extraperitoneal disease are the most important factors affecting outcome (32). Surgical resection of single brain metastasis followed by radiation therapy seems to improve survival, particularly if there is no evidence of metastatic spread elsewhere. Glucocorticoid and radiation therapy are the initial treatment when multiple cerebral metastases are present or when there is widespread metastatic disease. Some responses have been achieved in the treatment of cerebral metastases with systemic administration of chemotherapeutic agents that are active against ovarian cancer (cisplatin and carboplatin). However, survival times do not improve by combining chemotherapy and brain irradiation (33).

## B. Neoplastic Meningitis

A few cases of carcinomatous meningitis as a complication of epithelial ovarian cancer have been reported. The clinical manifestations are indistinguishable from meningeal involvement by other solid tumors. The diagnosis is confirmed with a positive cerebrospinal fluid (CSF) cytology. Although CSF measurement of CA 125 may be helpful for diagnosis and follow-up, the sensitivity and specificity of this marker in this context is unknown. Treatment with whole-brain radiation therapy and intraventricular methotrexate via an Ommaya reservoir may improve the prognosis (34).

## C. Paraneoplastic Syndromes

Ovarian cancer is the GU primary most frequently related to paraneoplastic syndromes, especially to subacute cerebellar degeneration.

### 1. Paraneoplastic Cerebellar Degeneration

This is a rare entity, which most frequently occurs in patients with undiagnosed epithelial ovarian cancer. The detection of serum and CSF antibodies against antigens shared by the primary tumor and the cerebellum suggest the etiology is autoimmune, although exact pathogenetic mechanisms are unclear. Usually, ovarian cancer associated with paraneoplastic cerebellar degeneration is a poorly differentiated carcinoma, presenting as stage II at diagnosis.

The clinical profile is a middle-aged woman with a rapidly progressing and symmetrical cerebellar syndrome. In most patients, the neurological manifestations precede or coincide with the diagnosis of ovarian cancer. In those with known cancer, the neurological syndrome may be the first indication of recurrence or progression of the neoplastic disease (35). Surprisingly, although they have poor prognostic features, patients with ovarian cancer and paraneoplastic cerebellar degeneration have a lower metastatic volume and often lack peritoneal implants, compared with patients without the neurological syndrome (36).

Several autoantibodies have been identified in patients with paraneoplastic cerebellar degeneration, but the most typical is the anti–Purkinje cell antibody, also called anti-Yo, which has a unique value as a marker of underlying cancer, either ovarian or breast primary. Occasionally, high titers of anti–Purkinje cell antibodies are present in the serum of neurologically normal patients with ovarian cancer (35). The detection of CSF anti-Yo is more specific than serum detection anti-Yo for diagnosis of the paraneoplastic syndrome.

Despite aggressive treatment of the primary neoplasm combined with plasmapheresis and corticosteroid therapy, the neurological damage is usually irreversible.

### 2. Dermatomyositis

The association between dermatomyositis and occult malignancy has been controversial and so has the impression of a disproportionately high number of ovarian cancers among patients with dermatomyositis. The clinical profile of the neurological syndrome associated with ovarian primary neoplasm consists of a more acute course, development of both diseases within 1 year of each other, and a poor response to steroid therapy. Cricopharyngeal achalasia, an otherwise rare finding with dermatomyositis, is common in patients with ovarian cancer and this paraneoplastic syndrome (37).

## V. KIDNEY

Brain metastases and epidural spinal cord compression are the most frequent neurological complications of renal carcinoma. Metastases from kidney cancer have been considered less sensitive to radiation therapy than metastases from many other primaries.

### A. Brain Metastases

The incidence of brain metastases from renal cancer is 4%, and the median interval between diagnosis of the primary cancer and neurological involvement is

12 months (range: 0–84 months) (38). Cerebral metastases usually develop in patients with advanced renal carcinoma who have metastases to other sites outside the brain. Only 3% of neurologically asymptomatic patients with kidney cancer have brain metastases on CT scan.

The clinical manifestations are the same as brain metastases from other primary malignancies. On noncontrast cerebral CT scan, renal metastases may be hyperdense or have intratumoral hemorrhage because they are hypervascularized. Some difficulty arises when renal carcinoma metastasizes to the posterior fossa because histologically the metastatic lesion may be indistinguishable from an hemangioblastoma. Immunohistochemical techniques help to make the distinction. Renal carcinomas stain strongly with epithelial membrane antigen, but hemangioblastomas do not (39).

Without treatment, the median survival after diagnosis is 2 months. With whole-brain radiation therapy, in approximately 30% of patients' symptoms are ameliorated or performance is recovered and the median survival improves to 4 months (38). Because of these unsatisfactory results, surgery followed by radiation therapy has been proposed for patients with one or two accessible metastases from renal cell carcinoma. In selected patients, combined surgery and radiotherapy results in a median survival of 21 months, with an operative mortality of 9% (40). The best survival after surgery occurs in patients who had the onset of cerebral metastases more than 1 year following nephrectomy, who had mild or no preoperative neurological deficit, and whose metastatic lesions were infratentorial.

Although the need for adjuvant radiotherapy after surgical excision of brain metastases from renal cancer has been questioned, in most instances, postoperative radiation should be offered.

## B. Spinal Cord Compression

Kidney cancer is the second most common GU malignancy causing epidural spinal cord compression. The median survival after diagnosis of cord compression from renal cancer is less than 4 months. Because of poor radioresponsiveness, the treatment outcome and survival time after radiotherapy may not be as good as with other primary neoplasms.

Surgery has been advocated to improve the results for solitary spinal metastases from kidney cancer, even if there is no evidence of cord compression. The surgical approach, either anterior decompression with vertebral body resection and stabilization or posterior decompression by laminectomy, depends on the location of the metastases. Even in experienced hands, the operative mortality is 6%. Prior radiation and prolonged high-dose steroids increase the likelihood of operative morbidity. Postoperative hemorrhage is a significant complication, which may be avoided by presurgical embolization (41). For most patients the primary treatment is radiation therapy.

## VI. GESTATIONAL TROPHOBLASTIC CARCINOMA

### A. Brain Metastases

Between 9% and 18% of patients with gestational trophoblastic tumors have central nervous system metastases (42). Neurological involvement by choriocarcinoma is responsible for 50% of deaths from this tumor. Two-thirds of those who die have cerebral metastases.

The presence of pulmonary metastases at the time of diagnosis is a high risk factor for developing intracranial metastases. Therefore, routine cranial CT scan and CSF human chorionic gonadotropin (HCG) measurement is recommended in all patients with lung metastases, even if there are no neurological symptoms and signs. Approximately 4% of patients with brain metastases from choriocarcinoma have clinically silent lesions.

Intratumoral hemorrhage is a common finding on noncontrast CT scan because metastases of choriocarcinoma are prone to bleed. Computed tomography and MRI scans are sensitive tests for detection of cerebral metastases. In certain patients, these tests may be more helpful than HCG measurement. The measurement of serum/CSF HCG ratio is a sensitive indicator of CNS metastases. A ratio of less than 60:1 is considered positive (43).

Patients with poor prognosis are those who present with intratumoral hemorrhage, who develop brain metastases while receiving systemic chemotherapy, or who have evidence of metastases to other organs besides lung and brain. The prognosis is better than for brain metastases from many other primaries. Most patients have long-term survivals after aggressive treatment with chemotherapy and whole-brain irradiation. The combination of systemic methotrexate, actinomycin D, and chlorambucil with intrathecal methotrexate plus whole-brain irradiation to a total dose of 3000 cGy over 10 fractions is the recommended treatment. Serum and CSF HCG should be in the normal range for at least 12 weeks before stopping chemotherapy (43).

### B. Neoplastic Intracranial Aneurysms

Neoplastic embolus from choriocarcinoma may invade an intracerebral vessel wall, with subsequent weakening and aneurysmal dilatation. Although it is a rare condition, the incidence of this complication may be higher than reported. Probably neoplastic aneurysms are underdiagnosed because of lack of clinical suspicion, destruction of the aneurysm by the resulting hemorrhage, or lack of histological examination. The majority of patients have only one aneurysm, but multiple aneurysms may occur. Clinical manifestations are produced by intracerebral or subarachnoid hemorrhage secondary to rupture of the aneurysm. These aneurysms occur in patients with advanced gestational trophoblastic disease and cardiac metastases involving the left ventricle, presumably the origin of the neoplastic emboli. However, in some cases cerebral hemorrhage may be the first manifestation of metastatic choriocarcinoma (44).

## VII. TESTICLE

### A. Brain Metastases

The incidence of clinically symptomatic brain metastases in patients with disseminated germ cell tumors of the testis is between 12 and 15% (45). However, 31% of patients who die with testicular cancer have brain metastases at autopsy. Cerebral involvement is a late occurrence in this disease, frequently associated with pulmonary metastases. Choriocarcinoma and endodermal sinus tumors are the most common histological types metastasizing to the brain. Brain metastases from apparently pure seminomas may show nonseminomatous histological features.

On presentation, most patients have multiple lesions, a characteristic that correlates with a poor prognosis. The suggestion that single lesions are more chemoresponsive than multiple lesions has not been confirmed. The appearance of cerebral metastases after failing chemotherapy for systemic disease is also a poor prognostic indicator. Alpha fetoprotein (AFP) and HCG are elevated in 60% of the patients with advanced germ cell tumors and may be valuable markers for diagnosis and follow-up of CNS involvement. Cerebrospinal fluid HCG measurement is very sensitive for the presence of tumors that produce this marker, while CSF AFP measurement has many false negatives.

Treatment results with only whole-brain radiation therapy have been disappointing. Combined radiotherapy and chemotherapy have been recommended for patients without prior therapy because germ cell tumors are very sensitive to cisplatin-based chemotherapy. This combined approach has resulted in prolonged survivals. Therefore, chemotherapy alone has been proposed as initial therapy for new patients presenting with cerebral metastases from germ cell tumors (46).

### B. Epidural Spinal Cord Compression

Testicular cancer frequently involves the retroperitoneal lymph nodes and from there directly grows into the spinal canal. Rarely, it metastasizes to the vertebral bone. Cisplatin-based chemotherapy, as primary treatment modality for epidural metastases from germ cell tumors, is effective in patients without vertebral body dislocation who are previously untreated or who previously responded to chemotherapy (47). Chemotherapy is also an alternative for patients with recurrent cord compression who have already received full doses of radiation therapy. Radiation therapy and surgery may be considered when the disease is not chemoresponsive, when the diagnosis is in doubt, or a fracture dislocation of the vertebral body exists.

## C. Lumbosacral Plexopathy

Lumbosacral plexus involvement occurs in patients with germ cell tumors of the testes. Back pain is considered an early symptom of retroperitoneal para-aortic lymph node metastases and is sometimes the initial manifestation of testicular cancer. Low back pain as the initial complaint of testicular cancer in young men results in a significant delay in the diagnosis, when compared with testicular symptoms without back pain. Testicular abnormalities should be sought in any young man with persistent, progressive low back pain (48).

## VIII. BLADDER
### A. Brain Metastases

Brain metastases from transitional cell carcinoma of the bladder are rare and usually associated with disseminated disease. The incidence of brain metastases may be increasing, due to improved survival achieved with cisplatin-based combination chemotherapy regimens for advanced high-grade disease (49). Most brain metastases from bladder cancer are solitary and therefore susceptible to surgical excision. Combined with whole-brain irradiation, many patients experience significant palliation.

### B. Neoplastic Meningitis

Similarly, the incidence of leptomeningeal carcinomatosis increased after the introduction of M-VAC (methotrexate, vinblastine, doxorubicin, and cisplatin) chemotherapy for advanced bladder cancer. Prolonged survival after diagnosis, selection of tumor cells resistant to treatment, and poor penetration of chemotherapeutic agents to the CNS are some of the explanations proposed for increased neurological complications in recent years (50). Early and aggressive treatment with intrathecal methotrexate and whole-brain irradiation may improve symptoms and prolong survival.

## REFERENCES

1. Saphner T, Gallion HH, Van Nagell JR, Kryscio R, Patchell RA. Neurologic complications of cervical cancer: a review of 2261 cases. Cancer 1989; 64:1147–51.
2. Reddy S, Hendrickson FR, Hoeksema J, Gelber R. The role of radiation therapy in the palliation of metastatic genitourinary tract carcinomas: a study of the Radiation Therapy Oncology Group. Cancer 1983; 52:25–9.
3. Delattre JY, Krol G, Thaler HT, Posner JB. Distribution of brain metastases. Arch Neurol 1988; 45:741–4.
4. Greenwald HP, Bonica JJ, Bergner M. The prevalence of pain in four cancers. Cancer 1987; 60:2563–9.

5. Kuban DA, El-Mahdi AM, Sigfred SV, Schellhammer PF, Babb TJ. Characteristics of spinal cord compression in adenocarcinoma of prostate. Urology 1986; 28:364–9.
6. Hoffman MS, Roberts WS, Cavanagh D. Neuropathies associated with radical pelvic surgery for gynecologic cancer. Gynecol Oncol 1988; 31:462–6.
7. Foley KM. Pain syndromes in patients with cancer. Med Clin N Am 1987; 71: 169–84.
8. Stryker JA, Sommerville K, Perez R, Velkley DE. Sacral plexus injury after radiotherapy for carcinoma of cervix. Cancer; 66: 1488–92.
9. Feistner H, Weissenborn K, Munte TF, Heinze HJ, Malin JP. Post-irradiation lesions of the caudal roots. Acta Neurol Scand 1989; 80:277–81.
10. van der Hoop RG, van der Burg MEL, ten Bokkel Huinink WW, van Houwelingen JC, Neijt JP. Incidence of neuropathy in 395 patients with ovarian cancer treated with or without cisplatin. Cancer 1990; 66:1697–702.
11. Boogerd W, Huinink WWB, Dalesio O, Hoppenbrowers WJJF, van del Sande JJ. Cisplatin induced neuropathy: central, peripheral and autonomic nerve involvement. J Neurooncol 1990; 9:255–63.
12. Mollman JE, Hogan WM, Glover DJ, McCluskey LF. Unusual presentation of cisplatinum neuropathy. Neurology 1988; 38:488–90.
13. Melamed LB, Selim MA, Schuchman D. Cisplatin ototoxicity in gynecologic cancer patients. Cancer 1985; 55:41–3.
14. Lipton RB, Apfel SC, Dutcher JP, Rosenberg R, Kaplan J, Berger A, Enzig AJ, Wiernik P, Schaumburg HH. Taxol produces predominantly sensory neuropathy. Neurology 1989; 39:368–73.
15. Castellanos AM, Glass JP, Yung WKA. Regional nerve injury after intra-arterial chemotherapy. Neurology 1987; 37:834–7.
16. Hanash KA. Neurologic complications of ketoconazole therapy for advanced prostate cancer. Urology 1989; 33:466–7.
17. Jacobs DH, McFarlane MJ, Holmes FF. Female patients with meningioma of the sphenoid ridge and additional primary neoplasms of the breast and genital tract. Cancer 1987; 60:3080–2.
18. Goodbody RA, Gamlen TR. Cerebellar hemangioblastoma and genitourinary tumours. J Neurol Neurosurg Psychiatry 1974; 37:606–9.
19. Bonnin JM, Rubinstein LJ, Palmer NF, Beckwith JB. The association of embryonal tumors originating in the kidney and the brain. Cancer 1984; 54:2137–46.
20. Chou SM, Anderson JS. Primary CNS malignant rhabdoid tumor (MRT): report of two cases and review of literature. Clin Neuropathol 1991; 10:1–10.
21. Senoh H, Iwatsubo H, Ichikawa Y, Kumahara Y, Matsuda M, Sagawa S. Remarkable effect of endocrine therapy on brain metastasis from prostatic carcinoma. Urology 1989; 33:243–6.
22. Flynn DF, Shipley WU. Management of spinal cord compression secondary to metastatic prostatic carcinoma. Urol Clin N Am 1991; 18:145–52.
23. Gupta SR, Zdonczyk DE, Rubino FA. Cranial neuropathy in systemic malignancy in a VA population. Neurology 1990; 40:997–9.
24. Seymore CH, Peeples WJ. Cranial nerve involvement with carcinoma of prostate. Urology 1988; 31:211–3.

25. Greenberg HS, Deck MDF, Vikram B, Chu FCH, Posner JB. Metastasis to the base of the skull: clinical findings in 43 patients. Neurology 1981; 31:530–7.
26. Ransom DT, Dinapoli RP, Richardson RL. Cranial nerve lesions due to base of the skull metastases in prostate carcinoma. Cancer 1990; 65:586–9.
27. Minette SE, Kimmel DW. Subdural hematoma in patients with systemic cancer. Mayo Clin Proc 1989; 64:637–42.
28. Lynes WL, Bostwick DG, Freiha FS, Stamey TA. Parenchymal brain metastases from adenocarcinoma of prostate. Urology 1986; 28:280–7.
29. Taylor HG, Lefkowitz M, Skoog SJ, Miles BJ, McLeod DG, Coggin JT. Intracranial metastases in prostate cancer. Cancer 1984; 53:2728–30.
30. Tetu B, Ro JY, Ayala AG, Ordoñez NG, Logothetis CJ, von Eschenbach AC. Small cell carcinoma of prostate associated with myasthenic (Eaton-Lambert) syndrome. Urology 1989; 33:148–52.
31. Kottke-Marchant K, Estes ML, Nunez C. Early brain metastases in endometrial carcinoma. Gynecol Oncol 1991; 41:67–73.
32. LeRoux PD, Berger MS, Elliott JP, Tamimi HK. Cerebral metastases from ovarian cancer. Cancer 1991; 67:2194–9.
33. Plaxe SC, Dottino PR, Lipsztein R, Dalton J, Cohen CJ. Clinical features and treatment otucome of patients with epithelial carcinoma of the ovary metastatic to the central nervous system. Obstet Gynecol 1990; 75:278–81.
34. Gordon AN, Kavanagh JS, Wharton JT, Rutledge FN, Obbens EAMT, Bodey GP. Successful treatment of leptomeningeal relapse of epithelial ovarian carcinoma. Gynecol Oncol 1984; 18:119–24.
35. Posner JB, Furneaux HM. Paraneoplastic syndromes. In: Waksman BH, ed. Immunologic mechanisms in neurologic and psychiatric diseases. New York: Raven Press, 1990:187–200.
36. Hetzel DJ, Stanhope CR, O'Neill BP, Lennon VA. Gynecologic cancer in patients with subacute cerebellar degeneration predicted by anti–Purkinje cell antibodies and limited in metastatic volume. Mayo Clin Proc 1990; 65:1558–63.
37. Peters WA, Andersen WA, Thornton N. Dermatomyositis and coexistent ovarian cancer: a review of the compounding clinical problems. Gynecol Oncol 1983; 15: 440–6.
38. Maor MH, Frias AE, Oswald MJ. Palliative radiotherapy for brain metastases in renal carcinoma. Cancer 1988; 62:1912–7.
39. Gouldesbrough DR, Bell JE, Gordon A. Use of immunohistochemical methods in the differential diagnosis between primary cerebellar hemangioblastoma and metastatic renal carcinoma. J Clin Pathol 1988; 41:861–5.
40. Badalament RA, Gluck RW, Wong GY, Gnecco C, Kreutzer E, Herr HW, Fair WR, Galicich JH. Surgical treatment of brain metastases from renal cell carcinoma. Urology 1990; 36:112–7.
41. Sundaresan N, Choi IS, Hughes JEO, Sachdev VP, Berenstein A. Treatment of spinal metastases from kidney cancer by presurgical embolization and resection. J Neurosurg 1990; 73:548–54.
42. Weed JC, Woodward KT, Hammond CB. Choriocarcinoma metastatic to the brain: therapy and prognosis. Semin Oncol 1982; 9:208–12.

43. Athanassiou A, Begent RHJ, Newlands ES, Parker D, Rustin GJS, Bagshawe KD. Central nervous system metastases of choriocarcinoma: 23 years' experience at Charing Cross Hospital. Cancer 1983; 52:1728–35.
44. Seigle JM, Caputy AJ, Manz HJ, Wheeler C, Fox JL. Multiple oncotic intracranial aneurysms and cardiac metastasis from choriocarcinoma: case report and review of the literature. Neurosurgery 1987; 20:39–42.
45. Logothetis CJ, Samuels ML, Trindade A. The management of brain metastases in germ cell tumors. Cancer 1982; 49:12–8.
46. Raghavan D, MacIntosh JF, Fox RM, Rogers J, Duval P, Besser M. Improved survival after brain metastases in non-seminomatous germ cell tumours with combined modality treatment. Br J Urol 1987; 60:364–7.
47. Cooper K, Bajorin D, Shapiro W, Krol G, Sze G, Bosl GJ. Decompression of epidural metastases from germ cell tumors with chemotherapy. J Neurooncol 1990; 8:275–80.
48. Cantwell BMJ, Mannix KA, Harris AL. Back pain—a presentation of metastatic testicular germ cell tumours. Lancet 1987; i:262–4.
49. Kabalin JN, Freiha FS, Torti FM. Brain metastases from transitional cell carcinoma of the bladder. J Urol 1988; 140:820–4.
50. Bishop JR, Moul JW, Maldonado L, McLeod DG. Transitional cell carcinomatous meningitis after M-VAC (methotrexate, vinblastine, doxorubicin, and cisplatin) chemotherapy. Urology 1990; 36:373–7.

# 18

## Neurological Complications of Gastrointestinal Cancers

**Neil A. Hagen**

*University of Calgary, Tom Baker Cancer Centre, Calgary, Alberta, Canada*

## I. OVERVIEW

In 1991, cancer of the gastrointestinal (GI) tract accounted for over 20% of new cancers and almost one-quarter of cancer deaths in the United States (1) (Table 1). There were over 150,000 patients diagnosed with colorectal cancer alone in 1991. Gastrointestinal neoplasms are responsible for four of the ten most common causes of cancer deaths. Gastrointestinal tumors are prevalent, and neurological involvement is correspondingly frequent.

Direct metastatic involvement of the nervous system is the most common neurological complication of cancer. However, direct metastatic involvement of the nervous system from GI neoplasms is much less prevalent than in tumors of other viscera such as lung (2) (Table 2). Because most metastases from GI neoplasms are hematogenous in origin and almost all of the GI tract is subserved by the portal venous system, central nervous system (CNS) metastasis tends to occur in patients with liver or lung metastases. Bulky regional metastases tend to be quite symptomatic in this population of patients, often overshadowing coexistent neurological abnormalities.

The incidence of brain metastases is lower in patients with GI tumors than other malignancies (3). Whereas brain metastases tend to be multiple in patients with melanoma, lung cancer, and cancer of unknown primary, patients with gastrointestinal, pelvic, and breast cancer more commonly have single brain metastases.

**Table 1** Causes of Cancer Death

| Primary tumor | Percent of cancer deaths |
|---|---|
| 1. Lung | 27.8% |
| 2. Colorectal | 11.8 |
| 3. Breast | 8.7 |
| 4. Prostate | 6.2 |
| 5. Pancreas | 4.9 |
| 6. Non-Hodgkin's lymphoma | 3.6 |
| 7. Leukemia | 3.5 |
| 8. Stomach | 2.6 |
| 9. Ovary | 2.4 |
| 10. Hepatobiliary | 2.4 |

Cancers of the gastrointestinal tract cause about one-quarter of cancer deaths (23.9%), and include four of the ten most common causes of cancer death (estimated figures, United States, 1991). (From Ref. 1.)

The anatomic distribution of brain metastasis from most malignancies is roughly proportional to the weight or blood supply to various nervous tissue regions (4). There is a tendency for metastasis to lodge in watershed blood flow areas in the cerebral hemispheres, such as the temporal-parietal and fronto-parietal gray-white junction (5). Although 90% of all brain metastases occur in the cerebral hemispheres and 10% in the cerebellum, there is a curious predilection of tumors of the

**Table 2** Prevalence of Central Nervous System Metastasis

| Primary | Number of patients | Number with CNS involvement | Percent with CNS involvement |
|---|---|---|---|
| Melanoma | 11 | 10 | 91% |
| Lung | 437 | 122 | 37.4 |
| Breast | 27 | 10 | 37 |
| Kidney | 30 | 7 | 23 |
| Prostate | 95 | 9 | 9.5 |
| Pancreas | 71 | 5 | 7 |
| Esophagus | 59 | 4 | 7 |
| Colon | 115 | 7 | 6.1 |
| Stomach | 99 | 4 | 4.4 |

Of 1096 autopsies performed on cancer patients, 200 (18.25%) demonstrated central nervous system (CNS) metastasis. Gastrointestinal malignancies were associated with direct CNS metastasis much less frequently than other tumor types. (From Ref. 2.)

gastrointestinal tract and pelvis to metastasize to the posterior fossa. Up to half of brain metastases from GI and pelvic primaries are to the cerebellum. This observation has clinical application: patients with gastrointestinal malignancies in whom brain metastases are suspected require particular attention to the posterior fossa.

Batson's plexus consists of epidural spinous veins which are in continuity with the cerebral dural sinuses. One explanation for the unusual distribution of brain metastasis in gastrointestinal and pelvic malignancies is that venous tumor emboli ascend to the brain through Batson's plexus during episodes of increased abdominal pressure and compression of the vena cava. Although Posner and colleagues have observed a preference of gastrointestinal and pelvic tumors to metastasize to the posterior fossa, they have found no increased incidence of spinal epidural and skull metastasis in this population, a finding that appears to argue against the Batson plexus route hypothesis (5). A more appealing explanation is the "fertile soil" hypothesis, which is based on both clinical and experimental evidence. Although tumors embolize to a wide variety of tissues, metastases develop in only certain tissues (6). Presumably, GI and pelvic neoplasms find the posterior fossa a more favorable environment, although the cellular mechanism for this preference is obscure.

Leptomeningeal metastases from GI neoplasms are relatively infrequent. Only one of 90 patients reported by Wasserstrom had a known GI malignancy (7). The clinical manifestations of leptomeningeal metastasis from a GI primary are similar to those seen from other solid tumors.

Malignant plexopathies can occur with a variety of neoplasms (Chap. 10). Adenocarcinomas of the GI tract are a relatively common cause of lumbosacral plexopathy. Distinction between malignant and radiation plexopathy can be difficult. However, lumbosacral plexopathy in patients with GI malignancy is usually due to tumor invasion and not radiation therapy (8).

Neurological complications not due to direct nervous system metastasis are prevalent in patients with GI neoplasms. Tumor replacement of hepatic parenchyma can result in liver failure and encephalopathy. Nutritional deficiency related to cancer can also cause encephalopathy. Neurological sequelae of nutritional deficiency are particularly common in GI tumors, for three reasons. First, some conditions which are risk factors for gastrointestinal malignancies can by themselves be associated with nutritional deficiency, such as alcoholism or inflammatory bowel disease. Second, tumors directly involving the alimentary tract are frequently associated with anorexia and vomiting, with resultant poor nutritional status. Finally, some tumors of the GI tract may elaborate large quantities of hormones which can result in depletion of essential metabolic substrates, such as tryptophan deficiency from carcinoid, with resultant pellagra.

The prevalence of Wernicke's disease in association with gastrointestinal cancers is of particular interest. Wernicke's first case concerned a woman who developed pyloric stenosis and stomach ulceration after swallowing sulfuric acid; she was not an alcoholic (9). Other patients have subsequently been described as having Wernicke's disease in association with carcinoma of the stomach and pancreas. Malnutrition from a large variety of causes has been implicated in the pathogenesis of Wernicke's disease (10). In one series, only four of 22 patients had chronic alcoholism as the underlying cause; six of 22 had an associated malignancy, including one patient with carcinoma of the stomach and another with carcinoma of the esophagus (11). In another series, the diagnosis of Wernicke's disease was made prior to death in only one-third of patients. While the presentation of the classic triad of ophthalmoplegia, ataxia, and encephalopathy is readily recognized, 33 of 97 patients with pathologically proven Wernicke's disease had encephalopathy as the only manifestation of thiamine deficiency (12). Encephalopathy remains a prevalent condition in patients with gastrointestinal cancers, mandating that thiamine deficiency be considered in the differential diagnosis.

Paraneoplastic effects of GI tumors are relatively common and include hormonal, electrolyte, and neurological abnormalities. Hormonal paraneoplastic syndromes arise from elevated blood levels of insulin, gastrin, glucagon, vasoactive intestinal polypeptide (VIP), and the various hormones which result in the carcinoid syndrome. While hypoglycemia is characteristic of secreting β cell tumors (insulinoma), symptoms of hypoglycemia have also been described in carcinoid as well as large retroperitoneal and bulky visceral tumors. Ectopic corticotropin production has been described in a number of GI tumors, most commonly in patients with pancreatic islet cell tumors.

There is a spectrum of exceedingly uncommon neoplastic neurological syndromes which have been described in gastrointestinal neoplasms, including encephalomyelitis, cerebellar degeneration, necrotizing myelopathy, sensory neuropathy, sensorimotor neuropathy, motor neuron disease, myasthenic syndrome, and dermatomyositis (see Chap. 8). There is a propensity for adenocarcinoma of the GI tract to be associated with disorders of coagulation (see Chap. 6).

While the above general principles are relevant to most GI tumors, each segment of the GI tract presents different tumors with their own particular neurological complications.

## II. CANCER OF THE ESOPHAGUS

Cancer of the esophagus is common and usually presents at an advanced stage. Local control is difficult to achieve, and local recurrence is the usual cause of death. Neurological complications are uncommon and relate primarily to contiguous thoracic spinal column spread, brain metastasis, or neurological consequences of malnutrition, which are at least as common as brain metastases in this population of patients.

Greater than 90% of malignant primary tumors of the esophagus are squamous cell. Other tumor types arising in this area include adenocarcinoma, adenoid cystic carcinoma, carcinoid, melanoma, sarcoma, and others. In 1991 there were 10,900 patients diagnosed with cancer of the esophagus in the United States, with the incidence being almost three times greater in men than women (1). Cancer of the esophagus is the thirteenth commonest cause of cancer death in the United States. The most significant risk factors for squamous cell carcinoma of the esophagus in the western world are alcohol and tobacco consumption. In other parts of the world, dietary factors have been implicated (13).

The typical clinical presentation is that of a man in his sixth or seventh decade of life who develops dysphagia and weight loss. Other frequent complaints include odynophagia, hematemesis or melena, and aspiration. Treatment of cancer of the esophagus includes surgery and radiation therapy; chemotherapy is of modest benefit.

Patients can present with neurological symptoms as the first evidence of cancer of the esophagus. Dysphonia is usually a manifestation of direct invasion of the left recurrent laryngeal nerve. Diaphragmatic paralysis is usually unilateral and rarely causes symptoms. Invasion of the sympathetic chain in the paraspinal area or within the spinal cord can result in Horner's syndrome.

A fistula develops in about 15% of patients due to direct tumor invasion; fistulae are usually between the esophagus and the respiratory tree. An aorto-esophageal fistula can result in fatal hemorrhage. Posterior extension of a fistula into the epidural space also is disastrous. Therapeutic interventions for such a lesion should consider the likelihood that the malignant fistula is superinfected.

The median survival following diagnosis of esophageal carcinoma is about 6 months. Based on cell doubling time, it seems highly likely that extent of disease at autopsy reflects the extent of disease at the time of initial presentation. Autopsy studies indicate that lymph node metastases are present in about 75% of patients, visceral metastases are present in 50%, and central nervous system metastases are present in 2–7% (2,14). The cause of death is usually extensive local and regional disease, resulting in aspiration pneumonia and cachexia. Hepatic failure is present in about one-fifth of patients.

Chronic alcoholism is prevalent in the esophageal cancer patient population. One report indicated that more than 90% of 111 patients had a history of alcoholism (14). Eighteen percent of patients had alcohol-related liver disease and 47% had evidence of pancreatitis. Of patients with neurological complaints, more had pathological changes consistent with alcoholism than had brain metastasis. Nutritional difficulties due to dysphagia and cachexia only compound the problem. Cancer of the esophagus is a common malignancy with a poor prognosis, primarily due to extensive regional disease at the time of initial diagnosis. Although neurological complications are uncommon, they serve to highlight the

**Table 3** Neurological Complications of Cancer of the Esophagus

| | |
|---|---|
| Neurological Manifestations of Locally Advanced Disease | |
| *Manifestation* | *Cause* |
| Dysphonia | Left recurrent laryngeal nerve invasion |
| Hypoxia | Fistula with aspiration |
| | Diaphragmatic paralysis (usually asymptomatic) |
| Horner's sign | Invasion of sympathetic chain in paraspinal area |
| Back pain | Epidural invasion by tumor, abscess, or both |
| Wernicke's disease | Dysphagia |
| | Cancer-related anorexia |
| | Alcoholism |
| Complications of Metastatic Disease (uncommon) | |
| Brain metastasis | |
| Metastasis elsewhere in the neuroaxis | |
| Paraneoplastic Syndromes (rare) | |

While direct CNS metastasis can occur in patients with esophageal carcinoma, neurological manifestations of locally advanced disease are particularly prominent.

importance of nutritional complications of cancer and neurological complications of regionally advanced malignancy (Table 3).

## III. CANCER OF THE STOMACH

Cancer of the stomach is common; in 1991 there were 23,800 patients diagnosed with this malignancy in the United States. It is the eighth most common cause of cancer death (1). The incidence is declining in recent decades. In other countries, gastric cancer is much more prevalent. Gastric malignancy is responsible for 40% of cancer deaths in Japan. Environmental factors have been implicated, including cured foods and aflatoxin (13).

Ninety-five percent of malignant gastric tumors are adenocarcinoma. Other pathological types include leiomyosarcoma, lymphoma, squamous cell, and carcinoid. Gastric lymphoma is increasing in frequency.

Most adenocarcinomas occur in the antrum, or distal one-third of the stomach. Extensive lymphatic drainage in three directions (left gastric chain, splenic chain, and hepatic chain) and close proximity to other tissues (hepatobiliary system, liver, diaphragm, esophagus, spleen, blood vessels) account for the tendency for disease to present at an advanced stage (15,16). Achlorhydria is associated with gastric cancer (17). Pernicious anemia is a condition which has been reported to result in a 20-fold increased risk of gastric cancer, although this issue remains controversial (13,18). Sensory complaints in a patient with gastric cancer should prompt an evaluation for vitamin $B_{12}$ deficiency.

The typical history in a patient with adenocarcinoma of the stomach is that of an adult in his or her sixties who presents with vague, nonlocalizing symptoms such as "tiredness," "stomach bloating," or weight loss. Treatment of gastric cancer can include surgery, radiation therapy, and chemotherapy. The selection of treatment modality depends on the goal of the intervention, whether palliative or cure. The only chance for cure is definitive surgery. Only 30% of patients have surgical specimens with margins free of tumor (15,16). Radiation therapy can be administered intraoperatively or by external beam. Chemotherapy can include single or multiple agents. The overall 5-year survival is about 7.5%.

Dumping syndrome can develop following surgery for gastric cancer. This consists of spells of postprandial bloating, epigastric discomfort, cramps, sweating, palpitations, and dizziness. It is due to fluid shift from the intravascular space into the lumen of the small bowel, caused by too rapid filling of the small intestine following a meal. All patients will become $B_{12}$ deficit following gastric resection unless parenteral $B_{12}$ is administered. Malabsorption can occur because of bacterial overgrowth in a blind loop of bowel, causing degradation of bile salts.

Direct metastatic involvement of the CNS by gastric carcinoma is uncommon. Involvement at the time of surgery or autopsy has been reported to be 4% or less in various series (2,15,16) (Table 4). The most common type of CNS spread is brain metastasis. Early reports based on small numbers of patients wrongly suggested that gastric carcinoma had a propensity to metastasize to the leptomeninges.

**Table 4**  Sites of Metastasis of Carcinoma of the Stomach

|  | Percent involved[a] ($n = 348$) | Percent involved[b] ($n = 250$) |
|---|---|---|
| Liver | 54% | 40% |
| Peritoneum | 24 | 17 |
| Lungs | 22 | 19 |
| Adrenals | 15 | 12 |
| Bone | 1 | 9 |
| CNS | 0.3 | 2.0 |
| No metastasis | 11 | N/A |
| One-year survival | N/A | 40.4 |

[a]From Ref. 15
[b]From Ref. 16

Sites of metastasis of carcinoma of the stomach at surgery or autopsy are most commonly to the liver, lung, and within the abdomen; metastases outside these areas are unusual.

Subsequent large series have indicated that leptomeningeal carcinomatosis from gastric cancer is decidedly uncommon (7,19).

## IV. CANCER OF THE PANCREAS

Malignancies of the pancreas are the fourth most common cause of cancer death in the United States. In 1991, there were 28,200 patients diagnosed with cancer of the pancreas (1). The prognosis following diagnosis remains among the most dismal in oncology. The incidence of cancer of the pancreas is similar in men and women and increases with age. Associated factors have been implicated to varying degrees, including chronic pancreatitis, tobacco use, and alcohol (13).

Pain is the commonest initial symptom and is soon followed by bloating, anorexia, and weight loss (20). Thrombophlebitis or other symptoms of hypercoagulability can be seen. Median survival is 6 months following diagnosis. Surgery is rarely curative, but gastroenterostomy is palliative. Radiation therapy with chemotherapy results in modest improvement in survival. The poor prognosis of cancer of the pancreas relates to the presence of microscopic metastases at the time of presentation in most patients: 40% of patients have locally advanced disease and 40% have distant metastases. The prevalence and nature of neurological complications are similar to those described for adenocarcinoma of the stomach.

Therapeutic efforts are focused on symptom control (21). Pain is an early, progressive, and prominent symptom throughout the course of disease in the majority of patients. The cause is likely due to invasion of the splenic nerve plexus and retroperitoneum by tumor. Prophylactic celiac plexus blockade at the time of surgery has been advocated because of the frequency of cancer-related pain, although this issue currently is under investigation.

Percutaneous chemical neurolysis is highly efficacious. The technique of celiac plexus blockade has been reviewed by workers from Memorial Sloan-Kettering Cancer Center (21). The celiac plexus receives fibers subserved by thoracic nerve roots T5 through T12. The right and left celiac ganglia are usually located 1.5 cm anterior to L1 vertebral body. The use of fluoroscopic or computed tomography (CT) guidance increases the accuracy and outcome of this intervention. Serious complications are uncommon and include neuritis with pain, weakness; bladder, bowel, or sexual dysfunction; visceral or blood vessel puncture; and seizures. Orthostatic hypotension is common, primarily in elderly patients. It generally resolves in 2 to 3 days because of compensatory extrasplanchnic vasoconstriction. Relief of pain occurs in about 85% of patients. Radiation therapy of the abdomen intraoperatively or by external beam can also produce pain relief.

One survey assessed the prevalence of pain in cancer of the lung, prostate, uterine cervix, and pancreas (22). Pancreatic cancer was the most painful, with about half of patients having "moderate" or "very bad pain" on average.

Symptom control remains a prominent and challenging aspect in the overall management of cancer of the pancreas.

## V. ENDOCRINE TUMORS OF THE GI TRACT

### A. Carcinoid

Carcinoid tumors are remarkable because they have a relatively benign pattern of growth and yet can metastasize widely and can be associated with paraneoplastic symptoms (13). The cell of origin of carcinoid tumor is the enterochromaffin cell, which is distributed widely in the body, predominantly in the submucosa of the intestine and main bronchi. Enterochromaffin cells are neural crest in origin. The site of origin of carcinoid tumors reflects the general distribution of enterochromaffin cells in the body. Carcinoid tumors most commonly arise in the appendix (44%), rectum (15%), ileum (11%), and bronchus (10%). They can also arise in a variety of other locations including colon, stomach, pancreas, duodenum, jejunum, biliary tract, esophagus, cervix, and ovaries (23). While carcinoid represents a small proportion of all tumors at most of these locations, carcinoid tumors make up one-third of small-intestine tumors and three-fourths of appendix tumors. Carcinoid tumors constitute about one-third of tumors of the endocrine pancreas but only a small proportion of all pancreatic neoplasms. Most carcinoid tumors are asymptomatic and are found incidentally at the time of appendectomy. However, carcinoid tumors may elaborate a wide variety of substances, including 5-hydroxytryptamine, 5-hydroxytryptophan, neurotensin, substance P, bombesin and insulin, among others.

Clinical features of carcinoid tumors vary according to material(s) secreted and the site of origin. Symptoms from carcinoid tumors are usually due to mass effect, not the carcinoid syndrome. For example, ileal tumors typically present with intermittent abdominal pain, other symptoms of small-bowel obstruction, or symptoms due to liver metastases. Age at presentation varies depending on the site of origin of the tumor, but generally is in the sixth or seventh decade of life (23). Foregut tumors, especially those arising in the bronchus, do not have portal vein drainage with hepatic inactivation of their secretory products. Therefore, they are often associated with the carcinoid syndrome. In contrast, midgut tumors, which arise in the ileum and appendix, frequently secrete serotonin. However, the carcinoid syndrome appears almost exclusively in association with metastases to liver and beyond. Hindgut carcinoid tumors, arising in the rectum or left colon, less commonly result in carcinoid syndrome. Carcinoid syndrome can be associated with other tumors, including small-cell carcinoma of the lung and islet cell tumors of the pancreas.

Carcinoid syndrome is a striking clinical entity which is seen in only about

10% of patients with malignant carcinoid tumor. Patients complain of spells of flushing and lightheadedness. Wheezing due to bronchospasm may develop. Diarrhea is common and usually but not always occurs in patients who have flushing spells. The clinical presentation may be highly suggestive of the disorder or may be more obtuse. Rarely reported complications include confusion, ophthalmic vessel occlusion, and pellagralike skin changes. Endocardinal fibrosis occurs late in the illness in a significant minority of patients and typically involves the right side of the heart with tricuspid insufficiency, pulmonary stenosis, and heart failure. About two-thirds of patients with the carcinoid syndrome have evidence on physical exam of palpable tumor, such as hepatomegaly. Treatment is primarily surgical. Radiation therapy and chemotherapy are less frequently used.

Symptom control remains an important aspect in the overall care of patients with carcinoid. Carcinoid syndrome is managed with a variety of agents. Initial interventions for mild symptoms include dietary nicotinamide supplementation and avoiding precipitants, which can include alcohol, various foods, or stress. Codeine or other hypomotility agents can help diarrhea. Other pharmacological agents used to treat symptoms of carcinoid include phenoxybenzamine, $H_1$ and $H_2$ blockers, and bronchodilators and steroids for wheezing. Beta-adrenergic agents for asthma should be avoided. A long-acting somatostatin analog (octreotide) has been found to be highly efficacious in relieving symptoms, moderately effective in reducing urinary 5-HIAA excretion, and occasionally associated with objective tumor regression (24).

Although the term "carcinoid" was chosen to reflect the relatively benign nature of the tumor, the natural history can be far from benign. Untreated, most carcinoid tumors other than appendix tumors will metastasize. Neurological complications associated with carcinoid occur in a significant minority of patients and are similar in prevalence and character to neurological abnormalities associated with other malignancies (Table 5). In a careful review of the clinical experience at Memorial Sloan-Kettering Cancer Center, Patchell and colleagues found that neurological complications occurred in 16% of 219 patients with carcinoid, all of whom had advanced (metastatic) carcinoid (25). Most neurological complications are due to metastases.

The most prevalent site of carcinoid metastases involving the nervous system is to the spinal column with continguous spread to the epidural space, causing spinal cord compression. Epidural spinal cord compression can be the first manifestation of carcinoid. Perhaps because carcinoid is a slowly growing tumor, patients are frequently ambulatory at the time of diagnosis of spinal cord compression. Pain is the first symptom in most patients with this complication. Radiation therapy is effective in over 90% of patients in preventing loss of ambulation. Surgery has also been effective. However, cord compression is associated with advanced metastatic disease and with a median survival of about 6 months.

The second most common neurological manifestation of carcinoid is cranial

**Table 5** Neurological Complications of Carcinoid

| | |
|---|---|
| Metastatic | |
|   Epidural spinal cord compression | |
|   Intracranial metastasis | Brain |
| | Dura |
| | Base of skull |
|   Leptomeningeal metastases | |
| Nonmetastatic | |
|   Metabolic encephalopathy | Liver failure |
| | Nutritional deficiency |
| | Other |
|   Herpes zoster | |
|   Cerebrovascular | Intracranial venous thrombosis |
| | Septic emboli |
|   Paraneoplastic | Myopathy |
| | Neuropathy |
|   Seizure | |

While metastatic complications of carcinoid are significant, nonmetastatic effects, including paraneoplastic syndromes, are prominent. (From Ref 25.)

metastases including single or multiple cerebral hemisphere metastases, pituitary metastasis, or base of skull metastases. Frequency of brain metastases in carcinoid is similar to that observed with other gastrointestinal tumors. The usual route of spread to the brain in carcinoid is hematogenous. Most patients have underlying liver or lung metastases. Radiation therapy is palliative (26).

Leptomeningeal involvement by carcinoid is uncommon either in isolation or in association with leptomeningeal spread from brain metastasis. While leptomeningeal metastases have been reported in up to 5% of all cancer patients, this complication occurs in only about 0.5% of patients with carcinoid tumor. Prognosis is dismal, and the optimal approach to therapy remains to be defined.

Malignant brachial plexopathy can occur by direct spread from contiguous lung deposits. Radiation therapy is effective treatment (26).

A number of neurological complications not due to nervous system metastasis have been reported in patients with carcinoid. The most common such complication is metabolic encephalopathy, usually due to hepatic failure from massive liver metastases. Treatment of hepatic encephalopathy by medical management in this setting can be successful. Encephalopathy also may be related to nutritional deficiency associated with carcinoid. Reported cerebral vascular complications include saggital sinus thrombosis and septic emboli. Although sometimes seen in patients with metabolic disorders, seizures in a carcinoid patient should alert the clinician to look for a serious underlying structural or vascular cause, such as brain metastasis or septic embolus.

Carcinoid myopathy is observed occasionally but the pathophysiology remains unclear. Pathological findings which have been reported include type 2 muscle fiber atrophy, central nuclei, mitochondrial changes, and fiber necrosis. Mildly elevated muscle enzymes have been noted. Clinical and animal experience has implicated serotonin in a similar myopathy. Indeed, patients with carcinoid myopathy have been found to have elevated urinary 5-HIAA levels. However, the vast majority of patients who have elevated urinary 5-HIAA levels never develop symptoms of myopathy. The myopathy has been successfully treated by the serotonin antagonist cyproheptadine.

Tryptophan and niacin are used in the biosynthesis of serotonin, and deficiency states associated with overproduction of serotonin by carcinoid have been reported. Serotonin does not cross the blood-brain barrier, resulting in the paradox of high serum and potentially low CNS levels of serotonin. Low brain levels of serotonin or norepinephrine have been felt to be associated with depression. While there are published reports of carcinoid patients who have depression, there is no convincing evidence that the prevalence of depression is above that expected in a general cancer population (25). Carcinoid syndrome has features in common with panic attack, and this psychiatric diagnosis is commonly given before the correct oncological diagnosis becomes evident. While encephalopathy is most commonly due to bulky liver metastases with hepatic failure, a trial of dietary supplementation should be considered because striking examples of encephalopathy responsive to dietary tryptophan or niacin have been reported. Pellegra has been rarely observed in the carcinoid population.

## B. Insulinoma

Insulinoma is the most common islet cell tumor. Symptoms are predominantly related to secretion of insulin. The tendency to metastasize is much lower for insulinoma than carcinoid or gastrinoma. Only about 10% of insulinomas demonstrate malignant potential (13). The tumor can occur at any age, although most usually in the fifth to seventh decade of life. Only half of insulinomas are seen on CT scan, but even quite small tumors are able to produce clinical symptoms. The treatment is by surgical resection although medical therapy (diazoxide, octreotide) may be used to control hypoglycemia.

Clinical presentation classically includes Whipple's triad of low blood sugar, symptoms of hypoglycemia, and relief of symptoms after administration of glucose. Patients frequently gain weight because of relief of symptoms upon eating and development of symptoms with even short-term fasting. Symptoms of hypoglycemia include headache, slurred speech, personality change, confusion, and ultimately coma and death. Associated with hypoglycemia is a secondary increase in serum catecholamines. This results in characteristic symptoms of tremulousness, sweating, and palpitations. However, a sixth of insulinoma patients never develop adrenergic symptoms during symptomatic hypoglycemia and present with isolated spells of focal or diffuse neurological dysfunction. Such spells can be clinically indistinguishable from transient ischemia attacks. The unanticipated laboratory finding of hypoglycemia during the spell leads to the correct diagnosis (27). Initially symptoms are intermittent and mild, occurring mainly after fasting (such as during the night) or exercise. Later in the course of the illness, symptoms may occur at any time.

The spectrum of neurological symptoms associated with insulinoma have been reviewed (28). Eighty-five percent of patients had spells that included diplopia, blurred vision, sweating, palpitations, or weakness. Confusion or abnormal behavior occurred in 80% of patients. Electroencephalogram (EEG) recording concurrent with confusion and hypoglycemia showed generalized slowing which was partially corrected with intravenous glucose. Amnesia for events occurring during spells was seen in 53% of patients. Twelve percent of patients had generalized convulsions. Neurological examination revealed no abnormalities except during spells of hypoglycemia, when confusion, altered consciousness, or focal neurological deficits were noted.

Insulinoma has been very rarely reported to be associated with peripheral neuropathy (29). None of 60 insulinoma patients reported by Service had the disorder (28). Patients develop neuropathy over a period of months, in association with spells of hypoglycemia during which CNS symptoms are prominent. Usually no single episode of hypoglycemia is responsible for the neuropathy. Neuropathy symptoms are mainly or exclusively motor and involve the hands more than the feet. Dysesthesias are common but are not usually associated with loss of sensation. Following resection of the insulinoma, sensory symptoms resolve completely and strength improves to a lesser degree. Wasting is usually permanent. Neuropathological information is sparse. Some data indicate that the underlying neuropathy is axonal, but anterior horn cell destruction has also been reported.

## C. Gastrinoma

Gastrinoma can produce Zollinger-Ellison syndrome, which is characterized by severe peptic ulcer disease, gastric acid hypersecretion, and elevated serum gastrin levels (13,30). Gastrinoma is the third most prevalent secretory GI tumor after insulinoma and carcinoid. Two-thirds or more of gastrinomas occur in the pancreas or duodenum. At the time of presentation, one-third of patients have metastatic disease. Metastases are most commonly to regional lymph nodes or the liver. Gastrinoma is a slowly growing tumor with a 5- and 10-year survival of 42% and 30%, respectively.

While gastrinoma is usually sporadic, in 25% of patients the tumor is part of an inherited endocrine neoplasia disorder which has an autosomal dominant inheritance. Multiple endocrine neoplasia type one (MEN-1) is of neurological importance because of the development of pituitary tumors in more than half of patients with the disorder. Other associated endocrine tumors include parathyroid tumors, insulinoma, and adrenal adenoma.

Clinical symptoms in gastrinoma relate primarily to gastric acid hypersecretion, with painful peptic ulcer disease, peptic esophagitis, and diarrhea. However, medical treatment of gastric hypersecretion is so effective that the incidence of morbidity due to ulcer disease is decreasing and morbidity due to progressive tumor growth is correspondingly increasing. Tumor metastases are usually limited to regional lymph nodes and the liver. Bone metastases have been described in patients who have extensive underlying hepatic metastases. The pattern of bony involvement has predominantly included the axial skeleton and, occasionally, resulted in radicular pain or neurological deficit (31). Radiation therapy is palliative.

## VI. SMALL INTESTINE NEOPLASMS

### A. Adenocarcinoma of the Small Intestine

Tumors of the small intestine are relatively uncommon, representing only 3–6% of gastrointestinal neoplasms (13). Next to carcinoid, the most common tumor of the small intestine is adenocarcinoma. The incidence of adenocarcinoma of the small intestine increases with age. The duodenum is more frequently involved than the jejunum, and the ileum is the least common site of adenocarcinoma of the small intestine. Symptoms at presentation consist of abdominal pain, jaundice, bloating or other GI symptoms, and weight loss. Treatment is by surgery, but the extent of disease is usually advanced at the time of laparotomy. Radiation therapy can be palliative and may increase survival, although results have generally been discouraging.

While metastases distant to the liver do occur, local and regional tumor growth is responsible for most symptoms. The spectrum of neurological involvement is similar to that from adenocarcinomas elsewhere.

### B. Lymphoma of the Small Intestine

Lymphoma represents about one-fifth of primary small-bowel neoplasms and 1% of all GI neoplasms. Only 1.5% of all non-Hodgkin's lymphomas originate in the small intestine (13). About half of GI lymphomas originate in the stomach and one-third in the small intestine. There is an increased risk of small-intestine lymphoma in patients with underlying celiac sprue, Crohn's disease, immunosuppression, or AIDS. Symptoms at onset are similar to those described for adenocarcinoma of the small intestine. Treatment is with surgery plus chemotherapy. There is frequently intra-abdominal spread at the time of initial laparotomy. The 5-year survival is about 75% if the extent of disease is localized at the time of diagnosis and is only 25% if patients present with unresectable tumor. Neurological complications of lymphomas are discussed in Chapter 21.

## VII. COLORECTAL CANCER

Malignancy involving the colorectal region is the most common cancer of the gastrointestinal tract. It is the second most common visceral malignancy, next to cancer of the lung. There were 60,500 deaths in the United States due to large-bowel cancer in 1991 (1). Colorectal cancer is much more common in North America than other areas such as Africa or Japan. Studies have implicated several dietary factors as being associated with the higher risk of colon cancer, including high dietary fat and low dietary fiber (13). Several heritable conditions are associated with a greatly increased risk of adenocarcinoma of the colon.

At least 90% of cancers of the colon are adenocarcinoma; other less common tumors include carcinoid and sarcoma. Symptoms of colon cancer are frequently vague and are typified by the patient over 40 years of age with abdominal pain, nausea, change in bowel habit, hematochezia, and symptoms of anemia. About 5–10% of patients have liver metastasis at the time of initial diagnosis. Rectal carcinoma presents with tenesmus, red blood per rectum, and if advanced, perineal pain, bladder symptoms, or symptoms of sacral nerve root or plexus irritation.

The liver is the most common site of distant metastasis in adenocarcinoma of the lower intestine owing to the portal venous system which subserves all of the colon and most of the rectum. The lower rectum has venous drainage by two routes: superiorly into the portal system and inferiorly into the systemic venous system. A third potential route is the vertebral venous system. It is thought to be under higher pressure than either the portal or the systemic venous system, but it may receive rectal blood during defecation.

Prognosis and treatment for colorectal cancer is related to extent of disease at the time of initial presentation. Surgery can be curative. Radiation therapy and chemotherapy can be effective. Rectosigmoid surgery is associated with a variety of postoperative neurological sequelae and includes neurogenic bladder (usually mild), retrograde ejaculation, impotence, and anal sphincter dysfunction. Neurotoxicity due to radiation therapy of the abdomen and pelvis can be serious; it is reviewed in Chapter 10. One chemotherapeutic agent often used in colon cancer, 5-fluorouracil (5-FU), has a well-described cerebellar toxicity, which is discussed in Chapter 11.

Colon cancer is associated with brain metastasis infrequently, compared with other malignancies. In one series of 183 cancer patients with brain metastasis only 11 (6%) had colon primaries (32). Colon metastases enhance on head CT or magnetic resonance imaging (MRI). Unenhanced CT frequently demonstrates a mass of increased density (33). This finding is likely related to the dense cell structure of adenocarcinoma and can be seen in brain metastasis from other primary sites. It is distinctly uncommon for brain metastasis to be the presenting symptom of colon cancer. Eighty percent of colon cancer patients with brain metastasis have regional lymph node metastases and more than 90% have extensive systemic metastases at time of neurological presentation. Whether patients are treated surgically or with radiation therapy, prognosis remains poor for both control of recurrent brain metastasis and survival. However, radiation therapy and, in selected patients, surgery are palliative and should be considered despite the poor overall prognosis. While colon cancer is considered relatively radiation resistant, radiation therapy can relieve symptoms and prolong life. The extent of systemic disease at the time of brain metastasis remains the single most reliable prognostic indicator, and treatment of brain metastasis should be tempered accordingly (34). See Chapter 1 for management of brain metastases.

The clinical presentation and management of leptomeningeal metastases from colon cancer is similar to that of other malignancies and is discussed in Chapter 3. Carcinoembryonic antigen (CEA) is a tumor marker which, if present in the CSF, can be helpful in the diagnosis of leptomeningeal carcinomatosis related to colon cancer. Carcinoembryonic antigen is not usually present in cerebrospinal fluid even if the serum CEA is elevated. However, there is evidence of a blood-CSF threshold, particularly with serum CEA levels above 100 ng/ml. In such cases the concentration of CSF CEA is less than 2% of the serum CEA level unless CNS metastases are present (35). Cerebrospinal fluid CEA can be elevated due to leptomeningeal carcinoma from tumors other than colon. If CSF CEA is elevated in a patient with a prior history of colon cancer, leptomeningeal metastasis should be suspected.

Involvement of the peripheral nervous system by colorectal carcinoma is common. Colorectal carcinoma was the most common tumor to cause lumbosacral plexopathy in one large series (36). Metastases also can involve nerves beyond the retroperitoneum, including the brachial plexus and nerve roots. Radiation therapy can provide significant palliation of symptoms in these patients.

Signs and symptoms of liver failure are unusual in colon metastasis until very late in the disease process. Generally less than half of hepatic function is needed to prevent signs and symptoms of hepatic failure. Rapidly progressive hepatomegaly predicts a poor overall survival. Several heritable conditions are associated with a greatly increased risk of adenocarcinoma of the colon, including Gardner's syndrome, familial adenomatosis syndrome, Olfield syndrome, and Turcot syndrome. Mortality and diseases associated with familial adenomatous polyposis have been reviewed (37). Eighty-five percent of deaths in 110 patients were due to cancer. The eight patients with brain tumors died at a median age of 15.5 years (range: 6–59 years). Pathological diagnoses included medulloblastoma (four patients), glioblastoma (two patients), astrocytoma (one patient) and uncertain histology (one patient). There is ongoing work to further delineate genetic and cytokinetic aspects of the syndrome (38). Turcot syndrome is a rare and usually recessively inherited disorder of polyposis and malignant central nervous system tumors (39,40). Autosomal dominant and sporadic cases have also been reported. One recent review included 50 patients with Turcot syndrome and a brain tumor (39).

A deletion of a segment of the short arm of chromosome 17 has been reported in patients with cancer of the colon (41). Interestingly, the short arm of chromosome 17 has been reported to have loss of alleles in medulloblastoma (42), as well as cerebral astrocytomas (43), adrenal cortical carcinomas (44), and cervical carcinomas (45). A tumor-suppressing gene has been implicated.

One long-term survivor of glioblastoma who also underwent resection of colon carcinoma was treated with *cis*-retinoic acid (46). Retinoids have been reported to promote tumor cell differentiation in hematological malignancies. Their usefulness in treating malignant glioma is currently undergoing clinical investigation.

A second malignancy occurring in a cancer patient can be related to treatment of the first tumor, an underlying predisposition to cancer, or a combination of the two. Primary central nervous system lymphoma has been reported as a secondary malignancy in a long-term survivor of colon cancer as well as long-term survivors of breast cancer, adenocarcinoma of the thyroid, Hodgkin's disease, and systemic lymphoma. The median interval from diagnosis of the first primary to diagnosis of the primary CNS lymphoma was 10 years (47).

## VIII. HEPATOBILIARY NEOPLASMS

Hepatobiliary carcinoma is relatively uncommon in North America. There were 15,000 hepatobiliary cancers diagnosed in 1991 in the United States, and it is the 10th most common cause of cancer death (1).

### A. Hepatoma

Although much less common in North America, hepatoma may be the most common cause of cancer death worldwide. The highest incidence is noted in areas of Asia and Africa, which parallels the geographic distribution of hepatitis B infection. The relative risk of hepatocellular carcinoma in hepatitis B carriers is over 200.

In industrialized countries, both hepatitis B infection and alcohol abuse are etiologically related to hepatocellular carcinoma. Hemochromatosis is also a predisposing factor. Hepatocellular carcinoma occurs twice as commonly in men as in women. Most patients present with dull aching right upper quadrant pain which may radiate to the right shoulder. Other associated clinical features are fever, ascites, jaundice, and encephalopathy. Late and unusual nonmetastatic effects include hypoglycemia, hypercalcemia, and carcinoid syndrome. Metastases are most commonly to local contiguous areas such as the bile duct, porta hepatis, inferior vena cava, and stomach. Brain, skull, and other bone metastases have been described but are uncommon.

Median survival is only 4 months. Cause of death in one extensive autopsy series was liver failure (one-third), hemorrhage (one-third), and advanced cancer (one-third) (48). Neurological involvement beyond encephalopathy includes brain metastasis, bone metastasis with spinal cord or nerve compression, and sensorimotor neuropathy. Brain metastases were present in 13 of 771 patients (1.7%). Radiation therapy has palliative benefit for both brain and bone metastasis.

## B. Biliary Tumors

Biliary tree carcinoma includes tumors of the gallbladder as well as tumors of the ducts proximal and distal to the gallbladder. Carcinoma of the gallbladder is the fifth most common GI cancer, after colorectal, pancreas, stomach, and esophagus. It is slightly more common than hepatocellular carcinoma in North America. Women are at least three times more likely to develop this tumor than men, and 75% or more of patients have gallstones at the time of discovery of gallbladder cancer. Most patients are over the age of 60 years at the time of diagnosis. The prognosis is dismal. Patients who survive 5 years usually have tumors found incidentally at the time of cholecystectomy.

Tumors of the biliary tree spread extensively to contiguous organs including liver, stomach, duodenum, pancreas, transverse colon, and diaphragm. Distant metastases to supraclavicular nodes, lungs, adrenals, ovaries, and vertebral column have been reported. Radiation therapy is palliative. Obstructive jaundice develops in most patients prior to death. Cause of death is tumor growth (60%), liver failure (29%), or hemorrhage (11%). One autopsy study found lung metastases in 54% of patients, bone metastases in 17%, and brain metastases in none of 55 patients (48).

## IX. CONCLUSION

Gastrointestinal neoplasms are common and can lead to a variety of neurological complications. Nervous system metastases are characteristically associated with locally and regionally advanced abdominal tumor and have a predilection for brain metastasis in the posterior fossa. The high frequency of encephalopathy, the presence of several unique paraneoplastic syndromes, and the high prevalence of neurological sequelae of nutritional deficiency are additional neurological complications.

# REFERENCES

1. Boring CC, Squires TS, Tong T. Cancer statistics 1991. CA 1991; 41:19–36.
2. Chason JL, Walker FB, Landers JW. Metastatic carcinoma in the central nervous system and dorsal root ganglia. Cancer 1963; 16:781–7.
3. Posner JP, Chernik NL. Intracranial metastasis form systemic cancer. Adv Neurol 1978; 19:579–92.
4. Ask-Upmark E. Metastatic tumors of brain and their localization. Acta Med Scand 1956; 154:1–9.
5. Delattre JY, Kvol G, Thaler HT, Posner JB. Distribution of brain metastases. Arch Neurol 1988; 45:741–4.
6. Brunson KW, Beattie G, Nicolson GL. Selections and altered properties of brain colonizing metastatic melanoma. Nature 1978; 272:543–5.
7. Wasserstrom WR, Glass PJ, Posner JB. Diagnosis and treatment of leptomeningeal metastases from solid tumors: experience with 90 patients. Cancer 1982; 49:759–72.
8. Thomas JE, Cascino TL, Earle JD. Differential diagnosis between radiation and tumor plexopathy of the pelvis. Neurology 1985; 35:1–7.
9. Vonderahe AR. Sequelae of severe disease of the abdominal viscera. JAMA 1941; 116:390–5.
10. Reuler JB, Girade DE, Cooney TG. Wernike's encephalopathy. N Engl J Med 1985; 312:1035–9.
11. Ebels EJ. Underlying illness in Wernike's encephalopathy. Eur Neurol 1974; 12:226–8.
12. Harper CG, Giles M, Finlay-Jones R. Clinical signs in the Wernike-Korsakoff complex: a retrospective analysis of 131 cases diagnosed at necropsy. J Neurol Neurosurg Psychiatry 1986; 49:341–5.
13. DeVita VT, Hellman S, Rosenberg SA, eds. Cancer. Philadelphia: JB Lippincott, 1989:725–964, 1303–44.
14. Manard AM, Chasle J, Marnay J, et al. Autopsy findings in 111 cases of esophageal cancer. Cancer 1981; 48:329–35.
15. Dupont JB, Lee JR, Burton GR, et al. Adenocarcinoma of the stomach: review of 1497 cases. Cancer 1978; 41:941–7.
16. Clarke JS, Cruze K, El Farra S, et al. The natural history and results of surgical therapy for carcinoma of the stomach: an analysis of 250 cases. Am J Surg 1961; 102:143–52.
17. Hitchcock CR, Scheiner SL. Early diagnosis of gastric cancer. Surg Gynecol Obstet 1961; 113:665–72.
18. Hoffman NR. The relationship between pernicious anemia and cancer of the stomach. Geriatrics 1970; 25:90–5.
19. Olson ME, Chernik NL, Posner JB. Infiltration of the leptomeninges by systemic cancer. Arch Neurol 1974; 30:122–37.

20. Gudjonsson B, Livstone EM, Spiro HM. Cancer of the pancreas: diagnostic accuracy and survival statistics. Cancer 1978; 42:2494–2506.
21. Saltzburg D, Foley KM. Management of pain in pancreatic cancer. Surg Clin N Am 1989; 69:629–49.
22. Greenwald HP, Bonica JJ, Bergner M. The prevalence of pain in four cancers. Cancer 1987; 60:2563–9.
23. Godwin JD. Carcinoid tumors; an analysis of 2837 cases. Cancer 1975; 36:560–9.
24. Kvols L, Moertel CG, O'Connell MJ, et al. The treatment of malignant carcinoid syndrome; evaluation of a long-acting somatostatin analogue. N Engl J Med 1986; 315:663–6.
25. Patchell RA, Posner JB. Neurologic complications of carcinoid. Neurology 1986; 36: 745–9.
26. Schupak KD, Wallner KE. The role of radiation therapy in the treatment of locally unresectable or metastatic carcinoid tumors. Int J Radiat Oncol Biol Phys 1991; 20:489–95.
27. Fajan SS, Vinik AI. Insulin-producing islet cell tumors. Endocrinol Metab Clin N Am 1989; 1:45–74.
28. Service FJ, Dale AJD, Elveback LR, Jiang NS. Insulinoma: clinical and diagnostic features of 60 consecutive cases. Mayo Clin Proc 1976; 51:417–29.
29. Jaspan JB, Wollman RL, Bernstein L, Rubenstein AH. Hypoglycemic peripheral neuropathy in association with insulinoma: implication of glucopenia rather than hyperinsulinism. Case report and review of the literature. Medicine 1982; 61:33–44.
30. Friesen SR. Tumors of the endocrine pancreas. N Engl J Med 1982; 306:580–90.
31. Barton JC, Hirschowitz BI, Naton P, Jensen LT. Bone metastases in gastrinoma. Gastroenterology 1986; 91:1179–85.
32. Cairncross JG, Kim JH, Posner JB. Radiation therapy for brain metastases. Ann Neurol 1980; 7:529–41.
33. Cascino TL, Leavengood JM, Kemeny N, Posner JB. Brain metastases from colon cancer. J Neurooncol 1983; 1:1203–9.
34. DeAngelis LM, Mandell LR, Thaler HT, et al. The role of postoperative radiotherapy after resection of single brain metastases. Neurosurgery 1989; 24:798–805.
35. Schold SC, Wasserstrom WR, Pleisher M, et al. Cerebrospinal fluid biochemical markers of central nervous system metastases. Ann Neurol 1980; 8:597–604.
36. Jaeckle KA, Young DF, Foley KM. The natural history of lumbosacral plexopathy in cancer. Neurology 1985; 35:8–15.
37. Arvanitis ML, Jagelman DG, Fazio VW, Laverty IC, McGannon E. Mortality in patients with familial adenomatous polyposis. Dis Colon Rectum 1990; 33:639–42.
38. Newton HB, Rosenblum MK, Malkin MG. Turcot's syndrome: flow cytometric analysis. Cancer 1991; 61:1636–9.
39. Mastronardi L, Ferrante L, Lunardi P, Cervoni L, Fortuna A. Association between neuroepithelial tumor and multiple intestinal polyposis (Turcot's syndrome): a report of a case and critical analysis of the literature. Neurosurgery 1990; 28:449–52.
40. Turcot J, Despres JP, St Pierre F. Malignant tumors of the central nervous system associated with familial polyposis of the colon: report of two cases. Dis Colon Rectum 1959; 2:465–8.

41. Fearon ER, Hamilton SR, Vogelstein B. Clonal analysis of human colorectal tumors. Science 1987; 238:193–7.
42. Cogen PH, Daneshvar L, Metzger AK, Edwards MSB. Deletion mapping of the medulloblastoma locus on chromosome 17P. Genomics 1990; 8:279–85.
43. James CD, Carlbom E, Nordenskjold M, Collius VP, Cavenee WK. Mitotic recombination of chromosome 17 in astrocytomas. Proc Natl Acad Sci U S A 1989; 86: 2858–62.
44. Yano T, Linehan M, Anglard P, et al. Genetic changes in human adrenocortical carcinomas. J Natl Cancer Inst 1989; 81:518–23.
45. Atkin NB, Baker MC. Chromosome 17p loss in carcinoma of the cervix uteri. Cancer Genet Cytogenet 1989; 37:229–33.
46. Rutz HP, Tribolet N, Calmes JM, Chapuis G. Long-time survival of a patient with glioblastoma and Turcot's syndrome. J Neurosurg 1991; 74:813–15.
47. DeAngelis . Primary central nervous system lymphoma as a secondary malignancy. Cancer 1991; 67:1431–5.
48. Takahashi Y, Kameda H, Kasai Y, et al. Primary liver cancer in Japan. Cancer 1987; 60:1400–11.

# 19
# Neurological Complications of Sarcomas

**Patricia T. Molloy**

*University of Pennsylvania Medical School, and Children's Hospital of Philadelphia, Philadelphia, Pennsylvania*

**Peter C. Phillips**

*Children's Hospital of Philadelphia, Philadelphia, Pennsylvania*

## I. INTRODUCTION

Sarcomas are cancers of embryonic mesenchymal origin representing 15–20% of all pediatric solid tumors and 5–10% of all childhood malignancies. By contrast, soft tissue sarcomas are uncommon in adults, with an estimated incidence of only 5600 per year in the United States. Osseous sarcomas in adults are also rare, although uncommon entities such as fibrosarcoma occur more frequently during the fourth and fifth decades.

Neurological complications of sarcomas have received little attention, overshadowed by the severity of the primary disease and limited responses to therapy. Recently, greater recognition of the frequency and importance of neurological complications has resulted from published studies from large single institutions or cooperative groups (Graus et al., 1983; Lewis et al., 1986; Baram et al., 1988; Kramer et al., 1989; Klein et al., 1991). These studies indicate that nearly 27% of children with soft tissue and osseous sarcomas develop neurological complications; the most common include metastatic spinal cord compression (11%), symptomatic peripheral neuropathy (10%), intracranial metastatic disease (7.5%), seizures (6%), and acute and chronic methotrexate-related neurological dysfunction (2.5%) (Kramer et al., 1989). (See Table 1.)

Three factors have contributed to the increased recognition of neurological complications of sarcomas. First, prolonged patient survival due to improved

**Table 1** Neurological Complications in Children with Sarcomas

| | |
|---|---|
| Epidural spinal cord compression | 11% |
| Symptomatic peripheral neuropathy | 10% |
| Intracranial metastases | 7.5% |
| Seizures | 6% |
| Acute/chronic methotrexate-related neurotoxicity | 2.5% |

Experience of 162 children with soft tissue and osseous sarcomas at the Children's Hospital of Philadelphia (1980–1987).
Source: Kramer (1989).

therapy has increased the occurrence of late CNS metastatic complications, Second, the use of computed tomography (CT) and magnetic resonance imaging (MRI) has increased the identification of tumor- and treatment-related complications. Third, efforts to increase therapeutic efficacy by use of new agents, higher drug doses, and aggressive multimodality therapies has increased the incidence of treatment-related neurotoxicity among sarcoma patients.

This chapter will present an initial overview of the two most important tumor-associated neurological complications of soft tissue and osseous sarcomas—intracerebral metastases and epidural spinal cord compression—followed by review of the incidence, range, and significance of neurological complications for each of the most common sarcomas: rhabdomyosarcoma (RMS), osteosarcoma, and Ewing's sarcoma (see Table 2). Because these tumors characteristically occur during childhood and adolescence, this chapter will emphasize the clinical features of pediatric soft tissue and osseous sarcomas.

## II. OVERVIEW

### A. Intracerebral Metastases

Early studies of soft tissue and osseous sarcoma found intracerebral metastases to be an infrequent complication; recent estimates suggest that brain metastases may occur in 7.5–14% of patients with sarcoma (Kramer et al., 1989; Graus et al., 1983). (See Table 3.) A survey of brain metastases in postmortem studies of children with solid tumors at Memorial Sloan-Kettering Cancer Center from 1973 to 1982 revealed an incidence of 13% in patients younger than 21 years (Graus et al., 1983). This represented a twofold increase in brain metastases compared with a prior autopsy series at the same institution reported by Vanucci and Baten (1974).

The clinical features of intracranial metastatic sarcoma are indistinguishable from other CNS mass lesions and include headache, increased intracranial pressure, cranial neuropathies, seizures, hemiparesis, and change in mental status.

Lewis and coworkers summarized 94 cases of sarcoma metastatic to the brain (Lewis, 1988). In this review, 50 patients had pathological verification and analyzable clinical data. The presentation during the illness varied from the time of diagnosis to incidental discovery at autopsy. The onset of neurological signs was the first manifestation of sarcoma in 12% of patients with intracerebral metastases. In 26% of patients studied, neurological symptoms from intracranial lesions occurred as a preterminal event and were frequently associated with hemorrhage into the tumor bed. In an additional 15 patients (30%), the presence of intracranial metastases was determined only at autopsy.

The neurological manifestations in children and adolescents differ from those of adults in two ways: a higher incidence of seizures and a more abrupt onset of symptoms. Seizures are more often seen in patients with germ cell tumors and in children less than 15 years old. Abrupt onset of neurological symptoms occurred in 20% of children with intracranial metastases (Graus et al., 1983). Brain metastases less frequently (10%) present with an acute or catastrophic onset in adults (Cairncross et al., 1980).

Graus and coworkers reviewed the records of 31 children with parenchymal brain metastases diagnosed by CT scan (13) or necropsy (18) (Graus et al., 1983). They identified intracerebral metastases at autopsy in 14% (10 of 71 patients) with osteosarcoma, RMS, and Ewing's sarcoma. In their review, RMS and osteogenic sarcoma were the most frequent primary tumors causing brain metastases in children less than 15 years of age, with testicular germ cell tumors more commonly causing intracerebral metastases from age 15 to 21 years. Pulmonary metastases were present in 90% of patients with intracerebral metastases and the interval from pulmonary metastases to the development of brain metastases was about 10 months. They also reported that of 18 postmortem examinations, hemorrhagic brain metastases were found in nine: two with osteogenic sarcoma, two with Ewing's sarcoma, one with RMS, and four with germ cell tumors. In all but two patients with hemorrhagic metastases, the platelet count was greater than 50,000 mm$^3$.

In a review of 162 consecutive children with soft tissue and osseous sarcomas seen at Children's Hospital of Philadelphia, Kramer and coworkers found intracranial metastatic disease in 7% of patients; 5% had soft tissue sarcomas; and 2% had osseous sarcomas. Consistent with the previous findings of Graus and coworkers (1983), pulmonary metastases were noted in a high percentage of patients (58%) with brain metastases. These and other studies have demonstrated that intracerebral metastases usually are found late in the course of the disease and rarely as the initial presentation of soft tissue and osseous sarcomas (Graus et al., 1983; Baram et al., 1988; Kramer et al., 1989).

Graus and investigators (1983) reported a median survival of 4 months in 15 patients with intracerebral metastases treated with radiation but no surgery. By

**Table 2** Common Neurological Complications by Sarcoma Type

| Neurological complications | Incidence | Method of dissemination | Symptoms | Diagnosis | Treatment |
|---|---|---|---|---|---|
| *Rhabdomyocarcoma* | | | | | |
| Intracerebral involvement | 13–26% | Direct infiltration (most common) Hematogenous spread (increased with pulmonary metastases) | Headache Seizure Focal deficits | MRI with gadolinium (coronal views most helpful) | Resection when appropriate Radiation therapy and chemotherapy |
| Epidural spinal cord compression | 5.3–13% | Direct extension from paravertebral sites | Back pain, weakness, sensory complaints Late bowel/bladder complaints | MRI with gadolinium (sagittal and axial views) | Decompression laminectomy and/or radiotherapy and chemotherapy |
| Leptomeningeal dissemination | 35–50% | Parameningeal sites | Cranial nerves palsies | CT for bone erosion. MRI for intracranial extension. CSF cytology useful if positive (low yield). | Radiotherapy and intrathecal chemotherapy |

# Sarcomas

| | | | | | |
|---|---|---|---|---|---|
| *Osteosarcoma* | | | | | |
| Intracerebral involvement | 2–13.5% | Hematogenous | Headache/seizures Focal deficits Slight increased incidence in intratumoral hemorrhage | MRI with gadolinium Screening MRI of patients with pulmonary metastases of possible usefulness | Resection when appropriate Radiotherapy and chemotherapy |
| Epidural spinal cord compression | 4–6.5% | Same as RMS | Same as RMS | Same as RMS | Same as RMS |
| *Ewing's Sarcoma* | | | | | |
| Intracerebral involvement | 4.3–16.6% | Direct extension with dural involvement Hematogenous dissemination (uncommon) | Same as RMS | MRI with gadolinium | Same as RMS |
| Epidural spinal cord compression | 17–21.7% | Same as RMS | Same as RMS | Same as RMS | Same as RMS |

CT = Computed tomography, MRI = Magnetic resonance imaging, RMS = Rhabdomyosarcoma

**Table 3** Intracerebral Metastases

| Tumor type | Number of Patients with Brain Metastases vs. Tumor Type | | |
|---|---|---|---|
| | BCRC (1971–1977) | MSKCC (1973–1982) | CHOP (1980–1987) |
| Osteosarcoma | 7% (1/14) | 13.5% (5/38) | 2% (1/50) |
| Rhabdomyosarcoma | 26% (4/15) | 14.3% (3/21) | 13% (7/53) |
| Ewing's sarcoma | — (0/3) | 16.6% (2/12) | 4.3% (1/23) |

BCRC = Baltimore Cancer Research Center
MSKCC = Memorial Sloan-Kettering Cancer Center
CHOP = Children's Hospital of Philadelphia

contrast, the median survival of six patients treated with surgical excision for solitary brain metastases followed by radiotherapy was 7 months. The slightly longer survival in patients who underwent surgery may reflect selection bias or better overall clinical condition. The optimal management of intracerebral metastases remains controversial and is discussed in Chapter 1.

Intracerebral metastases, an infrequent neurological complication of sarcomas, are usually secondary to metastases from lungs. Routine neuroimaging (head MRI or CT) at diagnosis is not justified currently; however, cranial imaging may be warranted when pulmonary metastases are discovered.

## B. Epidural Spinal Cord Compression and Myelopathy

Metastatic spinal cord compression occurs in 2.7–5.0% of children with cancer (Chien et al., 1982; Klein et al., 1991) and 5–10% of adults (Barron et al., 1959). Soft tissue and osseous sarcomas are the most common tumors associated with metastatic spinal cord disease in children. The comparative incidence of this complication in sarcomas is presented in Table 4. Approximately 10–12% of patients with sarcomas develop epidural spinal cord compression compared with 7% of patients with neuroblastoma and 3–4% of patients with lymphoma (Chien et al., 1982). The pathogenesis is most often direct vertebral spread or extension of tumor through intravertebral foramina. Accordingly, nearly all cases begin as epidural spinal cord compression. Intradural tumor is uncommon but may occur by infiltration or erosion of the dura. Intramedullary metastatic soft tissue or osseous sarcoma has not (to our knowledge) been reported. Spinal cord injury also may arise from compressive or invasive occlusion of the anterior spinal artery or myelopathies associated with intrathecal chemotherapy or radiation therapy.

Investigators at St. Jude's Children's Research Hospital (SJCRH) reported their 17-year experience with spinal cord compression in children with systemic cancer

**Table 4** Epidural Spinal Cord Compression

*Number of Patients with Spinal Cord Compression vs. Tumor Type*

| Tumor type | CHOP (1980–1987) | SJCRH (1962–1987) |
|---|---|---|
| Osteosarcoma | 4% (2/50) | 6.5% (16/243) |
| Rhabdomyosarcoma | 13.2% (7/53) | 4.9% (14/287) |
| Ewing's sarcoma | 21.7% (5/23) | 17.9% (30/168) |

CHOP = Children's Hospital of Philadelphia
SJCRH = St. Jude's Children Research Hospital

(Chien et al., 1982). The overall frequency of cord compression was 2.7% (81 of 2967 patients) with solid tumors and leukemias. The most common initial symptoms of cord compression were back pain and limb weakness. Bowel and bladder dysfunction were late occurrences. While spinal cord dysfunction may occur throughout the course of the primary malignancy, cord compression in Ewing's sarcoma often presented earlier in the clinical course than RMS and osteosarcoma. In this study, pretreatment neurological status and early treatment were predictive of neurological outcome. Only 18% of patients became ambulatory after presenting with paraplegia, complete loss of sphincteral tone, and sensory loss for greater than 48 h. By contrast, 67% of patients became ambulatory after partial loss of spinal cord function and when treatment began in the first 48 h.

To assess the role of decompressive laminectomy in the treatment of metastatic spinal cord compression in children, Klein et al. reexamined the St. Jude's experience of 2259 consecutive patients with malignant solid tumors between 1962–1987 (Klein et al., 1991). Epidural spinal cord compression was found in 5% of these patients, of which osteosarcoma accounted for 6.5%, Ewing's sarcoma for 17.9%, and RMS for 4.9%. Sarcoma patients with cord compression were evaluated according to treatment approach: 21 patients received medical but not surgical treatment; 31 patients were treated by decompressive laminectomy. No significant differences were found between the two groups with respect to age at diagnosis, interval to spinal cord compression, pretreatment neurological function, survival after cord compression, or total survival time. These investigators found that neurological outcome in sarcoma patients treated by laminectomy was significantly better than nonsurgical treatment. Nineteen of 20 patients with moderate to severe neurological impairment prior to treatment had significant improvement after decompressive laminectomy, the majority of whom became ambulatory. Childhood sarcoma patients did not show the same improvement with chemotherapy and irradiation as did patients with neuroblastoma and other small-cell tumors. It has been suggested that decompressive laminectomy was effective because sarcomas tend to invade the spinal canal, causing circumferential spinal cord compression.

In the evaluation of patients suspected of epidural spinal cord compression, magnetic resonance imaging (MRI) has been found superior to myelography and computed tomography (CT) scan. Magnetic resonance imaging is significantly better than CT scan without contrast and compares favorably to CT scan with intrathecal contrast for soft tissue abnormalities involving the thecal sac, nerve roots, and spinal cord.

Outcome of epidural spinal cord compression due to osseous and soft tissue sarcomas is optimal if diagnosis is made early by emergent MRI while the patient is still ambulatory. Although treatment depends on tumor type and presentation, there is evidence for better neurological outcome with surgical decompression.

## III. RHABDOMYOSARCOMA

### A. Introduction

Rhabdomyosarcoma (RMS) is a malignant tumor derived from embryonal mesenchyme with the potential to differentiate into striated skeletal muscle. It is the most common soft tissue sarcoma of childhood, representing between 5 and 15 percent of all malignant solid tumors of childhood (Young and Miller, 1975). The peak incidence of the disease occurs between the ages of 2 and 5 years, with about 70% of cases presenting before age 10 years (Maurer, 1988). Rhabdomyosarcomas in patients older than 20 years are uncommon. In a review of the experience at the Armed Forces Institute of Pathology with 558 cases of RMS, only 15% occurred in patients older than 20 years of age (Enzinger and Weiss, 1988).

The clinical presentation of RMS is that of a painless mass that grows steadily and metastasizes via lymphatic and hematogenous routes. The four major histological types of RMS include embryonal, alveolar, leiomyomatous, and other. Histological subtypes vary according to both age and site. Primary tumor sites include the orbit, head and neck, cranial-parameningeal, genitourinary, trunk, extremity, pelvis, and retroperitoneum. Embryonal RMS is the most common histological type in children, and head and neck is the most frequent location in children less than 5 years of age. Orbital tumors present with proptosis; middle ear involvement results in pain and chronic otitis media. Nasopharyngeal tumors cause nasal voice, dysphagia, pain, epistaxis, and obstruction of the airways. Parameningeal lesions may present with cranial neuropathies and meningeal symptoms.

The most important prognostic factors in RMS are site and invasiveness. Patients are staged pretreatment or at diagnosis; they are grouped postsurgically by criteria established by the Intergroup Rhabdomyosarcoma Study (IRS). These groups include: group I—localized or completely resected tumor; group II—grossly resected regional or local disease with microscopic residual; group III—

local or regional disease after biopsy only or gross residual tumor; group IV—distant metastatic disease to the lungs, bones, or bone marrow. The overall survival rate of patients with RMS is nearly 80% in groups I and II, but only 25–30% in group IV (Malogalowkin and Ortega, 1988; Ruymann, 1987). Radiation therapy plays an important role in local disease control; vincristine, actinomycin, cyclophosphamide, and doxorubicin are the best-established chemotherapeutic agents.

The neurological complications of RMS are predominantly related to the primary tumor site and intracranial or intraspinal extension of disease. Head and neck RMS arising in parameningeal sites gain access to the epidural space by direct extension through cranial foramina and fissures, by erosion of the skull base, or by extension of tumor along the cranial nerves (Gaiger et al., 1981) to the leptomeninges, brain, and ventricular system (Tefft et al., 1978; Raney et al., 1987). Patients with parameningeal embryonal or undifferentiated RMS have an increased risk of CNS relapse (see Sec. III.B) either related to the recurrence of the primary tumor or as meningeal sarcomatosis (Brown et al., 1975; Chan et al., 1979; Tefft et al., 1978). Intracranial involvement can be secondary to direct extension, metastatic disease from hematogenous dissemination, or rarely primary RMS of the cerebrum. Orbital RMS infrequently involves the epidural or subarachnoid space. Epidural spinal cord compression from direct extension of paravertebral RMS is discussed in detail below.

## B. Leptomeningeal Spread of Parameningeal Rhabdomyosarcoma

Leptomeningeal dissemination of embryonal or undifferentiated RMS is a well-recognized neurological complication. The most important predisposing factor for meningeal involvement is the presence of tumor adjacent to or contiguous with the meninges, i.e., parameningeal RMS. Common sites of parameningeal RMS include the middle ear, mastoids, paranasal sinuses, nasal cavity, nasopharynx, and pterygopalatine and infratemporal fossae (Fig. 1). Parameningeal sites invade the meninges in 35–55% of cases (Tefft et al., 1978; Berry et al., 1981). Bone erosion occurs in 18% of all parameningeal RMS and in up to 67% of middle ear rhabdomyosarcomas (Dehner et al., 1978; Tefft et al., 1978). The specific criteria used by the IRS to categorize patients with probable or definite CNS involvement are described in Table 5.

Tefft et al. reported the first clinical IRS–I trial (1972–1976) that included 141 patients with head and neck embryonal RMS from 409 RMS patients (Tefft et al., 1978). Fifty-seven patients had parameningeal tumors, 35% of whom had direct evidence of meningeal extension at the time of diagnosis or developed such evidence within 12 months. Clinical evidence of meningeal disease included cranial neuropathies in eight patients and increased intracranial pressure in five

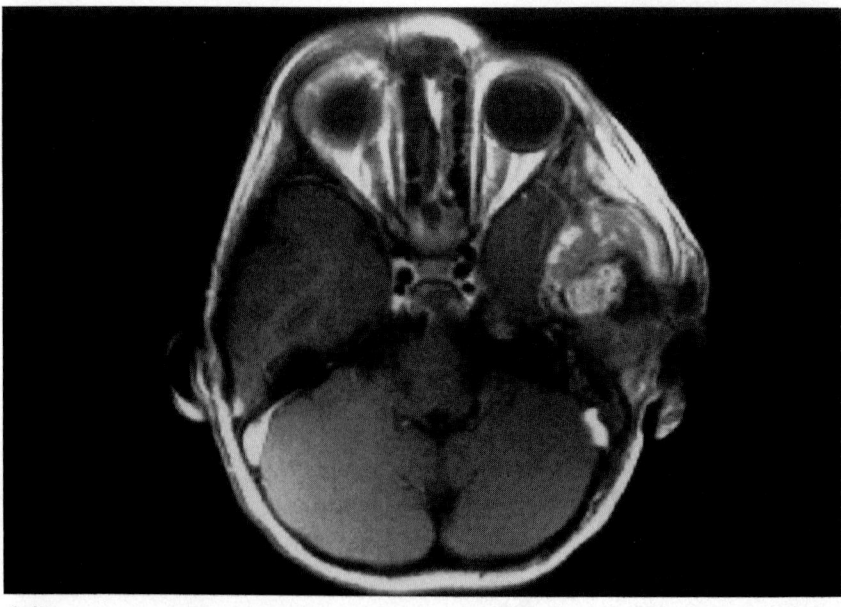

**(a)**

**Figure 1** Intracranial extension of rhabdomyosarcoma. $T_1$-weighted (600/22) magnetic resonance imaging (MRI) with gadolinium enhancement demonstrates rhabdomyosarcoma of the infratemporal fossa with skull base extension and intracranial invasion. Seen on (a) axial MRI but better demonstrated on (b) coronal view.

additional cases. Leptomeningeal dissemination was found by cell cytology or myelography in 10 patients with spinal cord block; however, cerebrospinal fluid was positive in only two patients. Cerebrospinal fluid is rarely positive in RMS. Concurrent evidence of bony erosion at the base of the skull was found in 10 patients.

Meningeal infiltration from parameningeal RMS is an important negative prognostic factor (Hutchinson et al., 1977; Tefft et al., 1978). A median survival of 9 months was reported in 90% of patients with meningeal extension from parameningeal RMS (Tefft et al., 1978). Poor survival in patients with meningeal involvement may have been due to inadequate radiation doses or treatment volumes. Although the adequacy of radiation treatment plans could be assessed in only 33% of IRS–I patients with parameningeal RMS, approximately 42% were treated with radiation doses below 4000 cGy and 58% with an irradiated tumor volume too small to encompass all known primary disease with a 2-cm margin of meninges.

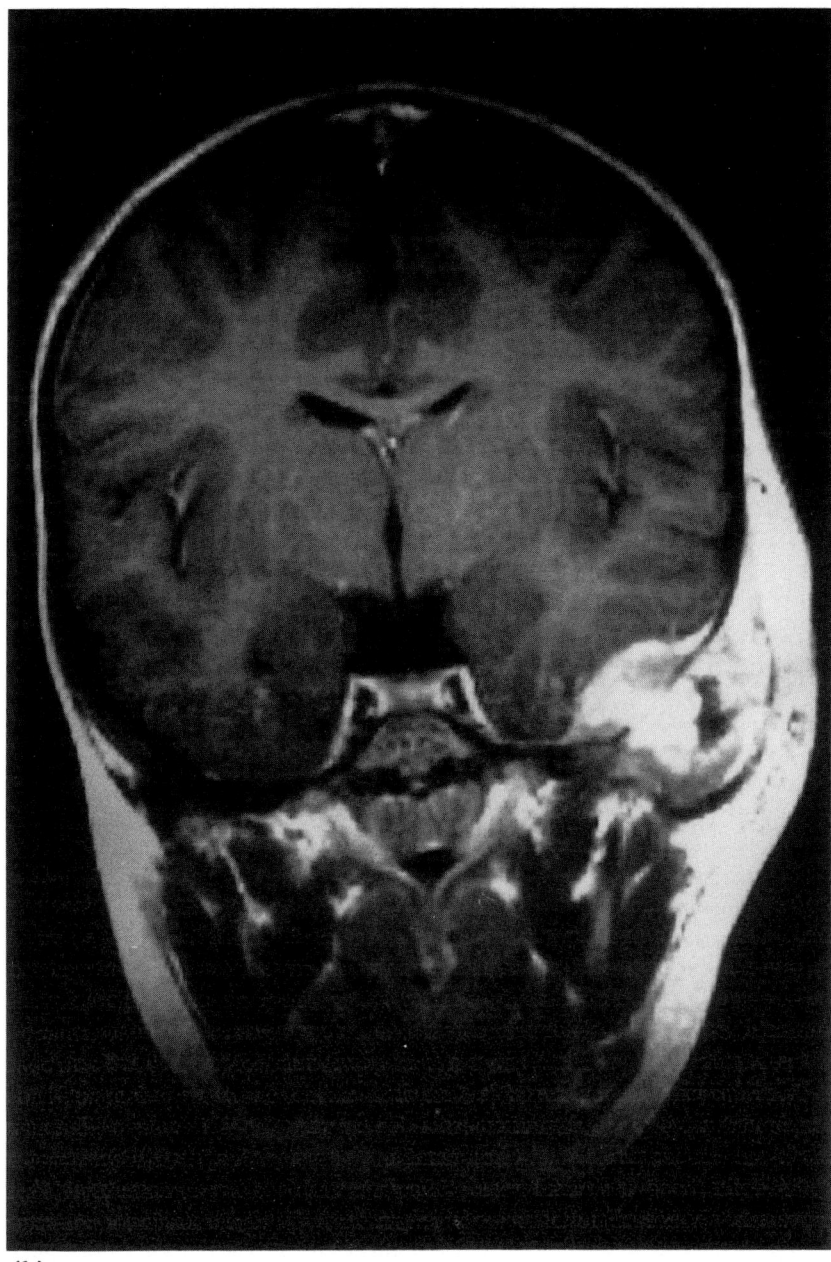
(b)

**Table 5** Head and Neck Rhabdomyosarcoma: Criteria of CNS Involvement[a]

*High Risk of Involvement*
    Primary in nasopharynx-nose, paranasal sinus, or middle ear–mastoid, or pterygoid-infratemporal fossa
    Abnormal cranial nerve function
    Enlargement of neural foramina
    Radiological evidence of eroded bone at cranial base
*Definite Involvement*
    Intracranial tumor by CT scan and/or arteriogram
    Tumor cells in CSF
    Spinal cord extension documented by myelogram

CT = Computed tomography, CSF = Cerebrospinal fluid
[a]Intergroup Rhabdomyosarcoma Study Specification

A different conclusion concerning the prognostic importance of meningeal involvement by parameningeal RMS was reported by Berry and Jenkins. In this review of 40 patients with parameningeal RMS treated at Princess Margaret Hospital, Toronto, from 1960–1977, 50% had pretreatment evidence of meningeal involvement based on at least one of the following IRS criteria: cranial nerve palsies; lytic destruction of bone adjacent to the meninges; intracranial extension demonstrated radiographically or directly visualized with exploration; malignant cells in the cerebrospinal fluid (CSF); intradural seeding by myelogram or increased intracranial pressure (Berry and Jenkins, 1981). These authors cautioned, however, that the true incidence of meningeal disease may have been overestimated, as bony destruction and cranial nerve palsies do not necessarily indicate meningeal involvement. In this series, all patients were treated with postoperative radiation therapy and 16 were treated with adjuvant chemotherapy. Meningeal involvement occurred in six of 35 patients at first or second relapse either as a local recurrence or as an isolated event with distant meningeal seeding. In contrast with the findings of the first IRS study, the 5-year survival rate for patients with meningeal involvement at initial presentation was not significantly different from patients without meningeal involvement (30% vs. 41%, respectively) (Berry and Jenkins, 1981). However, the small patient numbers and treatment differences may obscure a true difference between patients with parameningeal tumors with or without meningeal extension.

In an effort to improve the treatment outcome for patients with parameningeal RMS, the IRS protocol was modified. The Intergroup Rhabdomyosarcoma Study (IRS) conducted a second clinical trial (IRS–II) from 1977–1982 in which all patients with a high risk of meningeal involvement, defined by intracranial extension of tumor, bony erosion at the cranial base, and cranial nerve palsy, received CNS prophylactic therapy: whole brain radiotherapy and intrathecal chemotherapy with methotrexate, hydrocortisone, and arabinosylcytosine. Adjuvant chemotherapy consisted of vincristine and actinomycin D with or without cyclophosphamide and doxorubicin. Non–high-risk patients received local radiation therapy and the identical adjuvant systemic chemotherapy.

Results from this study, reported by Raney et al. (1987), indicated that high-risk parameningeal RMS patients who received intensive CNS prophylaxis had significantly better progression-free (57%) and total (68%) survival than less intensively treated patients in the first IRS clinical trial (33% and 41% for progression-free and total survival, respectively). The improved survival for high-risk patients seen in IRS–II was attributed to whole-brain radiation therapy. These encouraging results from IRS–II received further support from the German Cooperative Group in the CWS-81 study which also employed intrathecal chemotherapy and craniospinal radiation. These investigators reported a 50% relapse-free survival in 35 high-risk patients with parameningeal RMS after 60 months of observation (Kardos et al., 1989).

Conclusions from these studies have been extended to justify the use of widefield or whole-brain radiation in parameningeal RMS patients with any evidence of meningeal involvement. However, the improved survival in these studies may have been due to various other factors including (1) insufficient radiation treatment volumes and doses employed in IRS–I; (2) earlier initiation of radiation therapy in IRS–II; (3) use of intrathecal chemotherapy and more intensive parenteral chemotherapy in IRS–II; or (4) increased use of CT scanning in IRS–II, which allowed more accurate definition of tumor volume and intracranial extension, assuring improved radiation treatment planning.

Despite the encouraging results demonstrated in the IRS–II trial and by Kardos et al., the relative benefit of aggressive CNS prophylaxis for parameningeal RMS has been questioned in light of its significant neurotoxicity in children. The role of prophylactic CNS irradiation to prevent meningeal extension from parameningeal RMS was therefore prospectively studied by Gasparini and other investigators (Gasparini et al., 1990). Fifteen patients with meningeal extension were treated with a combination of systemic and IT chemotherapy and irradiation of total tumor volume, including a 2-cm tumor-free margin. These authors compared their results to their previous study which used similar chemotherapy in addition to wholebrain radiation therapy (Gasparini et al., 1983). The 3-year progression-free survival was not different for groups treated with local vs. whole-brain radiation therapy (59% vs. 64%, respectively) (Gasparini et al., 1983; Gasparini et al., 1990). These investigators concluded that CNS prophylaxis was questionable in the treatment of parameningeal RMS with meningeal extension, but both studies were nonrandomized and limited by low statistical power.

In IRS–III, the volume of radiotherapy was significantly reduced in patients with parameningeal tumors without intracranial extension (see review, Ruymann, 1987). Guidelines for the treatment of parameningeal RMS based on results of prior IRS studies are outlined in Table 6. For patients with intracranial extension and positive CSF cytology, management included radiation to the primary site and craniospinal axis with dose adjustment for age and triple intrathecal chemotherapy. For patients with intracranial extension and negative CSF cytology, radiation therapy was directed to the primary site, whole brain, and meninges, dropping spinal irradiation but including triple intrathecal chemotherapy. For patients without intracranial extension but with bone erosion or cranial neuropathy, radiotherapy is directed against the primary site, skull base, and adjacent meninges. If no bone erosion or cranial neuropathy is demonstrated, radiotherapy is limited to the primary site.

In summary, patients with parameningeal RMS are at high risk for intracranial tumor extension. With improved neuroradiological techniques, earlier diagnosis and intervention may be possible. Cerebrospinal fluid cytology is rarely positive in meningeal disease. Current IRS–IV guidelines for management of parameningeal RMS attempt to improve survival while judiciously using CNS irradiation in children. Patients with intracranial extension from parameningeal RMS receive craniospinal radiotherapy and intrathecal chemotherapy. Patients with cranial neuropathies and/or skull erosion and no intracranial extension are currently treated with radiation to the primary site, skull base, and adjacent meninges and with intrathecal chemotherapy. If there is no evidence of cranial nerve involvement or skull erosion, intrathecal chemotherapy is eliminated.

**Table 6** Guidelines for Management of Parameningeal Rhabdomyosarcoma

| (+) Parameningeal Intracranial Tumor Extension | | (−) Parameningeal Intracranial Tumor Extension | |
|---|---|---|---|
| (+) CSF cytology (rare) | (−) CSF cytology | (+) Skull erosion/ cranial neuropathy | (−) Skull erosion/ cranial neuropathy |
| Radiotherapy<br>(1) Primary site<br>(2) Craniospinal axis (dose varies with age) | Radiotherapy<br>(1) Primary site<br>(2) Whole brain and meninges (3000 cGy) | Radiotherapy<br>(1) Primary site<br>(2) Skull base and adjacent meninges with adequate margins | Radiotherapy<br>(1) Primary site with adequate margins |
| Triple intrathecal chemotherapy | Triple intrathecal chemotherapy | Triple intrathecal chemotherapy | |

## C. Orbital Rhabdomyosarcoma

Orbital RMS, the most common primary malignant orbital tumor of childhood, classically presents with proptosis, progressing rapidly over days to weeks. While the most common location of orbital RMS is the superomedial aspect of the orbit, it can also arise in adjacent paranasal sinuses, invading the bony walls of the orbit. The current standard treatment is biopsy followed by radiotherapy (4000 to 4500 cGy) delivered to all bony limits of the orbit. Orbital exenteration is reserved for recurrence. Survival rates in patients treated by this regimen are greater than 90%, with dissemination (3%) at the time of diagnosis and recurrence fairly uncommon (Hayes, 1986). Invasion of a parameningeal site at diagnosis has been found to substantially reduce the survival rate (Abramson et al., 1979). Irradiation-induced eye changes occur in a significant proportion of children with orbital RMS (Fromm et al., 1986; Heyn et al., 1986). In a series of 42 patients with orbital RMS, 32 patients (80%) had cataracts at a median age of 2.6 years, with decreased or complete loss of vision in most patients with cataracts (Heyn et al., 1986). Overall, patients with orbital RMS usually have long-term survival with few CNS complications.

## D. Cranial Neuropathies

Cranial nerve deficits are frequent neurological complications of head and neck RMS both at orbital and parameningeal sites. Seventh nerve palsies are frequently seen with parameningeal primaries or with compression of the facial nerve as it courses through the floor of the middle ear. Parotid primaries are also associated with peripheral facial nerve palsies. Entrapment of cranial nerves III, IV, and VI can result from tumor invasion of the cavernous sinus. This can occur with RMS located in the pterygoid fossa with intracranial extension through foramina in the petrous bone. Changes in phonation and difficulty swallowing may also result from tumor in the posterior nasopharynx (Ruymann, 1987).

## E. Epidural Spinal Cord Compression and Myelopathy

The reported incidence of epidural spinal cord compression (ESSC) with RMS ranges from 5.3% to 13% (Chien et al., 1982; Kramer et al., 1989). In contrast to other solid tumors in which ESSC is often a late event, spinal cord compression may be an early or the initial sign of malignancy in RMS. Kramer et al. (1989) found metastatic spinal cord compression in 13% of patients with RMS. In patients with RMS and ESSC, 57% had spinal cord compression as the presenting sign of their tumor (Kramer et al., 1989). The most common mechanism for ESSC in RMS was by direct extension of tumor from a paravertebral site. Conclusions about neurological outcome by treatment (surgical vs. radiotherapy or both) could not be determined from this review. However, in the SJCRH report, a trend toward improved neurological status with decompressive laminectomy was noted (Klein et al., 1991). The average posttreatment neurological outcome was better in six patients receiving decompressive laminectomy versus nine patients treated with radiation and chemotherapy for ESSC from RMS. (See Sec. II.B.)

Ascending myelitis after intensive chemotherapy and radiation therapy (RT) in children with high-risk cranial parameningeal sarcoma was reported by Raney et al. (1992). Five of 149 (3.4%) patients enrolled in IRS trials from 1977 to 1987 developed an ascending myelitis within 1 year of initiation of combined irradiation and chemotherapy. Four patients progressed from lower extremity weakness and loss of sphincter control to severe flaccid quadriparesis which necessitated long-term ventilatory support. Three had diffuse swelling of the cervical cord demonstrated by myelography. Pathology revealed necrosis of the lower medulla and spinal cord consistent with radiation damage in one patient. All patients had received 4770–5500 cGy to the primary tumor and four received 3000 cGy of cranial RT. All patients received four to seven courses of intrathecal (IT) chemotherapy. Three patients died: one with local and disseminated CNS tumor and two without known recurrence. As a result of the neurological deterioration noted in these patients, the IRS–III protocol was amended to reduce the intensity of intrathecal chemotherapy.

Epidural spinal cord compression is a frequent neurological complication of RMS and is treated either with decompressive laminectomy or radiation and chemotherapy. Ascending myelitis as a complication of intrathecal chemotherapy and radiation also may occur.

## F. Intracranial Rhabdomyosarcoma

The incidence of intracerebral involvement with RMS is 13%–27% (Kramer et al., 1989; Espana et al., 1980). It typically develops by direct infiltration of the cranial cavity, especially the posterior fossa. The incidence of intracranial RMS metastases from hematogenous dissemination, once felt to be rare, has increased together with increased pulmonary metastases.

In an early review of sarcomatous brain metastases, no RMS metastases were found (Willis, 1971). Gercovich reported three cases of intracranial RMS but two cases were head and neck primaries and thought to be contiguous not hematogenous spread (Gercovich et al., 1975). By contrast, from a series of 114 patients with systemic sarcomas, four of fifteen RMS patients (27%) had intracerebral metastases (Espana et al., 1980). The higher estimated incidence of intracerebral metastases with RMS was supported by other investigators in more recent studies. In a review of 139 children with solid tumors and postmortem examinations, 28% of children with RMS had brain metastases (Graus et al., 1983).

By comparison, primary RMS of the CNS is extremely rare. Fifteen cases have been described in the literature, 11 originating in the cerebellum and four in the cerebrum. (For review, see Min et al., 1975.)

Computed tomography (CT scan) and magnetic resonance imaging (MRI) are the primary imaging modalities for patients with parameningeal tumors (Scotti and Harwood-Nash, 1982; Yousem et al., 1990). In a recent neuroradiological review by Yousem et al., intracranial spread of tumor was detected in 12% of the 13 patients with head and neck RMS and in 33% of patients with tumors in parameningeal sites (Yousem et al., 1990). They suggested that coronal MRI was the best method for showing the extent of intracranial RMS.

In summary, intracranial extension of RMS is a frequent neurological complication, best visualized on coronal MRI. Hematogenous dissemination is rare but increasing with prolonged patient survival and in association with development of pulmonary metastases.

## G. Neurotoxicity of Rhabdomyosarcoma Chemotherapy

A detailed discussion of the neurotoxicity of chemotherapeutic agents is beyond the scope of this chapter and is addressed in Chapter 13. Of the various drugs that have shown significant activity against RMS, only ifosfamide and vincristine are associated with significant neurotoxicity. In a review by Pratt and coworkers, acute neurotoxicity developed in 11 of 50 patients treated with ifosfamide/Mesna (Pratt et al., 1986). Reversible neurological toxicity included encephalopathy, motor and cerebellar dysfunction, cranial neuropathies, and seizures. The putative mechanism of this neurotoxicity is the accumulation of high concentrations of the metabolite chloroacetaldehyde (Goren et al., 1986). Predisposing factors for ifosfamide neurotoxicity include high dose levels (e.g., $>4$ g/m$^2$/day) and renal impairment (Pratt et al., 1986; Antmann et al., 1989). The sensorimotor peripheral neuropathy and rare occurrence of seizures due to vincristine therapy are reviewed in Chapter 13.

## IV. OSTEOSARCOMA

### A. Introduction

Osteosarcoma constitutes 20–25% of all primary malignant osseous tumors. This malignant spindle-cell tumor produces osteoid and, at times, cartilage and collagen (Dahlin and Unni, 1977). There are many pathological subdivisions of osteosarcoma including osteoblastic, chondroblastic, fibroblastic, and telangiectatic types, as well as the more recently described small-cell osteosarcoma and the rare multifocal sclerosing osteosarcoma. This chapter will consider only the most common form—conventional osteosarcoma. The peak incidence of this type occurs between the ages of 10 and 25 years, coincident with the period of maximum growth velocity. A second peak in adults over age 40 years may be associated with preexistent conditions such as irradiated bones, Paget's disease, or polyostotic fibrous dysplasia (Wilner, 1982). Overall, 80–90% of osteosarcomas occur in the long bones, with rare involvement of the axial skeleton. A painful mass fixed to the underlying bone is the most common presenting condition.

After diagnostic biopsy, most patients receive preoperative chemotherapy and a limb salvage procedure. When limb salvage is not possible, tumor extirpation is accomplished by amputation or disarticulation. Prior to the era of adjuvant chemotherapy, early metastases to lungs and long bones limited the overall survival rate to less than 20% at 2 years (Marcove et al., 1970). Now preoperative chemotherapy, although still controversial, has been advocated to treat pulmonary micrometastases and improve the likelihood of tumor-free margins (see review, Jaffe, 1991). By contrast, postoperative chemotherapy is no longer a controversial issue (see review, Picci et al., 1988). The Multi-Institutional Osteosarcoma Study (MIOS) conducted a randomized controlled trial between 1982 and 1984 to assess the role of adjuvant chemotherapy for osteosarcoma (Link et al., 1986). Patients treated with multi-agent chemotherapy, including cyclophosphamide, bleomycin, dactinomycin, adriamycin, cisplatin, and high-dose methotrexate with leucovorin rescue did significantly better than patients treated with surgery alone. The projected disease-free survival for patients treated with adjuvant chemotherapy in the MIOS was 64% at 2 years and 60% at 4 years and was the same whether randomized or nonrandomized patients were considered. Currently most postoperative chemotherapeutic regimens yield disease-free survival rates that exceed 50% (Jaffe, 1989; Goorin et al., 1985).

Modern chemotherapy for osteosarcoma has altered the natural history of this disease. However, with prolonged survival, new targets for relapses include the brain (Danziger et al., 1979), heart (Das et al., 1983), and other sites. As a result, neurological complications with osteosarcoma have become more common. While treatment-associated toxicities such as seizures and acute encephalopathy caused by high-dose ifosfamide or methotrexate may complicate osteosarcoma therapy, the major neurological complications are intracerebral metastases and epidural spinal cord compression. These problems are more frequently encountered in patients with advanced disease and in patients with primary tumors of the skull or spine.

## B. Intracerebral Metastases

The increased incidence of intracerebral metastases is clearly related to increased patient survival. In early studies, lung and bone remained the primary targets of hematogenous metastasis and central nervous system metastases were rare. In 1967, Dahlin and Coventry reported an autopsy series of 152 patients with osteosarcoma, 95% of whom had lung metastases and 50% had bony metastases at relapse (Dahlin and Coventry, 1967). Only three patients (1.5%) in this study had cerebral involvement. Prior to the routine use of chemotherapy for osteosarcoma in the early 1970s, brain metastases were reported only as preterminal events or part of an autopsy series (McKenna et al., 1966; Dahlin and Coventry, 1967). At the present time, brain metastases are most typically found in the setting of widely metastatic disease with pulmonary involvement (Graus et al., 1983; Baram et al., 1988; Kramer et al., 1989).

In a series of 87 patients with osteosarcoma reported by Baram and coworkers at MD Anderson Hospital, 39 had pulmonary metastases, of which five (13%) developed intracerebral metastases (Baram et al., 1988). The clinical presentation of osteogenic sarcoma brain metastases in these patients was acute and severe: two had massive intracranial hemorrhage and three had status epilepticus. Surgical intervention in two patients provided dramatic but temporary clinical improvement. These investigators advocated periodic neuroradiological screening for early detection of CNS lesions in osteosarcoma patients with pulmonary metastases.

Intracerebral metastases with osteosarcoma increase with prolonged patient survival and development of pulmonary metastases. Treatment options include surgical resection, radiation therapy, and chemotherapy.

## C. Primary Intracerebral Osteosarcoma

Extraskeletal osteosarcoma, defined as a malignant mesenchymal tumor that produces any combination of osteoid, bone, or chondroid material and is not directly attached to the skeleton (Chung and Enzinger, 1987), may occur as a primary intracranial tumor. Reznik and Levelle reported a case of primary intracerebral osteosarcoma in an elderly man who presented with a left hemiparesis (Reznik and Levelle, 1991). A CT scan revealed a right-sided intrathalamic mass and the patient underwent a right-sided temporoparietal craniectomy and gross total resection of tumor. No attachment to the dura was seen. The patient died postoperatively from acute pulmonary edema. Postmortem examination did not demonstrate tumor at any other site. Only one additional case of primary intracerebral osteosarcoma has been reported, underscoring the rarity of this tumor (Jacques et al., 1976). Distinction of this tumor from metastatic osteosarcoma or primary osteosarcoma of the skull with intraparenchymal extension requires a careful search for an extraneural bony or soft tissue primary tumor.

## D. Epidural Spinal Cord Compression

The bony spine is an uncommon primary site for osteogenic sarcoma; however, osseous metastases to the spine are not rare in patients with end-stage disease or as an autopsy finding (Sundaresan et al., 1988) (Fig. 2). Thus, epidural spinal cord compression increases in frequency with advanced disease. In the St. Jude's

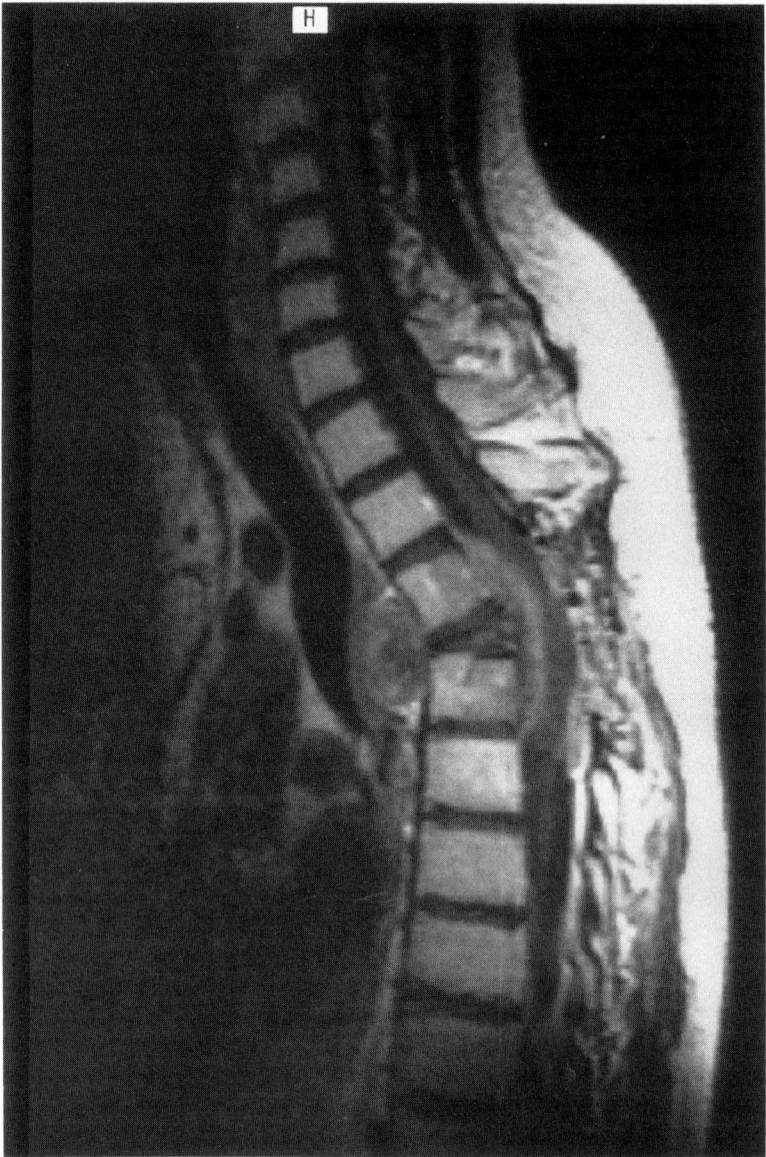

**Figure 2** Epidural spinal cord compression with osteosarcoma. $T_1$-weighted (600/15) magnetic resonance imaging (MRI) with gadolinium enhancement demonstrates epidural spinal cord compression from $T_3$–$T_5$ by osteosarcoma with vertebral body involvement and compression fracture of $T_4$ as well as prevertebral tumor.

Children's Research Hospital experience reported by Klein and coworkers, 6.5% of patients with osteogenic sarcoma developed epidural spinal cord compression (Klein et al., 1991). In this series, patients with metastatic osteosarcoma to the spine and epidural spinal cord compression were thought to benefit from surgical decompression with posterior laminectomy.

## E. Neurotoxic Chemotherapy in Osteosarcoma

The CNS toxicity of intrathecal methotrexate is well-recognized, as is the synergistic toxicity of intravenous methotrexate and radiation therapy (for review, see Phillips, 1990). However, high-dose intravenous methotrexate (HDMTX) alone is capable of causing MRI abnormalities in asymptomatic patients (Lien et al., 1991), serious subacute encephalopathy (Allen and Rosen, 1978; Fritsch and Urban, 1982; Jaffe et al., 1985; Walker et al., 1984) as well as fatal necrotizing leukoencephalopathy (Allen et al., 1980; Glass et al., 1986). These treatment complications are especially significant for osteogenic sarcoma patients because HDMTX with leucovorin (LV) rescue is of proven value as a cytoreductive agent as well as improving long-term survival (Grem et al., 1988; Rosen, 1986).

Allen et al. at Memorial Sloan-Kettering Cancer Center described seven patients with osseous or soft tissue sarcomas but without CNS metastases, who developed a chronic leukoencephalopathy after HDMTX (8,000–15,000 mg/m$^2$) and leucovorin rescue (Allen et al., 1980). For each patient, approximately 12 HDMTX treatments were administered over a 3–7 month period. No patient had cranial irradiation. Several months after beginning chemotherapy, patients developed progressive neurological deficits, with subtle personality changes, followed by decreased mentation, focal seizures, pseudobulbar palsy, spastic quadriparesis, and stupor. Computed tomographic scans revealed diffuse white matter hypodensity and atrophic changes including sulcal or ventricular enlargement in most symptomatic patients. Although white matter anterior to the frontal horns was the first to appear hypodense, most cerebral white matter was affected eventually. This syndrome affected the quality of survival, with each patient retaining varying degrees of neurological deficit, despite some improvement with discontinuation of MTX-LV therapy. Progression of systemic disease, not leukoencephalopathy, resulted in a fatal outcome in five of seven patients treated with HDMTX.

Subacute transient HDMTX encephalopathy has been reported most frequently in adolescents with osteogenic sarcoma (Jaffe et al., 1985; Allen and Rosen, 1978; Packer et al., 1983; Walker et al., 1984). Transient cerebral dysfunction following HDMTX chemotherapy (8.0 to 9.0 g/m$^2$) was described by Allen and Rosen (1978). Four of 158 patients developed acute symptoms of neurological dysfunction approximately 10 days after HDMTX with resolution of symptoms 72 h after the onset. Two patients developed permanent mild hemiparesis. All patients later were treated with HDMTX without reappearance of neurological dysfunction. The low frequency of acute and transient neurological dysfunction reported in this study has been noted subsequently by others (Packer et al., 1983; Walker et al., 1984). In contrast, Jaffe and coworkers noted temporary neurological dysfunction in nine of 60 (15%) patients undergoing HDMTX and LV rescue for osteosarcoma with repeat episodes occurring in five of nine (55%) patients (Jaffe et al., 1985). In their study, the methotrexate dose was higher (12.5 g/m$^2$) and the interval before initiation of leucovorin rescue was increased to 12 h, with treatments administered more often; however, the LV dose and schedule was increased as well. No permanent neurological deficit was encountered in any patient in this series.

To determine the incidence of asymptomatic MRI abnormalities in patients treated with HDMTX, 22 patients with osteosarcoma were evaluated by MRI of the brain either during HDMTX therapy or after completion of all treatments (Lien et al., 1991). No patient received intrathecal MTX or cranial irradiation. Sixty-four percent (64%) of these patients had high signal intensity abnormalities in cerebral white matter on $T_2$-weighted images. These lesions were most frequently located either adjacent to the lateral ventricles or within the centrum semiovale. The corpus callosum was also involved in five patients. The time interval between last MTX therapy and MRI was shorter in patients with positive scans. Approximately 86% of patients imaged within 2 years of the completion of HDMTX treatment had white matter abnormalities. By contrast, white matter abnormalities were found in only 25% of patients imaged 2 or more years from treatment completion. These observations suggest that the white matter abnormalities in asymptomatic osteogenic sarcoma patients are self-resolving.

Neurotoxicity from intrathecal methotrexate or combined intravenous methotrexate and radiation therapy is well described (Phillips, 1990). Patients with osseous and soft tissue sarcomas treated with intravenous high-dose methotrexate alone have a range of neurological complications including MRI abnormalities in asymptomatic patients, subacute transient encephalopathy, and even fatal necrotizing leukoencephalopathy.

## IV. EWING'S SARCOMA

### A. Introduction

Ewing's sarcoma, the second most common primary bone tumor of childhood, is characteristically found in the midshaft of long bones with the femur as the most involved primary site. It occurs most frequently in the second decade of life and is rare before 5 or after 30 years of age. Ewing's sarcoma is an undifferentiated round cell tumor that is vascular, occasionally hemorrhagic, and has no unique morphological markers. The diagnosis is often made by exclusion, after other "small, round, blue cell tumors" of childhood such as neuroblastomas, rhabdomyosarcomas, and primary sarcomas of bone are considered.

Recent cytogenetic studies have identified an 11,22 translocation in Ewing's sarcoma. This translocation is also found in malignant neuroepithelioma, a neural tumor arising outside the CNS (see review, Womer, 1991) and suggests that Ewing's sarcoma, primitive neuroectodermal tumors, and perhaps other small round cell tumors may be closely related and originate from embryonic neural crest cells.

The clinical presentation of Ewing's sarcoma is similar to that of osteosarcoma with localized pain and swelling. Systemic symptoms of fatigue, fever, and weight loss may be present, especially in patients with metastatic disease. Less common neurological presentations include primary vertebral tumor with spinal cord compression and/or symptoms of nerve root involvement, sacral primaries with neurogenic bladder and mandibular lesions presenting with lip and chin paresthesias. Currently, there is no uniformly accepted staging system for Ewing's sarcoma. Favorable prognostic factors include distal site of primary tumor and absence of metastatic disease at diagnosis. Poor prognostic indicators include pelvic and sacral sites for primary tumors and metastatic disease.

Prior to the introduction of adjuvant chemotherapy, the 5-year survival rate in patients with localized Ewing's sarcoma was only 10% to 25%. Subsequent prospective clinical trials demonstrated a significant benefit to intensive multi-agent adjuvant chemotherapy (see review, Meyers, 1987). The Intergroup Ewing's Sarcoma Study (IESS) reported a 74% 2-year disease-free survival in patients with localized tumor treated with whole-bone radiation and adjuvant chemotherapy (vincristine, dactinomycin, cyclophosphamide, and doxorubicin). After surgery, local control is best achieved by radiation therapy to this relatively radiosensitive tumor. Current treatment regimens require 3000 cGy to 4000 cGy to the whole bone with a boost to the tumor bed bringing the primary tumor dose to 5000–5500 cGy (see review, Meyers, 1987).

The incidence of metastatic disease at the time of presentation in patients with Ewing's sarcoma ranges from 10% to 30% (see review, Meyers, 1987). The lungs and skeleton represent the most frequent sites for metastatic disease. Although Ewing's sarcoma rarely originates in the vertebral column, spinal metastases have been reported (Pritchard et al., 1975). Unlike osteosarcoma, Ewing's sarcoma spreads to the marrow with the development of spinal metastases. At time of diagnosis, CNS involvement by Ewing's sarcoma is detected in less than 1% of patients and the CNS is an uncommon site for first relapse (Marsa and Johnson, 1971; Yu et al., 1990). Central nervous system metastases can occur late in the natural history of disease and in the setting of systemic metastases (see review, Trigg et al., 1981). More commonly, the CNS is involved by direct intracranial or intraspinal extension of metastatic disease.

## B. Epidural Spinal Cord Compression

Metastatic spinal cord compression is the most common neurological complication in Ewing's sarcoma. Myelopathy from epidural spinal cord compression in Ewing's sarcoma may manifest itself early in the course of the disease or even as a first indication of underlying cancer (Chien et al., 1982). Ewing's sarcoma tends to invade the spinal canal, compressing the spinal cord in a circumferential manner from vertebral metastases (see Fig. 3).

Epidural spinal cord compression was found in 17.9% of patients (30 of 168) with Ewing's sarcoma at St. Jude's Children's Research Hospital (Klein et al., 1991). Twenty of these patients underwent decompressive laminectomy while nine received only chemotherapy and/or radiation therapy. Patients treated by laminectomy had a superior neurological outcome compared with patients receiving chemotherapy. Although not statistically different, patients in the surgical group survived an average of 3 years longer after spinal cord compression than the medically treated group.

Kaspars and coworkers described a case of primary spinal epidural extraosseous Ewing's sarcoma (EES) and reviewed another fifteen cases in the literature (Kaspars et al., 1991). Patients presented with typical symptoms of spinal cord compression including back or radicular pain, paresis of one or both legs, sensory disturbances, and bladder and bowel dysfunction. Although all patients underwent decompressive laminectomy, complete resection was not possible in over 50% of cases. Most patients also received chemotherapy and/or radiation therapy. Ten of 16 patients (63%) died a mean of 16 months after diagnosis. Both local recurrences and distant metastases were common in spinal EES.

## C. Intracerebral Metastases

Intracerebral metastases from Ewing's sarcoma are uncommon and occur by direct intracranial extension of dural tumor (Fig. 4). In 1970, Kulick and Mones reported a series of 100 patients with Ewing's sarcoma and found only one documented case of intracerebral metastasis (Kulick and Mones, 1970). The following year, Marsa and Johnson reported the first case of "isolated" meningeal relapse in a Ewing's patient without evidence of systemic metastases. A second patient included in this report had pulmonary relapse prior to brain metastases (Marsa and Johnson, 1971).

Mehta and Hendrickson (1974) reported neurological symptoms in half of their patients with Ewing's sarcoma and extensive dural metastases in about one-fifth. This series predated the availability of CT or MRI neuroimaging, so it is unclear whether these were dural metastases or bone metastases with dural invasion. Kies and Kennedy noted this pattern of contiguous intracranial tumor extension from dural metastasis in Ewing's sarcoma (Kies and Kennedy, 1978). In this series, 16%

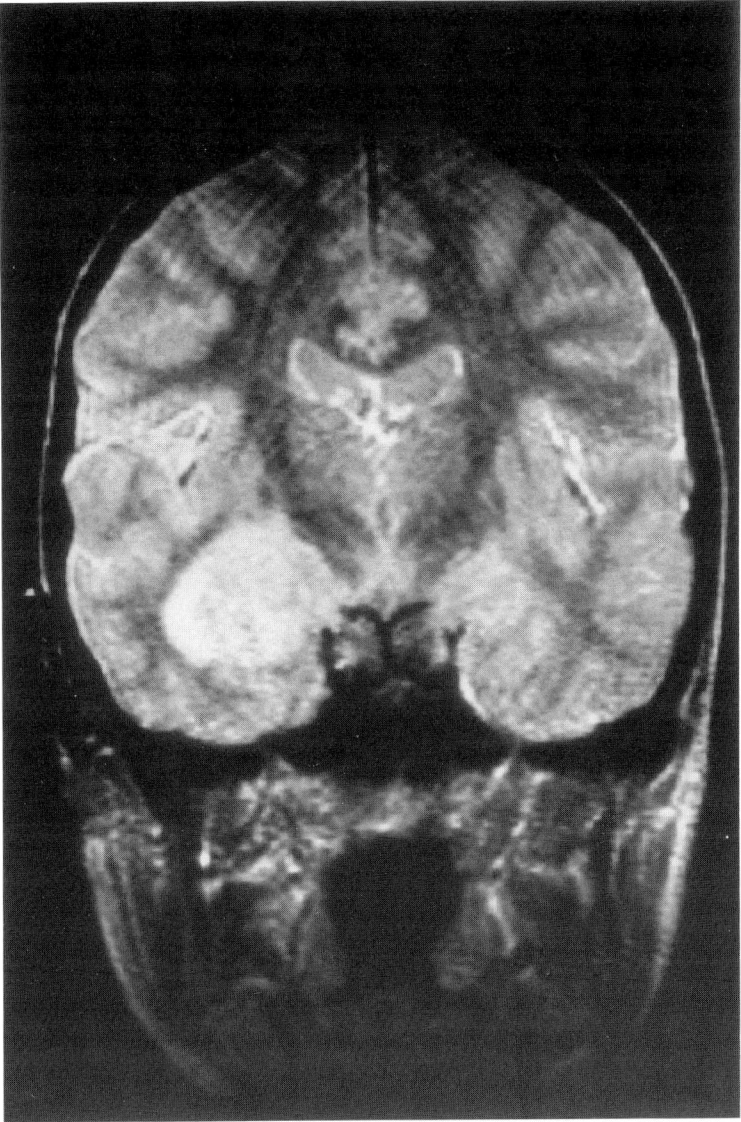

**Figure 3** Intracranial Metastases from Ewing's Sarcoma. Proton density (3000/30) coronal MRI demonstrates a mass in the right temporal lobe medially involving the area of the choroidal fissure and parahippocampal gyrus.

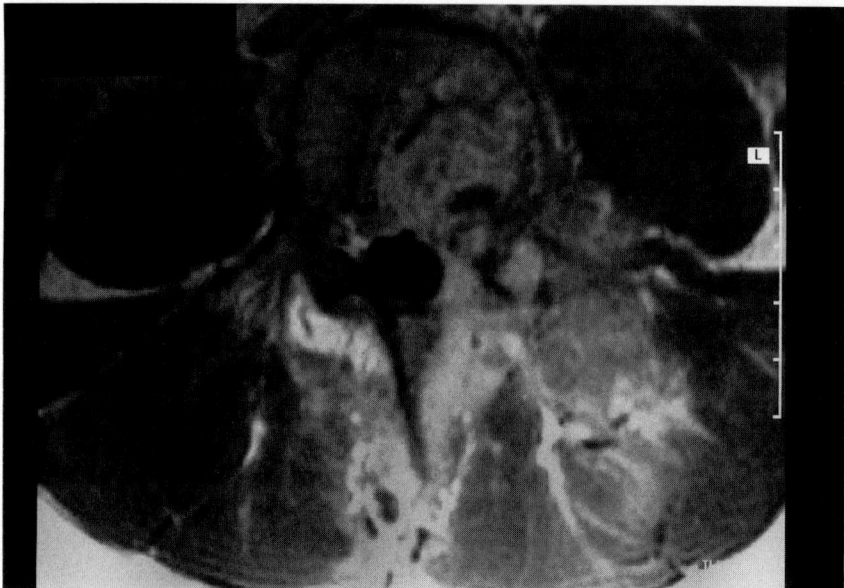

**Figure 4** Circumferential epidural Ewing's sarcoma. $T_1$-weighted (600/15/2) magnetic resonance image (MRI) with gadolinium enhancement after decompression with enhancing tumor in the vertebral body and epidural space (left greater than right) with extensive paravertebral soft tissue involvement.

(22 of 134) with Ewing's sarcoma had intracranial or meningeal involvement, but radiological documentation varied. Of the 13 patients with proven intracerebral tumor, three had intraparenchymal lesions without extension from the skull, suggesting hematogenous dissemination.

The occurrence of intracerebral metastases without adjacent bone or dural involvement was addressed by Trigg et al. (1982), who reviewed 161 patients with Ewing's sarcoma treated at the National Cancer Institute (NCI) and 284 patients from the Intergroup Ewing's Sarcoma Study I. The incidence of intracerebral metastases from Ewing's sarcoma was 2.2% (Trigg et al., 1982). No patient with Ewing's sarcoma had intracerebral tumor at diagnosis. However, in 0.7% of patients, the brain was the initial site of relapse. Cortical mass lesions were documented in 1.8% of patients and seven of these eight patients had a previous relapse at another site or simultaneous appearance of disseminated disease. Interestingly enough, four of the NCI patients with CNS involvement were part of a study group of 93 patients who had been previously treated with prophylactic

CNS irradiation (2000 cGy) and one dose of intrathecal methotrexate (12 mg/m$^2$). Currently, CNS prophylaxis is not included either in current treatment regimens at the NCI or Intergroup Ewing's Sarcoma Study protocols because of the low incidence of isolated CNS disease in Ewing's sarcoma.

Intracerebral involvement with Ewing's sarcoma occurs late in the history of the disease, usually in the setting of dissemination, and continues to be an uncommon site for first relapse.

## D. Leptomeningeal Dissemination in Ewing's Sarcoma

Leptomeningeal dissemination in patients with Ewing's sarcoma is rare and usually limited to case reports (Marsa and Johnson, 1971; Yu et al., 1990). In the series by Trigg et al., meningeal disease was uncommon, occurring in two of 445 patients (Trigg et al., 1982). Yu et al. (1990) reported two patients who developed CNS disease as the initial site of recurrence despite aggressive adjuvant chemotherapy. In one patient, leptomeningeal involvement was confirmed by CSF cytology. In the second patient, who presented with an intradural mass from $L_2$ to $S_1$, a diagnosis of leptomeningeal disease was confirmed by biopsy. Both patients remained in complete remission 24 months after detection of CNS disease and treatment with craniospinal irradiation or cranial irradiation with intrathecal chemotherapy. These investigators suggested that leptomeningeal dissemination with Ewing's sarcoma can be responsive to chemotherapy and radiotherapy and may not be a preterminal event (Yu et al., 1990).

## VI. SUMMARY

The importance of neurological complications in sarcoma patients is underscored by several factors. First, improved neurodiagnostic techniques, such as MRI and CT, have identified neurological involvement in cases that would only be confirmed at autopsy. Second, the true incidence of these complications appears to be increasing and may be due to improved therapy with increased survival.

The management of sarcomatous intracerebral metastases, single or multiple, remains controversial. Surgical approaches to single brain metastases in children and adolescents requires further study. Although patients with sarcoma and epidural spinal cord compression appear to benefit from decompressive spinal cord laminectomy, this too awaits prospective clinical trials. Finally, a greater awareness of the transient and permanent neurological sequelae of cancer therapy will aid rational treatment planning and reduce the risk of severe neurotoxicity that may seriously impair the quality of life for long-term survivors of systemic sarcomas.

# REFERENCES

Abramson DH, Ellsworth RM, et al. The treatment of orbital rhabdomyosarcoma with irradiation and chemotherapy. Ophthalmology 1979; 86:1330–5.

Allen JC, Rosen G. Transient cerebral dysfunction following chemotherapy for osteogenic sarcoma. Ann Neurol 1978; 3:441–4.

Allen, JC, Rosen G, Mehta BM, Horten B. Leukoencepathy following high-dose methotrexate chemotherapy with leucovorin rescue. Cancer Treat Rep 1980; 64:1261–73.

Antmann KH, Ryan L, et al. Response to ifosfamide and Mesna: 124 previously treated patients with metastatic or unresectable sarcoma. J Clin Oncol 1989; 7:126–31.

Baram TZ, Van Tassel P, Jaffe NA. Brain metastases in osteosarcoma: incidence, clinical and neuroradiologic findings and management options. J Neurooncol 1988; 6:47–52.

Barron KD, Hirono A, et al. Experiences with metastatic neoplasma involving the spinal cord. Neurology 1959; 9:91–106.

Baten M, Vanucci RC. Intraspinal metastastic disease in childhood cancer. J Pediatr 1977; 90:207–12.

Berry MP, Jenkins RDT. Parameningeal rhabdomyosarcoma in the young. Cancer 1981; 48: 281–8.

Brown MR, Sherry WE, Menkes JW, Feig FA. Occult recurrence of nasopharyngeal rhabdomyosarcoma manifesting as isolated increased intracranial pressure. Pediatrics 1975; 56:115–19.

Cairncross JG, Kim JH, Posner JB. Radiation therapy for brain metastases. Ann Neurol 1980; 7:529–41.

Chan RC, Sutow W, Lindberg RD. Parameningeal rhabdomyosarcoma. Radiology 1979; 131:211–14.

Chien LT, Kalwinsky DK, Peterson G, et al. Metastatic epidural tumor in children. Med Pediatr Oncol 1982; 10:455–62.

Chung EB, Enzinger FM. Extraskeletal osteosarcoma. Cancer 1987; 60:1132–42.

Dahlin DC, Unni KK. Osteosarcoma of bone and its important recognizable variables. Am J Surg Pathol 1977; 1:61–72.

Dahlin DC, Coventry MB. Osteogenic sarcoma: A study of 600 cases. J Bone Joint Surg [Am] 1967; 49:101–10.

Danziger J, Wallace S, Handel SF, deSantos LA. Metastatic osteogenic sarcoma to the brain. Cancer 1979; 43:707–10.

Das L, Farooki ZQ, Hakimi MN, et al. Asymptomatic intracardiac metastasis from osteosarcoma: a case report with literature review. Med Pediatr Oncol 1983; 11:164–6.

Dehner LP, Chen KTK. Primary tumors of the external and middle ear. Arch Otolaryngol 1978; 104:399–403.

Enzinger FM, Weiss SW. Soft tissue tumors. 2nd ed. St. Louis: CV Mosby, 1988; 448–88.

Espana P, Chang P, Wiernik P. Increased incidence of brain metastases in sarcoma patients. Cancer 1980; 45:377–80.

Fritsch G, Urban C. Transient encephalopathy during the late course of treatment with high-dose methotrexate. Cancer Treat Rep 1982; 66:1719–22.

Fromm M, Littman P, Raney RB. Late effects after treatment of twenty children with soft tissue sarcomas of the head and neck. Cancer 1986; 57:2070–6.

children with cranial soft tissue sarcomas arising in nonorbital sites. Cancer 1987; 59:147–55.

Raney RB. Spinal cord "drop metastases" from head and neck rhabdomyosarcoma: proceedings of the Tumor Board of the Children's Hospital of Philadelphia. Med Pediatr Oncol 1978; 4:3–9.

Reznik M, Levelle J. Primary intracerebral osteosarcoma. Cancer 1991; 68:793–7.

Rosen G. Role of chemotherapy in the treatment of osteogenic sarcoma. A five year follow-up on $T_{10}$ neoadjuvant chemotherapy. In: Kimura K, Wang Y-M, eds. Methotrexate in cancer therapy. New York: Raven Press, 1986:227–38.

Ruymann RB. Rhabdomyosarcoma in children and adolescents: a review. Hematol Oncol Clin North Am 1987; 1:621–54.

Scotti G, Harwood-Nash DC. Computed tomography of rhabdomyosarcoma of the skull base in children. J Comput Assist Tomogr 1982; 6:33.

Sundaresan N, Rosen G, Huvos AG, Krol G. Combined treatment of osteosarcoma in the spine. Neurosurgery 1988; 23:714–19.

Tefft M, Fernandez C, Donaldson M, Newton W, Moon TE. Evidence of meningeal involvement by rhabdomyosarcoma of the head and neck in children: a report of the Intergroup Rhabdomyosarcoma Study (IRS). Cancer 1978; 42:253–8.

Trigg ME, Glaubiger D, Nesbit ME. The frequency of isolated CNS involvement in Ewing's sarcoma. Cancer 1982; 49:2404–9.

Vanucci RC, Baten M. Cerebral metastatic disease in childhood. Neurology 1974; 24: 981–7.

Walker RW, Allen JG, Rosen G, Caparros B. Acute and transient cerebral dysfunction following high dose intravenous methotrexate. Proc Am Soc Clin Oncol 1984; 20:84.

Willis RA. Pathology of the nervous system. Vol. 2. New York: McGraw-Hill, 1971: 2178–96.

Wilner D. Osteogenic sarcoma (osteosarcoma). In: Wilner D, ed. Radiology of bone tumors and allied disorders. Philadelphia: WB Saunders, 1982:1897–2005.

Womer RB. The cellular biology of bone tumors. Clin Orthop 1991; 262:12–21.

Young JL, Miller RW. Incidence of malignant tumors in U.S. children. J Pediatr 1975; 86:254–8.

Yousem DM, Lexa FJ, et al. Rhabdomyosarcomas in the head and neck: MR imaging evaluation. Radiology 1990; 177:683–6.

Yu L, Craver R, Boliga M, et al. Isolated CNS involvement in Ewing's sarcoma. Med Pediatr Oncol 1990; 18:354–8.

Kulich SA, Mones RJ. The neurologic complications of Ewing's sarcoma: incidence of neurologic involvement and value of radiotherapy. Mt Sinai J Med 1970; 37:40–50.

Lewis AJ. Sarcoma metastatic to the brain. Cancer 1988; 61:593–601.

Lewis DW, Packer RJ, Raney B, Rak IW, Belasco J, Lange B. Incidence, presentation, and outcome of spinal cord disease in children with systemic cancer. Pediatrics 1986; 3: 438–42.

Lien HH, Blomlie V, Saetar G, et al. Osteogenic sarcoma: MR signal abnormalities of the brain in asymptomatic patients treated with high-dose methotrexate. Radiology 1991; 179:547–50.

Link MP, Goarin AM, Miser AW, et al. The effect of adjuvant chemotherapy on relapse-free survival in patients with osteosarcoma of the extremity. N Engl J Med 1986; 314: 1600–6.

McKenna RG, Schwinn CP, Soong KY, Higinbottom NL. Sarcomata of the osteogenic series: an analysis of 552 cases. J Bone Joint Surg 1966; 48:4–26.

Malogolowkin MH, Ortega JA. Rhabdomyosarcoma of childhood. Pediatr Ann 1988; 17:251–68.

Marcove RV, Mike V, Hajack JV, et al. Osteogenic sarcoma under the age of twenty-one. J Bone Joint Surg 1970; 52:411–23.

Marsa GW, Johnson RE. Altered pattern of metastasis following treatment of Ewing's sarcoma with radiotherapy and chemotherapy. Cancer 1971; 27:1051–4.

Maurer HM. Rhabdomyosarcoma. Pediatr Ann 1979; 8:11.

Maurer HM, Beltangady M, Gehan EA, Crist W, Hammond D, Hays DM, Heyn R, Lawrence W, Newton W, Ortega J. The intergroup rhabdomyosarcoma study—I. A final report. Cancer 1988; 61(2):209–20.

Mehta Y, Hendrickson FR. CNS involvement in Ewing's sarcoma. Cancer 1974; 33: 859–62.

Meyers P. Malignant bone tumors in children: Ewing's sarcoma. Hematol Oncol Clin North Am 1987; 1(4):667–73.

Min KW, Gyorkey F, Halpert B. Primary rhabdomyosarcoma of the cerebrum. Cancer 1975; 35:1405–11.

Packer RJ, Grossman RI, Belasco J. High dose systemic methotrexate: associated acute neurologic dysfunction. Med Pediatr Oncol 1983; 11:159–61.

Phillips PC. Methotrexate neurotoxicity. In: Rottenberg DA, ed. Neurologic Complications of Cancer Treatment. London: Butterworths, 1990:115–130.

Picci P, Bacci G, Capanna R, et al. Neoadjuvant chemotherapy for osteosarcoma: results of the prospective study. In: Ryan JR, Baker LO, eds. Recent concepts in sarcoma treatment. Dordrecht: Kluwer Academic Publishers, 1980; 291–5.

Pratt CB, Green AA, et al. Central nervous system toxicity following the treatment of pediatric patients with ifosfamide/Mesna. J Clin Oncol 1986; 4:1253–61.

Pritchard DJ, Dahlin DC, Dauphine RT, et al. Ewing's sarcoma: a clinicopathological and statistical analysis of patients surviving 5 years or longer. J Bone Joint Surg (Am) 1975; 57:10–16.

Raney B, Tefft M, et al. Ascending myelitis after intensive chemotherapy and radiation therapy in children with cranial parameningeal sarcoma. Cancer 1992; 69:1496–1506.

Raney RB, Tefft M, Newton WA, et al. Improved prognosis with intensive treatment of

Gaiger AM, Soule EH, Newton WA. Pathology of a rhabdomyosarcoma, experience of the intergroup rhabdomyosarcoma study, 1972–1978. Natl Cancer Inst Monograph 1981; 56:19–27.

Gasparini M, Lombardi F, Gianni C, et al. Childhood rhabdomyosarcoma with meningeal extension: results of a combined therapy including central nervous system prophylaxis. Am J Clin Oncol 1983; 6:393–8.

Gasparini M, Lombardi MC, Massimino M, et al. Questionable role of CWS radioprophylaxis in the therapeutic management of childhood rhabdomyosarcoma with meningeal extension. J Clin Oncol 1990; 8:1854–7.

Gercovich FG, Luna MA, Gottlieb JA. Increased incidence of cerebral metastases in sarcoma patients with prolonged survival from chemotherapy. Cancer 1975; 36: 1843–51.

Glass JP, Lee YY, Buner J, et al. Treatment-related leukoencephalopathy. Medicine 1986; 65:154–62.

Goorin AM, Abelson HT, Frei E. Osteosarcoma: fifteen years later. N Engl J Med 1985; 26:1637–43.

Goren MP, Wright RK, et al. Dechloroethylation of ifosfamide and neurotoxicity. Lancet 1986; 1219–20.

Grauss F, Walker RW, Allen JC. Brain metastases in children. J Pediatr 1983; 103:558–61.

Grem JL, King SA, Wittes RE, et al. The role of methotrexate in osteosarcoma. J Natl Cancer Inst 1988; 80:626–56.

Hays DM. Rhabdomyosarcoma: management in children and young adults. Curr Concepts Oncol 1986; 3–10.

Heyn R, Ragab A, Raney RB (for the IRS Committee). Late effects of therapy in orbital rhabdomyosarcoma in children. Cancer 1986; 57:1738–43.

Hutchinson RT, Raney RB, Littman P. Meningeal extension of head and neck rhabdomyosarcoma. J Pediatr 1977; 91:516–17.

Jacques S, Freshwater DB, et al. Primary osteogenic sarcoma of the brain. J Neurosurg 1976; 44:92–5.

Jaffe N. Osteosarcoma. Pediatr Rev 1991; 12(11):333–43.

Jaffe N. Chemotherapy for malignant bone tumors: bone tumor evaluation and treatment. Orthop Clin North Am 1989; 20:487–503.

Jaffe N, Takave Y, Anzai Y, et al. Transient neurologic disturbances induced by high dose methotrexate treatment. Cancer 1985; 56:1356–60.

Kardos G, Koscielniak E, Trenner J. Treatment results of parameningeal rhabdomyosarcoma in the CWS-81 study. SIOP XXI Meeting. Med Pediatr Oncol 1989; 17:313 (abstr 136).

Kaspars GJ, Kamphorst W, et al. Primary spinal epidural extraosseous Ewing's sarcoma. Cancer 1991; 68:648–54.

Kies MS, Kennedy PS. Central nervous system involvement in Ewing's sarcoma. Ann Intern Med 1978; 9(2):226–7.

Klein SL, Sanford RA, Muhlbauer MS. Pediatric spinal epidural metastases. J Neurosurg 1991; 74:70–5.

Kramer ED, Lewis D, Raney B, Womer R, Packer RJ. Neurologic complications in children with soft tissue and osseous sarcoma. Cancer 1989; 64:2600–3.

## C. Epidural Lymphoma

Approximately 5% of all lymphoma patients develop epidural spinal cord compressions secondary to their primary disease (37). This incidence is similar for both HD and NHL. Although it may unusually be the first symptom of lymphoma (38–40), most epidural lesions are diagnosed when extranodal or extensive nodal disease exists (37). With lymphomas, as with other tumors, the thoracic cord is the most frequently involved part of the spine. In contrast to other solid cancers, however, lymphomas frequently spread from paraspinous regions into the epidural space via intervertebral foramina. This sometimes results in a spinal cord compression despite normal plain films and bone scans, an important point for the clinician to remember in evaluating a lymphoma patient with spinal cord dysfunction (5,37).

The presenting symptoms and signs of epidural lymphoma are similar to those produced by other cancers. Although technically epidural lymphoma produces symptoms by compression rather than direct CNS invasion, ML frequently coexists. Because it will alter the therapeutic approach (i.e., exclusively local therapy for ML will likely result in eventual relapse at another CNS site), it is important to characterize exactly the pathological process. In a patient with suspected epidural lymphoma, a CSF examination is an essential part of the workup along with MRI or myelographic imaging of the entire spine.

The approach to treating lymphomatous epidural compression is similar to that delineated for other neoplasms (41,42, Chap. 3). Because the administration of steroids can cause a brisk oncolytic response, a lesion may be missed if undue delays occur before diagnostic testing is performed. Most lymphomatous lesions respond effectively to irradiation. Surgery is reserved for tissue diagnosis when the diagnosis is uncertain (such as when epidural lymphoma is the first manifestation of disease). Due to the radiosensitivity of lesions, therapeutic results in epidural lymphoma are favorable. Severity of weakness at time of diagnosis and treatment remains the most important prognostic factor of outcome. Therefore, the physician must maintain a high index of suspicion and be prepared to act before major dysfunction occurs. Effectively treated epidural lymphoma probably has little impact on the prognosis of these patients (43).

## D. Neoplastic Angioendotheliomatosis (Intravascular Lymphoma)

A unique, very rare complication of NHL involving the CNS is neoplastic angioendotheliomatosis (NAE). This entity is characterized by the presence of neoplastic cells within the lumina of small- and intermediate-sized blood vessels. The skin and CNS are preferentially involved. Clinical features are related to vascular occlusion by neoplastic cells which accumulate in small arterioles, outcome is not invariably fatal. Up to 25% of patients presenting with ML can attain long-term survivals (>18 mo) with intensive treatment (8).

## B. Intracranial Mass Lesions

While primary CNS lymphomas typically present as intraparenchymal mass lesions, discrete masses are less frequently encountered when systemic NHL invades the CNS. Nevertheless, approximately one-quarter of patients with CNSL will develop either one or multiple intraparenchymal lesions (5,16,30,32). Masses develop because of expansion and overgrowth of meningeal deposits as well as hematogenous spread. Certain lymphoma types such as mycosis fungoides, although rarely invading CNS, produce a disproportionately high incidence of mass lesions (33). Unusually, Hodgkin's disease can also produce intraparenchymal lesions (34). In addition, there is a correlation between the presence of intraocular NHL and CNS lymphomatous mass lesions which may represent either a multicentric or metastatic disease process (35,36).

In the patient who is at risk for ML, contrast-enhanced CT or MRI should be performed before spinal fluid examination if symptoms or signs suggest a mass lesion. Single or multiple periventricular lesions strongly suggest a diagnosis of lymphoma, especially in the presence of progressive systemic disease. However, the possibility that a mass lesion might represent another disease process, such as infection, must also be considered. In the instances where the diagnosis cannot be made with confidence, stereotactic biopsy may be indicated.

Lymphomatous parenchymal lesions are responsive to the effects of radiation therapy and will almost always respond to the standard regimen for intracranial metastasis (30 grays [Gy] delivered in 10 fractions). Because it is likely that small undetectable foci of ML exist in these patients, at least the entire brain should be irradiated. Sometimes, the administration of steroids results in a brisk lysis of tumor masses secondary to its oncolytic effects on this neoplasm. There are two corollaries to this observation. First, the rapid disappearance of an intraparenchymal lesion after steroid administration supports the diagnosis of lymphoma. Second, undue delays between initiation of steroids and surgery may obscure biopsy results.

When not contraindicated, a lumbar puncture should also be performed to assess whether ML is present. If the presence of ML is confirmed, some form of additional CNS therapy (systemic or intrathecal chemotherapy) should be considered after irradiation is completed. However, there are no data indicating that this is the optimal approach to this problem. An alternative strategy could be to defer CSF examination and any CNS-directed chemotherapy until after irradiation is finished. If no evidence of ML exists at that time, then further therapy can be deferred and the patient closely followed.

**Table 3** Useful Therapeutic Modalities for Meningeal Lymphomas

| Radiotherapy | Intrathecal or intraventricular therapy | Systemic |
|---|---|---|
| Whole brain[a] | MTX[a,b,c] | Steroids |
| Focal[c] | Ara-C[a,b,c] | High-dose Ara-C[d] |
| Craniospinal | | High-dose MTX[e] |
| | | Combination chemotherapy |

MTX = Methotrexate
[a]Ref. 7
[b]Ref. 8
[c]Ref. 30
[d]Ref. 26
[e]Ref. 27

Although systemic chemotherapy using high-dose methotrexate (MTX) or arabinosylcytosine (ara-C) has been used to treat ML with some success (25–27), most patients receive chemotherapy by intrathecal (IT) or intraventricular infusion. Either MTX or ara-C can be administered either along with or instead of radiation therapy (RT). Lymphomas respond to both agents more frequently than do other solid neoplasms. Although guidelines for administering intra-CSF chemotherapy are variable, the most widely used approach in adults is to administer either MTX 6.25 mg/M$^2$ (up to 15 mg per dose) with supplemental leucovorin (9 mg orally every 12 h for 4 days) or ara-C 50 mg twice per week. Once CSF cytologies revert to negative, the interval between doses can be gradually increased. Although it has been difficult to demonstrate a clear superiority of intraventricular over IT therapy in treating ML (8), utilization of an Ommaya reservoir combines the practical advantage of ease of administration with the theoretical one of better penetration into the entire neuraxis (28). Furthermore, in experienced hands, complications of Ommayas are infrequent (8,29). For these reasons, we prefer early placement of Ommaya reservoirs to deliver intra-CNS chemotherapy.

Using such an approach, both quantity and quality of life can be markedly improved in ML patients. Therefore, utilizing steroids, focal irradiation, and local chemotherapy, neurological symptoms are controlled in approximately 80% of patients (8,9,19,30), although median patient survival still is short, ranging from 1–8 months (7–9,15,19,30,31). Death usually ensues from progressive systemic disease. Favorable prognostic factors are young age, CNS involvement occurring as an isolated event, and receiving combined intra-CNS chemotherapy and whole-brain irradiation (7). Furthermore, when ML is present at onset of disease, the

Other radiographic examinations can also be helpful. The appearance of subependymal intraparenchymal masses or noncommunicating hydrocephalus on computed tomography (CT) or magnetic resonance imaging (MRI) scans suggests a meningeal process. Similarly, visualizing discrete nodules on nerve roots in the cauda equina on myelography or gadolinium-enhanced MRI also supports a diagnosis of ML. Even when cytologies are negative, patients may be clinically diagnosed as having ML with reasonable certainty if other features are strongly suggestive (Table 2).

The development of ML during lymphoma is associated with a very poor prognosis. Without treatment, median survivals after diagnosis are usually measurable in weeks. Therefore, an aggressive therapeutic approach using some combination of steroids, radiation therapy, and either local or systemic chemotherapy is warranted (Table 3).

Although symptoms and signs frequently exist which suggest a focal disorder, ML is a diffuse process. The entire CNS axis needs to be treated to ensure that all tumor is eradicated. Unlike its effects on most other neoplasms, steroids are more than just palliative when used in lymphoma patients. Sometimes, brisk oncolytic effects can be observed. Radiation therapy may be administered to the entire neuraxis to treat ML. However, this can be associated with increased neurological morbidity and myelosuppression that limits further systemic chemotherapy. For this reason, our preferred approach combines focal irradiation to areas of maximal neurological involvement (as assessed clinically and radiographically) with intrathecal or intraventricular chemotherapy.

**Table 2** Criteria for Diagnosis of CNS Lymphoma in Patients at Risk[a]

Definite (start treatment):
  Biopsy-proven CNS lymphoma
  Identification of lymphoma cells in CSF
Highly probable (can start treatment if clinical features otherwise consistent):
  Demonstration of thickened roots and/or nodules on spine MRI or myelographic studies in symptomatic patient
  Contrast-enhancing lesion(s) on CT or MRI scan in afebrile patient
Probable (should have both criteria present or abnormal CSF fluid profile before treatment considered):
  Communicating hydrocephalus
  Multiple cranial nerve palsies, multiple radiculopathies, multifocal CNS symptomatology, meningeal signs
Suspicious (consider further confirmatory tests before initiating treatment):
  Abnormal cell count or increased protein content in CSF without malignant cells

[a]Patients at risk are those with diffuse NHL histological subtypes (not well-differentiated lymphocytic lymphoma).

tissue, which may result in visible intraparenchymal tumor masses. The infiltrate in the basal meninges is most abundant around blood vessels and at the points of exit of cranial nerves in the subarachnoid space. The pathological findings suggest that the leptomeninges are often involved by extension from the medullary bone marrow cavity along perforating vessels through dura into the subarachnoid space (9,15). The frequent association of ML with leukemic conversion of lymphoma suggests CNS involvement may also occur as a result of hematogenous spread of tumor cells (6).

Meningeal lymphoma can occur at any time in the lymphomatous disease process. It may be present at time of diagnosis, can be clinically asymptomatic, can occur as a manifestation of relapse after a complete remission, or, most commonly, develop in the setting of progressive systemic disease (7–9,16). It may even be the sole manifestation of NHL, although this is distinctly unusual (17). Any neurological symptom may be associated with ML. Most commonly, patients present with a combination of symptoms involving cerebral dysfunction (i.e., headache, altered mental status), cranial nerve abnormalities (most often, the facial nerve), or spinal cord dysfunction (8,14). More unusual syndromes can occur. For example, bilateral optic neuritis has been reported in NHL patients otherwise in complete remission (18). Therefore, the clinician is well advised to maintain a high index of suspicion for the presence of ML and to have a low threshold for confirmatory testing when a NHL patient at risk develops neurological symptoms.

The diagnosis of ML is best made by identification of neoplastic cells in the cerebrospinal fluid (CSF). At least one CSF parameter is abnormal in virtually all patients with ML (19). Cytological examinations should yield lymphoma cells in more than 90% of ML patients if three examinations are performed and an adequate volume of CSF (10 ml or more) is obtained (8,14). Because ML may be present at the onset of disease and associated with no symptoms (8,20), all patients with newly diagnosed NHL of diffuse histologies should have a lumbar puncture performed as part of their staging procedure.

Although it occurs rarely, a characteristic eosinophilic meningitis is observed when HD invades the meninges (2,3). Thus, HD should be in the differential of any patient who develops an eosinophilic CSF pleocytosis.

Sometimes, identification of neoplastic cells cannot be made despite a high index of suspicion that ML is present. In these cases, other laboratory testing can be helpful. An elevated β-2-microglobulin level in serum and CSF can be an early indicator of ML. It is also a useful way to monitor the clinical course of patients with ML (21,22). Lymphocyte markers may also be useful in expediting the evaluation of ML if a monoclonal population of lymphocytes can be demonstrated (23). Recently, in vitro gene amplification by the polymerase chain reaction (PCR) has also been utilized to demonstrate chromosome translocations on CSF material. This test may have future application in ML, especially when the number of recoverable cells for analysis is small (24).

In this chapter, the neurological complications of adult systemic lymphomas are grouped according to whether they result from either direct invasion of tumor or a remote effect of tumor or treatment (Table 1). Primary CNS lymphomas are discussed.

## II. DIRECT INVOLVEMENT OF THE CNS BY LYMPHOMA

Lymphomas can invade the CNS at any time during the disease. Patients may have CNS involvement at presentation, develop it during progression of disease, or, most distressingly, develop CNS symptoms when the disease is otherwise in remission. Central nervous system invasion by lymphoma (CNSL) occurs frequently in NHL and is one of the more commonly involved extranodal sites. Approximately 10% of NHL patients will develop this complication. In patients with AIDS, CNSL occurs even more frequently (up to 25%) and is more aggressive and harder to treat than when it occurs in otherwise normal individuals (1). Lymphomas produce CNS symptoms directly by some combination of leptomeningeal infiltration, intraparenchymal mass lesions, epidural masses, or infiltration of blood vessels or peripheral nerves. More than one complication may be present in an individual patient.

### A. Leptomeningeal Involvement by Lymphoma

Lymphomatous infiltration of the meninges [meningeal lymphoma (ML)] occurs almost exclusively in NHL. Only occasional reports exist of its occurrence in Hodgkin's disease (2–4). The likelihood of developing ML varies as a function of the particular NHL histology. Diffuse histologies are much more commonly associated with ML than nodular ones (5–8). Even among diffuse histologies, the incidence of ML varies. Patients with well-differentiated cell types have a low incidence of ML. In more undifferentiated neoplasms such as lymphoblastic and Burkitt's lymphoma, the risk of developing ML may be as high as 25% over the course of the disease (7,9–11). Involvement of either bone marrow, testes, or leukemic transformation increases further the risk of developing ML in NHL patients (7,9,10,12). In addition, prior chemotherapy and young age also correlate with ML development (6).

Tumor implants are inhomogeneously distributed along the meninges. Infiltration is usually most pronounced at the base of the brain and surrounding the spinal cord (13,14). Tumor deposits result in gross thickening of the meninges and are often large enough to be identified macroscopically. In most patients, there is infiltration of lymphoma cells into the Virchow-Robin (superficial perivascular) spaces. Less commonly, tumor cells infiltrate beyond this into the parenchymal

**Table 1** Neurological Complications of Lymphoma: Summary Table

| Neurological complication | Signs/symptoms | Histological subtypes | Therapies |
|---|---|---|---|
| *Direct Effects of Lymphoma* | | | |
| Leptomeningeal lymphoma | Headache<br>Encephalopathy<br>Cranial neuropathies<br>Spinal cord dysfunction<br>Radiculopathies | NHL >> HD<br>More common in more undifferentiated NHL | Steroids<br>Radiation therapy<br>IT or intraventricular chemotherapy<br>Systemic chemotherapy<br>Combinations |
| Intraparenchymal masses | Headache<br>Hydrocephalus<br>Focal symptomatology | NHL >> HD | Steroids<br>Radiation therapy<br>Systemic chemotherapy<br>Combinations |
| Epidural lymphoma | Back pain, local and radicular weakness; myelopathy<br>Sensory level<br>Sphincter disturbance | NHL = HD | Steroids<br>Radiation therapy<br>Surgery (laminectomy vs. anterior approaches) |
| Intravascular lymphoma | Variable and fluctuating CNS or myelopathic symptoms/signs | B-cell lymphoma | Uncertain |
| Neurolymphomatosis | Painful neuropathy | NHL | Uncertain |
| *Indirect Effects of Lymphoma* | | | |
| Infections | Meningitis (*Cryptococcus; Listeria*)<br>Shingles (Herpes zoster) | HD = NHL<br>HD > NHL | Antibiotics<br>Acyclovir |
| Iatrogenic hazards | Cerebellar dysfunction (Ara-C)<br>Leukoencephalopathy (MTX + RT)<br>Infections (Ommaya reservoir) | NHL > HD | Symptomatic therapy |
| Paraneoplastic syndromes | Subacute motor neuronopathy<br>Acute idiopathic polyradiculopathy (GBS) | NHL = HD<br>HD > NHL | Symptomatic therapy<br>Plasmapheresis |

GBS = Guillain-Barré syndrome; HD = Hodgkin's disease; IT = Intrathecal; MTX = Methotrexate; NHL = Non-Hodgkin's lymphoma; RT = Radiation therapy

# 21
# Neurological Complications of Lymphoma

**Lawrence D. Recht**

*University of Massachusetts Medical Center, Worcester, Massachusetts*

## I. INTRODUCTION

The term lymphoma denotes a heterogeneous group of malignant neoplasms derived from lymphoreticular tissues. Approximately 30% of lymphomas are Hodgkin's disease (HD), which is distinguished by the presence of characteristic Reed-Sternberg cells. The remainder is a diverse group of neoplasms which are classified as non-Hodgkin's lymphoma (NHL). This subdivision is neurologically important because HD only rarely infiltrates the central nervous system (CNS) directly. By contrast, this phenomenon occurs frequently in certain types of NHL.

NHLs can be further subdivided according to the tumor's characteristic pathological features. Unfortunately, a uniform classification system has not been universally agreed upon. All classifications, however, are based on the characteristic architecture of the lymph node and the malignant cell type. From the viewpoint of neurological complications, it is useful to distinguish *nodular* from *diffuse* lymph node architectures because direct CNS involvement is much more common in the latter. Also, the less differentiated the cell type, the more likely the occurrence of CNS infiltration. Lymphoblastic and undifferentiated lymphomas are associated with meningeal involvement much more frequently than the less aggressive histologies such as well and poorly differentiated (small-cleaved cell) lymphocytic lymphomas.

chronic graft-versus-host disease (GVHD). Although uncommon, both inflammatory myopathy and myasthenia gravis have developed in such patients (62–64). Since genetically different donor lymphoid cells attack host tissues in GVHD, organ-specific antibodies may be the common underlying cause of these two disorders.

## REFERENCES

1. Wiernik PH, Canellos GP, Kyle RA, Schiffer CA, eds. Neoplastic diseases of blood. New York: Churchill Livingstone, 1991.
2. Thomas LB. Pathology of leukemia in the brain and meninges: postmortem studies of patients with acute leukemia and of mice given inoculations of L1210 leukemia. Cancer Res 1965; 25:1555–71.
3. Bleyer WA. Central nervous system leukemia. Pediatr Clin North Am 1988; 35: 789–814.
4. Stewart DJ, Smith TL, Keating MJ, Maor M, Leavens M, Hurtubise M, McCredie KB, Bodey GP, Freireich E. Remission from central nervous system involvement in adults with acute leukemia. Cancer 1985; 56:632–41.
5. Hardisty RM, Normal PM. Meningeal leukemia. Arch Dis Child 1967; 42:441–7.
6. Cash J, Fehir KM, Pollack MS. Meningeal involvement in early stage chronic lymphocytic leukemia. Cancer 1987; 59:798–800.
7. Bleyer WA. Leptomeningeal cancer in leukemia and solid tumors. Curr Probl Cancer 1988; 185–237.
8. Peterson BA, Brunnig RD, Bloomfield CD, Hurd DD, Gau JA, Peng GT, Goldman AI. Central nervous system involvement in acute nonlymphocytic leukemia: a prospective study of adults in remission. Am J Med 1987; 83:464–70.
9. Sheehan T, Cutubert RJG, Parker AC. Central nervous system involvement in hematological malignancies. Clin Lab Haematol 1989; 11:331–8.
10. Glass JP, Van Tassel P, Keating MJ, Cork A, Trujillo J, Holmes R. Central nervous system complications of a newly recognized subtype of leukemia: AMML with a pericentric inversion of chromosome 16. Neurology 1987; 37:639–44.
11. Bezu M, Pinaudeau Y, Poirier J, Dreyfus B. Involvement of the nervous system in hairy-cell leukemia (letter). Arch Neurol 1986; 43:432.
12. Fritz RD, Forkner CE, Freireich EJ, Frei E, Thomas LB. The association of fatal intracranial hemorrhage and "blastic crisis" in patients with acute leukemia. N Engl J Med 1959; 261:59–64.
13. Freireich EJ, Thomas LB, Frei E, Fritz RD, Forkner CE. A distinctive type of intracerebral hemorrhage associated with "blastic crisis" in patients with leukemia. Cancer 1960; 13:146–54.
14. Ernst E, Hammerschmidt DE, Bagge V, Matrai A, Dormandy JA. Leukocytes and the risk of ischemic diseases. JAMA 1987; 257:2318–24.
15. Creutzig V, Ritter J, Budde M, Sutor A, Schellong G, and German BFM Study Group. Early deaths due to hemorrhage and leukostasis in childhood acute myelogenous leukemia. Cancer 1987; 60:3071–9.
16. Cuttner J, Holland JF, Norton L, Ainbinder E, Button G, Meyer RJ. Therapeutic leukapheresis for hyperleukocytosis in acute myelocytic leukemia. Med Pediatr Oncol 1983; 11:76–8.

17. Grund FM, Armitage JO, Burns CP. Hydroxyurea in the prevention of the effects of leukostasis in acute leukemia. Arch Intern Med 1977; 137:1246–7.
18. Sigsbee B, Deck MDF, Posner JB. Nonmetastatic superior sagittal sinus thrombosis complicating systemic cancer. Neurology 1979; 29:139–46.
19. Nagpal RD. Dural sinus and cerebral venous thrombosis. Neurosurg Rev 1983; 6: 155–60.
20. Lockman LA, Mastir A, Priest JR, Nesbit M. Dural venous sinus thrombosis in acute lymphoblastic leukemia. Pediatrics 1980; 66:943–7.
21. David RB, Hadfield MG, Vines FS, Maurer HM. Dural sinus occlusion in leukemia. Pediatrics 1974; 56:793–6.
22. Feinberg WM, Swenson MR. Cerebrovascular complications of L-asparaginase therapy. Neurology 1988; 38:127–33.
23. Graus F, Rogers LR, Posner JB. Cerebrovascular complications in patients with cancer. Medicine (Baltimore) 1981; 64:16–35.
24. Minette SE, Kimmel DW. Subdural hematoma in patients with systemic cancer. Mayo Clin Proc 1989; 64:637–42.
25. Pitner SE, Johnson WW. Chronic subdural hematoma in childhood acute leukemia. Cancer 1973; 32:185–90.
26. Case records of the Massachusetts General Hospital (Case 7-1988). N Engl J Med 1988; 318:427–40.
27. Kimmel DW, Hermann RC, O'Neill BP. Neurologic complications of hairy cell leukemia. Arch Neurol 1984; 41:202–3.
28. Salata RA, Kling RE, Gose F, Pearson RD. Listeria monocytogenes cerebritis, bacteremia, and cutaneous lesions complicating hairy cell leukemia. Am J Med 1986; 81:1068–72.
29. Foreman NK, Molt MG, Parkyr TM, Moss G. Mycotic intracranial abscesses during induction treatment for acute lymphoblastic leukemia. Arch Dis Child 1988; 63:436–8.
30. Dykes A, Baraff LJ, Herzog P. Listeria brain abscess in an immunosuppressed child. J Pediatr 1979; 94:72–4.
31. Case records of Massachusetts General Hospital (Case 33-1991). N Engl J Med 1991; 325:494–504.
32. Wiernik PH, Serpick AA. Granulocytic sarcoma (chloroma). Blood 1970; 35:361–9.
33. Kim FSC, Rutka JT, Bernstein M, Resch L, Warner E, Pantalony D. Intradural granulocytic sarcoma presenting as a lumbar radiculopathy. J Neurosurg 1990; 72: 663–7.
34. Vinters HV, Gilbert JJ. Multifocal chloromas of the brain. Surg Neurol 1982; 17: 47–51.
35. Llena JF, Kawamoto K, Hirano A, Feiring EH. Granulocytic sarcoma of the central nervous system: initial presentation of leukemia. Acta Neuropathol (Berl) 1978; 42:145–7.
36. Barnett MJ, Zussman WV. Granulocytic sarcoma of the brain: a case report and review of the literature. Radiology 1986; 160:223–5.
37. Stillman MJ, Christensen W, Payne R, Foley KM. Leukemic relapse presenting as sciatic nerve involvement by chloroma (granulocytic sarcoma). Cancer 1988; 62: 2047–50.

38. Nickels J, Koivunieri A, Heiskanen D. Granulocytic sarcoma (chloroma) of the cerebellum and meninges: a case report. Acta Neurochir (Wien) 1979; 46:297–301.
39. Demaray MJ, Coladonato JP, Parker JC, Rosonoff HL. Intracerebellar chloroma (granulocytic sarcoma): a neurological complication of acute myelocytic leukemia. Surg Neurol 1976; 6:353–6.
40. Petersson SR, Boggs DR. Spinal cord involvement in leukemia: A review of the literature and a case of Ph+ acute myeloid leukemia presenting with a conus medullaris syndrome. Cancer 1981; 47:346–50.
41. Shalev O, Siew F, Yaar I, Rachmilewitz EA. Intracerebral tumor and diffuse central nervous system infiltration complications of acute myelogenous leukemia. Cancer 1979; 44:1066–9.
42. Krishnamurthy M, Nussbacher N, Elguezabal A, Seligman BR. Granulocytic sarcoma of the brain. Cancer 1977; 39:1542–6.
43. Henson JW, Wiley RG. CNS chloromas in patients presenting with eosinophilia. Neurology 1989; 39:1386–8.
44. Ripp DJ, Davis JW, Rengachary SS, Lotvaco LG, Watanabe IS. Granulocytic sarcoma presenting as an epidural mass with cord compression. Neurosurgery 1989; 24:125–8.
45. Hurwitz BS, Sutherland JC, Walker MD. Central nervous system chloromas preceding acute leukemia by one year. Neurology 1970; 20:771–5.
46. Mason TE, DeMaree RS, Margolis CI. Granulocytic sarcoma (chloroma), two years preceding myelogenous leukemia. Cancer 1973; 31:423–32.
47. Case records of the Massachusetts General Hospital (Case 45-1988). N Engl J Med 1988; 319:1268–80.
48. Pittella JEH, Fonseca de Castro LP. Wernicke's encephalopathy manifested as Korsakoff's syndrome in a patient with promyelocytic leukemia. South Med J 1990; 83:570–73.
49. Sharp RA, Lang CC. Hyperammonaemic encephalopathy in chronic myelomonocytic leukaemia (letter). Lancet 1987; 805.
50. Mitchell RB, Wagner JE, Karp JE, Watson AJ, Brusilow SW, Przepiorka D, Storb R, Santos GW, Burke PJ, Saral R. Syndrome of idiopathic hyperammonemia after high-dose chemotherapy: review of nine cases. Am J Med 1988; 85:662–7.
51. Currie JN, Lessell S, Lessell IM, Weiss JS, Albert DM, Benson EM. Optic neuropathy in chronic lymphocytic leukemia. Arch Ophthalmol 1988; 106:654–60.
52. Lossos A, Siegal T. Numb chin syndrome in cancer patients: etiology, response to treatment, and prognostic significance. Neurology 1992; 42:1181–4.
53. Fenaux P, Lai JL, Miaux O, Zandecki M, Jouet JP, Bauters F. Burkitt cell acute leukemia ($L_3$ALL) in adults: a report of 18 cases. Br J Haematol 1989; 71:371–6.
54. Kuroda Y, Fujiyama F, Ohyama T, Watanabe T, Endo C, Neshige R, Kakigi R. Numb chin syndrome secondary to Burkitt's cell acute leukemia. Neurology 1991; 41:453–4.
55. Case records of the Massachusetts General Hospital (Case 36-1989). N Engl J Med 1989; 321:663–75.
56. Kawai H, Nishda Y, Takagi M, Nakamura K, Masuda K. Saito S, Shirakami A. HTLV-associated myelopathy with adult T-cell leukemia. Neurology 1989; 39:1120–31.

57. Yasvi C, Fukaya T, Koizumi H, Kobayashi H, Ohkawara A. HTLV-associated myelopathy in a patient with adult T-cell leukemia. J Am Acad Dermatol 1991; 24:633–7.
58. Kurosawa M, Machii T, Kitani T, Tokumine Y, Kawa K, Maekawa I, Kawamura T, Miyake T, Kanda M. HTLV-associated myelopathy (HAM) after blood transfusion in a patient with $CD_2+$ hairy cell leukemia. Am J Clin Pathol 1991; 95:72–6.
59. Haberland C, Cipriani M, Kucuk O, Sarpel G, Ezdinli EZ, Ro JO. Fulminant leukemic polyradiculoneuropathy in a case of B-cell promyelocytic leukemia: a clinicopathologic report. Cancer 1987; 60:1454–8.
60. Phanthumchinda K, Intragumtornchai T, Kasantikul V. Guillain-Barré syndrome and optic neuropathy in acute leukemia. Neurology 1988; 38:1324–6.
61. Krendel DA, Albright RE, Graham, DG. Infiltrative polyneuropathy due to acute monoblastic leukemia in hematologic remission. Neurology 1987; 37:474–7.
62. Urbano-Marquez A, Estruch R, Grav JM, Grañena A, Martin-Oregg E, Palou J, Roznan C. Inflammatory myopathy associated with chronic graft-versus-host disease. Neurology 1986; 36:1091–3.
63. Bolger GB, Sullivan KM, Spence AM, Appelbaum FR, Johnston R, Sanders JE, Deeg HJ, Witherspoon RP, Doney KC, Nims J, Thomas ED, Storb R. Myasthenia gravis after allogenic bone marrow transplantation: relationship to chronic graft-versus-host disease. Neurology 1986; 36:1087–91.
64. Smith CIE, Aarli JA, Biberfeld P, Bolme P, Christensson B, Gahrton G, Hammarstrm L, Lefvert A-K, Lnngvist B, Mattell G, Pirskanen R, Ringdn O, Svanborg E. Myasthenia gravis after bone marrow transplantation: evidence for a donor origin. N Engl J Med 1983; 309:1565–8.

## IV. HTLV$_1$-ASSOCIATED MYELOPATHY (HAM)

Tropical spastic paraparesis (TSP) or HAM is a demyelinating myelopathy which presents with sphincter impairment, few sensory signs, and a progressive spastic paraparesis evolving over months to years. Initially described in Japan, it is now found in the Caribbean, South America, Hawaii, and in the southern United States among blacks. Retroviral infection with HTLV$_1$ is believed to cause the demyelination and perivascular cuffing seen in this disorder (55).

HTLV$_1$ also causes adult-T-cell leukemia (ATL), which is a rare malignancy of mature T lymphocytes with a predilection for skin involvement such that it has been misdiagnosed as mycosis fungoides. Though HAM and adult T-cell leukemia are both caused by HTLV$_1$ infection, they rarely coexist. Prevalence figures for HAM and ATL are estimated as 1 in 2000–3000 patients with HTLV$_1$ infection. This low rate, coupled with the longer incubation rate for ATL, is thought to account for the paucity of patients with both disorders (56,57).

One case of HAM has been described in a patient with hairy-cell leukemia but the HTLV$_1$ infection in that case was iatrogenic, from a blood transfusion used for the treatment of hemolytic anemia complicating the leukemia (58).

## V. LEUKEMIC POLYRADICULONEUROPATHY

Peripheral nervous system complications in leukemic patients are rare and generally due to tumor invasion of roots in the leptomeninges. Scattered case reports over the past 20 years have discussed patients who present with ascending a reflexic paralysis that mimics Guillain-Barré syndrome (GBS) (59–61). Many patients had active leukemia at the time of their GBS diagnosis, but it also has occurred in a patient in hematological remission (61).

Cerebrospinal fluid examination in most of the cases did not show the usual albuminocytological dissociation found in GBS. Often the CSF either was normal (60,61) or revealed elevated white counts with positive cytology (59).

The course can be fulminant and fatal within 2 months. Pathological findings have been diverse, ranging from a prominent dense malignant lymphocytic infiltration of dorsal and ventral nerve roots (59) to normal leptomeninges with infiltration of multiple peripheral nerves (61).

In one case, an 18-year-old boy presented with otherwise typical GBS, normal spinal fluid, anemia, and bone marrow infiltration with monoblasts. At autopsy there was loss of myelin sheaths in most cranial and spinal nerves without any inflammatory or leukemic cell infiltration. This case was felt to be an example of a remote effect or paraneoplastic syndrome (60).

## VI. BONE MARROW TRANSPLANTATION

Leukemic patients often go on to allogeneic bone marrow transplantation for treatment of their underlying disease. Of those who survive, 20–40% will develop

Treatment requires aggressive, early intubation, hemodialysis, and the use of ammonia-trapping agents, though their relative benefits have yet to be clearly proven. Hyperammonemic encephalopathy should be considered in any leukemia patient undergoing active chemotherapy who develops a metabolic encephalopathy—particularly if out of proportion to drug use or end-organ damage.

## II. CRANIAL NERVE SYNDROMES

### A. Optic Neuropathy

Progressive monocular or binocular visual loss as part of the presentation of acute leukemic meningitis is common, occurring in 30% of acute leukemia patients with CNS involvement (3). Pathological studies have shown diffuse infiltration of the optic nerve by leukemic cells with subsequent papillitis in the involved eye.

However, optic neuropathy is rarely reported in association with CLL. Three cases, one of which came to autopsy, were described in 1988 (51). All patients had previously asymptomatic CLL diagnosed 2 to 12 years before the onset of visual loss. Patients developed transient visual obscurations followed by central scotoma with decreased acuity and disk edema. Computed tomography scan revealed thickened optic nerves in all patients, and CSF contained 15–25 white cells with normal protein and glucose.

An autopsied case revealed a monoclonal B-cell population infiltrating nerves in a perivascular fashion. As a result of this finding, patients were treated with 2400 cGy to the optic nerves in six divided doses, with good return of vision.

Though uncommon, and easily confused with ischemic optic neuropathy, this highly treatable cause of visual loss must be considered in patients with CLL.

### B. Numb Chin Syndrome

Facial numbness in the distribution of the mental nerve occurs in many malignancies, particularly breast cancer and lymphoma (52). Of the leukemias, the rare Burkitt or $L_3$ALL is peculiarly associated with this disorder.

Representing 3% of ALL in both children and adults, $L_3$ALL has a very high incidence of CNS involvement at presentation, ranging from 35–83% (53). In a series of 18 patients with Burkitt cell acute leukemia, 10 had a mental neuropathy which in eight patients was the only neurological symptom. Cerebrospinal fluid was abnormal (positive cytology) in 50% of these patients. Why the mental nerve would be preferentially involved is unclear, though there has been autopsy demonstration of direct leukemic involvement of the trigeminal ganglion in the cavernous sinus with normal CSF and only scattered leptomeningeal deposits (54).

Whole-brain radiotherapy and intrathecal chemotherapy are routine but reported median survival has been only 6 months (53).

ated with white matter disease on CT or MRI scanning. There is no known effective treatment.

## H. Wernicke-Korsakoff Syndrome

Acute memory deficit for recent events (Korsakoff's syndrome) associated with ophthalmoparesis and gait ataxia makes up the clinical triad of Wernicke's encephalopathy. Myelin destruction and petechial hemorrhage are found at autopsy in the mamillary bodies, hypothalamus, thalamus, and periaqueductal gray matter. Thiamine is the only treatment known to reverse the disorder, and is usually given as 50–100 mg parenterally.

While strongly associated with alcoholism and starvation, this disorder does not often come to mind for patients being treated with chemotherapy. In 1990, Pitella reviewed cases of leukemia associated with Wernicke's encephalopathy and found four, three of which were autopsy proven (48). The most common symptoms were nonspecific mental status changes—stupor, confusion, and a short-term memory deficit. One patient exhibited the classic triad, which was promptly reversed with thiamine. All patients were felt to be nutritionally deficient and had been exposed to carbohydrate loading by intravenous glucose solutions without supplemental vitamins.

Because of the high frequency of confusional states in sick leukemic patients undergoing chemotherapy, it is likely that this disorder is underdiagnosed. Routine administration of thiamine in this setting is strongly encouraged.

## I. Hyperammonemic Encephalopathy

Unexplained coma in chronic and acute leukemic patients due to hyperammonemia is now well described (49,50). Beginning with insidious lethargy, patients develop coma and tachypnea leading to respiratory alkalosis and respiratory arrest. Increased intracranial pressure and seizures occur in association with plasma ammonia levels that can be elevated 20-fold (range 100–1500 µmol/L) above normal. Reviewed in 1988, hyperammonemic encephalopathy was diagnosed in 2.4% of patients on the acute leukemia service and in 1.2% of bone marrow transplant patients at Johns Hopkins Hospital. All patients had only mildly abnormal liver function tests at the onset of the hyperammonemia and only liver congestion or fatty infiltration at autopsy.

The mechanism for the development of hyperammonemia is unknown though it is associated in most patients with intensive cytoreductive therapy and profound neutropenia. Death rates from cerebral herniation are high (66%). Brains from seven autopsy cases showed diffuse cerebral edema and tonsillar herniation. The clinical and pathological changes have not been reproduced by any animal model. It is thought that the cerebral edema may be produced by an osmotic effect from accumulated intracellular glutamine, a byproduct of ammonia metabolism (50).

lung biopsy of a suspicious infiltrate and serial angiograms revealing progressive growth of the aneurysmal sac. Amphotericin B, flucytosine, and aneurysm clipping can all be tried, although, once again, outcome has been uniformly fatal (26).

## F. Granulocytic Sarcoma

Solid tumors composed of early myeloid cell lines have been called chloromas since they were first described in 1823 in a patient with proptosis from green retro-orbital masses. The color is thought to occur because of the presence of a certain myeloperoxidase. Since this feature is not always present, the term "granulocytic sarcoma," proposed in 1966, now is preferred (32).

Virtually all cases of granulocytic sarcoma are reported in children and young adults with the myelocytic or monocytic varieties of ANLL, with a reported incidence of 3–8% (33).

The tumor is thought to arise in the bone marrow and usually presents in periosteal sites such as the dura. The orbit and spinal extradural sites are favored, although chloromas have also been reported in the cerebrum (34–36), peripheral nerve (37), and cerebellum (38,39).

Spinal cord compression, lumbar radiculopathy, or cauda equina syndromes have all been described but are quite rare (40). Extradural leukemic infiltration and subsequent compression is the usual presentation, though intradural nodular deposits also can occur (33). The tumors are highly radiosensitive; therefore, local radiotherapy and systemic chemotherapy are the preferred treatment modalities, with little role for surgery.

Most intracranial chloromas reported in the literature are attached to the dura as extra-axial masses, but there have been isolated reports of intraparenchymal tumors, often in association with a positive CSF cytology and bone marrow relapse (34,38,39,41,42). Peripheral eosinophilia of 5–79% is also a recognized association (43).

When chloromas are the initial presentation of leukemia, diagnosis can be extremely challenging and the pathology confused with other small-cell tumors such as undifferentiated carcinoma or lymphoma (35,44). There are a handful of cases, in addition, where central nervous system chloromas *preceded* the development of acute leukemia by 1 or more years (45,46).

## G. Progressive Multifocal Leukoencephalopathy (PML)

Infection of the brain by the JC virus was, until recently, seen almost exclusively in patients with CLL (47). Progressive multifocal leukoencephalopathy is now more commonly associated with human immunodeficiency virus (HIV) infection, but should be considered in chronic leukemia patients with subacute dementia associ-

Gait abnormalities, headache, encephalopathy, and focal neurological signs suggest the diagnosis, which is usually easily proved by CT or MRI scanning. Focal signs may be subtle or unapparent.

Abnormalities of prothrombin time (PT)/partial thromboplastin time (PTT), platelet count, bleeding time, and DIC screens occur in the majority of leukemic patients with acute SDH (24,14). Because of the abnormal clotting parameters, surgery is often not possible and, even when accomplished without incident, can be accompanied by recurrent SDH. Dural biopsy searching for underlying leukemic infiltration should always be a part of the surgery, with additional radiotherapy given if discovered.

Chronic subdurals have been found in 10% of children with ALL at autopsy (25). These children often presented with focal seizures many months after their diagnosis of leukemia and without abnormalities of clotting parameters. Because of the improved survival of childhood ALL and the low morbidity of surgical intervention, chronic subdurals should be sought aggressively in such a clinical setting.

## E. Brain Abscess/Mycotic Aneurysms

Infection is very common during the prolonged course of immunosuppression associated with chemotherapy for leukemia and, as in other types of cancers, many organisms have been implicated (see Chap. 7).

Within the first 100 days after bone marrow transplantation, *Aspergillus* brain abscess is a common central nervous system infection and has a very characteristic clinical presentation. Associated manifestations include pulmonary infiltrates, paranasal sinusitis, and persistent fevers.

Patients with *Aspergillus* brain abscess often present in a strokelike fashion with focal neurological deficits within a single vascular territory, so the true nature of the initial illness may not be suspected. Unlike the patient with a simple ischemic infarct, however, these patients worsen rapidly over a few days.

Despite early diagnosis, which usually requires a brain biopsy and treatment with amphotericin B, outcome in reported cases has been uniformly fatal (26,27). Adequate tissue diagnosis is important, because there have been patients with *Listeria* and *Candida* brain abscesses, clinically indistinguishable from aspergillosis, who have had a complete recovery from their CNS infection (28–30). Aspergillosis, like mucormycosis, can also present as an orbital apex syndrome or cavernous sinus thrombosis with rapid invasion of adjacent structures in the immunocompromised host (31).

True fungal mycotic aneurysms also can occur, leading to rupture and subarachnoid hemorrhage. Pathological studies have revealed vascular invasion, thrombosis in neighboring arteries and aneurysms, often multiple, on large proximal arteries, commonly the basilar. Diagnosis sometimes can be made by leukocyte counts in the chronic leukemias are well tolerated (14,15). Both oral hydroxyurea (50–100 mg per kg) and leukapheresis (16) have been effective in rapidly lowering blast counts, often as much as 50% within days (17).

Other causes of hemorrhage are thrombocytopenia and disseminated intravascular coagulation (DIC). Acute promyelocytic leukemia may cause a bleeding diathesis, including bruising, DIC, and intracerebral hemorrhage. Symptomatic leukemic patients with platelet counts less than 20,000 should be treated with platelet transfusions in order to reduce the risk of intracerebral bleeding.

## C. Venous Sinus Thrombosis

Sagittal sinus or cortical vein thrombosis can be very difficult to diagnose. Patients present with headache or focal seizures and can go on to develop lethargy, hemiplegia, visual field deficits, or coma.

Pathological studies have shown venous sinuses occluded with organizing thrombus and subsequent hemorrhagic infarctions that often occur symmetrically around the superior sagittal sinus, typically in the occipital and parietal lobes (18). Concomitant leukemic infiltration through the dura forming the walls of the sinuses has been demonstrated at autopsy (19), though this disorder can also occur in the setting of dehydration, petrositis, or L-asparaginase chemotherapy (20,21). Venous stasis, slow blood flow near the torcula, and abnormalities in the fibrinolytic pathways all contribute to the development of decreased venous drainage, increasing intracranial pressure and eventual venous infarction.

Diagnosis is aided by finding an increased opening pressure and red blood cells on a spinal tap. Computed tomography scan can show subtle areas of decreased attenuation within the brain posteriorly and symmetrically around an "empty delta sign" (fresh thrombus seen as a negative image within a triangle of contrast in the sinus). Magnetic resonance imaging scan reveals an absence of the usual flow void in the sinus and angiography show lack of filling in the late venous phase. In all the radiological studies mentioned, findings can be very subtle and easily missed by the radiologist unless the clinician specifically suggests the possibility of sagittal sinus thrombosis.

Many patients make an uneventful recovery after spontaneous recanalization but others go on to progressive decline and death. Therapy consists of mannitol and dexamethasone to decrease elevated intracranial pressure (22). Although there have been recent attempts to recanalize occluded sinuses with streptokinase (23), the use of anticoagulants is controversial, and probably best avoided, because of the concern about augmenting the risk of serious hemorrhage.

## D. Subdural Hematoma

Acute subdural hematoma (SDH) occurs more often in patients with hematological malignancies than with solid tumors, though, as a symptomatic clinical problem, it remains uncommon.

types to identify a monoclonal, and therefore malignant, population of lymphocytes can increase diagnostic yield (6).

Magnetic resonance imaging (MRI) of the head with gadolinium or computed tomography (CT) of the head with contrast can identify nodular leptomeningeal deposits or subtle meningeal enhancement, a finding that helps solidify the diagnosis. Staging myelography or spinal MRI scanning with gadolinium can identify nodular nerve root disease or frank spinal cord compression that should be treated with focal radiotherapy, in addition to whole-brain radiotherapy and intrathecal chemotherapy.

Placement of an Ommaya reservoir optimizes delivery of drug to the cranial compartment and is better tolerated by the patient than multiple lumbar spinal taps (7). The usual regimen is 12 mg of preservative-free methotrexate placed in the intrathecal space every 3 to 4 days until the CSF clears of malignant cells. Maintenance therapy consists of additional doses of intrathecal methotrexate once a month.

As noted, ALL is so commonly associated with leptomeningeal disease that patients are now routinely treated prophylactically prior to the development of symptoms or a positive CSF cytology. Leptomeningeal leukemia, much less common in ANLL, is most often of the acute myelomonocytic subtype (M4). Bone marrow eosinophilia and pericentric inversion of chromosome 16 may increase the risk of CNS involvement in ANLL (8–10).

Though extremely rare, meningeal involvement can occur in CLL (chronic lymphocytic leukemia) (6) and hairy-cell leukemia (11).

## B. Intracerebral Hemorrhage

Intracerebral hemorrhage may present with sudden loss of consciousness and catastrophic neurological sequela or, more subtly, with headache, confusion, and focal neurological deficits. Patients with acute leukemia and blast crisis who have markedly elevated leukocyte counts (greater than $300,000/\mu l$) have a 60% chance of dying from intracranial hemorrhage in the first few weeks following the peak of their white counts (12). This complication is much more common in ANLL, particularly the acute myelocytic form, than in ALL. The clinical situation that calls for urgent therapy, therefore, is a patient with ANLL and a white count greater than 300,000 presenting with hyperleukocytic symptoms of dizziness, tinnitus, blurred vision, stupor, papilledema, and distention of retinal veins or "box car" formation. Pathological studies have clearly demonstrated thin-walled cerebral vessels distended with leukemic cells, the formation of intracerebral leukemic nodules, and subsequent peritumoral hemorrhage (13). This produces a rather characteristic cerebral hemorrhage which is sharply demarcated and confined to the white matter.

White cell diffusion studies have suggested that it is the large, nondeformable myeloblasts and lymphoblasts that prevent proper blood flow through the microvasculature and lead to this phenomenon. This may explain why similar high

| Condition | Sx | Diagnosis | Leukemia type | Rx |
|---|---|---|---|---|
| Wernicke-Korsakoff | Anorexia Prolonged IV glucose + chemotherapy | Clinical diagnosis | ANLL > ALL | Thiamine IV, 50–100 mg |
| Hyperammonemic encephalopathy | Unexplained coma Respiratory alkalosis | Plasma Ammonia > 2× normal | Any leukemia + cytoreductive therapy or s/p BMT | Intubation Dialysis Ammonia-trapping agents |
| Optic neuropathy | Progressive optic atrophy with loss acuity + VF 2° leukemic infiltrates into optic nerve | Clinical diagnosis ⊕ CSF cytology Enlarged optic nerves on CT/MRI scan | CLL ALL | Optic nerve irradiation |
| Numb chin syndrome | Uni- or bilateral chin numbness | Mandibular x-ray + CSF cytology | Burkitt's cell ALL ($L_3$ ALL) | Radiotherapy |
| Lumbar radiculopathy or cauda equina syndrome 2° granulocytic sarcoma | Back pain Bowel/bladder complaints | Uni- or bilateral radicular weakness/sensory findings in lumbosacral roots | ANLL | Radiotherapy Systemic chemotherapy |
| $HTLV_1$-associated myelopathy (HAM) | Subacute spastic paraparesis in black or Japanese patient | ⊕ $HTLV_1$ Ab blood/CSF Otherwise normal CSF | T-cell leukemia | Steroids |
| Leukemic polyneuritis | Areflexic paralysis (GBS) | Acute sensorimotor neuropathy | CLL (B-cell prolymphocytic) ANLL | Intrathecal therapy if CSF cytology ⊕ |
| Inflammatory myopathy | Subacute proximal weakness | Muscle biopsy | Leukemia s/p BMT with chronic GVHD | Prednisone Cyclosporine |
| Myasthenia gravis | Generalized fluctuating weakness | ⊕ Ach Rab | Leukemia s/p BMT with chronic GVHD | Prednisone Cyclosporine |

Abbreviations: ⊕: Positive; ALL: Acute lymphocytic leukemia; ANLL: Acute nonlymphocytic leukemia; Sx: Symptoms; RT: Radiotherapy; IT: Intrathecal; HA: Headache; WM: White matter; ICP: Intracranial pressure; CLL: Chronic lymphocytic leukemia; SAH: Subarachnoid hemorrhage; WBRT: Whole-brain radiotherapy; CSF: Cerebrospinal fluid; BMT: Bone marrow transplant; GVHD: Graft-versus-host disease; $HTLV_1$: Human T-cell lymphoma virus; Ab: Antibody; VF: Visual field; GBS: Guillain-Barré syndrome; Ach Rab: Acetylcholine receptor antibody; RBC: Red blood cell; CT: Computed tomography; MRI: Magnetic resonance imaging; SDH: Subdural hematoma; Rx: Therapy; XRT: Local radiotherapy; q: Every; N/V: Nausea/vomiting; S/P: status/post.

**Table 2** Diagnosis and Treatment of Common Clinical Syndromes Associated with Leukemia

| Neurological disorder | Presenting symptoms and signs | Diagnosis | Tumor type | Therapeutic options |
|---|---|---|---|---|
| Leukemic meningitis | Asymptomatic (or see Chapter 3) | CSF ↓ glucose, ↑ protein, ⊕ cytology, Immunohistochemical staining ⊕ clonal B population | ALL > ANLL (M4) >> Chronic leukemias | Pre-sx: cranial RT 18 Gy + IT Mtx × 5 q 3–4 days (12 mg) [*ALL only*] Sx: craniospinal RT 24 Gy + IT Mtx 12 mg (Ommaya if possible) |
| Intracerebral hemorrhage (intracerebral leukostasis) (thrombocytopenia) | Acute HA plus obtundation with focal cerebral signs | Large WM hemorrhage >200,000 blasts/µl <20,000 platelets | ANLL (especially acute promyelocytic M3) | Urgent hydroxyureas Leukapheresis *prior to* symptoms Platelet transfusion |
| Dural venous sinus thrombosis (idiopathic, leukemic, infiltrative, L-asp.) | Fever, HA, ↑ ICP, seizures | ↑ CSF protein, ↑ RBCs, ↑ Opening pressure ⊕ Angio (venous phase) or MRI | ALL > ANLL | Decadron, mannitol to ↓ICP |
| Chronic SDH | HA, ↑ICP | CT: extra-axial mass | ALL (>10% incidence) | Surgical evacuation (+ dural biopsy) |
| Brain abscess (aspergillosis, candida, listeria) | HA, abrupt focal weakness, pulmonary infiltrate | Ring-enhancing lesion on CT/MRI Brain biopsy | Hairy-cell ALL any S/P BMT | Amphotericin Flucytosine |
| Mycotic aneurysms (aspergillosis) | HA, SAH | Serial angiography | ANLL | Craniotomy + clipping vs. amphotericin + flucytosine |
| Intracranial chloroma | HA, N/V | Papilledema, hypereosinophilia | ANLL $M_2$, $M_4$ subtypes | XRT Systemic chemotherapy |
| Progressive multifocal leukoencephalopathy | Subacute dementia + visual defects | White matter disease on CT/MRI Brain biopsy | CLL | None |

Because of these observations, routine prophylactic treatment of the central nervous system for ALL patients was instituted in the 1970s (3). Subsequent recognition of the potential for neurotoxicity from early brain radiotherapy has led to individualized treatments for high-, intermediate-, and low-risk groups. Patients now are stratified at diagnosis into risk groups using a variety of prognostic variables. Age at diagnosis (2–10 years) and leukocyte count ($<5000/\mu l$) are the most reliable indices of a low-risk patient.

*High-risk* patients are more likely to develop central nervous system (CNS) leukemia and so are treated more intensively at diagnosis. High leukocyte count, lymphadenopathy, hepatosplenomegaly, and T-cell subset increase the risk of this complication. High-risk patients are further stratified, with 1800 cGy whole-brain radiotherapy and intrathecal chemotherapy if cerebrospinal fluid (CSF) cytology is negative, 2400 cGy to the whole neuraxis with intrathecal therapy if CSF cytology is positive.

*Good-risk* patients are treated at induction with intrathecal methotrexate and *intermediate-risk* patients with triple intrathecal therapy or combined intravenous and intrathecal methotrexate.

The prognosis for *symptomatic* central nervous system leukemia is dependent on the degree of pretreatment of the central nervous system and the time from induction therapy to first relapse. Patients who relapse more than 1 year off therapy have the best prognosis. In adult patients treated intensively for leukemic meningitis with cranial radiotherapy and triple intrathecal therapy (12 mg methotrexate, 15 mg hydrocortisone, 100 mg arabinosylcytosine through an Ommaya reservoir), an initial response rate to treatment of 70–80% is typical. Factors associated with prolonged meningeal remission are a diagnosis of ANLL, a low CSF white blood cell count (0–99 WBC/$\mu l$), and rapid attainment of CNS remission (1–2 weeks) (4).

The clinical presentation of symptomatic central nervous system leukemia is no different than for other leptomeningeal involvement by malignancies (5) (see Chap. 5). Confusion, cranial nerve palsies, and cauda equina syndromes are common and reflect the tendency for widespread invasion of the neuraxis with a predilection for tumor cells to grow at the base of the brain and in the distal thecal sac. Radicular pain is a fairly common, and probably underappreciated, presentation of leptomeningeal disease, particularly in the young patient, and may be misdiagnosed as bone pain because of its intensity and diffuse, appendicular presentation.

Although a positive CSF cytology is the gold standard for the diagnosis of leptomeningeal leukemia, this is often not possible to obtain even with repeated spinal taps. The diagnosis often rests upon the clinical presentation of multifocal cranial nerve and root lesions in a leukemic patient, with one or more of the following CSF abnormalities: elevated CSF protein, hypoglycorrhachia, leukocytosis, "suspicious" cytology, or elevated opening pressure. For the lymphocytic leukemias, sending CSF for immunohistochemical staining for cell surface pheno-

**Table 1** Classification of Leukemias

|  | Type | Acute Leukemia Subtype | Childhood | Adult |
|---|---|---|---|---|
| ALL | Lymphocytic | L1 | 80% | 30% |
|  |  | L2 | 17% | 67% |
|  |  | L3 | 3% | 3% |
|  |  | (B cell or Burkitt) |  |  |
| ANLL | Myelocytic | M1 |  | 20% |
|  |  | M2 |  | 30% |
|  |  | M3 (Promyelocytic) |  | 10% |
|  | Myelomonocytic | M4 (AMML) |  | 25% |
|  |  | M5 |  | 10% |
|  |  | M6 |  | 5% |

ALL = Acute lymphocytic leukemia
ANLL = Acute nonlymphocytic leukemia
AMML = Acute myelomonocytic leukemia
Source: Ref. 1.

characteristics and cytochemical staining (see Table 1) (1). In addition to leptomeningeal leukemia in ALL, there is a high incidence of neurological involvement in the L3, M3, and M4 subtypes.

Leukemic patients who have been treated with bone marrow transplantation are a very special group. Their presentations are largely encephalopathic or infectious.

Table 2 is organized anatomically, with cerebral presentations first, followed by cranial nerve, spinal, and peripheral nervous system problems. This is done with the expectation that the neurologist confronted with a leukemic patient will localize the lesion as usual before proceeding to diagnostic testing.

## II. MENINGITIC AND ENCEPHALOPATHIC SYNDROMES

### A. Leukemic Meningitis

Infiltration of the leptomeninges by leukemic cells is by far the most common complication of leukemia. As surveillance techniques and prophylactic therapies have improved, this complication is often identified and treated in the individual patient long before the arrival of the neurologist.

In the 1960s, as improved systemic treatments led to increased survival, leukemic meningitis was identified at autopsy in 70% of patients with ALL and 40% of patients with ANLL (2). Clinical studies showed a 75% incidence of central nervous system relapse in patients who had achieved remission with initial systemic therapy.

# 20
# Neurological Complications of Leukemia

**Lynne P. Taylor**

*Virginia Mason Clinic, University of Washington, and Fred Hutchinson Bone Marrow Transplant Center, Seattle, Washington*

## I. INTRODUCTION

The neurological complications of leukemia are protean and merge seamlessly with the complications associated with its treatment. The challenge at the bedside, therefore, is to sort carefully through types and doses of neurotoxic agents used in treatment (particularly vincristine, Ara-C, and methotrexate), doses and ports of radiotherapy, and the likelihood of neurological disease as a direct effect of leukemia based on the tumor type. This information, logically ordered, can then be compared to the neuranatomical localization of the lesion in the individual patient and a likely diagnosis made.

For the neurologist, several points deserve emphasis. Childhood acute leukemias are 75% ALL (acute lymphocytic leukemia) and 25% ANLL (acute nonlymphocytic leukemia), almost the reverse of the presentation for the adult leukemias (15% ALL, 85% ANLL). Because ALL patients, particularly children, are at high risk to develop CNS involvement, they receive nervous system treatment prophylactically at diagnosis. Patients with ANLL are more likely to develop space-occupying lesions, or granulocytic sarcomas, near the periosteum in dura, orbit, and brain. Chronic leukemics, on the other hand, rarely develop neurological difficulty, and, when they do, the complications are usually infectious.

Over the past 15 years the French-American-British (FAB) Cooperative Group has established a classification scheme for leukemias based on histological

43,51). Furthermore, up to 35% of patients with diffuse histiocytic lymphoma (DHL) and bone marrow involvement developed intracerebral lymphoma, suggesting that this too represented a group at high risk (5). When multivariate analyses were performed, the three most important factors that predicted CNSL were histology (lymphoblastic and noncleaved cell), younger age (<40 yrs), and advanced stage. The estimated probability of developing meningeal involvement was as high as 60% when all three risk factors were present (6,52).

Therefore, although NHL is a heterogeneous group of neoplasms, it is possible to define a subgroup at especially high risk who might benefit from CNS prophylaxis. However, despite the ability to define such a high-risk patient, the case for CNS prophylaxis is not as clearcut in NHL as it is in leukemia, primarily because patients with NHL usually develop their CNS complications in the setting of progressive disease. Isolated CNS relapse is an unusual presentation of CNSL in NHL patients and accounts for less than 10% of ML presentations (7,8,16,19). Data accrued from two large trials of the Eastern Cooperative Oncology Group which indicate that only 1% of patients with DHL (the most common form of NHL) develop isolated CNS relapses (53). Since CNS prophylaxis administered in the form of either RT, chemotherapy, or both is associated with potential complications, the morbidity of treatment may outweigh any minimal benefits. In addition, CNS prophylaxis will obviously not affect development of epidural lymphoma, one of the more common manifestations of CNSL.

Few previous studies have addressed the benefits of CNS prophylaxis in NHL and all suffer from either analyzing too few patients or being retrospective. Not surprisingly, they have yielded differing conclusions. The observation that administering the chemotherapy regimen M-BACOD, which includes high-dose MTX (3 gm/$M^2$) and leucovorin rescue, decreased the incidence of CNSL at recurrence was felt by the investigators to support CNS prophylaxis, although CNS involvement still occurred in 5% of patients with DHL and diffuse undifferentiated lymphoma (54). Another study indicated a lower incidence of CNSL in patients with diffuse NHL at high risk for CNSL who received IT MTX and intermediate-dose intravenous MTX when compared to a historical control group (55). Other studies have been less supportive of a role for CNS prophylaxis, however. For example, retrospective studies analyzing larger groups of NHL patients suggest that the incidence of CNS lymphoma is similar whether or not CNS prophylaxis (delivered as either RT or intrathecal chemotherapy) is administered (8,51). At present, therefore, the question remains unanswered; a reasonable approach would provide CNS prophylaxis only for those patients at very high risk for ML, i.e., younger patients with lymphoblastic or undifferentiated lymphomas and bone marrow involvement. Although the optimal prophylactic regimen has not been elucidated, these patients may be treated with a combination of IV and IT MTX without irradiation (55).

capillaries, and venules. Neurological involvement is usually associated with a rapidly progressive, albeit fluctuating, course.

The name is somewhat misleading. Originally, the condition was felt to be a disorder of endothelial cells (44). However, recent immunohistochemical and molecular evidence indicate that the proliferative cells are actually of lymphocytic, primarily B cell, origin. Therefore, the condition is more properly designated intravascular lymphoma or angiotropic large-cell lymphoma (45,46).

Because clinical and radiographic features are nonspecific, diagnosis is rarely made during the patient's lifetime. When NAE is suspected, the only definitive method of diagnosis is by brain and meningeal biopsy. Anecdotal reports suggest that NAE may respond to steroids or chemotherapy (47). These assertions are difficult to interpret, however, because few patients are available for analysis.

## E. Neurolymphomatosis

Another rare manifestation of NHL affecting the nervous system is a rapidly progressive and fatal painful neuropathy which cannot be attributed to chemotherapy, Guillain-Barré syndrome (GBS), or a paraneoplastic syndrome (see below). The CSF profile is unremarkable except for slightly increased protein and a few cells. Cerebrospinal fluid cytology is negative. At autopsy, predominant and exclusive infiltration of peripheral nerves by lymphoma is seen (48,49). Antemortem diagnosis of this rare condition is extremely difficult. No treatment has been reported to be effective.

## F. Should CNS Prophylaxis Be Administered to Lymphoma Patients?

Soon after the first systemic remissions from acute lymphoblastic leukemia were obtained, it was observed that up to 10% of relapses occurred exclusively in the meninges. Presumably this occurred because of limited CNS penetration of systemically administered chemotherapeutic agents. This observation led to the practice of treating the CNS with prophylactic radiation or chemotherapy. This strategy has improved patient outcome and increased cure rates in this disease.

Similar to treatment of the leukemias, early initial therapies of aggressive NHLs did not include any CNS-directed treatment. Subsequent development of CNS lymphoma (CNSL) was noted to be significant (50). Because CNSL was associated with a short survival and serious morbidity, a rationale existed for administering CNS prophylaxis to NHL patients. To this end, a characteristic profile of a patient at high risk for development of CNSL was drawn. Central nervous system involvement occurred with significant frequency in more aggressive NHLs such as lymphoblastic, Burkitt's, or undifferentiated types (8,16,

## III. INDIRECT COMPLICATIONS OF LYMPHOMA

Besides directly infiltrating CNS, lymphomas may produce neurological symptoms via indirect mechanisms. These indirect complications are important because they are frequently treatable and because mistaking them for tumor progression may result in the administration of incorrect treatments (which in turn may produce more neurological problems). Many of these complications are similar to those produced by other cancers and can be found detailed in other chapters of this book. In the following paragraphs, however, we will concentrate on those complications that occur with increased frequency or exclusively in lymphoma patients.

### A. Infectious Complications

Patients with lymphomas are susceptible to infections for several reasons. Staging splenectomies predispose patients to infections by encapsulated bacteria. Furthermore, especially in HD patients, cell-mediated immunity is deficient, which increases susceptibility to opportunistic infections. The frequent use of steroid medications further compounds any underlying immunosuppression in these patients.

Approximately 40% of CNS infections are due to bacteria, most commonly *Listeria*, *pneumococcus*, and gram-negative organisms (56,57). Although their symptoms are occasionally fulminant, immunosuppressed patients usually present more subacutely, with milder symptoms than their normal counterparts. Fungal infections, especially *Cryptococcus*, constitute another 40% of CNS infections (56). These infections can also be insidious in onset, presenting only as a headache and subtle change in mental status. More than 85% of patients with cryptococcal meningitis will have capsular antigen demonstrable in the CSF, making this a useful confirmatory diagnostic test.

Lymphoma patients, especially those with HD, are also prone to viral infections, most commonly to herpes zoster (HZ). Incidence figures suggest up to 15–25% of HD and 10% of NHL patients will have at least one herpes zoster infection during their disease (58).

Herpes zoster infections may occur at any time during the disease process, and disseminated disease can occur in up to 20% of patients (59). Usually, these infections are relatively self-limited in the normal host. When disseminated skin involvement occurs, visceral, ophthalmic, or neurological involvement develops in up to 50% of patients. The neurological complications of herpes zoster include encephalitis, meningitis, peripheral neuropathy, and acute and postherpetic pain syndromes. Besides persistent pain, motor neuropathies are the most common neurological complication (60). Weakness typically involves the myotome corresponding to the area of rash. Prognosis for recovery is usually favorable. A more disabling sequela of HZ infection is a chronic meningoencephalitis which may persist and lead to a progressive encephalopathy (61). Another complication which may result in serious dysfunction is a unique syndrome of contralateral hemiparesis complicating ophthalmic zoster. This syndrome is presumably secondary to a vasculopathy (62). Intravenous acyclovir is recommended when zoster infections occur in immunosuppressed patients (63).

## B. Vascular Complications

Neurological symptoms may also develop in lymphoma patients as a result of cerebrovascular events. In an autopsy series in which vascular complications of cancer were analyzed, 22 cases were accrued from lymphoma patients. Of these, two-thirds had cerebral infarctions that were caused by such diverse etiologies as disseminated intravascular coagulation, nonbacterial thrombotic endocarditis, septic embolism, and venous occlusions (64). In the other third, cerebral hemorrhages were noted, usually secondary to coagulopathies (64).

## C. Iatrogenic Hazards

Neurological dysfunction may develop as a result of the numerous therapies that lymphoma patients receive. Specifically patients may develop complications from (1) systemic chemotherapies (see Chap. 11); (2) intra-CNS chemotherapies; (3) combined effects of radiation and intra-CNS chemotherapy (see Chap. 10); and (4) surgical procedures such as Ommaya reservoir placement.

Systemic administration of either ara-C or MTX in high doses can result in neurological complications. High-dose ara-C produces cerebral or cerebellar symptoms (65, 66). Neurological toxicity is related both to increased age (67) and renal insufficiency (65). Usually, neurological dysfunction attenuates with time and withdrawal of medication. Damage to Purkinje cells and the dentate nucleus can be seen histopathologically. Methotrexate in high doses can also produce temporal cerebral dysfunction characterized by behavioral changes and focal sensorimotor signs (68,69). This complication tends to occur more frequently in children (70).

Intrathecal or intraventricular administration of MTX is also associated with neurological complications. Pharmacokinetic studies show that clearance of MTX from CSF is slower in patients with ML than in those who are administered this therapy for CNS prophylaxis. This may predispose the ML patient to the development of complications (71). Intrathecal MTX can acutely produce a reversible myelopathy or encephalopathy, especially when given frequently as it is when treating ML (72). Ara-C can also result in an acute paraparesis which may be related to utilization of benzoyl alcohol as a diluent (73). Delayed neurological toxicities are uncommon if only chemotherapy is administered (as opposed to when it is utilized in combination with RT; see below) (74).

The neurological effects of cranial irradiation are described in Chapter 10. The combination of radiation and intra-CNS chemotherapy in lymphoma patients can produce delayed sequelae ranging from a mild intellectual deficit to a fatal necrotizing leukoencephalopathy (75,76). Studies in children confirm that it is the combination of radiation and chemotherapy, rather than either therapy alone, that causes these effects (77). Current data indicate that large doses of MTX given after cranial irradiation produce greater neurotoxicity. Judicious use of these agents in CNSL is obviously necessary; however, exact guidelines are not available for maximal amounts of intra-CNS chemotherapy that can be tolerated by the patient after irradiation.

Central nervous system prophylaxis may also result in neuropsychological morbidity. Although sequelae are common when RT is prophylactically administered to children (78,79), few effects are noted in adult lymphoma patients who receive either RT or IT chemotherapy prophylactically (80). For unclear reasons, this latter reported experience differs from that noted in small-cell lung cancer patients, in whom prophylactic RT results in significant long-term sequelae (81).

Complications of Ommaya reservoirs are infrequent and self-limited. Complication rates in centers where Ommaya reservoirs are routinely utilized range from 5–10% and usually are secondary either to infection (usually *Staphylococcus epidermidis*) or reservoir malfunction (29). Seizures, leukoencephalopathy, and pericatheter necrosis can also occasionally be seen in patients who receive chemotherapy via intraventricular catheters (82), particularly if CSF circulation is impaired.

## D. Paraneoplastic Syndromes

Several syndromes which occur in cancer patients have been termed "paraneoplastic." These syndromes by definition are not due to either the cancer or any known treatment, infection, or vascular or metabolic aberration. In the past, they were assumed to be of idiopathic nature. In recent years, however intensive research into these fascinating syndromes has indicated that many of them probably occur secondary to autoimmune mechanisms (83) (Chap. 8). Virtually any paraneoplastic syndrome can occur in a patient with lymphoma. Certain ones are particularly frequent, however, and will be discussed below.

A reported association exists between paraneoplastic cerebellar degeneration and HD (84) (see Chap. 8). A peculiar syndrome almost exclusively associated with lymphoma is subacute motor neuropathy. In both HD and NHL patients, it is usually noted while the patient is in remission and its manifestations occur independent of the underlying neoplasm's activity. Painless and often patchy weakness of lower motor neuron variety is encountered which occurs subacutely and is progressive; sensory loss is mild. The electromyogram (EMG) reveals denervation. Pathologically, degeneration of anterior horns and demyelination of anterior nerve roots is seen. The course is benign and stabilizes or improves spontaneously (85–87). A syndrome which approximates more closely actual motor neuron disease with both upper and lower motor neuron signs has been recently reported in patients with both HD and NHL, frequently in association with a coexistent paraproteinemia (88).

Remote syndromes involving peripheral nerves are common in patients with either lymphoma or related diseases such as myeloma (see Chap. 22). An acute polyradiculopathy indistinguishable from classic GBS has been associated with HD. It may occur at any stage of the disease (89,90). Hodgkin's disease has also been associated with a painful brachial neuritis (91). A rare association between lymphoblastic lymphoma and myasthenia gravis has also been reported where elevated anti–acetylcholine receptor antibody levels disappeared with successful treatment of the lymphoma (92). For a more detailed discussion of peripheral nerve disorders, see Chapter 4.

## IV. PRIMARY CNS LYMPHOMA (PCNSL)

When Shaumberg and coworkers (93) first characterized the reticulum cell sarcoma/microglioma as a primary CNC lymphoma, it was considered a rare curiosity. In fact, up until recently PCNSLs accounted for no more than 800–1000 cases of brain tumor in the United States per annum. It has become a more important problem primarily because of its association with AIDS, which alone accounted for more than 1800 cases in 1991 (94). Even with exclusion of these patients, the incidence of PCNSL is also apparently increasing in the general population for as yet unexplained reasons (95).

### A. Clinical Characteristics

Primary CNS lymphoma usually presents as a subacute mass lesion; men are more commonly afflicted, with peak incidence of PCNSL occurring in the sixth decade of life (96). It commonly manifests as a single bulky mass in the hemispheric white or deep gray matter, but multiple tumors occur in more than 25% of patients (97,98). The subarachnoid space is involved in approximately one-quarter and ocular lymphoma is a frequent accompaniment (36,97). Therefore, a careful ophthalmological examination should be performed in these patients.

Primary CNS lymphoma occurs much more frequently in AIDS patients. As many as 3% of patients will develop this tumor during their disease (94,97). Patients with AIDS-associated PCNSL are significantly younger than their immunocompetent counterparts. In addition, they are more likely to have B symptoms and a lower performance status (99).

In AIDS patients, it is frequently difficult to differentiate PCNSL from the more commonly occurring toxoplasmosis. No specific CT or MRI pattern distinguishes with a high degree of confidence (99). Nevertheless, over 70% of solitary lesions as seen on MRI were determined to be PCNSL in a retrospective study (100). Therefore, in patients with single lesions on MRI, empiric toxoplasmosis therapy is not likely to be effective, and early biopsy may be advisable to ensure accurate diagnosis.

## B. Pathology

No significant pathological difference exists between visceral and primary CNS lymphomas (93). Diffuse histiocytic and immunoblastic lymphomas are most commonly encountered (96). The majority of these are B-cell neoplasms that exhibit aggressive histologic features (101). T-cell PCNSLs are very unusual (102,103). Pathological specimens from AIDS-associated PCNSL are not significantly different from those obtained in immunocompetent hosts. Angiocentric, high-grade large-cell tumors expressing B-cell markers are most common. Evidence of necrosis is frequent (104).

## C. Pathogenesis

Soon after the original description of this lymphoma, the observation was made that PCNSL developed more frequently in the setting of chronic immunosuppression (105). Thus the incidence of PCNSL was noted to be approximately 300 times greater in organ transplant recipients than in the general population. In the AIDS population this incidence is even higher.

More recent data suggest that the induction of PCNSL may be related in some way to Epstein-Barr virus (EBV) infection (102). Epstein-Barr virus infection, demonstrable by in situ hybridization or PCR, is particularly evident in immunosuppressed (i.e., AIDS) patients. Such evidence is unusual in immunocompetent hosts (103,106). Although this observation is highly suggestive, it remains uncertain whether this explains the more frequent occurrence of PCNSL in the immunocompromised patient.

## D. Treatment

Although PCNSL can occasionally be associated with an unusual course characterized by repeated transient remissions and unusual regrowth patterns (107,108), a rapidly progressive course reminiscent of glioblastoma multiforme (GBM) is more common. If left untreated, death from PCNSL frequently ensues within weeks of diagnosis. Several unusual properties differentiate PCNSL from GBM. One is the propensity of PCNSL to respond dramatically to steroids, with remissions lasting as long as 18 months without further therapy (109–111). This characteristic is important when placing a patient with a possible PCNSL on steroids because steroid therapy may obscure pathological results (112).

Another aspect of therapy for PCNSL which differentiates it from GBM is that extensive surgery is not indicated. If anything, large resections correlate negatively with outcome (113–115). Therefore, CT-guided stereotaxic biopsies are preferable and can be safely done with a high diagnostic yield (114,116).

Radiation therapy forms the foundation of PCNSL treatment. PCNSL often responds to conventional courses (i.e., 4000–5000 cGy) of whole-brain radiation therapy (WBRT). Nevertheless, median survival is still only in the range of 12–18 months. Attempts have therefore been made to increase survival using chemotherapy. Controlled prospective studies do not exist which attest to the superiority of chemotherapy-treated patients. Several studies suggest a survival benefit for patients treated with chemotherapy, especially when administered pre-irradiation (114,116–120). For the immunocompetent patient, therefore, pre-irradiation chemotherapy using one of the published regimens is recommended. Simultaneous administration of RT may be necessary to treat symptomatic lesions within the spinal axis or intraocular region (121).

Because of their overall poor prognosis, patients with AIDS represent a special subset of PCNSL patients. This does not mean that therapy should be withheld, however. AIDS-associated PCNSLs respond well both clinically and radiographically to WBRT of 40 Gy or more. Furthermore, although survival is still poor (in the range of 3 months), recent studies indicate that patients who do not receive RT succumb to their lymphoma, compared with treated patients who survive significantly longer and die of opportunistic infections (94,104). Thus, although no firm recommendations can be made concerning aggressive treatment of these patients, the data do suggest that these tumors can be controlled and survival lengthened, albeit modestly. Steroids and RT are recommended after biopsy confirmation of PCNSL in AIDS patients who are not terminally ill.

## REFERENCES

1. Lowenthal DA, Straus DJ, Campbell SW, et al. AIDS-related lymphoid neoplasia: the Memorial Hospital experience. Cancer 1988; 61:2325–37.
2. Cervantes F, Montserrat E, Rozman C. Eosinophilic meningitis in Hodgkin's disease. Ann Intern Med 1979; 91:930.
3. Dillman RO, Mueh J, Greco CM, Green MR. Leptomeningeal Hodgkin's disease. Ann Intern Med 1980; 92:714–5.
4. Patchell R, Perry MC. Eosinophilic meningitis in Hodgkin's disease. Neurology 1981; 31:887–8.
5. Levitt LJ, Dawson DM, Rosenthal DS, Moloney WC. CNS involvement in the non-Hodgkin's lymphomas. Cancer 1980; 45:545–52.
6. Litam JP, Cabanillas F, Smith TL, et al. Central nervous system relapse in malignant lymphomas: risk factors and implications for prophylaxis. Blood 1979; 54:1249–57.

7. Mackintosh FR, Colby TV, Podolsky WJ, et al. Central nervous system involvement in non-Hodgkin's lymphoma: an analysis of 105 cases. Cancer 1982; 49:586–95.
8. Recht L, Straus DJ, Cirrincione C, et al. Central nervous system metastases from non-Hodgkin's lymphoma: treatment and prophylaxis. Am J Med 1988; 84:425–35.
9. Bunn PA, Schein PS, Banks PM, DeVita VT. Central nervous system complications in patients with diffuse histiocytic and undifferentiated lymphoma: leukemia revisited. Blood 1976; 47:3–10.
10. Jellinger K, Radaszkiewicz T. Involvement of the central nervous system in malignant lymphomas. Virchows Arch [A] 1976; 370:345–62.
11. Sariban E, Edwards B, Janus C, Magrath I. Central nervous system involvement in American Burkitt's lymphoma. J Clin Oncol 1983; 1:677–82.
12. Law IP, Dick FR, Blom J, Bergevin PR. Involvement of the central nervous system in non-Hodgkin's lymphoma. Cancer 1975; 36:225–31.
13. Cairncross JG, Posner JB. Neurological complications of malignant lymphoma. In Vinken PJ, Bruyn GW, eds. Handbook of clinical neurology. Vol. 39. Amsterdam: North Holland Publishing Co., 1980:27–62.
14. Lokich J, Galbo C. Leptomeningeal lymphoma: perspectives on management. Cancer Treat Rev 1981; 8:103–10.
15. Griffin JW, Thompson RW, Mitchinson MJ, et al. Lymphomatous leptomeningitis. Am J Med 1971; 51:200–08.
16. Wolf MM, Cooper IA, Olver IN, et al. Non-Hodgkin's lymphoma involving the central nervous system. Aust N Z J Med 1985; 15:16–20.
17. Lachance DH, O'Neill BP, MacDonald DR, et al. Primary leptomeningeal lymphoma: report of 9 cases, diagnosis with immunocytochemical analysis, and review of the literature. Neurology 1991; 41:95–100.
18. Holte H, Saeter G, Dahl I, Abrahamsen AF. Progressive loss of vision in patients with high-grade non-Hodgkin's lymphoma. Cancer 1987; 60:2521–23.
19. Young RC, Howser DM, Anderson T, et al. Central nervous system complications of non-Hodgkin's lymphoma: the potential role for prophylactic therapy. Am J Med 1979; 66:435–43.
20. Monfardini S, Ficarra G, Giardini R, Santoro A. Central nervous system involvement in non-Hodgkin's lymphomas: value of lumbar puncture as initial staging procedure. Tumori 1981; 67:197–202.
21. Koch TR, Lichtenfeld KM, Wiernik PH. Detection of central nervous system metastasis with cerebrospinal fluid beta-2-microglobulin. Cancer 1983; 52:101–04.
22. Mavlight GM, Stuckey SE, Cabanillas FF, et al. Diagnosis of leukemia or lymphoma in the central nervous system by beta$_2$-microglobulin determination. N Engl J Med 1980; 303:718–22.
23. Goodson JD, Strauss GM. Diagnosis of lymphomatous leptomeningitis by cerebrospinal fluid lymphocyte cell surface markers. Am J Med 1979; 66:1057–9.
24. Shibata D, Nichols P, Sherrod A, et al. Detection of occult CNS involvement of follicular small cleaved lymphoma by the polymerase chain reaction. Mod Pathol 1990; 3:71–5.
25. Amadori S, Papa G, Avvisati G, et al. Sequential combination of systemic high-dose

ara-C and asparaginase for the treatment of central nervous system leukemia and lymphoma. J Clin Oncol 1984; 2:98–101.
26. Shipp MA, Takvorian RC, Canellos GP. High-dose cytosine arabinoside: active agent in treatment of non-Hodgkin's lymphoma. Am J Med 1984; 77:845–50.
27. Skarin AT, Zuckerman KS, Pitman SW, et al. High-dose methotrexate with folinic acid in the treatment of advanced non-Hodgkin's lymphoma including CNS involvement. Blood 1977; 50:1039–47.
28. Shapiro WR, Young DF, Mehta BM. Methotrexate: distribution in cerebrospinal fluid after intravenous, ventricular and lumbar injections. N Engl J Med 1975; 293:161–6.
29. Obbens E, Leavans ME, Beal JW, Lee YY. Ommaya reservoirs in 387 patients: a 15 year experience. Neurology 1985; 35:1274–8.
30. Raz I, Siegal T, Siegal T. Polliack A. CNS involvement by non-Hodgkin's lymphoma: response to a standard therapeutic protocol. Arch Neurol 1984; 41: 1167–71.
31. Venables GS, Proctor SJ, Bates D, et al. Intracranial disease in non-Hodgkin's lymphoma. Q J Med 1980; 49:111–31.
32. Herman TS, Hammond N, Jones SE, et al. Involvement of the central nervous system by non-Hodgkin's lymphoma: The Southwest Oncology Group Experience. Cancer 1979; 43:390–7.
33. Hallahan D, Griem M, Griem S, et al. Mycosis fungoides involving the central nervous system. J Clin Oncol 1986; 4:1638–44.
34. Sapozink MD, Kaplan HS. Intracranial Hodgkin's disease: a report of 12 cases and review of the literature. Cancer 1983; 52:1301–7.
35. Qualman SJ, Mendelsohn G, Mann RB, Green WR. Intraocular lymphomas: natural history based on a clinicopathologic study of eight cases and review of the literature. Cancer 1983; 52:878–86.
36. Rockwood EJ, Zakov ZN, Bay JW. Combined malignant lymphoma of the eye and CNS (reticulum-cell sarcoma): report of three cases. J Neurosurg 1984; 61:369–74.
37. Friedman M, Kim TH, Panahon AM. Spinal cord compression in malignant lymphoma: treatment and results. Cancer 1976; 37:1485–91.
38. DiMarco A, Campostrini F, Garusi GF. Non-Hodgkin lymphomas presenting with spinal epidural involvement. Acta Oncol 1989; 28:485–8.
39. Eeles RA, O'Brien PO, Horwich A, Brada M. Non-Hodgkin's lymphoma presenting with extradural spinal cord compression: functional outcome and survival. Br J Cancer 1991; 63:126–9.
40. Goffinet DR, Warnke R, Dunnick NR, et al. Clinical and surgical (laparotomy) evaluation of patients with non-Hodgkin's lymphomas. Cancer Treat Rep 1977; 61: 981–92.
41. Gilbert RW, Kim J-H, Posner JB. Epidural spinal cord compression from metastatic tumor: diagnosis and treatment. Ann Neurol 1978; 3:40–51.
42. Slatkin NE, Posner JB. Management of spinal epidural metastases. Clin Neurosurg 1983; 30:698–715.
43. Sheehan T, Cuthbert RJG, Parker AC. Central nervous system involvement in hematological malignancies. Clin Lab Haematol 1989; 11:331–8.

44. Fulling KH, Gersell DJ. Neoplastic angioendotheliomatosis: histologic, immunohistochemical, and ultrastructural findings in two cases. Cancer 1983; 51:1107–18.
45. Abe S, Kumanishi T, Yoshida Y, et al. Neoplastic angioendotheliosis: demonstration of immunoglobulin gene rearrangements by the Southern blot hybridization technique. Virchows Arch [B] 1990; 58:241–4.
46. Clark WC, Dohan FC, Moss T, Schweitzer JB. Immunocytochemical evidence of lymphocytic derivation of neoplastic cells in malignant angioendotheliomatosis. J Neurosurg 1991; 74:757–62.
47. Williams DB, Lyons MK, Yanagihara T, et al. Cerebral angiotropic large cell lymphoma (neoplastic angioendotheliosis): therapeutic considerations. J Neurol Sci 1991; 103:16–21.
48. Guberman A, Rosenbaum H, Braiciale T, Schlaepfer W. Human neurolymphomatosis. J Neurol Sci 1978; 36:1–12.
49. Schoenfeld Y, Aderka D, Sandbank U, et al. Fatal peripheral neurolymphomatosis after remission of histiocytic lymphoma. Neurology 1983; 33:243–5.
50. Skarin AT, Rosenthal DS, Moloney WC, Frei E. Combination chemotherapy of advanced non-Hodgkin lymphoma with bleomycin, adriamycin, cyclophosphamide, vincristine, and prednisone (BACOP). Blood 1977; 49:759–70.
51. Hoerni-Simon G, Suchaud JP, Eghbali H, et al. Secondary involvement of the central nervous system in malignant non-Hodgkin's lymphoma: a study of 30 cases in a series of 498 patients. Oncology 1987; 44:98–101.
52. Ersboll J, Schultz HB, Thomsen B, et al. Meningeal involvement in non-Hodgkin's lymphoma: symptoms, incidence, risk factors and treatment. Scand J Haematol 1985; 35:487–96.
53. Johnson GJ, Oken MM, Anderson JR, et al. Central nervous system relapse in unfavourable-histology non-Hodgkin's lymphoma: is prophylaxis indicated? Lancet 1984; 2:685–7.
54. Skarin AT, Canellos GP, Rosenthal DS, et al. Improved prognosis at diffuse histiocytic and undifferentiated lymphoma by use of high dose methotrexate alternating with standard agents (M-BACOD). J Clin Oncol 1983; 1:92–8.
55. Perez-Soler R, Smith TL, Cabanillas F. Central nervous system prophylaxis with combined intravenous and intrathecal methotrexate in diffuse lymphoma of aggressive histologic type. Cancer 1986; 57:971–7.
56. Chernik NL, Armstrong D, Posner JB. Central nervous system infections in patients with cancer. Medicine 1973; 52:563–81.
57. Lukes SA, Posner JB, Nielsen S, Armstrong D. Bacterial infections of the CNS in neutropenic patients. Neurology 1984; 34:269–75.
58. Goffinet DR, Glatstein EJ, Merigan TC. Herpes zoster-varicella infections and lymphoma. Ann Intern Med 1972; 76:235–40.
59. Mazur MH, Dolin R. Herpes zoster at the NIH: a twenty year experience. Am J Med 1978; 65:738–44.
60. Weiss S, Streifler M, Weiser HJ. Motor lesion in herpes zoster. Eur Neurol 1975; 13:332–8.
61. Horton B, Price RW, Jimenez D. Multifocal varicella-zoster virus leukoencephalitis temporally remote from herpes zoster. Ann Neurol 1981; 9:251–66.

62. Hilt DC, Buchholz D, Krumholz A, et al. Herpes zoster ophthalmicus and delayed contralateral hemiparesis caused by cerebral angiitis: diagnosis and management approaches. Ann Neurol 1983; 14:543–53.
63. Croen KD. Latency and the consequences of reactivation of the varicella-zoster virus. In: Straus SE, moderator. Varicella-zoster virus infections: biology, natural history, treatment, and prevention. Ann Intern Med 1988; 108:221–37.
64. Graus F, Rogers LR, Posner JB. Cerebrovascular complications in patients with cancer. Medicine 1985; 64:16–35.
65. Damon LE, Mass R, Linker CA. The association between high-dose cytarabine neurotoxicity and renal insufficiency. J Clin Oncol 1989; 7:1563–68.
66. Lazarus HM, Herzig RH, Herzig GP, et al. Central nervous system toxicity of high-dose systemic cytosine arabinoside. Cancer 1981; 48:2577–82.
67. Gottlieb D, Bradstock K, Koutts J, et al. The neurotoxicity of high-dose cytosine arabinoside is age-related. Cancer 1987; 60:1439–41.
68. Jaffe N, Takaue Y, Anzai T, Robertson R. Transient neurologic disturbances induced by high-dose methotrexate treatment. Cancer 1985; 56:1356–60.
69. Walker RW, Allen JC, Rosen G, et al. Transient cerebral dysfunction secondary to high-dose methotrexate. J Clin Oncol 1986; 4:1845–50.
70. Yap HY, Blumenschein GR, Yap BS, et al. High-dose methotrexate for advanced breast cancer. Cancer Treat Rep 1979; 63:757.
71. Ettinger LJ, Chervinsky DS, Freeman AI, Creavan PJ. Pharmacokinetics of methotrexate following intravenous and intraventricular administration in acute lymphocytic leukemia and non-Hodgkins lymphoma. Cancer 1982; 50:1676–82.
72. Gagliano RG, Costanzi JJ. Paraplegia following intrathecal methotrexate: report of a case and review of the literature. Cancer 1976; 37:1663–8.
73. Hahn AF, Feasby TE, Gilbert JJ. Paraparesis following intrathecal chemotherapy. Neurology 1983; 33:1032–8.
74. Allen JC. The effects of cancer therapy on the nervous system. J Pediatr 1978; 93:903–9.
75. Bleyer WA. Neurologic sequelae of methotrexate and ionizing radiation: a new classification. Cancer Treat Rep 1981; 65(Suppl 1):89–98.
76. Glass JP, Lee YY, Bruner J, et al. Treatment-related leukoencephalopathy: a study of three cases and literature review. Medicine 1986; 65:154–62.
77. Fallovollita J, Bleyer A, Robison L, et al. Intellectual dysfunction after cranial irradiation in young children with acute lymphoblastic leukemia: concurrent intrathecal methotrexate is a contributing factor (abs). Proc Am Soc Clin Oncol 1987; 6:257.
78. McIntosh S, Fischer DB, Rothman S, et al. Chronic neurologic disturbance in childhood leukemia. Cancer 1976; 37:853–7.
79. Peylan-Ramu N, Poplack D, Pizzo P, et al. Abnormal CT scans of the brain in asymptomatic children with acute lymphocytic leukemia after prophylactic treatment of the central nervous system with radiation and intrathecal chemotherapy. N Engl J Med 1978; 298:815–8.
80. Tucker J, Prior PF, Green CR, et al. Minimal neuropsychological sequelae following

prophylactic treatment of the central nervous system in adult leukemia and lymphoma. Br J Cancer 1989; 60:775–80.
81. Craig JB, Jackson DV, Moody D, et al. Prospective evaluation of changes in computed cranial tomography in patients with small cell lung carcinoma treated with chemotherapy and prophylactic cranial irradiation. J Clin Oncol 1984; 2:1151–6.
82. Lemann W, Wiley RG, Posner JB. Leukoencephalopathy complicating intraventricular catheters: clinical, radiographic and pathologic study of 10 cases. J Neurooncol 1988; 6:67–74.
83. Anderson NE, Cunningham JM, Posner JB. Autoimmune pathogenesis of paraneoplastic neurological syndromes. Crit Rev Neurobiol 1987; 3:245–99.
84. Brazis PW, Biller J, Fine M, et al. Cerebellar degeneration with Hodgkin's disease: computed tomographic correlation and literature review. Arch Neurol 1981; 38: 253–6.
85. Rowland LP, Schneck SA. Neuromuscular disorders associated with malignant neoplastic disease. J Chronic Dis 1963; 16:777–95.
86. Schold SC, Cho ES, Somasundaram M, Posner JB. Subacute motor neuronopathy: a remote effect of lymphoma. Ann Neurol 1979; 5:271–87.
87. Walton JN, Tomlinson BE, Pearce GW. Subacute "poliomyelitis" and Hodgkin's disease. J Neurol Sci 1968; 6:435–45.
88. Younger DS, Rowland LP, Latov N, et al. Lymphoma, motor neuron diseases, and amyotrophic lateral sclerosis. Ann Neurol 1991; 29:78–86.
89. Julien J, Vital C, Aupy G, et al. Guillain-Barre syndrome in Hodgkin's disease. Ultrastructural study of a peripheral nerve. J Neurol Sci 1980; 45:23–7.
90. Lisak RP, Mitchell M, Zweiman B, et al. Guillain-Barre syndrome and Hodgkin's disease: three cases with immunological studies. Ann Neurol 1977; 1:72–8.
91. Pezzimenti JF, Bruckner HW, DeConti RC. Paralytic brachial neuritis in Hodgkin's disease. Cancer 1973; 31:626–9.
92. Mortimer JE, Kidd P. Myasthenia gravis and lymphoblastic lymphoma antiacetylcholine receptor antibody as a tumor marker—a case report. Cancer Invest 1989; 7:327–31.
93. Schaumburg HH, Plank CR, Adams RD. The reticulum cell sarcoma-microglioma group of brain tumours. Brain 1972; 95:199–212.
94. Baumgartner JE, Rachlin JR, Beckstead JH, et al. Primary central nervous system lymphomas: natural history and response to radiation therapy in 55 patients with acquired immunodeficiency syndrome. J Neurosurg 1990; 73:206–11.
95. Eby NL, Grufferman S, Flannelly CM, et al. Increasing incidence of primary brain lymphoma in the US. Cancer 1988; 62:2461–5.
96. Helle TL, Britt RH, Colby TV. Primary lymphoma of the central nervous system: clinicopathological study of the experience at Stanford. J Neurosurgery 1984; 60: 94–103.
97. Hochberg FH, Miller DC. Primary central nervous system lymphoma. J Neurosurgery 1988; 68:835–53.
98. O'Neill BP, Illig JJ. Primary central nervous system lymphoma. Mayo Clin Proc 1989; 64:1005–20.

99. Remick SC, Diamond C, Migliozzi JA, et al. Primary central nervous system lymphoma in patients with and without the acquired immune deficiency syndrome: a retrospective analysis and review of the literature. Medicine 1990:69; 345–60.
100. Ciricillo SF, Rosenblum ML. Use of CT and MR imaging to distinguish intracranial lesions and to define the need for biopsy in AIDS patients. J Neurosurg 1990; 73: 720–4.
101. Morgello S, Maiese K, Petito CK. T-cell lymphoma in the CNS: clinical and pathologic features. Neurology 1989; 39:1190–6.
102. Hochberg FH, Miller G, Schooley RT, et al. Central-nervous-system lymphoma related to Epstein-Barr virus. N Engl J Med 1983; 309:745–8.
103. Bashir RM, Harris NL, Hochberg FH, Singer RM. Detection of Epstein-Barr virus in CNS lymphomas by in-situ hybridization. Neurology 1989; 39:813–17.
104. Goldstein JD, Dickson DW, Moser FG, et al. Primary central nervous system lymphoma in acquired immune deficiency syndrome: a clinical and pathologic study with results of treatment with radiation. Cancer 1991; 67:2756–65.
105. Matas AJ, Hertel BF, Rosai J, et al. Post-transplant malignant lymphoma: distinctive morphologic features related to its pathogenesis. Am J Med 1976; 61:716–20.
106. Rouah E, Rogers BB, Wilson DR, et al. Demonstration of Epstein-Barr virus in primary central nervous system lymphomas by the polymerase chain reaction and in situ hybridization. Hum Pathol 1990; 21:545–50.
107. Sugita Y, Shigemori M, Yuge T, et al. Spontaneous regression of primary malignant intracranial lymphoma. Surg Neurology 1988; 30:148–52.
108. Yamasaki T, Kikuchi H, Yamashita J, et al. Intracerebral malignant lymphoma with fluctuating regression and spatial evolution. Surg Neurol 1990; 34:235–44.
109. Pohl P, Oberhuber G, Dietze O, et al. Steroid-induced complete remission in a case of primary cerebral non-Hodgkin's lymphoma. Clin Neurol Neurosurg 1989; 91: 247–51.
110. Singh A, Strobos RJ, Singh BM, et al. Steroid-induced remissions in CNS lymphoma. Neurology 1982; 32:1267–71.
111. Geppert M, Ostertag CB, Seitz G, Kiessling M. Glucocorticoid therapy obscures the diagnosis of cerebral lymphoma. Acta Neuropathol 1990; 80:629–34.
112. Williams RS, Crowell RM, Fisher CM, et al. Clinical and radiologic remission in reticulum cell sarcoma of the brain. Arch Neurol 1979; 36:206–10.
113. Bogdahn U, Bogdahn S, Mertens HG, et al. Primary non-Hodgkin's lymphomas of the CNS. Acta Neurol Scand 1986; 73:602–14.
114. DeAngelis LM, Yahalom J, Heinemann M-H, et al. Primary CNS lymphoma: combined treatment with chemotherapy and radiotherapy. Neurology 1990; 40: 80–6.
115. O'Neill BP, Kelly PJ, Earle JD, et al. Computer-assisted stereotaxic biopsy for the diagnosis of primary central nervous system lymphoma. Neurology 1987; 37: 1160–4.
116. Neuwelt EA, Frenkel EP, Gumerlock MK, et al. Developments in the diagnosis and treatment of primary CNS lymphoma: a prospective series. Cancer 1986; 58: 1609–20.

117. Chamberlain MC, Levin VA. Adjuvant chemotherapy for primary lymphoma of the central nervous system. Arch Neurol 1990; 47:1113–16.
118. Gabbai AA, Hochberg FH, Linggood RM, et al. High-dose methotrexate for non-AIDS primary central nervous system lymphoma. J Neurosurg 1989; 70:190–4.
119. Shibamoto Y, Tsutsui K, Dodo Y, et al. Improved survival rate in primary intracranial lymphoma treated by high-dose radiation and systemic vincristine-doxorubicin-cyclophosphamide-prednisolone chemotherapy. Cancer 1990; 65: 1907–12.
120. Socie G, Piprot-Chauffat C, Schlienger M, et al. Primary lymphoma of the central nervous system: an unresolved therapeutic problem. Cancer 1990; 65:322–6.
121. Hochberg FH, Loeffler JS, Prados M. The therapy of primary brain lymphoma. J Neurooncol 1991; 10:191–201.

# 22

# Neurological Complications of Plasma Cell Dyscrasias

## J. Peter Glass

*Duke University Medical Center, Durham, North Carolina*

## I. THE NEUROLOGICAL COMPLICATIONS OF PLASMA CELL DYSCRASIAS

Plasma cell dyscrasias are a group of related disorders with many different names (dysproteinemias, gammopathies, immunoglobulinopathies, paraproteinemias), each of which is associated with proliferation and accumulation of immunoglobulin-secreting cells that are derived from the B-cell series of lymphocytes (1). The most important malignancy of plasma cells is multiple myeloma.

The clinical characteristics of a particular plasma cell dyscrasia depend upon the level of B-lymphocyte maturation and the nature of the secretory products. The predominant tumor cell in myeloma is the bone marrow–based plasma cell. In myeloma, tumor infiltration of soft tissues can also produce isolated or multiple plasmacytomas.

In Waldenström's macroglobulinemia, an important plasma cell dyscrasia, the predominant cell is a plasmacytoid lymphocyte that secretes IgM molecules. The major neurological complications of plasma cell dyscrasias will be discussed in this chapter. Their underlying pathophysiology and management will also be addressed.

## II. NEUROPATHIES IN PLASMA CELL DYSCRASIAS

The overall incidence of polyneuropathy in plasma cell dyscrasias approximates 10% (2). In some cases, the plasma cell dyscrasia or the M protein may cause the neuropathy.

In the only controlled statistical analysis to date, published by Kelly et al. (3) in 1981, the frequency of monoclonal gammopathy in patients with idiopathic polyneuropathy was 10%. Monoclonal gammopathy of undetermined significance (MGUS) was the most frequent plasma cell dyscrasia encountered, occurring in 50–60% of cases. Primary amyloidosis occurred in 30–40% and multiple myeloma in 5–10%.

### A. Amyloid Polyneuropathy

Amyloid in plasma cell dyscrasias comes from the variable portion of the Ig light chain. The mechanism by which amyloid is deposited is not clear (4,5). Primary amyloidosis occurs both with and without plasma cell dyscrasias (6). Typically, the polyneuropathy occurs in men over 60. It is mainly sensory and autonomic. Patients frequently complain of pain in the lower extremities, often described as "stabbing" or "burning." Small cutaneous nerve fibers are affected initially with marked loss of pain and temperature sensation but preservation of vibratory and joint position sensation. As the polyneuropathy progresses, weakness becomes more of a factor. The clinical findings are most prominent distally and are symmetric, with a slow proximal spread.

Autonomic dysfunction is a major component of the polyneuropathy in primary amyloidosis associated with plasma cell dyscrasias. Patients complain of orthostatic dizziness, lightheadedness or syncope, impotence, urinary incontinence, and decreased sweating.

Electrophysiological studies, according to Kelly (2), reveal reduced or absent sensory nerve action potentials, mild slowing of motor nerve conduction velocities, and symmetric neurogenic changes upon needle examination. This is a pattern characteristic of distal axonal degeneration. Amyloid deposits are found in sural nerve biopsies in 90% of cases, often with the changes of axonal degeneration. Biopsy of any organ system cannot differentiate primary amyloidosis from amyloidosis associated with plasma cell dyscrasia unless there are bony lesions or bone marrow proliferation of plasma cells.

The pathogenesis of amyloid polyneuropathy is felt to be most likely due to infiltration of nerves leading to ischemia of nerve fibers. Amyloid is also deposited in dorsal root and autonomic ganglia.

The prognosis for patients with amyloid polyneuropathy in plasma cell dyscrasias is poor. Effective treatment does not exist. Fifty percent of patients die within 1 year of the diagnosis and 80% within 3 years. Death is due to multiple organ involvement. Symptomatic treatment is frequently helpful, including the use of elastic stockings, fluorinated steroids to increase intravascular volume, and medications such as carbamazepine, phenytoin, or amitriptyline to control pain. Definitive treatment has met with little success. The use of melphalan and prednisone as well as plasmapheresis to reduce the proteins produced by plasma cells has been of limited value. Long-term therapy by this approach is not recommended because of its poor efficacy.

## B. Myeloma Neuropathy

Myeloma neuropathy is heterogeneous and more difficult to diagnose clinically than amyloid polyneuropathy. It has little direct relationship to the status of the underlying plasma cell dyscrasia. There are two groups of patients; those with multiple myeloma–associated polyneuropathy and those with osteosclerotic plasmacytoma (also referred to as solitary plasmacytoma) and polyneuropathy.

Multiple myeloma polyneuropathy occurs in 3–5% of patients with typical lytic multiple myeloma. Kelly et al. (3) in 1981 demonstrated that almost 50% of patients with myeloma polyneuropathy were actually associated with amyloidosis. The polyneuropathy in these patients resembled amyloid polyneuropathy without myeloma. Additional features were due to the presence of bony involvement by myeloma. Some patients appeared to have distal polyneuropathy and a superimposed mononeuritis multiplex. However, careful workup of the mononeuritis revealed radiculopathies secondary to local vertebral body or epidural disease.

Multiple myeloma patients with amyloidosis may also develop another polyneuropathy manifested by areflexia, significant ataxia secondary to loss of joint position sensation, and little or no motor involvement. This sensory neuropathy represents a mild distal axonal neuropathy resembling the sensory neuropathy syndrome of Denny-Brown, a remote effect of the underlying malignancy.

The polyneuropathy in patients with osteosclerotic myeloma has distinctive features (7). Osteosclerotic lesions on skeletal surveys occur in less than 3% of untreated myeloma patients. One-half of osteosclerotic patients have polyneuropathy. The patients are younger than most myeloma patients and are usually not systemically ill. They present because of indirect effects of the plasmacytoma upon peripheral nerves and other organs. The neuropathy is slowly progressive with distal to proximal spread. Weakness is a major factor, with associated absence of reflexes and large fiber sensory loss. Demyelination is suggested by the marked reduction in nerve conduction velocities. Nerve biopsies reveal both demyelination and loss of axons. Cerebrospinal fluid (CSF) protein levels are usually very high.

Aside from the polyneuropathy in osteosclerotic myeloma, a major clue to its diagnosis may be the presence of multisystem involvement referred to as POEMS syndrome (8,9). POEMS is an acronym for polyneuropathy, organomegaly, endocrinopathy, M protein, and skin lesions. Organomegaly is manifested by hepatosplenomegaly and lymphadenopathy. Endocrinopathy and cutaneous signs include decreased testosterone and increased estrogen levels, impotence, hyperglycemia, hyperprolactinemia, hyperpigmentation, and hypertrichosis. The majority of patients have only a few manifestations of the entire syndrome. Histochemical studies of POEMS have revealed a specific antibody against the pituitary (10).

Bone lesions are solitary in 50% of patients with osteosclerotic myeloma and multiple in 50%. They involve primarily the vertebral bodies but may affect the skull and proximal long bones. The M protein is also characteristic. Since it may not appear on routine serum protein electrophoresis, immunoelectrophoresis is essential. The M protein is made up of a lambda light chain with either an IgG or IgA heavy chain. There is an argument that the tumor secretes a substance, perhaps the M protein itself, which has secondary manifestations. The substance recognizes a receptor and binds to it. However, efforts to identify such a receptor have, to date, been unsuccessful.

The polyneuropathy in osteosclerotic myeloma responds to treatment of the malignancy. Patients with solitary plasmacytomas are given local radiation therapy. After treatment, there is usually slow but progressive improvement for up to 2 years with reversal of the nonneurological features of the disease as well. Radiation is contraindicated in patients with multiple lesions. Chemotherapy with such agents as melphalan and prednisone has led to improvement of the neuropathy in patients with multiple lesions, though not as successfully as the treatment of solitary plasmacytomas.

A third type of polyneuropathy seen in patients with multiple myeloma is a Guillain-Barré–like syndrome with motor involvement, slowed nerve conduction velocities, and high CSF protein (11). This syndrome evolves slowly, may stabilize, and even improve. It is much like the Guillain-Barré syndrome seen in patients with lymphoma. The results of plasmapheresis have been inconsistent.

## C. The Polyneuropathy of Waldenström's Macroglobulinemia

Waldenström's macroglobulinemia can present with a polyneuropathy in several ways. These include typical amyloid neuropathy, mild sensorimotor neuropathy, Guillain-Barré syndrome, or pure large fiber sensory neuropathy. In these patients, the M protein is found deposited on myelin sheaths and reacts with MAG (myelin-associated glycoprotein), resulting in a demyelinating neuropathy. Treatment is the same as that for the various polyneuropathies associated with multiple myeloma as described above.

## D. Neuropathy in MGUS

Patients with MGUS have an M protein without a specific plasma cell proliferative disorder. When these patients are initially seen, it cannot be determined whether they will develop a more serious plasma cell disorder such as multiple myeloma or

Waldenström's macroglobulinemia. In a series of 241 such patients reported by Kyle (12) in 1978 and followed for more than 10 years, 14% developed myeloma, macroglobulinemia, or amyloidosis. Only 37% had no significant increase in M protein, representing true benign monoclonal gammopathy. Patients with MGUS and polyneuropathy represent the largest but least well-defined group. They are divided into IgM and non-IgM (IgA and IgG) associated neuropathies.

Fifty percent of patients with IgM-MGUS and neuropathy present with a sensory polyneuropathy. There is sensory loss, ataxia, loss of deep tendon reflexes, a reduction in conduction velocities, and a very high CSF protein level. This neuropathy is invariably mild and chronic. Immunofluorescent studies demonstrate deposits of IgM kappa M proteins on the myelin sheaths of biopsied peripheral nerves, and immunological studies show that these proteins react with MAG antigen on the surface of the myelin sheaths. This suggests that the polyneuropathy is caused by autoantibody activity directed at the myelin sheath. The polyneuropathies in patients with non-IgM gammopathies are both motor and sensory, and it is not clear if the M proteins in these patients are related to pathogenesis.

In a recent double-blind study, Dyck et al. (13) randomly assigned 39 patients with MGUS and neuropathy to plasmapheresis or a sham procedure twice a week for 3 weeks. Those who initially underwent the sham procedure later underwent plasmapheresis in an open trial. Improvement was assessed in terms of muscle strength, sensation, deep tendon reflexes, and electrophysiological testing.

Plasmapheresis was effective in improving the neuropathy in MGUS. Those patients with non-IgM–associated neuropathies did better than those with IgM-associated neuropathy. Some patients who could not walk before treatment were able to walk afterward. However, improvement was only transient, lasting from 7–20 days. Improvement was attributed to either remyelination of nerve fibers or the removal of antibodies, relieving the conduction block of motor fibers.

Table 1 summarizes the peripheral neuropathies in plasma cell dyscrasias.

A uniform approach should be taken in patients with idiopathic polyneuropathy (2,14). A thorough search for a monoclonal protein is in order, starting with a serum protein electrophoresis. If the electrophoresis is negative and the patient has a very mild neuropathy not suggestive of one of the previously described syndromes, no further testing is necessary. The patients are treated symptomatically and followed. More extensive testing is carried out if the neuropathy evolves.

Extensive testing should be undertaken initially in those patients who present with severe neuropathy. This includes serum and urine protein electrophoresis and immunoelectrophoresis looking for the presence, nature, and amount of any monoclonal protein. If a monoclonal protein is found, a full hematological workup is necessary, including bone marrow aspiration and biopsy, skeletal survey, and biopsy of appropriate tissue for amyloidosis and myeloma. According to Kelly (2), ". . . sural nerve biopsy should be performed when inflammation, vasculitis, amyloid, or tumor infiltration is considered or when immunofluorescent studies are indicated."

## III. THE HYPERVISCOSITY SYNDROME

The hyperviscosity syndrome occurs in 50% of patients with Waldenström's macroglobulinemia and fewer than 5% of patients with multiple myeloma (1,15). Hyperviscosity results from protein-protein interactions of either very large, long molecules with high intrinsic viscosity (IgM, M component) or when there are high concentrations of specific IgG or IgA M components that have a tendency to form multimolecular aggregates (16–18). Patient-to-patient variation in concentration of M components and viscosity make the prediction of plasma viscosity difficult without direct measurement.

The symptoms and signs of hyperviscosity syndrome are not seen unless the relative viscosity is greater than 4.0. The classic syndrome is not seen unless the viscosity is greater than 5.0. Normal viscosity is 1.4–1.8. The syndrome consists of a triad of bleeding, visual signs and symptoms, and neurological manifestations. Bleeding disorders include bruising, purpura, and recurrent mucosal hemorrhage from such sites as the nose and uterus. Ocular findings include marked dilatation of retinal veins with segmentation called the "box car" sign, retinal hemorrhages, and in some cases papilledema. The neurological manifestations are secondary to transient ischemia of the central nervous system and have not been reported to involve hemorrhage. They range from fatigue and generalized numbness to headache, vertigo, nystagmus, confusion, stupor, and coma. Macular edema producing diminished visual acuity also occurs in hyperviscosity syndrome. The edema is felt to be secondary to immunoglobulin deposits within the retinal layers and subretinal space (19).

The initial approach to patients with hyperviscosity syndrome is plasmapheresis. This can be followed by systemic chemotherapy to reduce the M-component production or tumor burden. In drug-resistant cases, satisfactory long-term control of hyperviscosity can be obtained with intermittent plasmapheresis alone at 2- to 3-week intervals.

## IV. LEPTOMENINGEAL METASTASIS IN MYELOMA

Leptomeningeal metastasis (meningeal myelomatosis) is a rare complication of multiple myeloma (20). Only 10 such cases have been reported in the literature. The immunoglobulin types have included IgG, IgA, IgD, and the Bence Jones type.

The most frequent symptom in meningeal myelomatosis is weakness, especially weakness of the lower extremities. Headaches and changes in mental status are next in line. Various cranial nerve pareses have been described. Sensory disturbances are rare. Of the 10 reported cases of meningeal myelomatosis, six were accompanied by either plasma cell leukemia or an increase in circulating plasma cells. Subarachnoid spread is suspected to originate from the hematogenous dissemination of circulating plasma cells.

The treatment of meningeal myelomatosis is not established. Patients have received total neuraxis irradiation instead of focal irradiation as in solid tumors. This has resulted in disappearance of plasma cells from the cerebrospinal fluid and symptomatic relief for no longer than 2 months. None of the patients has had the placement of an Ommaya device, but six received intrathecal methotrexate which was effective for only a few weeks.

Disturbances in consciousness in meningeal myelomatosis resemble those of hypercalcemia and the hyperviscosity syndrome. Clinicians should be aware of this consideration, especially in patients with circulating plasma cells or plasma cell leukemia.

## V. MOTOR NEURON DISEASE IN MYELOMA

In a report by Shy et al. (21) in 1986, M proteins were found in 10 patients with motor neuron disease (MND) out of a total group of 206. The frequency of paraproteins was 5.3%. In every decade of life from age 30 to 79, the frequency of plasma cell dyscrasias was higher in patients with MND than in age-matched controls. It was calculated that 1.7 cases of plasma cell dyscrasias would have been expected by chance alone in this series of 206. The occurrence of 10 cases was statistically significant.

Autopsy findings in patients with MND and plasma cell dyscrasias have demonstrated the typical changes of loss of anterior horn cells alone and with degeneration of corticospinal tracts, and also myelomatous infiltration of nerve roots with perivascular lymphocytic infiltration.

The frequency of paraproteinemias in patients with MND indicates that the association is probably not just coincidental. However, this as yet has not been proven by a prospective study. Whether or not the association is causal also remains unproven.

Patients with MND do not have anti-MAG activity. However, there has been a report of two patients in whom the serum monoclonal IgM protein bound specifically to gangliosides $G_{M1}$ and $G_{D1b}$ (22). This binding was present at serum dilutions up to 1:100,000. Absorption with lacto-$n$-tetraose–bovine serum albumin (LNT-BSA) completely removed the M protein from the sera of these patients as determined by serum protein electrophoresis. This indicated that it was the M protein that bound to $G_{M1}$, $G_{D1b}$, and LNT-BSA. The sera of patients without IgM who had MND and those with other neurological conditions, including Eaton-

**Table 1** Peripheral Neuropathies in Plasma Cell Dyscrasias

| Systemic disorder | Abnormal protein | Symptoms | Signs | Therapy |
|---|---|---|---|---|
| Amyloidosis | Ig light chains | "Burning feet" Lightheadedness Impotence Distal weakness | Decreased pain and temperature Orthostatic hypotension Distal axonopathy | Elastic hose Fluorinated steroids Carbamazepine Amitriptyline |
| Multiple myeloma with amyloidosis 1 | Ig light chains M protein | Same as above | Same as above | Same as above |
| Multiple myeloma with amyloidosis 2 | Ig light chains M protein | Unsteady gait | Loss of JPS Sensory ataxia Areflexia | Same as above |
| Multiple myeloma | M protein | Weakness Unsteady gait | Areflexia Decreased NCV Increased CSF protein | Melphalan and prednisone |
| Osteosclerotic myeloma (plasmacytoma) | Lambda light chain + IgG or IgA heavy chain | Polyneuropathy Organomegaly Endocrinopathy M protein Skin lesions | Weakness distal > proximal Decreased NCV Increased CSF protein | XRT or surgery Melphalan and prednisone |

## Plasma Cell Dyscrasias

| | | | | |
|---|---|---|---|---|
| Waldenström's macroglobulinemia with amyloidosis | IgM | Same as amyloidosis | Same as amyloidosis | Chemotherapy plasmapheresis |
| Waldenström's macroglobulinemia | IgM Anti-MAG | Distal numbness Mild weakness Gait instability | Impaired pain and temperature Areflexia Weakness Increased CSF protein Sensory ataxia Decreased NCV | Same as above |
| MGUS | IgM kappa (anti-MAG) | Numbness Gait difficulty | Areflexia Decreased vibration and proprioception Ataxia Decreaseed NCV Increased CSF protein | Plasmapheresis or chemotherapy or both |
| MGUS | IgG or IgA | Weakness Sensory loss | Same as above | Same as above |

CSF = Cerebrospinal fluid; JPS = Joint position sensation; MAG = Myelin-associated glycoprotein; MGUS = Monoclonal gammopathy of undetermined significance; NCV = Nerve conduction velocities; XRT = Local radiation therapy

Lambert syndrome, paraneoplastic cerebellar degeneration, and multiple sclerosis, as well as normal subjects had antibodies to $G_{M1}$ or $G_{D1b}$ in serum dilutions of not greater than 1:80. Absorption with LNT-BSA in these patients did not decrease anti-$G_{M1}$ activity (22,23).

In one patient treated with multiple plasma exchanges and chlorambucil, the reduction in serum IgM concentration was associated with clinical improvement of MND. Therefore, it is possible that autoantibodies can cause MND.

There may be several different etiologies for MND. Thus far only two patients have been reported to have autoantibodies that reacted with $G_{M1}$, $G_{D1b}$, and LNT-BSA. However, these antibodies may be present in a significant number of patients who have MND and other plasma cell dyscrasias in which IgM monoclonal antibodies may be found. If MND can be shown to be caused by M proteins, then other antibodies that react with different components of motor neurons might cause MND in other patients.

## VI. PARANEOPLASTIC SYNDROMES IN MYELOMA

"Paraneoplastic syndromes" with nervous system involvement have been reported in association with multiple myeloma. These include a patient with peripheral neuropathy, polymyalgia, and arthralgias (24); Eaton-Lambert syndrome (25); a pancerebellar syndrome (26); and three cases of progressive limb-girdle dystrophy who were found to have a monoclonal gammopathy (27).

## VII. CRANIAL NERVE AND EYE FINDINGS IN PATIENTS WITH MYELOMA

Cranial neuropathies have been described in multiple myeloma patients, most commonly secondary to bony involvement at the base of the skull (28–30). There have also been a few cases of "numb chin syndrome" secondary to mental nerve compression (31). Lam et al. (32) reported a patient who developed a cavernous sinus syndrome as the initial manifestation of extramedullary myeloma.

Total ophthalmoplegia associated with biopsy-proven amyloid infiltration of extraocular muscles has been described in a patient with multiple myeloma (33). Treating the myeloma had no effect upon the ophthalmoplegia. Physicians should be aware that ophthalmoplegia and amyloidosis may indicate an underlying myeloma rather than primary systemic amyloidosis. A patient with multiple myeloma who was being treated with steroids (dexamethasone 40 mg orally every day) for more than 6 months developed weakness of both upper and lower extremities as well as diplopia. On examination, he had moderate to severe proximal muscle weakness, and ocular motility was limited in all fields of gaze. A lumbar puncture was unremarkable. It was felt that the patient had developed a steroid-induced myopathy including extraocular muscles. Taking him off steroids for 3 months resulted in complete resolution of his signs.

## VIII. EPIDURAL SPINAL CORD COMPRESSION

The incidence of spinal cord compression from isolated (solitary) plasmacytoma or multiple myeloma is approximately 10% (34,35). In these patients, spinal cord compression most commonly results from vertebral body collapse, less commonly secondary to epidural extension from an adjacent vertebral body, and least commonly from epidural tumor without local bony disease.

In Brenner's study (36) of 114 patients with multiple myeloma followed for 10 years, there were 21 cases of central nervous system involvement. Nineteen episodes of spinal cord compression occurred in 17 patients. Spinal cord compression was the presenting symptom in eight patients and developed during the course of the disease in nine.

In a series of 32 patients with plasma cell dyscrasias and neurological complications out of 110 unselected patients with myelomatous disease, Camacho and coworkers (37) reported 12 cases of spinal cord compression. In nine cases, this represented the presentation of the underlying dyscrasia. In 11 cases, it was caused by isolated plasmacytoma affecting the thoracic spinal cord. The presentation of spinal cord compression in patients with solitary plasmacytomas or multiple myeloma is no different from that of any other malignancy (see Chap. 4). If any controversy exists, it concerns therapy in these patients. At the present time, the treatment of choice for solitary plasmacytoma is that of anterior decompression followed by radiation therapy, despite the fact that 25–50% of the cases go on to develop multiple myeloma. The treatment of choice in multiple myeloma is radiation therapy alone. If a patient progresses in spite of radiation therapy or has previously been irradiated to the maximum cord tolerance, surgical decompression may be considered.

Sinoff and Blumsohn (36) published a series of five cases of multiple myeloma with spinal cord compression and paraparesis, all of whom improved to ambulation without assistance after treatment only with systemic chemotherapy.

The best predictor of outcome is the neurological status of patients before treatment, i.e., whether or not they are ambulatory. Overall survival is dependent upon the underlying disease. Long-term survival after spinal cord compression is not uncommon for patients with multiple myeloma. In the group findings published by Spiess et al. (35), the median survival was 37 months and the 1-year survival was 100%.

## IX. INTRACRANIAL PLASMACYTOMA

Brenner et al. (36) reported four cases of intracranial plasmacytoma. The intracranial tumor was the presenting symptom of multiple myeloma in one patient. In three, it appeared during the course of myeloma. A large mass growing inward from the skull preceded neurological signs by 4–6 months. Neurological signs included hemiparesis, seizures, and altered mental status. Treatment consisted of craniotomy followed by radiation therapy.

## X. SUMMARY

Nervous system involvement is a small but important aspect of plasma cell dyscrasias. Most often this involvement is the result of direct extension of the malignancy. Less frequently, it is the result of an indirect effect or what has been described as a paraneoplastic syndrome. The earlier the involvement is recognized, the earlier treatment can be instituted and the patient spared the consequences.

## ACKNOWLEDGMENT

We express our gratitude to Ms. Kristina Koehler who persisted in the typing of this chapter.

## REFERENCES

1. Salmon SE, Cassady JR. Plasma cell neoplasms. In DeVita VT, Hellman S, Rosenberg SA, eds. Cancer: principles and practice of oncology. Philadelphia: J.B. Lippincott Company, 1989:1853–95.
2. Kelly JJ. Polyneuropathies associated with plasma cell dyscrasias. Semin Neurol 1987; 7:30–9.
3. Kelly JJ, Kyle RA, O'Brien PC, et al. Prevalence of monoclonal protein in peripheral neuropathy. Neurology 1981; 31:1480–3.
4. Durie BGM, Persky B, Soehnlen BJ, et al. Amyloid production in human myeloma stem cell culture, with morphologic evidence of amyloid secretion by associated macrophages. N Engl J Med 1982; 307:1689–92.
5. Verghese JP, Bradley WG, Nemni R, et al. Amyloid neuropathy in multiple myeloma and other plasma cell dyscrasias: a hypothesis of the pathogenesis of amyloid neuropathies. J Neurol Sci 1983; 59:237–46.
6. Kelly JJ, Kyle RA, O'Brien PC, et al. The natural history of peripheral neuropathy in primary systemic amyloidosis. Ann Neurol 1979; 6:1–7.
7. Kelly JJ, Kyle RA, Miles JM, et al. Osteosclerotic myeloma and peripheral neuropathy. Neurology 1983; 33:202–10.

8. Bisail M, Cossu A, Massarelli G, et al. POEMS syndrome; a case report. Haematologica 1990; 75:384–6.
9. Hyman BT, Westrick MA: Multiple myeloma and coagulopathy: a case report of polyneuropathy, organomegaly, endocrinopathy, M-protein, and skin changes POEMS syndrome. Arch Intern Med 1986; 146:993–4.
10. Meier C, Reulecke M, Kesselring, et al. Polyneuropathy, organomegaly, endocrinopathy, and skin changes in a case of solitary myeloma. Schweiz Med Wochenschr 1986; 116:1326–31.
11. Mactier RA, Khanna R. Guillain-Barre syndrome in kappa light chain myeloma. South Med J 1987; 80:1054–5.
12. Kyle RA. Monoclonal gammopathy of undetermined significance: natural history of 241 cases. Am J Med 1978; 64:814–26.
13. Dyck PJ, Low PA, Windebank AJ, et al. Plasma exchange in polyneuropathy associated with monoclonal gammopathy of undetermined significance. N Engl J Med 1991; 325:1482–6.
14. Kelly JJ. Peripheral neuropathies associated with monoclonal proteins: a clinical review. Muscle Nerve 1985; 8:138–50.
15. Tojo K, Morita A, Miki T, et al. IgA myeloma complicated by fractures of the bones and hyperviscosity syndrome; report of an autopsied case. Osaka City Med J 1990; 36:61–70.
16. MacKenzie MR, Babcock J. Studies in the hyperviscosity syndrome, II: Macroglobulinemia. J Lab Clin Med 1975; 35:227–34.
17. Somer T. Hyperviscosity syndrome in plasma cell dyscrasias. Adv Microcirc 1975; 6:1–70.
18. MacKenzie MR, Lee TK. Blood viscosity in Waldenstrom macroglobulinemia. Blood 1977; 49:507.
19. Bernard A, Rousselie F. Macular manifestations of monoclonal dysgammaglobulinemias: apropos of 3 cases. J Fr Ophthalmol 1986; 9:805–10.
20. Oda K, Egawa H, Okuhara T, et al. Meningeal involvement in Bence Jones multiple myeloma. Cancer 1991; 67:1900–2.
21. Shy ME, Rowland LF, Smith T, et al. Motor neuron disease and plasma cell dyscrasia. Neurology 1986; 36:1429–36.
22. Latov N, Hays AP, Donofrio PD, et al. Monoclonal IgM with unique specificity to ganglioside $G_M$, and $G_{D16}$ and to lacto-n-tetraose associated with human motor neuron disease. Neurology 1988; 38:763–8.
23. Steck AJ, Adams D. In: Rowland LP, ed. Advances in neurology, Vol. 56: Amyotrophic lateral sclerosis and other motor neuron diseases. New York: Raven Press, 1991:421–5.
24. Samanta A, Hilton D, Roy S. Peripheral neuropathy, polymyalgia, and arthralgia: a paraneoplastic syndrome associated with myeloma. Clin Rheumatol 1990; 9:246–8.
25. Portha C, Dupond JL, Monnier G, et al. Eaton-Lambert syndrome associated with multiple myeloma; resolution of the neuro-muscular block after chemotherapy. Sem Hop Paris 1983; 59:1337–9.
26. Prieto J, Leira R, de Toro FJ, et al. Cerebellar syndrome as the first manifestation of multiple myeloma. Neurologia 1987; 2:123–7.

27. Kissling D, Michot F. Multiple myeloma occurring in association with a pre-existing neuromuscular disease (progressive muscular dystrophy): a chance occurrence or a nosological entity? Acta Haematol 1984; 72:94–104.
28. Bellan LD, Cox TA, Gascoyne RD. Parasellar syndrome caused by plasma cell leukemia. Can J Ophthalmol 1989; 24:331–4.
29. Knapp AJ, Gartner S, Henkind P. Multiple myeloma and its ocular manifestations. Surv Ophthalmol 1987; 31:343–51.
30. Shone GR. Facial palsy due to myeloma of the temporal bone. J Laryngol Otol 1985; 99:907–8.
31. Massey EW, Moore J, Schold SC. Mental neuropathy from systemic cancer. Neurology 1981; 31:1277–81.
32. Lam S, Margo CE, Beck R, et al. Cavernous sinus syndrome as the initial manifestation of multiple myeloma. J Clin Neuro Ophthalmol 1987; 7:135–8.
33. Raflo GT, Farrell TA, Sioussat RS. Complete ophthalmoplegia secondary to amyloidosis associated with multiple myeloma. Am J Ophthalmol 1981; 92:221–4.
34. Colak A, Cataltepe O, Erbengi A. Spinal cord compression caused by plasmacytomas: a retrospective review of 14 cases. Neurosurg Rev 1989; 12:305–8.
35. Speiss JL, Adelstein DJ, Hines JD. Multiple myeloma presenting with spinal cord compression. Oncology 1988; 45:88–92.
36. Brenner B, Carter A, Tatarsky I, et al. Incidence, prognostic significance, and therapeutic modalities of central nervous system involvement in multiple myeloma. Acta Haematol 1982; 68:77–83.
37. Camacho J, Arnalich F, Anciones B, et al. The spectrum of neurological manifestations in myeloma. J Med 1985; 16:597–611.
38. Sinoff CL, Blumsohn A. Spinal cord compression in myelomatosis: response to chemotherapy alone. Br J Cancer Clin Oncol 1989; 25:197–200.

# 23

# Neurological Complications of Childhood Cancer

**Mark T. Jennings**

*Vanderbilt University School of Medicine, Nashville, Tennessee*

## I. INTRODUCTION

This chapter addresses the neurological complications of the common solid tumors of childhood and the toxicity of antineoplastic therapy for the developing central nervous system (CNS). The related topic, neurological complications of sarcomas, is discussed in Chapter 19.

## II. SPECIFIC NEUROLOGICAL COMPLICATIONS

### A. Encephalopathy

Acute mental status alterations, such as loss of consciousness, delirium, amnesia, hallucinations, obtundation, and ictal events, are reported in 11% (89/815) of children with systemic cancers (1). Seizure (60%), encephalopathy (27%), and a strokelike syndrome (13%) are the most common forms of acute mental status alterations. Encephalopathy may be the presenting sign of a malignancy in 3% of pediatric oncology patients. Risk factors for acute mental status alterations depend upon the type of neoplasm, its natural history, and therapy-related complications (Table 1). The causes of encephalopathy are multifactorial (Table 2). Pharmacological complications account for 25% of all cases of acute mental status alterations (Table 3) (1). Encephalopathy is an adverse prognostic variable with

**Table 1** Encephalopathy

*Incidence: 3% of Pediatric Cancer Patients*
Acute nonlymphoblastic leukemia: 18%
Acute lymphoblastic leukemia: 13%
Lymphoma: 11%
Sarcoma: 10%
Neuroblastoma: 9%

significant neurological morbidity (12.5%) and mortality (29–48%). Fifty-seven percent of encephalopathy-associated deaths are due to direct involvement of the CNS. The mortality may be greater than 70% in cases of encephalopathy associated with sepsis or intracranial hemorrhage (1,2).

A unique parkinsonian encephalopathy is described among children experiencing successful engraftment following bone marrow transplantation. The clinical features include the development of disorientation, dementia, bradykinesia, tremor, rigidity, myoclonus, and leukoencephalopathy (3). The encephalopathy can develop suddenly, within days, or subacutely over weeks. This neurological complication occurs both among autologous transplant as well as allogeneic transplant patients at risk for graft-versus-host disease (GVHD). Neither cranial irradiation or intrathecal chemotherapy are obligatory risk factors. The electroencephalogram reveals diffuse slowing, the cerebrospinal fluid (CSF) profile shows a variably elevated protein (range 20–198 mg/dl) with an increase in myelin basic protein. The neuropathological appearance is that of a macrophage infiltrate, hypertrophied astrocytes, pyknotic oligodendroglia with mild demyelination, and axonal preservation. Etiological considerations are drug reaction, GVHD, autoimmune disease, infection, or a complication of the induction regimen. High-dose steroids appear to be more effective therapy than carbidopa/levodopa (3).

## B. Seizures

Among children with systemic cancers, 6.5% (53/815) experience a seizure during their illness (1). Approximately 26% of these patients experience status

**Table 2** Encephalopathy

*Differential Diagnosis*
| | |
|---|---|
| Coagulopathy: 23% | Leukoencephalopathy: 9% |
| Shock: 19% | Brain/meningeal metastases: 6% |
| Pharmacological: 19% | Venous sinus thrombosis: 6% |
| CNS infection: 17% | Metabolic imbalance: 6% |

**Table 3** Encephalopathy

*Pharmacological Causes (25% of All Cases)*
L-Asparaginase: 59%   Intrathecal chemotherapy
Arabinosylcytosine    Amphotericin B
Methotrexate          Narcotics
Ifosfamide

epilepticus or repetitive seizures within the 24 h of first ictal event. Etiological and aggravating factors are many (Table 4). Hypoglycemia, hyponatremia, hypomagnesemia, hypocalcemia, and hypoxia are well-known epileptogenic insults that occur in stressed oncological patients or following therapy (1). Meningoencephalitis, cerebral abscesses, and "opportunistic" infections, especially *Aspergillus*, *Candida*, *Listeria*, and *Toxoplasmosis*, also may contribute to the development of seizures (see Chap. 3).

Systemic chemotherapy is associated with seizures in less than 1% of all patients treated (4). Convulsions occur in about 6% of pediatric sarcoma patients and are most commonly related to chemotherapy-induced electrolyte abnormalities (5,6). Chemotherapeutic drugs implicated in causing seizures are also associated with encephalopathy (Table 5) (5,7). Vincristine may provoke seizures through the induction of inappropriate antidiuretic hormone secretion and hyponatremia (8). Busulfan demonstrates dose-dependent neurotoxicity, principally seizures, which may be prophylactically controlled with clonazepam (9). Intrathecal chemotherapy may be epileptogenic (see Chap. 10). Seizures may herald neurotoxicity secondary to external-beam radiotherapy of the CNS (see Chap. 11).

Patients with early status epilepticus or repetitive seizures suffer from significant mortality (29% within the first week) and morbidity (60% of survivors require continued anticonvulsant therapy). Long-term neurological sequelae occur in 28% of children with repetitive or prolonged initial seizures and 11% of those with brief or single seizures. Approximately 13% of pediatric cancer patients who experience a seizure will require long-term antiepileptic therapy. Indications include a history of status epilepticus, initially repetitive seizures and patients with refrac-

**Table 4** Seizures

*Differential Diagnosis*
CNS metastases: 20%         Venous sinus thrombosis: 6%
Metabolic imbalance: 17%    Leukoencephalopathy: 6%
Coagulopathy: 17%           CNS infection: 5%
Cerebrovascular event: 15%  Septic shock: 3%
Hypertension: 8%            Pharmacological toxicity: 2%

**Table 5**  Seizures

*Pharmacological Causes: 1–6% of Patients*

| | |
|---|---|
| Methotrexate | Ifosfamide |
| Arabinosylcytosine | IA BCNU |
| L-Asparaginase | Vincristine (via SIADH) |
| Etoposide/VP 16 | Busulfan |
| Chlorambucil | |

IA = Intra-arterial; SIADH = Syndrome of inappropriate antidiuretic hormone secretion

tory early seizures, who have a higher incidence of cerebral metastases, leukoencephalopathy, and infarction (1).

## C. Cerebrovascular Disease

Four cerebrovascular syndromes are recognized complications of cancer in children (10). These include (1) disseminated intravascular coagulation (DIC) causing thrombosis; (2) acute arterial or venous sinus thrombosis secondary to L-asparaginase therapy; (3) a strokelike syndrome associated with high-dose methotrexate; and (4) encephalopathy, seizures, and focal neurological deficits due to compression of the cranial venous sinuses or torcular herophili by epidural metastases of neuroblastoma. Other forms of cerebrovascular accidents (CVA) include intraparenchymal and subarachnoid hemorrhage. The overall incidence of CVAs among children with systemic cancer is 3.7% (26/700). In 11.5% of these patients, the CVA represents the presenting sign of malignancy. For the majority, the CVA occurs a median of 5 months following diagnosis. The relative distribution by pathological diagnosis varies between solid and hematopoietic malignancies (Table 6). Acute promyelocytic leukemia is the subtype of pediatric leukemia with the highest relative incidence of CVA. Postmortem examination reveals hemorrhagic and/or ischemic vascular CNS lesions in 20% of children dying with systemic cancer. Cerebrovascular accidents are the direct cause of death in 23% of the pediatric cancer patients who are affected. The setting is frequently that of progressive intracranial DIC, especially in patients with acute promyelocytic leukemia (10).

Diffuse encephalopathy, superimposed upon an acute or fluctuating focal neurological deficit, is a common presentation for DIC and may precede laboratory evidence of the coagulopathy by 24–48 h. Fifteen percent of CVAs develop during bacterial sepsis complicated by DIC. Vasculitis secondary to varicella or fungal sepsis also may cause CVA. Intracerebral hemorrhage is associated with thrombocytopenia in 11.5% of pediatric patients who experience a CVA. Leukocytosis is not a significant risk factor for CVAs associated with childhood cancer.

**Table 6**  Cerebrovascular Complications

*Incidence:* 4%
Nonacute lymphoblastic leukemia:
　13% of these patients
Neuroblastoma: 6%
Bone sarcomas: 5%
Acute lymphoblastic leukemia: 4%
Lymphoma: 1%

Nonbacterial thrombotic endocarditis is a rare complication among children; however, cardiomyopathy due to vertebral irradiation or anthracycline therapy may be associated with embolic CVA (10).

L-Asparaginase and high-dose methotrexate are the pharmacological agents especially associated with CVA. Typically, CVAs due to L-asparaginase occur along with the development of seizures and encephalopathy late in induction therapy for acute lymphocytic leukemia (ALL). This usually develops after the seventh to ninth doses and as long as 2–3 weeks following L-asparaginase therapy. The diagnosis is confirmed by neuroradiological examination and evidence of a rebound hypercoagulable state (1,10,11). The strokelike syndrome associated with high-dose methotrexate frequently develops with sudden onset following the third to seventh courses and is associated with a gradual, complete recovery. Recurrence is uncommon with subsequent methotrexate therapy (10). The delayed vascular complications of cerebrospinal radiotherapy are discussed in Chapter 12.

## D. Pain

Of all the neurological complications of pediatric malignant disease, pain is probably the most common and least discussed. At least 62% of children with cancer present with pain, although the incidence may be 100% among diseases such as Ewing's sarcoma, osteogenic sarcoma, and neuroblastoma. Pain is the sole presenting symptom in 34%, while 28% experience pain in concert with other localizing symptoms (12). Poor functional status correlates with the severity of pain ($p_2 = 0.004$). Such children experience pain for a median of 74 days (3–821 days) prior to beginning therapy. As many as 29% of pediatric oncology referrals to the National Cancer Institute report moderate to severe pain that has not been treated adequately (12). Pain continues to be a problem in 54% of inpatients and 26% of the outpatient pediatric cancer population. Yet 40% of inpatients and 38% of outpatients experiencing pain do not receive appropriate analgesics (13). Once treated, the pain persists a median of 10 days for patients with either isolated primary or metastatic tumors (12). Appropriate analgesic and disease-control measures are available and effective. In part, the lack of appropriate pain management reflects the inadequacy of the physician's assessment of pain in the child. The discrepancy between physician-rated pain and patient-rated pain is greatest among younger children (13). These children are the least articulate and able to provide a localizing description of their pain to the physician. A small child is more likely to express distress with withdrawal, regression, and depression, rather than with spontaneous complaints (14).

In contrast to widely held assumptions, relapse is the cause of the pain in only 54% of pediatric oncologic inpatient hospital-days and 30% of outpatient visits (Table 7). Disease-related pain is due to skeletal invasion in 68% of cases, soft tissue involvement in 16%, spinal cord compression in 5%, and may be multifactorial in 11% (i.e., related to soft tissue disease with viscus obstruction, neuropathic compression, or bone metastasis, etc.). Other causes include chemotherapy-related dysesthesias, phantom-limb pain, post–lumbar puncture headache, abdominal pain related to refractory vomiting, and radiation dermatitis (13).

Pain is such a frequent accompaniment to other neurological complications that its presence is "taken for granted." Distinct syndromes are recognizable that require specific therapeutic approaches. Bone pain frequently occurs in a setting of diffuse metastases. Metastatic bone pain often is responsive to steroids, which may obviate the use of narcotics. Diagnosis is potentially difficult for metastases to the T1 vertebral body or the basicranium. However, cranial nerve deficits and radicular distribution of pain may be localizing for the examiner (15).

Headache and signs of increased intracranial pressure occur in 52% of children with CNS parenchymal metastases (16). Historical features of ominous significance include early-morning headache and vomiting which awakens the patient. "Gray-out" of vision occurring during the worst of the headache may represent a Lundborg pressure wave superimposed upon elevated baseline intracranial pressure. Pain is the first symptom of spinal cord compression secondary to epidural metastasis in as many as 96% of patients (15,17–19). The pain of spinal cord

**Table 7** Pain

*Differential Diagnosis*
Mucositis: 26%
Infection: 7%
Postoperative: 18%
Neuropathic: 8%
Tumor: 35%
   Bony metastases: 68%
   Soft tissue invasion: 16%
   Spinal cord compression: 5%

compression may also be radicular and exacerbated by the supine position. Lhermitte's sign (an electric shock–like dysesthesia associated with cervical flexion) may suggest epidural tumor (20). Pain may be a presenting complaint of leptomeningeal metastases in 24–76% of patients of all ages. The pain may be radicular (58% of the time), or present as headache (32%), neck, or back pain (17%) (21). Headache with intracerebral or subarachnoid hemorrhages is immediate, maximal at onset and potentially catastrophic. Subdural hemorrhage in the child with cancer may be asymptomatic and related to previous episodes of thrombocytopenia or the placement of a ventriculoperitoneal shunt. However, pediatric cancer patients with subdural hematomas often do not have a history of prior cranial trauma. Venous sinus occlusion associated with L-asparaginase therapy or calvarial metastases typically presents with a gradually evolving headache, papilledema or retinal hemorrhages, gait dysfunction, and spasticity of the lower extremities.

Pain also may occur as a neurological complication of surgery, radiation therapy, or chemotherapy. Headache may accompany cerebral radionecrosis of the "somnolence syndrome" which follows cranial radiotherapy (see Chap. 10). Steroids may be palliative. Painful symptoms associated with external-beam radiotherapy of the spinal cord include Lhermitte's sign, which may occur within the first 6–12 weeks of treatment. Delayed radiation myelopathy may be complicated by pain in 20% of affected patients (22). Pain in this setting necessitates evaluation for locally recurrent disease. Radionecrosis of craniofacial bones may be a long-term painful complication of radiotherapy. An important discriminating feature from recurrent tumor is the frequent occurrence of cranial nerve deficits with recurrent tumor. Tumor lysis secondary to chemotherapy may exacerbate the pain of bone marrow and skeletal metastases. Vincristine administration may cause diffuse dysesthesias or jaw pain. Procarbazine is a monoamine oxidase inhibitor that may produce intense headache related to hypertension precipitated by coincident use of phenothiazine anti-emetics, meperidine, and tyramine-containing foods such as cured cheeses and chocolate. Intrathecal chemotherapy can cause post–lumbar puncture headaches, headache from arachnoiditis secondary to chemical meningitis, and even communicating hydrocephalus leading to headache from increased intracranial pressure.

## E. Brain Metastases

The incidence of solid tumors of adulthood metastasizing to the brain ranges from 10–20% at postmortem examination. Metastatic lesions make up 13.5–37% of all intracranial tumors (23,24). Brain metastases are relatively less frequent among patients less than 21 years of age with solid tumors, being documented in 10% (1.8–13%) of postmortem examinations. The relative incidence of cerebral metastases is increasing over time, apparently related to prolongation of life by chemotherapy, especially among patients with sarcomas (16,25–27). In pediatric autopsy series, the incidence of brain metastases varies depending on the primary solid tumors (Table 8) (16,25,28). In the older literature, 12.9% of autopsied patients with Wilms' tumor had CNS metastases. The recent decreased incidence of CNS metastases from Wilms' tumor reflects improved disease control (25). The major predictor for brain metastases is the existence of pulmonary metastases. The latency between the development of lung and CNS metastatic disease ranges from 1–20 months, with sarcomas, carcinomas, and melanomas displaying shorter latencies (16,25).

The clinical presentations of children with brain metastases is summarized in Table 9 (16). Seizures are the presenting sign in 50% of those younger than 15 years and in children with metastatic germ cell tumor. Brain metastases may also present as an acute neurological catastrophe, which occurs in 20% of pediatric patients so afflicted. Such acute deterioration often is due to hemorrhage into metastases, especially metastases of sarcomas and germ cell tumors (16).

## F. Myelopathy

Twenty-five percent (15–40%) of the spinal tumors of childhood represent contiguous or distant metastatic spread from a systemic neoplasm (17). The incidence of spinal cord compression by an epidural metastasis is 5% (112/2259) among children with malignant solid tumors (29). However, less than 5% of cases of spinal cord compression due to neoplastic epidural compression occur in patients younger than 20 years of age (30). Neoplasms in this age group associated with myelopathy are shown in Table 10 (29). Sixty-nine percent of the children with spinal cord compression secondary to epidural metastases are known to have cancer. Myelopathy also may be the presenting sign of a malignancy in 10–31% of patients with unexplained spinal cord compression, particularly with neuroblastoma. The interval between onset and diagnosis of spinal cord compression among patients known to have cancer is a mean of 21 days (2–84 days). In contrast, for the children whose condition is without a known etiology, diagnosis is delayed to a mean of 44 days (21–84 days) ($p < 0.002$). Such patients are

**Table 8** Brain Metastases

Incidence: 10% (2–13% of
  Childhoood Cancers)
Osteogenic sarcoma: 6–14%
Rhabdomyosarcoma: 7–14%
Ewing's sarcoma: 2–16%
Germ cell tumors: 20–50%

**Table 9** Brain Metastases

| |
|---|
| *Clinical Presentation* |
| Headache, papilledema: 52% |
| Seizures: 36% |
| Hemiparesis: 36% |
| Encephalopathy: 16% |
| Catastrophic intratumoral hemorrhage: 20% |
|     Sarcomas |
|     Germ cell tumors |

frequently misdiagnosed as having primary orthopedic, rheumatoid, or infectious problems (17,29).

The clinical presentation of metastatic epidural spinal cord compression may be categorized by segmental level of involvement: spinal (C1-T10), conus medullaris (T10-L2), and cauda equina (L2-S5) (Table 11). Myelography reveals a complete block in 65% and high-grade block in 12%. Cerebrospinal fluid exhibits a pleocytosis ($> 5$ white blood cells/mm$^3$) (range 9–200 WBC/mm$^3$) in 22%. The mean CSF protein is 227 mg/dl; higher values correlate with complete obstruction. The CSF profile may be entirely normal in 38% (17).

The therapeutic approach to these children involves multimodality treatment. Neurosurgical indications include the need to establish a pathological diagnosis, the treatment for radioresistant tumors (such as sarcomas), and "small-cell tumors" (especially Ewing's sarcoma, neuroblastoma, lymphoma, and germ cell tumor) presenting with rapid neurological deterioration. Patients with metastatic sarcoma particularly benefit from decompressive posterior laminectomy. Survival time following surgical decompression is prolonged for patients with Ewing's sarcoma. Aggressive surgical and medical intervention is especially recommended for children presenting with severe motor deficits (29). Prompt neurosurgical intervention may not achieve complete neurological recovery among patients with small-cell tumors, which are likely to be radio- and/or chemoresponsive. Due to the relative incidence of spinal cord compression by these neoplasms during childhood, aggressive chemotherapeutic intervention may be considered

**Table 10** Myelopathy

| | |
|---|---|
| *Incidence:* 5% | |
| Ewing's sarcoma: 18% of patients with cord compression | Rhabdomyosarcoma: 5% |
| | Soft tissue sarcomas: 4% |
| Neuroblastoma: 8% | Germ cell tumors: 4% |
| Osteogenic sarcoma: 7% | Lymphoma: 2% |

**Table 11** Myelopathy

| Clinical Presentation | |
|---|---|
| Weakness: 69% | Vertebral tenderness: 23% |
| Reflex abnormalities: 58% | Sphincter incompetence: 23% |
| Hypotonia: 46% | Ataxia |
| + Babinski: 46% | Segmental sensory loss |

as an alternative, with or without adjunctive radiotherapy. Excellent results may be achieved in as many as 64% of patients, with 71–100% of survivors remaining ambulatory. Neurological recovery can occur within 8 days of initiation of chemotherapy (31,32). In contrast, surgical decompression and radiation therapy are associated with subluxation, scoliosis, and/or kyphosis in about 50% (20–78%) of long-term survivors (29,32). Risk factors for radiation-related complications include early age at diagnosis, asymmetric spinal column irradiation, and dosage prescriptions greater than 20 gray (Gy) (1 Gy = 100 rad) (33).

Spinal cord and/or radicular deficits may occur as a consequence of intrathecal or systemic chemotherapy (19). Two syndromes are recognized, one of which is the acute onset of a flaccid areflexic paraparesis, temporally related to the intrathecal chemotherapy injection. The mechanism is unknown but may include a toxic effect of the benzyl alcohol preservative on the spinal nerve roots. The prognosis for recovery is poor, even with immediate lavage of the thecal subarachnoid space (34). A second form occurs with high-dose nitrosourea chemotherapy for malignant gliomas characterized by progressive spastic-ataxic paraparesis, sphincter incompetence, and a fluctuating sensory level. Recovery may be limited and delayed. This is likely a toxic myelopathy. The neuropathological findings include demyelination, especially of the posterior columns, axonal swelling, and fibrillary gliosis with a macrophagic infiltration (reviewed by 19,35).

## G. Neoplastic Meningitis

Meningeal carcinomatosis was originally observed by Eberth (36). The mechanisms of dissemination include extension from a CNS parenchymal metastasis, hematogenous spread with seeding of the choroid plexus, or retrograde involvement of Batson's venous plexus from an infiltrated bone marrow (37). The incidence is difficult to determine among children with solid cancers but is probably more common among patients with leukemia. About 5% of children with ALL present with involvement of the meninges or brain parenchyma (38,39). At first relapse, 50% of patients develop CNS disease; the incidence at postmortem is 60–70% (40). Risk factors include younger age ($\leq$ 24 months), duration of diagnosis ($\geq$ 120 months), leukocytosis ($\geq$ 20,000), and organomegaly (41).

Cranial nerve deficits are an unfavorable prognostic sign in children with leukemia, implying occult meningeal disease (42).

The presenting symptoms of leptomeningeal metastases at any age are presented in Table 12 (19,21). Progression to myelopathy or a cauda equina syndrome is not uncommon. The diagnosis is based upon clinical findings, CSF pleocytosis, hypoglycorrhachia, a positive CSF cytology, or radiographic evidence of "drop" metastases. However, the CSF profile (cell count and protein) correlate poorly with cytological confirmation (21). Myelography may be nondiagnostic in 43–67% of patients with metastatic subarachnoid disease (21,43). Magnetic resonance imaging may be a convenient, noninvasive substitute for myelography, although its sensitivity may be further improved by postmyelography computed tomography of the spine (44). Evidence of intracranial subarachnoid spread and communicating hydrocephalus also should be sought. Newer intrathecal pharmacological approaches for disease control include diaziquone, 6-mercaptopurine, and mafosfamide (45).

## H. Paraneoplastic Disorders

Paraneoplastic effects on the nervous system are unusual among childhood cancers. A notable exception is the opsoclonus-myoclonus syndrome, which occurs in 2% of patients with ganglioneuroblastomas and neuroblastoma. Between 50–100% of pediatric patients with opsoclonus-myoclonus syndrome harbor a neural crest tumor (46–49). Transient opsoclonus-myoclonus syndrome is also described in a child with Beckwith-Wiedemann syndrome and hepatoblastoma (50). A similar condition in the adult is associated with neoplasms of the lung, breast, and ovary (51).

Opsoclonus refers to chaotic, periodic, irregular conjugate eye movements (52). The condition is also called the "myoclonic encephalopathy of infants," "dancing eyes; dancing feet," and "infantile polymyoclonia-opsoclonus" syndromes. Opso-myoclonus may develop as an acute or subacute syndrome, frequently as the presenting sign of a remote malignancy with a prediagnosis symptomatic interval of 2 weeks to 47 months (48,49). The older literature emphasizes the opsoclonus and myoclonus, while more recent reports describe the

**Table 12** Neoplastic Meningitis

| | |
|---|---|
| *Clinical Presentation* | |
| Encephalopathy: 31–52% | Ataxia: 22–36% |
| Cranioneuropathy: 49–88% | Sensory deficit: 27–51% |
| Weakness: 47–78% | Radiculopathy: ?–82% |
| Reflex abnormalities: 27–71% | |

subacute onset of inability to sit/stand, dysarthria, intention tremor, head titubation, and loss of head control. Anorexia, irritability, and spinocerebellar ataxia appear to be ubiquitous features (49,53). This movement disorder may continue during sleep (54) and be associated with seizures (55). Since opsoclonus-myoclonus syndrome may be associated with a mild CSF pleocytosis and respond to steroids, the clinical distinction from a parainfectious process may be difficult (49).

The opsoclonus and ataxia are often responsive to corticotropin (50–80 units/day) or prednisone (2 mg/kg/day). Some patients may become steroid-dependent (56). Intravenous immunoglobulin (IVIG) (1g/kg) is reported to improve the polymyoclonia and ataxia in 48 hs. There may be a role for maintenance therapy with IVIG (57). Unfortunately, the neurological disorder frequently develops a chronic, relapsing course which leaves the child severely developmentally delayed and disabled (49,53). Resection of the neuroblastoma may or may not ameliorate the symptoms. In contrast, the oncological prognosis is favorable because the patients typically present with low-stage disease (Stage I, II, or $IV_s$), favorable histopathology, and single copies of the *N-myc* oncogene (58,59).

Less well characterized paraneoplastic disorders of childhood include the syndrome of acute polyneuropathy, encephalopathy, pathological corticospinal tract signs, and dysautonomia in children treated for Hodgkin's lymphoma (60). This entity may overlap with the "encephalo-myelo-radiculo-neuropathy" syndrome described by Gamstorp (61). Cranial and proximal muscle weakness, areflexia, early atrophy, and absence of response to anti-acetylcholinesterases ("the Lambert-Eaton-Rooke myasthenic syndrome") rarely occurs as the heralding symptom of leukemia in children (62).

## III. CHILDHOOD NEOPLASMS
### A. Tumors of the Central Nervous System
### 1. Clinical Presentation

Brain cancers are the most common solid tumors of childhood. Intracranial neoplasms presenting during infancy are among the most difficult to diagnose. The symptoms that should initiate investigation include unexplained vomiting, increasing head circumference, seizures, lethargy, and focal neurological deficits. Frequent neurological signs at diagnosis are shown in Table 13 (63).

Between infancy and adolescence, CNS neoplasms are more frequently located infratentorially (56%) than supratentorially (44%) (64). The clinical paradigm of the posterior fossa neoplasm is headache, papilledema, and axial ataxia, secondary to obstructive hydrocephalus. Medulloblastoma constitutes about 25% of pediatric CNS neoplasms; most (76%) of these children are ill less than 3 months before the diagnosis is established (65). The typical presenting findings are shown

**Table 13** Brain Tumors of Infancy

| Clinical Presentation | |
|---|---|
| Macrocephaly: 45% | Encephalopathy: 16% |
| Bulging fontanel: 27% | Hyperreflexia: 16% |
| Cranioneuropathy: 25% | Hypotonia: 11% |
| Papilledema: 16% | Hemiparesis: 9% |
| Meningismus: 16% | Hypertonia: 9% |

in Table 14. Brainstem gliomas present with ataxia and cranial nerve deficits (Table 15). Although not common initially, hemiparesis is a nearly ubiquitous late finding (66).

For children with supratentorial astrocytomas, the mean prediagnosis symptomatic interval is 10–13 months (64,67). The clinical presentation is summarized in Table 16. In contrast, thalamic tumors typically (60–75%) present with symptoms of less than 6 months' duration. In addition to hemiparesis and increased intracranial pressure, the patient may demonstrate involuntary movements (tremor, choreathetosis, and dystonia) (Table 17) (68,69).

## 2. Seizures

Brain tumors are a rare cause of seizures among children, accounting for 1–2% of diagnoses (70). However, convulsions may be a presenting symptom in 25–76% of pediatric patients with supratentorial tumors. Another 15–20% will develop a seizure disorder later (67,71–73). Partial and partial complex seizures (46.9%) are the most common forms of seizure among children with CNS neoplasms (67,71,74,75). There is a bias toward low-grade, well-differentiated tumors among reported series on neurosurgical management of epilepsy (75).

## 3. Intratumoral Hemorrhage

Intratumoral, parenchymal, and/or subarachnoid hemorrhages bring 10% (1–16%) of pediatric patients with brain tumors to medical attention (76,77). In one series, 62% of cases of intratumoral hemorrhages occurred in children (78). During childhood, 41% of intratumoral bleeds are associated with primitive

**Table 14** Medulloblastoma

| Clinical Presentation | |
|---|---|
| Symptomatic < 3 months | Axial ataxia: 62% |
| Headaches: 65% | Nystagmus: 44% |
| Papilledema: 76% | Appendicular dysmetria: 35% |

**Table 15**   Brainstem Gliomas

| | |
|---|---|
| *Clinical Presentation* | |
| Axial ataxia: 49% | Dysarthria, dysphagia: 11% |
| Diplopia: 38% | Multiple cranioneuropathies: 52% |
| Head tilt: 20% | Late, progressive hemiparesis |
| Facial paresis: 17% | |

neuroectodermal tumors (PNET) (76,79,80). Microscopic evidence of hemorrhage may be found in 53% of glioblastomas, 57% of oligodendrogliomas, and 10% of astrocytomas in patients of all ages (81).

## 4. Neoplastic Meningitis

Leptomeningeal dissemination is evident at postmortem examination in 20–77% of primary brain tumors (82–84). The average age at diagnosis is 15.7 years (83). A recent review reports the antemortem diagnosis of neoplastic meningitis in 19% (60/314) of children with CNS neoplasms. Of these patients, 50% (30/60) are affected at the time of diagnosis, 28% as an isolated event or concurrent with local recurrent disease, and 22% late in disease progression (43). The majority of cases of "meningeal gliomatosis" are attributable to childhood PNET (47–55% of cases of neoplastic meningitis) (Table 18) (83,85–99). Medulloblastoma is notorious for the frequency of meningeal dissemination at recurrence, developing in 35% (13–78%) (43,65,100,101). In addition to a disease-specific predilection for subarachnoid dissemination, other risk factors include accessibility of the tumor to the ventricular system and a history of multiple craniotomies (99).

The incidence of meningeal involvement among *newly diagnosed* brain tumor patients of *all ages* is 0.01%, principally affecting patients with PNET (61%) and malignant gliomas (27%) (102). Prospective and retrospective analyses demonstrate CSF cytological and/or myelographic evidence of meningeal seeding in 28% (3–63%) of intracranial PNET and medulloblastoma patients at presentation (43,101,103–110). The wide range reported may reflect the vigor and technical methods with which the diagnosis is pursued. Diagnosis is based on CSF cyto-

**Table 16**   Supratentorial Gliomas

| | |
|---|---|
| *Clinical Presentation* | |
| Symptomatic 10–13 months | Visual disturbance: 30% |
| Headache and vomiting: 62% | Sensory deficit: 20% |
| Seizures: 55% | Cranioneuropathy: 20% |
| Papilledema: 85% | Aphasia: 15% |
| Hemiparesis: 40% | |

**Table 17** Thalamic Gliomas

| Clinical Presentation | |
|---|---|
| Symptomatic < 6 months: 70% | Involuntary movements: 22% |
| Headache: 68% | Dysphasia: 22% |
| Hemiparesis: 75% | Seizures: 17% |
| Increased intracranial pressure: 53% | Hemianopsia: 15% |
| | Anisocoria |

logical analysis and imaging studies (43). Subarachnoid and systemic dissemination among PNET correlate with earlier age of onset ($p < 0.01$) and an adverse prognosis ($p = 0.0002$) (43,101,104). The incidence is lower among other CNS neoplasms such as malignant glioma (12% of meningeal seeding) and ependymoma (5%) (43).

An inflammatory meningeal syndrome may be present in 7% of pediatric CNS neoplasms. This most commonly occurs as "aseptic meningitis" following posterior fossa craniotomies (111,112). A few cases of neoplastic meningitis are reported without an obvious primary tumor at the time of diagnosis. Connor and Cushing (113) described a case of medulloblastoma with extensive meningeal involvement, in which the primary cerebellar tumor was clinically silent and only discovered by postmortem microscopy. Three pediatric cases of meningeal gliomatosis are reported to have presented with hydrocephalus and multifocal and diffuse neurological findings. These patients died within months of diagnosis and were found to have diffuse leptomeningeal astrocytomas (114). Canady and Zakalik (115) report three children who presented with suspected tuberculous or recurrent aseptic meningitis that was proven related to suprasellar PNET, butterfly glioblastoma, and pontine epidermoid.

## 5. Systemic Metastases

Systemic metastatic spread of a CNS neoplasm is an unusual event, the overall incidence being 2.3% among childhood brain tumors (116–118). Extracranial and systemic metastases are more common among younger children and those with

**Table 18** Neoplastic Meningitis

| Incidence Among Brain Tumor Patients: 19% | |
|---|---|
| Primitive neuroectodermal tumors and medulloblastoma: 50% | Ependymoma: 12–16% |
| | Oligodendroglioma: 1–12% |
| Malignant gliomas: 7–61% | Astrocytomas (any site): 2–7% |
| Brainstem gliomas: 18–33% | |

PNET (104). About 10% (0–18%) of medulloblastoma and PNET patients suffer from extraneural spread (116,119). Medulloblastoma accounts for 27–77% of cases of childhood CNS tumors that disseminate systemically (116,117,119,120). Fifteen percent of recurrent medulloblastomas are associated with systemic dissemination. Extra-axial metastasis represents the only site of relapse in 8% of medulloblastoma recurrences (121). The mean time to metastasis is 17 months (9–83 months) after diagnosis (118). The most common sites of dissemination are shown in Table 19 (116,117,119,120). Peritoneal spread is hypothesized to occur via ventriculoperitoneal shunts, although this is controversial (110,116,119,122, 123). Glioblastoma is rarely reported during childhood to present with osseous metastases at diagnosis or in late relapse (124). There are anecdotal accounts of systemic metastases from low-grade astrocytomas (124,125). Recent reviews discuss systemic metastases of primary intracranial germ cell tumor (126,127). Survival among brain tumor patients with systemic dissemination is almost uniformly dismal (116,118).

## 6. *Neuropsychological Sequelae*

There is increasing concern with the "quality of life" of survivors of pediatric brain tumors. Historically, it was appreciated that 20–40% of survivors experienced long-term sequelae; of these, less than 10% were globally or severely impaired. More sophisticated psychometric studies demonstrate cognitive deficiencies in as many as 40–100% of treated patients. The problems relate to learning disabilities, memory deficits, visual-perceptual integration, and adaptability (128). The controversies regarding the pathogenesis of these long-term deficits, particularly those related to radiotherapy, are reviewed elsewhere (129,130, Chap. 10).

## 7. *Neurosurgical Complications*

Unusual postoperative complications of infratentorial tumors include the "posterior fossa postcraniotomy syndrome," which may complicate craniotomy for tumors of the brainstem, fourth ventricle, and vermis cerebelli. This syndrome is characterized by mutism, multiple cranial nerve deficits, hemiparesis or quadriparesis, as well as pseudobulbar palsy. The onset may occur within the immediate postoperative period or be delayed for hours to days. Recovery may be protracted and evolves through phases of dysarthria and spinocerebellar dysfunction

**Table 19** Systemic Metastases: 2–3%

| *Primitive Neuroectodermal Tumors: 10% (0–18%)* | |
|---|---|
| Skeleton: 71–93% of patients with metastases | Bone marrow: 31–61% |
| | Lymph nodes: 29–65% |
| Peritoneum: 30–43% | Lung: 7–30% |

(131,132). The pathogenesis is unknown. Neuroradiographic studies do not indicate frank vascular compromise, edema, or hemorrhage as a causative factor. Injury to the dentate nuclei appears to be an important and potentially preventable contributing factor (133). Another complication of pediatric posterior fossa surgery is the 3–10% risk of rostral brainstem herniation through the incisura of the tentorium cerebelli during the preoperative placement of ventriculoperitoneal shunts for obstructive hydrocephalus in patients with posterior fossa masses (134,135). The mechanism of herniation appears related to the reversed force gradient in which the posterior fossa pressure is higher (due to the space-occupying lesion) relative to supratentorial pressure that is abruptly lowered by CSF drainage. Intratumoral hemorrhage may be an additional complicating event (134,135).

## B. Neuroblastoma, Tumors of the Autonomic and Peripheral Nervous System

Neuroblastoma is narrowly defined to represent a neoplasm of the adrenal glands and/or sympathetic nervous system that arises predominantly in childhood. Clinical localization of the primary tumor within the cervicothoracic ganglia may be assisted by the finding of Horner's syndrome and heterochromia iridis (136). Urinary retention or a neurogenic bladder may be associated with presacral primary tumors arising from the organ of Zukerkandl. Unusual neurological presentations include the opsoclonus-myoclonus syndrome and the Verner-Morrison syndrome associated with ganglioneuroblastomas. This presents as a chronic watery diarrhea secondary to secretion of vasoactive intestinal peptide which enhances intestinal secretion and motility (137,138).

The most frequent neurological complication of neuroblastoma is epidural metastasis with spinal cord compression (36% of neuroblastoma patients who develop neurological symptoms) (139). Eight to thirty percent of the neoplastic compressive myelopathies of childhood are due to neuroblastoma (29,140–142). Often neuroblastoma spreads contiguously from a paravertebral primary site via an intervertebral foramen into the epidural space. Myelopathy may be the presenting sign of neuroblastoma, especially in infants under 12 months of age (18). These younger babies frequently have little metastatic disease burden at presentation; therefore, their prognosis is more favorable than the common situation of late-onset spinal cord compromise in an older child with Stage IV disease. Infants 1 year of age or younger with Stage II neuroblastoma may be treated with radiotherapy for the control of mediastinal and intraspinal disease. Doses of 0.9–18 Gy are associated with good local control and acceptable toxicity, in terms of kyphoscoliotic complications (143).

Tumor spread is evident in 60–70% of cases of neuroblastoma at presentation. Approximately 55% of newly diagnosed patients suffer from widely metastatic disease (Stage IV). This is age dependent. Sixty percent of children 2 years of age or older are Stage IV while only 25% of patients less than 1 year of age are so affected (144). Frequent sites of metastasis include the subcutaneous tissues (especially in the infant), bone marrow ($\geq$ 50%), the orbital basicranium, calvarium, and skeleton. Intracranial epidural metastases of neuroblastoma may be complicated by venous sinus obstruction (145). Ocular and oculomotor cranial nerve deficits, as well as proptosis, may result from mechanical distortion secondary to periorbital metastases. Parenchymal brain metastases and neoplastic meningitis from systemic neuroblastoma are exceedingly rare (139,146–150).

## C. Retinoblastoma

The annual incidence of retinoblastoma is $3.58/10^6$ children in the United States. Approximately 30–40% of these patients have bilateral disease and germ-line mutations. Retinoblastoma and associated malignancies account for about 1.5% of childhood cancer deaths. The neurological features of the clinical presentation include strabismus (20%), visual dysfunction (5%), anisocoria, and nystagmus (151). Visual loss may be due to macular involvement, vitreous dissemination, or retinal detachment. Proptosis or systemic signs of disease are uncommon at presentation (152). Patients with structural deletions of chromosome 13q may have associated mental retardation, microcephaly, holoprosencephaly, microophthalmos, and other congenital malformations (153). Independent neoplastic transformation within the pineal may occur among retinoblastoma patients with bilateral disease, producing a condition termed trilateral retinoblastoma (154).

Intraocular retinoblastoma is initially confined to the retina, vitreous, choroid, and/or sclera. Choroidal involvement (25–61%) probably serves as the source of dissemination. Scleral involvement (17–30%) is secondary to direct extension from the choroid or draining veins. Optic nerve extension occurs as in 72–77% of patients who develop metastatic disease (155–157). Ten to twelve percent of retinoblastoma patients develop extraocular disease that is present at diagnosis in 57% of this subgroup (151,158). The incidence is similar between patients with unilateral (14%) and bilateral disease (10.5%). However, late-onset metastatic disease is more frequent among younger patients and those with bilateral retinoblastoma. Age and bilaterality are also interrelated (151,159).

The most common signs of extraocular disease are an orbital mass (69%), cranial nerve deficits (39%), or evidence of bone marrow compromise (39%) (160). Extraocular lesions at presentation are primarily confined to the orbit or calvarium (92%) (151). Dissemination to the CNS can occur without local recurrence, 1–24 months after diagnosis (161). In 50% (22–100%) of those with extraocular disease, metastatic retinoblastoma ultimately invades the brain, spinal cord, meninges, or epidural space (158,160,161). The mechanism of spread may be via optic nerve, the lamina cribosa, or the periorbital veins that allow extension into the cavernous sinus, hence into the subarachnoid space (156). The survival of patients with metastatic retinoblastoma is virtually nil. At least 47% of deaths are directly attributable to the CNS involvement (155). Parenchymal brain metastases are found in 25–94% at postmortem examination (155,160,161). Systemic dissemination (65% of cases of extraocular retinoblastoma) is primarily hematogenous with a predilection for the bone marrow, skeleton, and lymph nodes. As many as 25% of those with metastases may have extracranial lesions without CNS disease (156).

Treatment of retinoblastoma may also be associated with neurological complications. Cryotherapy and irradiation are used in an attempt to forestall enucleation and spare vision. Radiotherapy of disease limited to the primary site utilizes doses of 35–50 Gy. Radiation therapy for postoperative, residual disease requires a wider field encompassing the orbit with doses of 50–55 Gy. The resulting radiation effects may include visual loss, inferior frontal leukoencephalopathy as well as retardation of development of the oculofacial skeleton (162).

Cranial nerve deficits and CNS metastases may result from secondary malignancies that develop among retinoblastoma patients with germ-line mutations. Patients with bilateral retinoblastoma have a 15–20% chance of developing a second nonocular neoplasm from 1–40 years later. The incidence is similar among treated and untreated patients (151). Osteogenic sarcoma is the most common second malignancy with relative excess risk of 200–500-fold. Within the irradiated field, the incidence of osteogenic sarcoma increases to 2000–5000-fold (163). Other radiation-associated neoplasms in retinoblastoma patients include fibrosarcoma, soft tissue sarcoma, squamous cell carcinoma, angiosarcoma, rhabdomyosarcoma, fibrous histiocytoma, neuroblastoma, and meningioma. Unrelated neoplasms with a higher incidence among retinoblastoma patients than the general population are melanoma, thyroid carcinoma, testicular carcinoma, liposarcoma, Ewing's sarcoma, and Wilms' tumor (151,163).

## D. Tumors of Viscera and Germ Cell Tumors

Neurological complications, such as encephalopathy, seizure, brain metastases, or spinal cord compression, may occur with any solid tumor of childhood. This section will address the predictably associated neurological findings of visceral neoplasms. Patients with Wilms' tumor and aniridia (1.4% of cases of Wilms') may have associated mental retardation and congenital anomalies related to chromosome 11p deletions (164). Wilms' tumor may metastasize to the brain; as previously noted, the incidence of this complication is decreasing (165).

Malignant germ cell tumor (germinoma, teratoma, embryonal carcinoma, endodermal sinus tumor, and choriocarcinoma) of childhood may be categorized by site of origin and age of onset, which correlate with histological subtype and natural history. Adult germ cell tumor primaries occur most often in the gonads, in contrast to the multiple sites of origin among pediatric cases; these sites include the sacrococcygeum, retroperitoneum, mediastinum, ovary, and diencephalon (166). Anticipated neurological deficits associated with sacrococcygeal germ cell tumor include pain, neurogenic bladder, lumbosacral plexopathy, radiculopathy, and spinal cord compression. Mediastinal germ cell tumor may be complicated by contiguous spread to the epidural space and myelopathy due to spinal cord compression. In addition, extragonadal germ cell tumors typically present at an advanced stage during childhood ($p < 0.01$) (167). Systemic germ cell tumors metastasize to the CNS in 20–40% of cases. The brain is the site of metastases 62% of the time, the spinal cord 15%, or both sites 23% (167,168). These complications typically occur (69% of the time) 2–16 months (median = 6 months) following pulmonary dissemination or via direct extension of paravertebral disease (31% of the time) (167). The histological subtypes most likely to spread hematogenously are the embryonal carcinoma and choriocarcinoma (168). Choriocarcinoma tends to develop multiple lesions; embryonal carcinoma often presents as a single metastatic lesion. Metastatic choriocarcinoma to the CNS may present as a neurological catastrophe due to the high incidence of intratumoral hemorrhage.

## E. The Histiocytoses

The history and nomenclature of "histiocytosis X" (eosinophilic granuloma, Letterer-Siwe disease, Hand-Schüller-Christian disease, and Langerhans' cell histiocytosis) are reviewed elsewhere (169,170). While the pathogenesis of histiocytosis X is not understood, it is a disease related to the proliferation of cells derived from the Langerhans' cell. Clinically histiocytosis X resembles other immunologically mediated diseases such as GVHD and certain immunodeficiencies (171,172).

The neurological complications of this disease may be classified as central (parenchymal, leptomeningeal) or peripheral. The classic clinical descriptions of Hand-Schüller-Christian disease emphasize polyuria, exophthalmos, and calvarial lesions (169). The most common example of CNS involvement by histiocytosis X is hypothalamic dysfunction causing diabetes insipidus. This is described in the older European literature as "Gagel's disease" (173,174). Diabetes insipidus affects 25–50% of patients and may be the presenting sign in about half, with the remainder developing it at the time of disease progression (175). In its most severe form, the patient may experience pan-hypopituitarism (176). Extension of the disease process into the third ventricle may cause obstructive hydrocephalus (177). Parenchymal histiocytosis X lesions may be solitary or multifocal, occurring within the cerebrum, basal ganglia, optic chiasm, brainstem, spinal cord, and cauda equina (169,178–181). A characteristic, if not pathognomonic, lesion

42. Ingram LC, Fairclough DL, Furman WL, et al. Cranial nerve palsy in childhood acute lymphoblastic leukemia and non-Hodgkin's lymphoma. Cancer 1991; 67: 2262–8.
43. Packer RJ, Siegel KR, Sutton LN, et al. Leptomeningeal dissemination of primary central nervous system tumors of childhood. Ann Neurol 1985; 18:217–21.
44. Kramer ED, Rafto SE, Packer RJ, Zimmerman RA. Comparison of myelography with CT followup versus gadolinium MRI for subarachnoid metastatic disease in children. Neurology 1991; 41:46–50.
45. Blaney SM, Balis FM, Poplack DG. Pharmacologic approaches to the treatment of meningeal malignancy. Oncology 1911; 5:107–16.
46. Cushing H, Wolback SB. The transformation of a malignant paravertebral sympathicoblastoma into a benign ganglioneuroma. Am J Pathol 1927; 3:203–20.
47. Solomon GE, Chutorian AM. Opsoclonus and occult neuroblastoma. N Engl J Med 1968; 279:475–77.
48. Boltshauser E, Deonna T, Hirt HR. Myoclonic encephalopathy of infants or "dancing eyes syndrome": report of 7 cases with long-term follow-up and review of the literature (cases with and without neuroblastoma). Helv Paediatr Acta 1979; 34:119–33.
49. Mitchell WG, Snodgrass SR. Opsoclonus-ataxia due to childhood neural crest tumors: a chronic neurologic syndrome. J Child Neurol 1990; 5:153–8.
50. Wilfong AA, Parke JT, McCrary JA, III. Opsoclonus-myoclonus with Beckwith-Wiedemann syndrome and hepatoblastoma. Pediatr Neurol 1992; 8:77–9.
51. Digre KB. Opsoclonus in adults: report of three cases and review of the literature. Arch Neurol 1986; 43:1165–75.
52. Kinsbourne M. Myoclonic encephalopathy of infants. J Neurol Neurosurg Psychiatry 1962; 25:271–9.
53. Senelick RC, Bray PF, Lahey E, et al. Neuroblastoma and myoclonic encephalopathy: two cases and a review of the literature. J Pediatr Surg 1973; 8:623–32.
54. Martin ES, Griffith JF. Myoclonic encephalopathy and neuroblastoma. Am J Dis Child 1971; 122:257–8.
55. Bale JF, Bray PF. Convulsions with an occult neuroblastoma. N Engl J Med 1979; 301:555–6.
56. Nickerson BG, Hutter JJ. Opsomyoclonus and neuroblastoma: response to ACTH. Clin Pediatr 1979; 18:446–8.
57. Petruzzi MJF, De Alarcon P. Treatment of a patient with opsoclonus-myoclonus syndrome and neuroblastoma with intravenous gammaglobulin. Pediatr Res 1992; 31:144A.
58. Altman AJ, Baehner RL. Favorable prognosis for survival in children with coincident opso-myoclonus and neuroblastoma. Cancer 1976; 37:816–52.
59. Cohn SL, Salwen H, Herst CV, et al. Single copies of the N-myc oncogene in neuroblastomas from children presenting with the syndrome of opsoclonus-myoclonus. Cancer 1988; 62:723–6.
60. Kurczynski TW, Choudhury AA, Horwitz SJ, et al. Remote effect of malignancy on the nervous system in children. Dev Med Child Neurol 1980; 22:205–22.
61. Gamstorp I. Encephalo-myelo-radiculo-neuropathy: involvement of the CNS in

21. Kaplan JG, DeSouza TG, Farkash A, et al. Leptomeningeal metastases: comparison of clinical features and laboratory data of solid tumors, lymphomas and leukemias. J Neurooncol 1990; 9:225–9.
22. Godwin-Austen RB, Howell DA, Worthington B. Observations on radiation myelopathy. Brain 1975; 98:557–68.
23. Stortebecker TP. Metastatic tumors of the brain from a neurosurgical point of view: a follow-up of 158 cases. J Neurosurg 1954; 11:84–111.
24. Posner JB. Brain metastases: a clinician's view. In: Weiss L, Gilbert HA, Posner JB, eds. Brain metastases. Boston: GK Hall, 1980:2–30.
25. Vanucci RC, Baten M. Cerebral metastatic disease in childhood. Neurology 1974; 24:981–5.
26. Gerkovich FG, Luna MA, Gottlieb JA. Increased incidence of cerebral metastases in sarcoma patients with prolonged survival from chemotherapy: report of cases of leiomyosarcoma and chondrosarcoma. Cancer 1975; 36:1843–51.
27. Espana P, Chang P, Wiernik PH. Increased incidence of brain metastases in sarcoma patients. Cancer 1980; 45:377–80.
28. Trigg ME, Glaubiger D, Nesbit NE. The frequency of isolated CNS involvement in Ewing's sarcoma. Cancer 1982; 49:2404–9.
29. Klein SL, Sanford RA, Muhlbauer MS. Pediatric spinal epidural metastases. J Neurosurg 1991; 74:70–5.
30. Constans JP, de Divitiis E, Donzelli R, et al. Spinal metastases with neurological manifestations: review of 600 cases. J Neurosurg 1983; 59:111–18.
31. Mones RJ, Dozier D, Berrett A. Analysis of medical treatment of malignant extradural spinal cord tumors. Cancer 1966; 19:1842–53.
32. Hayes FA, Thompson EI, Hvizdala E, et al. Chemotherapy as an alternative to laminectomy and radiation in the management of epidural tumor. J Pediatr 1984; 104:221–4.
33. Mayfield JK, Riseborough EJ, Jaffe N, et al. Spinal deformities in children treated for neuroblastoma. J Bone Joint Surg 1981; 63:183–93.
34. Hahn AF, Feasby TE, Gilbert JJ. Paraparesis following intrathecal chemotherapy. Neurology 1983; 33:1032–8.
35. Burger PC, Kamenar E, Schold SC, et al. Encephalomyelopathy following high-dose BCNU therapy. Cancer 1981; 48:1318–27.
36. Eberth CJ. Zur entwickelung des epitheliomas (cholesteatomas) der piaung der lunge. Virchows Arch [A] 1870; 49:51–60.
37. Kokkoris CP. Leptomeningeal carcinomatosis: how does cancer reach the pia-arachnoid? Cancer 1983; 51:154–60.
38. Evans AE, Gilbert ES, Zandstra A. The increasing incidence of central nervous system leukemia in children. Cancer 1970; 26:404–9.
39. Simone JV, Verzosa MS, Rudy JA. Initial features and prognosis in 363 children with acute lymphoblastic leukemia. Cancer 1975; 36:2099–108.
40. Price RA, Johnson WW. The central nervous system in childhood leukemia: I. the arachnoid. Cancer 1973; 31:520–33.
41. Graham Pole JR, Willoughby JLN. Leukemia in the nervous system: factors in pathogenesis. Mod Probl Pediatr 1975; 16:59–79.

# REFERENCES

1. DiMario FJ Jr, Packer RJ. Acute mental status changes in children with systemic cancer. Pediatrics 1990; 85:353–60.
2. Butt W, Barker G, Walker C, et al. Outcome of children with hematologic malignancy who are admitted to an intensive care unit. Crit Care Med 1988; 16:761–4.
3. Lockman LA, Sung JH, Krivit W. Acute parkinsonian syndrome with demyelinating leukoencephalopathy in bone marrow transplant recipients. Pediatr Neurol 1991; 7: 457–63.
4. Zaocara G, Muscas GC, Messori A. Clinical features, pathogenesis and management of drug-induced seizures. Drug Saf 1990; 5:109–51.
5. Stein DA, Chamberlain MC. Evaluation and management of seizures in the patient with cancer. Oncology 1991; 5:33–9.
6. Kramer ED, Lewis D, Raney B, et al. Neurologic complications in children with soft tissue and osseous sarcomas. Cancer 1989; 64:2600–3.
7. Weiss HD, Walker MD, Wiernik PH. Neurotoxicity of commonly used antineoplastic agents. N Engl J Med 1974; 291:75–81.
8. Legha SS. Vincristine neurotoxicity: pathophysiology and management. Med Toxicol 1986; 1:421–7.
9. Vassal G, Deroussent A, Hartmann O, et al. Dose-dependent neurotoxicity of high-dose busulfan in children: a clinical and pharmacological study. Cancer Res 1990; 50:6203–7.
10. Packer RJ, Rorke LB, Lange BJ, et al. Cerebrovascular accidents in children with cancer. Pediatrics 1985; 76:194–201.
11. Cairo MS, Lazarus K, Gilmore FL, Baehner RL. Intracranial hemorrhage and focal seizures secondary to use of L-asparaginase during induction therapy of acute lymphocytic leukemia. J Pediatr 1980; 97:829–33.
12. Miser AW, McCalla J, Dothage JA, et al. Pain as a presenting symptom in children and young adults with newly diagnosed malignancy. Pain 1987; 29:85–90.
13. Miser AW, Dothage JA, Wesley RA, Miser JS. The prevalence of pain in a pediatric and young adult cancer population. Pain 1987; 29:73–83.
14. Savedra M, Gibbons, P, Tesler M, et al. How do children describe pain? A tentative assessment. Pain 1982; 14:95–104.
15. Greenberg HS, Deck MD, Vikram B, et al. Metastases to the base of the skull: clinical findings in 43 cases. Neurology 1981; 31:530–7.
16. Graus F, Walker RW, Allen JC. Brain metastases in children. J Pediatr 1983; 103:558–61.
17. Baten M, Vanucci RC. Intraspinal metastatic disease in childhood cancer. J Pediatr 1977; 90:207–12.
18. Punt J, Pritchard J, Pincott JR, Till K. Neuroblastoma: a review of 21 cases presenting with spinal cord compression. Cancer 1980; 45:3095–101.
19. Choucair AK. Myelopathies in the cancer patient: incidence, presentation, diagnosis and management. Oncology 1991; 5:25–31.
20. Ventrafridda V, Caraceni A, Martini C, et al. On the significance of Lhermitte's sign in oncology. J Neurooncol 1991; 10:133–7.

involves the dentate nuclei of the cerebellum, which may appear calcified or hypodense on CT (169,178,182–184). Cerebellar findings may antedate other stigmata of histiocytosis X (182,183). A "meningo-encephalitic" syndrome is caused by extension of histiocytosis X lesions into the Virchow-Robin spaces. Frank leptomeningeal infiltration is particularly associated with Letterer-Siwe disease (185,186). A diffuse encephalitis-like process may occur, with attendant plaques or diffuse demyelination with axonal sparing (169,187,188). The choroid plexus may be infiltrated, especially within the glomus (169). Solitary or multiple subdural masses may cause neurological complications without calvarial radiographic abnormalities (189).

Peripheral neurological deficits are often related to basicranial or skeletal histiocytosis X lesions. Hypothalamic-pituitary dysfunction may also result from extension of the calvarial disease into the sella turcica. Possible cranial nerve deficits may include blindness and ophthalmoplegia from periorbital lesions (177). Epidural lesions may present with radiculopathy (190,191). Skeletal changes in the vertebral bodies can cause collapse and myelopathy (192). Critically placed lesions often require radiotherapy for disease control (193). The neurological sequelae of histiocytosis X may be increased over the long term by radiotoxicity, causing the development of learning disabilities, seizures, demyelination, blindness, and cranial nerve deficits as well as secondary malignancies (194,195).

## IV. CONCLUSIONS

Much work remains to be done to further delineate the neurological complications of childhood cancer. The spectrum of diseases varies from that of adults. Children are vulnerable to complications of the disease and its treatment during critical periods of cellular migration (for the cerebellum), glial proliferation, and myelination. Improvements in neoplastic disease control will contribute positively to the personal outcome and socioeconomic burden of neurotoxicity placed upon families of surviving children. Innovative application of therapies such as IVIG for opsoclonus-myoclonus syndrome, although not understood pathophysiologically, are to be encouraged and investigated. Pain control in pediatric cancer patients is an area in which improvement is needed by all caring for these children. This is one area where effective analgesic and disease control measures are available and immediately applicable.

## ACKNOWLEDGMENTS

This work was supported by the National Institutes of Neurological Disorders and Stroke (1 KO8 NS 00986), National Institutes of Health BRSG, and Vanderbilt University Research Council.

children with Guillain-Barré-Stohl syndrome. Dev Med Child Neurol 1974; 16: 654–8.
62. Shapira Y, Cividalli G, Szabo G, et al. A myasthenic syndrome in childhood leukemia. Dev Med Child Neurol 1974; 16:668–71.
63. Farwell JR, Dohrmann GJ, Flannery JT. Intracranial neoplasms in infants. Arch Neurol 1978; 35:533–7.
64. Mercuri S, Russo A, Palma L. Hemispheric supratentorial astrocytomas in children: long term results in 29 cases. J Neurosurg 1981; 55:170–3.
65. Park TS, Hoffmann HJ, Hendrick EB, et al. Medulloblastoma: clinical presentation and management. Experience at the Hospital for Sick Children, Toronto, 1950–1980. J Neurosurg 1983; 58:543–52.
66. Albright AL, Price RA, Guthkelch AN. Brain stem gliomas of children: a clinicopathologic study. Cancer 1983; 52:2313–19.
67. Hirsch J-F, Sainte Rose C, Pierre-Kahn A, et al. Benign astrocytic and oligodendrocytic tumors of the cerebral hemispheres in children. J Neurosurg 1989; 70: 568–72.
68. Hirose G, Lombroso CT, Eisenberg H. Thalamic tumors in childhood. Arch Neurol 1975; 32:740–4.
69. Bernstein M, Hoffmann HJ, Halliday WC, et al. Thalamic tumors in children: long-term follow-up and treatment guidelines. J Neurosurg 1984; 61:649–56.
70. Page LK, Lombroso CT, Mattson DD. Childhood epilepsy with late detection of cerebral glioma. J Neurosurg 1969; 31:253–61.
71. Aicardi J, Praud E, Bancaud J, et al. Epilepsies cliniquement primitives et tumeurs cerebrales chez l'enfant. Arch Fr Pediatr 1970; 27:1041–55.
72. Backus RE, Millichap JG. The seizure as manifestation of intracranial tumor in childhood. Pediatrics 1962; 29:978–84.
73. Hauser WA, Hesdorffer D. Epilepsy—frequency, causes and consequences. Epilepsy Foundation of America: Demos Publishing, 1990.
74. Blume WT, Girvin JP, Kaufmann JCE. Childhood brain tumors presenting as chronic uncontrolled focal seizure disorders. Ann Neurol 1982; 12:538–41.
75. Spencer SS, Spencer DD, Mattson RH, et al. Intracerebral masses in patients with intractable partial epilepsy. Neurology 1984; 34:432–6.
76. Laurent JP, Bruce DA, Schut L. Hemorrhagic brain tumors in pediatric patients. Childs Brain 1981; 8:263–70.
77. Yokota A, Kajiwara H, Matsuoka S, et al. Subarachnoid hemorrhage from brain tumors in childhood. Childs Nerv Syst 1987; 3:65–9.
78. Glass B, Abbott KH. Subarachnoid hemorrhage consequent to intracranial tumors. Arch Neurol Psychiatry 1955; 73:369–79.
79. Russell DS. The pathology of spontaneous intracranial haemorrhage. Proc R Soc Med 1954; 47:689–93.
80. Scott M. Spontaneous intracerebral hematoma caused by cerebral neoplasms: report of eight verified cases. J Neurosurg 1975; 42:338–42.
81. Liwnicz BS, Wu SZ, Tew JM Jr. The relationship between the capillary structure and hemorrhage in gliomas. J Neurosurg 1987; 66:536–41.

82. Cairns H, Russell DA. Intracranial and spinal metastasis in gliomas of the brain. Brain 1931; 54:377–402.
83. Polmeteer FE, Kernohan JW. Meningeal gliomatosis: a study of forty-two cases. Arch Neurol Psychiatry 1947; 57:593–616.
84. Nishio S, Korosue K, Tateishi J, et al. Ventricular and subarachnoid seeding of intracranial tumors of neuroectodermal origin—a study of 26 consecutive autopsy cases with reference with focal ependymal defect. Clin Neuropathol 1982; 1: 83–91.
85. Bryan P. CSF seeding of intra-cranial tumours: a study of 96 cases. Clin Radiol 1974; 25:355–60.
86. Erlich SS, Davis RL. Spinal subarachnoid metastasis from primary intracranial glioblastoma multiforme. Cancer 1978; 42:2854–64.
87. Yung WK-A, Horten BC, Shapiro WR. Meningeal gliomatosis: a review of 12 cases. Ann Neurol 1980; 8:605–8.
88. Packer RJ, Allen J, Nielsen S, et al. Brainstem glioma: clinical manifestations of meningeal gliomatosis. Ann Neurol 1983; 14:177–82.
89. Salazar OM. A better understanding of CNS seeding and a brighter outlook for postoperatively irradiated patients with ependymomas. Int J Radiat Biol Phys 1983; 9:1231–4.
90. Awad I, Bay JW, Rogers L. Leptomeningeal metastasis from supratentorial malignant gliomas. Neurosurgery 1986; 19:247–51.
91. Ludwig CI, Smith MT, Godfrey AD, Armbrustmacher VW. A clinicopathologic study of 323 patients with oligodendrogliomas. Ann Neurol 1986; 19:15–21.
92. Dropcho EJ, Wisoff JH, Walker RW, Allen JC. Supratentorial malignant gliomas in childhood: a review of fifty cases. Ann Neurol 1987; 22:355–64.
93. Civitello LA, Packer RJ, Rorke LB, et al. Leptomeningeal dissemination of low-grade gliomas in childhood. Neurology 1988; 38:562–6.
94. de Deizer RJW, de Wolff-Rouendaal, Bots GTAM, et al. Optic glioma with intraocular tumor and seeding in a child with neurofibromatosis. Am J Ophthalmol 1989; 108:717–25.
95. Kocks W, Kalff R, Reinhardt V, et al. Spinal metastasis of pilocytic astrocytoma of the chiasma opticum. Childs Nerv Syst 1989; 5:118–20.
96. Sposto R, Ertel IJ, Jenkins RDT, et al. The effectiveness of chemotherapy for treatment of high grade astrocytoma in children: results of a randomized trial. A report from the CCSG. J Neurooncol 1989; 7:165–77.
97. Yamagami T, Kikuchi H, Higashi K, et al. Intracranial metastasis of a spinal cord astrocytoma—case report. Neurol Med Chir (Tokyo) 1990; 30:69–73.
98. Bruggers CS, Friedman HS, Phillips PC, et al. Leptomeningeal dissemination of optic pathway gliomas in three children. Am J Ophthalmol 1991; 111:719–23.
99. Grabb PA, Albright AL, Pang D. Dissemination of supratentorial malignant gliomas via the cerebrospinal fluid in children. Neurosurgery 1992; 30:64–71.
100. McFarland DR, Horwitz H, Saenger EL, et al. Medulloblastoma—a review of prognosis and survival. Br J Radiol 1969; 42:198–214.
101. Deutsch M, Reigel DH. The value of myelography in the management of childhood medulloblastoma. Cancer 1980; 45:2194–7.

102. Perezeskhpour GH, Henry JM, Armbrustmacher VW. Spinal metastases: a rare mode of presentation of brain tumors. Cancer 1984; 54:353–6.
103. Dorwart RH, Wara WM, Norman D, Levin VA. Complete myelographic evaluation of spinal metastases from medulloblastoma. Neuroradiology 1981; 139:403–8.
104. Allen JC, Epstein F. Medulloblastoma and other primary malignant neuroectodermal tumors of the CNS: the effect of patients' age and extent of disease on prognosis. J Neurosurg 1982; 57:446–51.
105. George RE, Laurent JP, McCluggage CW, Cheek WR. Spinal metastasis in primitive neuroectodermal tumors (medulloblastoma) of the posterior fossa: evaluation with CT myelography and correlation with patient age and tumor differentiation. Pediatr Neurosci 1985–86; 12:157–60.
106. Kellie SJ, Kun LE, Kovnar EH, et al. Pediatric brain tumors with neuraxis dissemination at diagnosis: response to preirradiation chemotherapy. Pediatr Neurosci 1988; 14:154.
107. Stanley P, Suminski N. The incidence and distribution of spinal metastases in children with posterior fossa medulloblastomas. Am J Pediatr Hematol Oncol 1988; 10:283–7.
108. Flannery AM, Tomita T, Radkowski M, McLone DG. Medulloblastomas in childhood: postsurgical evaluation with myelography and cerebrospinal fluid cytology. J Neurooncol 1990; 8:149–51.
109. Evans AE, Jenkin DT, Sposto R, et al. The treatment of medulloblastoma: results of a prospective randomized trial of radiation therapy with and without CCNU, vincristine and prednisone. J Neurosurg 1990; 72:572–82.
110. Jenkin D, Goddard K, Armstrong D, et al. Posterior fossa medulloblastoma in childhood: treatment results and proposal for a new staging system. Int J Radiat Oncol Biol Phys 1990; 19:265–74.
111. Bernat JL. Glioblastoma multiforme and the meningeal syndrome. Neurology 1976; 26:1071–4.
112. Lunardi P, Missori P, Fraioli B. Chemical meningitis: unusual presentation of a cerebellar astrocytoma: case report and review of the literature. Neurosurgery 1989; 25:264–70.
113. Connor CL, Cushing H. Diffuse tumors of leptomeninges: two cases in which process was revealed only by microscope. Arch Pathol 1927; 3:374–92.
114. Whelan HT, Mastri AR. Primary diffuse meningeal gliomatosis in children. Ann Neurol 1984; 16:391.
115. Canady A, Zakalik K. Brain tumors presenting as meningitis. Presented at the First International Pediatric Neuro-Oncology Conference, June 1989.
116. Campbell AN, Chan HSL, Becker LE, et al. Extracranial metastases in childhood primary intracranial tumors: a report of 21 cases and review of the literature. Cancer 1984; 53:974–81.
117. Hoffman HJ, Duffner PK. Extraneural metastases of central nervous system tumors. Cancer 1985; 56:1178–82.
118. Chamberlain MC, Silver P, Edwards MSB, Levin VA. Treatment of extraneural metastatic medulloblastoma with a combination of cyclophosphamide, adriamycin and vincristine. Neurosurgery 1988; 23:476–9.

119. Kleinman GM, Hochberg FH, Richardson EP Jr. Systemic metastases from medulloblastoma: report of two cases and review of the literature. Cancer 1981; 48:2296–309.
120. Spencer CD, Weiss RB, Van Eys J, et al. Medulloblastoma metastatic to marrow: report of four cases and review of the literature. J Neurooncol 1984; 2:223–35.
121. Kun LE, D'Souze B, Gefft M. The value of surveillance testing in childhood brain tumors. Cancer 1985; 56:1818–23.
122. Hoffman HJ, Hendrick EB, Humphreys RP. Metastases via ventriculoperitoneal shunt in patients with medulloblastoma. J Neurosurg 1976; 44:562–6.
123. Berger MS, Baumeister B, Geyer JR, et al. The risks of metastasis from shunting in children with primary central nervous system tumors. J Neurosurg 1991; 74:872–7.
124. Gamis AS, Egelhoff J, Roloson G, et al. Diffuse bony metastases at presentation in a child with glioblastoma multiforme: a case report. Cancer 1990; 66:180–4.
125. Longee DC, Friedman HS, Phillips PC, et al. Osteoblastic metastases from astrocytomas: a report of two cases. Med Pediatr Oncol 1991; 19:318–24.
126. Balsitis M, Rothwell I, Pigott TJ, et al. Systemic metastases from primary intracranial germinoma: a case report and literature review. Br J Neurosurg 1989; 3: 717–23.
127. Pallini R, Bozzini V, Scerrati M, et al. Bone metastasis associated with shunt-related peritoneal deposits from a pineal germinoma: case report and review of the literature. Acta Neurochir 1991; 109:788–93.
128. Glauser TA, Packer RJ. Cognitive deficits in long-term survivors of childhood brain tumors. Childs Nerv Syst 1991; 7:2–12.
129. Cohen ME, Duffner PK. Long-term consequences of CNS treatment for childhood cancer, Part I: Pathologic consequences and potential for oncogenesis. Pediatr Neurol 1991; 7:157–63.
130. Duffner PK, Cohen ME. Long-term consequences of CNS treatment for childhood cancer, Part II: Clinical consequences. Pediatr Neurol 1991; 7:237–42.
131. Wisoff JH, Epstein FJ. Pseudobulbar palsy after posterior fossa operation in children. Neurosurgery 1984; 15:707–9.
132. Ammirati M, Mirzai S, Samii M. Transient mutism following removal of a cerebellar tumor: a case report and review of the literature. Childs Nerve Syst 1989; 5:12–14.
133. Dietze DD Jr, Mickle JP. Cerebellar mutism after posterior fossa surgery. Pediatr Neurosurg 1990–91; 16:25–31.
134. Epstein F, Murali R. Pediatric posterior fossa tumors: hazards of the "preoperative" shunt. Neurosurgery 1978; 3:348–50.
135. Raimondi AJ, Tomita T. Hydrocephalus and infratentorial tumors: incidence, clinical picture and treatment. J Neurosurg 1981; 55:174–82.
136. Jaffe N, Cassady R, Filler RM, et al. Heterochromia and Horner syndrome associated with cervical and mediastinal neuroblastoma. J Pediatr 1975; 87:75–7.
137. Rosenstein BJ, Engelman K. Diarrhea in a child with catecholamine secreting ganglioneuroma. J Pediatr 1963; 63:217–26.
138. Williams TH, House RF Jr, Burgert EO Jr, Lynn HB. Unusual manifestations of neuroblastoma: chronic diarrhea, polymyoclonia-opsoclonus and erythrocyte abnormalities. Cancer 1972; 29:475–80.

139. Alpert JN, Mones R. Neurologic manifestations of neuroblastoma. Mt Sinai J Med 1969; 36:37–47.
140. Giuffre R, Di Lorenzo N. Primary spinal cord tumors in infancy and childhood. In: Modern problems in paediatrics: neurosurgery. Basel: Karger, 1977; 18:231–5.
141. Le Pintre J, Schweisguth O, Labrune M, Lemerle J. Les neuroblastomes en sablier—etude de 22 cas. Arch Fr Pediatr 1969; 26:829–47.
142. Till K. Paediatric neurosurgery. Oxford: Blackwell Scientific Publications, 1975:200.
143. Jacobson HM, Marcus RB, Thor TL, et al. Pediatric neuroblastoma: postoperative radiation therapy using less than 2000 rad. Int J Radiat Oncol Biol Phys 1983; 9:501–5.
144. Evans AE. Staging and treatment of neuroblastoma. Cancer 1980; 45:1799–1802.
145. Szymula NJ, Lore JM Jr. Neuroblastoma in the head and neck. In: Pochedly C, ed. Neuroblastoma: clinical and biological manifestations. New York: Elsevier Biomedical, 1982:23–8.
146. Ringertz N, Lidholm SO. Mediastinal tumors and cysts. J Thorac Surg 1956; 31:458–87.
147. Russell DS, Rubinstein LJ. Pathology of tumors of the nervous system. Baltimore: Williams & Wilkins, 1972:309–11.
148. Dresler S, Harvey DG, Levisohn PM. Retroperitoneal neuroblastoma widely metastatic to the central nervous system. Ann Neurol 1979; 5:196–8.
149. Koizumi JH, Del Canto MC. Retroperitoneal neuroblastoma metastatic to brain: report of a case and review of the literature. Childs Brain 1980; 7:267–79.
150. Feldges AJ, Stanisic M, Morger R, Waidelich E. Neuroblastoma with meningeal involvement causing increased intracranial pressure and coma in two children. Am J Pediatr Hematol Oncol 1986; 8:355–7.
151. Grabowski EF, Abramson DH. Intraocular and extraocular retinoblastoma. Hematol Oncol Clin N Am 1987; 1:721–35.
152. Bedford MA, Bedotto C, MacFaul PA. Retinoblastoma: a study of 139 cases. Br J Ophthalmol 1971; 55:19–27.
153. Allerdice PW, Davis JG, Miller OJ, et al. The 13q deletion syndrome. Am J Hum Genet 1969; 21:499–512.
154. Bader JL, Meadows AT, Zimmerman LE, et al. Bilateral retinoblastoma with ectopic intracranial retinoblastoma: trilateral retinoblastoma. Cancer Genet Cytogenet 1983; 5:203–13.
155. Merriam GR Jr. Retinoblastoma: an analysis of 17 autopsies. Arch Ophthalmol 1950; 44:71–108.
156. Carbajal UM. Metastases in retinoblastoma. Am J Ophthalmol 1959; 48:47–69.
157. Stannard C, Lipper S, Sealy R, Sevel D. Retinoblastoma: correlation of invasion of the optic nerve and choroid with prognosis and metastases. Br J Ophthalmol 1979; 63:560–70.
158. Pratt CB, Crom DB, Howarth C. The use of chemotherapy for extraocular retinoblastoma. Med Pediatr Oncol 1985; 13:330–3.
159. Abramson DH, Ellsworth RM, Grumbach N, et al. Retinoblastoma: survival, age

at diagnosis and comparison 1914–1958, 1958–1983. J Pediatr Ophthalmol Strabismus 1985; 22:246–50.
160. MacKay CJ, Abramson DH, Ellworth RM. Metastatic patterns of retinoblastoma. Arch Ophthalmol 1984; 102:391–6.
161. Meli FJ, Boccaleri CA, Manzitti J, Lylyk P. Meningeal dissemination of retinoblastoma: CT findings in eight patients. Am J Neuroradiol 1990; 11:983–6.
162. Egbert PR, Donaldson S, Moazed K, Rosenthal AR. Visual results and ocular complications following radiotherapy for retinoblastoma. Arch Ophthalmol 1978; 97:1826–30.
163. Draper GJ, Saunders DM, Kingston JE. Secondary primary neoplasms in patients with retinoblastoma. Br J Cancer 1986; 53:661–7.
164. Riccardi VM, Sujansky E, Smith AC, et al. Chromosomal imbalance in the aniridia-Wilms' tumor association: 11p interstitial deletion. Pediatrics 1978; 61:604–10.
165. Movassaghi N, Leiken S, Chandra R. Wilms' tumor metastasis to uncommon sites. J Pediatr 1974; 84:416–17.
166. Jennings MT, Gelman R, Hochberg F. Intracranial germ cell tumors: natural history and pathogenesis. In: Neuwelt EA, ed. Diagnosis and treatment of pineal region tumors. Baltimore: Williams & Wilkins, 1984:116–38.
167. Brodeur GM, Howarth CB, Pratt CB, et al. Malignant germ cell tumors in 57 children and adolescents. Cancer 1981; 48:1890–8.
168. Vugrin D, Cvitkovic E, Posner JB, et al. Neurological complications of malignant germ cell tumors of testis: biology of brain metastasis (I). Cancer 1979; 44:2349–53.
169. Kepes JJ. Histiocytosis X. In: Vinken PJ, Bruyn GW, eds. Handbook of clinical neurology. Amsterdam: North Holland Publishing Company, 1977; 38:93–117.
170. Osband ME. Histiocytosis X: Langerhans cell histiocytosis. Hematol Oncol Clin N Am 1987; 1:737–51.
171. Nezelof C, Basset F, Rousseau MF. Histiocytosis-X. Histogenetic arguments for a Langerhans' cell origin. Biomed 1973; 18:365–71.
172. Nesbit ME Jr, O'Leary M, Dehner LP, Ramsay NKC. Histiocytosis continued: the immune system and the histiocytosis syndromes. Am J Pediatr Hematol Oncol 1981; 3:141–9.
173. Gagel O. Eine granulationsgeschwulst im gebiete des hypothalamus. Z ges Neurol Psychiatr 1941; 172:50–73.
174. Kepes JJ, Kepes M. Predominantly cerebral forms of histiocytosis X: a reappraisal of "Gagel's hypothalamic granuloma," "granuloma infiltrans of the hypothalamus" and "Ayala's disease" with a report of four cases. Acta Neuropathol 1969; 14:77–98.
175. Lieberman PH, Jones CR, Dargeon HWK, et al. A reappraisal of eosinophilic granuloma of bone, Hand-Schüller-Christian syndrome and Letterer-Siwe syndrome. Medicine 1969; 48:375–400.
176. Braunstein GD, Kohler PO. Endocrine manifestations of histiocytosis. Am J Pediatr Hematol Oncol 1981; 3:67–75.
177. Cureton RJR. A case of intracerebral xanthomatosis with pituitary involvement. J Pathol Bact 1949; 61:533–40.
178. Chiari H. Uber verandergungen im zentralnervensystem bei generalisierter xanthomatose vom typus Schuller-Christian. Virchows Arch [A] 1933; 288:527–53.

179. Beard W, Foster DB, Kepes JJ, Guillan RA. Xanthomatosis of the central nervous system. Clinical and pathological observations of a case with a posterior fossa syndrome. Neurology 1970; 20:305–14.
180. Salcman MD, Quest DO, Mount LA. Histiocytosis X of the spinal cord. J Neurosurg 1974; 41:383–6.
181. Hewlett RH, Ganz JC. Histiocytosis of the cauda equina. Neurology 1976; 26: 472–6.
182. Haslam RHA, Clark DB. Progressive cerebellar ataxia associated with Hand-Schüller-Christian disease. Dev Med Child Neurol 1971; 13:174–9.
183. Braunstein GD, Whitaker JN, Kohler PO. Cerebellar dysfunction in Hand-Schüller-Christian disease. Arch Intern Med 1973; 132:387–90.
184. Adornato BT, Eil C, Head GL, Loriaux L. Cerebellar involvement in multifocal eosinophilic granuloma: demonstration by computerized tomographic scanning. Ann Neurol 1980; 7:125–9.
185. Herzenberg H. Die skelettform der Niemann-Pickschen krankheit. Virchows Arch [A] 1928; 269:614–37.
186. Rube J, De La Pava S, Pickren JW. Histiocytosis X with involvement of the brain. Cancer 1967; 20:486–92.
187. Davison C. Xanthomatosis and the central nervous system (Schüller-Christian syndrome). Arch Neurol Psychiatry 1933; 30:75–98.
188. Rubens-Duval A, Lapresle J, Pardeau M, Amstutz PH. Les determinations nerveuses de la maladie de Hand-Schüller-Christian (etude d'une observation anatomo-clinique). Semin Hop Paris 1966; 42:1425–39.
189. Elian M, Bornstein B, Matz S, et al. Neurological manifestation of general xanthomatosis: Hand-Schüller-Christian disease. Arch Neurol 1969; 20:115–20.
190. Liebeskind A, Jacobson R, Anderson R, Schechter MM. Unusual neurologic and roentgenographic manifestations of eosinophilic granuloma. Arch Neurol 1973; 28: 131–3.
191. Eil C, Adornato BT. Radicular compression in multifocal eosinophilic granuloma: successful treatment with radiotherapy. Arch Neurol 1977; 34:786–7.
192. Cardozo LJ, Bailey IC, Billinghurst JR, Poltera AA. Non-osseous eosinophilic granuloma presenting as acute transverse myelitis. Br J Surg 1974; 61:747–9.
193. Richter MP, D'Angio GJ. The role of radiation therapy in the management of children with histiocytosis X. Am J Pediatr Hematol Oncol 1981; 3:161–3.
194. Nezelof C, Frileux-Herbet F, Cronier-Sachot J. Disseminated histiocytosis X: analysis of prognostic factors based upon a retrospective study of 50 cases. Cancer 1979; 44:1824–38.
195. Komp DM. Long-term sequelae of histiocytosis X. Am J Pediatr Hematol Oncol 1981; 3:165–7.

# Index

Adenoviral encephalitis, 162
Amyloid neuropathy with plasma cell dyscrasia, 490–491, 496
Aneurysm, intracranial with choriocarcinoma, 389–390
Angioendotheliomatosis, 466, 472–473
Antibiotics, in meningitis, 151
Arabinosylcytosine (Ara-C):
  aseptic meningitis with intrathecal, 251–252
  brachial plexopathy, 252
  cerebellar dysfunction, 252
  cranial neuropathy, 252
  encephalopathy, 251–252
  leptomeningeal metastases treatment, 60, 64
  lymphoma, side effects, 466, 476
  Parkinsonism, 252
  ocular toxicity, 252
  peripheral neuropathy, 252
  SIADH with, 252
  transverse myelopathy with intrathecal, 251–252

Ara-C (see Arabinosylcytosine)
Aseptic meningitis (see Meningitis, aseptic)
Asparaginase:
  brain hemorrhage, 130
  encephalopathy, 252
  venous thrombosis, cerebral, 252–253
*Aspergillus fumigatus*:
  brain abscess, 154–155
  with leukemia, 452, 456
Astrocytoma (see Brain tumor)
Autonomic dysfunction:
  paraneoplastic, 188–189
  with suramin, 255
  with taxol, 255
  with vincristine, 250

Bacterial meningitis, 152
Basal cell carcinoma, perineural spread, 346–347

**535**

BCNU (*see* Nitrosoureas)
Bell's palsy (*see* Mononeuropathy, facial)
Bone marrow transplantation:
 myasthenia gravis, 453, 461
 myopathy, 453, 461
Biliary carcinoma:
 brain metastases, 411
 vertebral metastases, 411
Bladder carcinoma:
 brain metastases, 391
 leptomeningeal metastases, 391
Brachial plexopathy:
 arabinosylcytosine (Ara-C), 252
 breast carcinoma, 322
 carcinoid, 405
 head and neck cancer, 366
 Hodgkin's disease, 478
 interleukin-2, 282, 283
 lung cancer, 303–305
 malignant melanoma, 344
 radiotherapy, 84, 92, 229–230, 326
Brachial plexus metastases (*see* Nerve metastases; Brachial plexus)
Brain abscess (*see* Infections, brain abscess)
Brain metastases:
 biliary carcinoma, 411
 bladder carcinoma, 391
 breast carcinoma, 312, 315–317
 carcinoid, 405
 choriocarcinoma, 389, 390
 colorectal carcinoma, 410
 computed tomography, 6–10
 diagnosis, 6–10
 differential diagnosis, 7
 distribution, anatomical, 2–4
 encephalopathy, 5–6
 epidemiology, 1–4
 Ewing's sarcoma, 441–443
 gastric carcinoma, 401–402
 gastrointestinal cancer, 395–397
 head and neck cancer, 360–361
 hemorrhage, 6
 hepatoma, 411
 incidence, 1–2
 lung cancer, 298–300

[Brain metastases]
 lymphoma, 466, 471
 malignant melanoma, 336–343
 management, 10–18
  algorithm, 11
  chemotherapy, 16–17
  glucocorticoids, 10–12, 201–206
  interstitial brachytherapy, 14
  magnetic resonance imaging, 6–10
  radiosurgery, 13–14
  radiotherapy, 12–13
  recurrences, 17–18
  surgery, 14–16
 mode of spread, 2
 multiple, 4
 osteosarcoma, 434–435
 pediatric cancer, 3, 509–510, 511
 primary sites, 2
 prostate carcinoma, 383
 renal carcinoma, 387–388
 rhabdomyosarcoma, 432–433
 sarcoma, 418–422
 seizures, 5
 signs, 5
 single, 4
 solitary, 4
 symptoms, 5
 testicular carcinoma, 390
 uterine cervical carcinoma, 384
 uterine endometrial carcinoma, 385
Brain plasmacytoma, 500
Brainstem glioma in children, 515, 516
Brain tumors, in adults:
 brainstem dysfunction, 111
 cerebellar dysfunction, 111
 chemotherapy, 115–116
 clinical manifestations, 104–112
 diagnostic tests, 112
 differential diagnosis, 112–113
 encephalopathy, 105
 epidemiology, 103–104
 false localizing signs, 112
 glucocorticoids, 116–117, 201–206
 headache, 105–107
 herniation, 117
 increased intracranial pressure, 108–109

# Index

[Brain tumors, in adults]
  management, 113–119
  metastases, 117–118
  motor symptoms, 109
  progressive symptoms, 104
  radiotherapy, 114–115
  seizures, 107–108, 117
  sensory loss, 109
  speech disorders, 109–110
  steroid receptors, 202
  surgery, 113–114
  thrombophlebitis, 118–119
  visual dysfunction, 110–111
Brain tumors, in children:
  clinical features, 514–515
  hemorrhage, cerebral, 515–516
  leptomeningeal metastases, 516
  neuropsychological sequelae, 518
  seizures, 515
  surgery, 518–519
  systemic metastases, 517–518
Breast cancer:
  brain metastases, 312, 315–317
  cerebrovascular complications, 328–329
  chemotherapy side effects, 324–325
  dural metastases, 312, 313–314
  encephalopathy, 324
  infections of nervous system, 230
  leptomeningeal metastases, 312, 314–315
  ocular metastases, 312, 317
  paraneoplastic syndromes, 330
  peripheral neuropathy, 312, 322–324
  pituitary metastases, 312, 317–318
  radiotherapy side effects, 326–327
  skull metastases, 311–324
  spinal metastases, 312, 318–321
  surgical complications, 326–328

*Candida albicans* brain abscess, 452, 456
Carboplatin neurotoxicity, 249
Carcinoid:
  brachial plexopathy, 405

[Carcinoid]
  brain metastases, 405
  carcinoid syndrome, 403–404
  clinical features, 403
  encephalopathy, 405–406
  leptomeningeal metastases, 405
  myopathy, 406
  niacin deficiency, 406
  pituitary metastases, 405
  skull metastases, 404–405
  spinal metastases, epidural, 404
  tryptophan deficiency, 406
Carcinomatous meningitis (*see* Leptomeningeal metastases)
Carotid artery rupture with head and neck cancer, 362
Carpal tunnel syndrome (*see* Mononeuropathy, median)
Cauda equina syndrome:
  leukemia, 453, 457
  testicular carcinoma, 377
CCNU (*see* Nitrosoureas)
Cerebrovascular disorders:
  epidemiology, 123–124
  head and neck cancer, 366
  hemorrhage, intracerebral, 124–130
    aneurysm, neoplastic, 125–126
    breast cancer, 328
    coagulopathy, 128–130
    hypertension, 130
    iatrogenic, 130
    intratumoral, 124–125
    leptomeningeal metastases, 126
    leukemia, 126–128
    myeloproliferative disorders, 130
    polycythemia, 130
    thrombocythemia, 130
    thrombocytopenia, 128–130
  Hodgkin's disease, TIA, 140–141
  infarction, cerebral, 130–141
    asparaginase, 507
    atherosclerosis, 140
    breast cancer, 329
    chemotherapy-related, 139
    disseminated intravascular coagulation, 132–134

[Cerebrovascular disorders]
  embolus, tumor, 137–138
  granulomatous angiitis, 140
  head and neck cancer, 366
  Herpes zoster, 136
  leptomeningeal metastases, 138
  leukemia, 506
  lymphoma, 476
  methotrexate, 306, 507
  nonbacterial endocarditis, 131–132
  radiotherapy-related, 139
  septic, 135–136
  thrombocytosis, 140
  venous thrombosis, 134–135
  pediatric cancer, 506–507
  subdural hematoma:
    breast cancer, 328
    leptomeningeal metastases, 126
    leukemia, 452, 455–456
    prostate cancer, 382–383
  venous occlusion by tumor, 137
Cerebellar degeneration:
  breast cancer, 330
  head and neck cancer, 361
  multiple myeloma, 498
  ovarian carcinoma, 386–387
  paraneoplastic, 169–174
Cerebellar dysfunction:
  arabinosylcytosine (Ara-C), 252
  fluorouracil (5-FU), 244–245, 367
Cerebellar hemangioblastoma and renal carcinoma, 379
Chemoembolization-associated lumbosacral plexopathy, 378–379
Chemotherapy complications:
  arabinosylcytosine (Ara-C), 251, 252
  asparaginase, 252–253
  carboplatin, 249
  cisplatin (DDP), 246–248
  etoposide (VP-16), 254
  fluorinated antipyrimidines, other, 246
  fluorouracil (5-FU), 244–245, 367
  levamisole, with 5-FU, 245
  methotrexate, 251–244, 324–325, 437–438, 466, 476 (*see also* Methotrexate)
  procarbazine, 253

[Chemotherapy complications]
  suramin, 255
  taxol, 254–255
  thio-TEPA, 255
  vincristine, 249–251
Chloroma, cerebral, 457
Choriocarcinoma:
  aneurysm, neoplastic, 389–390
  brain metastases, 389, 390
  hemorrhage, intracerebral, 389
Cisplatin (DDP) neurotoxicity:
  cranial neuropathy, 247
  focal brain dysfunction, 248
  gastrointestinal cancer, 378
  LHermitte's sign, 247–248
  herniation, cerebral, 248
  intra-arterial, 248
  ototoxicity, 378
  peripheral neuropathy, 246–247
CNS infections (*see* Infections)
CNS lymphoma (*see* Lymphoma, primary CNS)
Coagulopathy, hemorrhage, intracerebral, 128–130
Coma, vincristine, 251
Colorectal cancer:
  brain metastases, 410
  brain tumors, 411
  encephalopathy, 410
  familial syndromes, 411
  leptomeningeal metastases, 410
  lumbosacral plexopathy, 410
  radiotherapy, 409–410
  *cis*-retinoic acid, 411
  surgery, 409
Cortical blindness:
  vincristine, 251
Cranial neuropathy:
  arabinosylcytosine, 252
  cisplatin, 247, 248
  head and neck cancer, 361–362, 363
  histiocytosis, 523
  malignant melanoma, 344
  multiple myeloma, 498–499
  radiotherapy, 229–230, 363
  rhabdomyosarcoma, 431
  vincristine, 250

# Index

*Cryptococcus neoformans* meningitis, 148–150
   lymphoma, 466, 475
Cutaneous T-cell lymphoma, 348
Cyclosporine:
   encephalopathy, 270, 272–273
   myelopathy, 273
   myopathy, 271, 273
   paresthesias, 271, 273
   seizures, 269–272
   tremor, 269, 270
Cytomegalovirus (CMV) encephalitis, 161

Dermatomyositis (*see* Myopathy)
Dexamethasone (*see also* Glucocorticoids):
   animal data, spinal cord compression, 208
   anti-edema, 201–202
   bioavailability, 200–201
   brain tumors, 203–206
   spinal cord compression, 208
   toxicity, 205, 209–213
Diabetes insipidus with histiocytosis, 522–523
Disseminated intravascular coagulation:
   breast cancer, 328–329
   infarction, cerebral, 132–134
Disulfiram-like syndrome, with procarbazine, 253
Dural metastases:
   breast cancer, 312, 313–314
   Ewing's sarcoma, 441–443
Dysgeusia with levamisole, 268
Dysproteinemias (*see* Plasma cell dyscrasias)

Embryonal tumors of CNS, associated renal embryonal tumors, 380
Encephalopathy:
   asparaginase, 252

[Encephalopathy]
   BCNU, 254
   brain metastases, 5–6
   breast cancer, 328
   carcinoid, 405–406
   chemotherapy, 503, 505
   colorectal cancer, 410
   cyclosporine, 270, 272–273
   disseminated intravascular coagulation, 506
   drug-related, 504
   gastrointestinal cancer, 397–398
   hepatoma, 411
   ifosfamide, 253
   immunotoxins, 287–288
   insulinoma, 407
   interferon, 274–275, 277–279
   interleukin-2, 281–283
   ketoconazole, 379
   levamisole, 268–269
   leukemia, 453, 458–459
   lung cancer, 305
   methotrexate, 437–438
   pediatric cancers, 503–504
   procarbazine, 253
   uterine carcinoma, cervical, 385
Endodermal sinus tumors (*see* Testicular cancer)
Eosinophilic granuloma (*see* Histiocytosis)
Ependymoma (*see* Brain tumors)
Epidemiology:
   brain metastases, 1–4
   brain tumors, adult, 103–104
   cerebrovascular disorders, 123–124
   Ewing's sarcoma, 438–439
   gastrointestinal cancer, 395–398
   infections, 145–146
   leptomeningeal metastases, 50–51
   leukemias, 449–450
   lymphoma, leptomeningeal, 467
   lymphoma, primary CNS, 478
   lymphomas, 465–467
   osteosarcoma, 433–434
   paraneoplastic syndromes, 167–169
   rhabdomyosarcoma, 424
   sarcomas, 417–418
   spinal metastases, epidural, 23–24

Epidural spinal cord compression (*see* Spinal metastases, epidural)
Esophageal carcinoma, 396–397
Etoposide (VP-16) neurotoxicity, 254
Ewing's sarcoma:
  brain metastases, 441
  clinical features, 438–439
  dural metastases, 441–443
  epidemiology, 438–439
  gastrointestinal cancer, 373–374, 375
  leptomeningeal metastases, 443
  lung cancer, 295–298
  malignant melanoma, 334
  skull metastases, 441–443
  spinal metastases, epidural, 440–441

Familial adenomatosis syndrome, 411
Fluorinated antipyrimidines, 246
Fluorouracil (5-FU) neurotoxicity:
  cerebellar dysfunction, 244–245
  in head and neck cancer, 367
  with levamisole, 245
  with other agents, 245

Gamma knife (*see* Radiotherapy, stereotactic)
Gammopathy (*see* Plasma cell dyscrasias)
Ganglioneurolastoma, opsoclonus-myoclonus, 513–514
Gardner's syndrome, 411
Gastric carcinoma, 400–402
  brain metastases, 401–402
  leptomeningeal metastases, 402
  subacute combined degeneration, 400–401
Gastrinoma, 407–408
  MEA-I, 408
  pain, 408
  with pituitary tumors, 408

Gastrointestinal cancer:
  brain metastases, 395–397
  encephalopathy, 397–398
  leptomeningeal metastases, 397
  lumbosacral plexopathy, 397
  paraneoplastic syndromes, 398
Genitourinary cancer:
  associated CNS neoplasms, 379–380
  clinical presentation, 375
  pathogenesis of neurological complications, 374–375
  treatment modalities, 376–377
  treatment, neurological complications, 376, 377–379
    chemotherapy, 378–379
    radiotherapy, 377–378
    surgery, 377
Germ cell tumor, malignant in children, 521–522
Gestational trophoblastic carcinoma (*see* Choriocarcinoma)
Glioblastoma multiforme (*see* Brain tumors)
Gliomas (*see* Brain tumors)
Glucocorticoids:
  actions, 199–200
    animal data, spinal cord compression, 207–208
    in spinal cord compression, 206–207
  anti-edema, brain tumors, 201–202
  bioavailability, 200–201
  clinical use, brain tumors, 202–206
  clinical use, spinal cord compression, 208–209
  toxicity, 209–213
    discontinuation of treatment/withdrawal, 213
    drug interactions, 211–212
    pituitary-adrenal suppression, 212–213
    side effects, direct, 209–210
Granulocytic sarcoma (*see* Chloroma)
Guillain-Barré syndrome (acute inflammatory polyradiculo-neuropathy) (*see also* Peripheral neuropathy), 82, 186

# Index

[Guillain-Barré syndrome]
  Hodgkin's disease, 466, 478
  leukemia, 453, 460
  multiple myeloma, 492
  suramin, 255

HAM (see HTLV$_1$-associated myelopathy)
Hand-Schuler-Christian disease (see Histiocytosis)
Head and neck cancer:
  associated diseases, 357
  brachial plexopathy, 360
  brain metastases, 360–361
  chemotherapy, 366
  clinical features, squamous carcinoma, 355–367
  diplopia, 353, 354
  ear pain, 353–354
  facial numbness/paresthesias, 354
  facial weakness, 254–355
  hoarseness, 354
  leptomeningeal metastases, 359–360
  local metastases, 358–359
  management, 357–358
  paraneoplastic syndromes, 361
  radiotherapy, neurological complications, 362–366
  spinal metastases, epidural, 360
  squamous carcinoma, 355–367
  surgery, neurological complications, 361–362
Headache:
  brain metastases, 4
  interferon, intrathecal, 274
  pediatric cancer, 509
Hemangioblastoma (see Cerebellar hemangioblastoma)
Hemorrhage, brain (see also Cerebrovascular disorders):
  brain metastases, 6
  breast cancer, 328
  choriocarcinoma, 389

[Hemorrhage, brain]
  leukemia, 452, 454–455
  lymphoma, 476
  osteosarcoma, 435
Hepatoma, 411–412
Hepatobiliary cancer, 411–412
Herniation, cerebral, cisplatin, 248
*Herpes simplex* encephalitis, 161
*Herpes zoster*:
  cerebral infarction, 136
  lymphoma, 475–476
  shingles, 83
Histiocytoses, 522–523
Hoarseness:
  esophageal carcinoma, 399
  head and neck cancer, 354
Hodgkin's disease:
  cerebellar degeneration, 466, 477
  Guillain-Barré syndrome, 466, 478
  *Herpes zoster*, 475–476
  infections, nervous system, 466, 475–476
  leptomeningeal metastases, 466, 468
  motor neuronopathy, 466, 477
HTLV$_1$-associated myelopathy (HAM), 453, 460
Hydrocephalus, with histiocytosis, 522
Hyperammonemic encephalopathy, with leukemia, 453, 458–459
Hyperviscosity syndrome:
  multiple myeloma, 494
  Waldenstrom's macroglobulinemia, 494
Hypoglycemia, with insulinoma, 406–407
Hyponatremia, with vincristine, 250
Hypotension, paroxysmal with head and neck cancer, 359
Hypothalamic-pituitary dysfunction, 523

Ifosfamide neurotoxicity, 253
  in rhabdomyosarcoma, 433
Immunoglobulinopathy (see Plasma cell dyscrasias)

Immunotherapy:
  cyclosporine, 269–273
  immunotoxins, 286–288
  interferons, 273–280
  interleukin-2, 281–283
  interleukin-2/LAK cells, 280–281
  levamisole, 267–269
  OKT3 (anti-CD3), 284–286
  other monoclonal antibodies, 286
Immunotoxins, neurotoxicity, 286–288
Impotence, with surgery for colorectal cancer, 409
Infections, of nervous system:
  brain abscess, 154–160
    *Aspergillus fumigatus*, 154–155
    bacterial, 158
    *Candida albicans*, 157–158
    clinical approach, 158–160
    *Nocardia asteroides*, 155
    *Toxoplasma gondii*, 156–157
    *Zygomycetes*, 155–156
  encephalitis, 160–164
    adenovirus, 162
    cytomegalovirus, 161
    *Herpes simplex*, 161
    *Herpes zoster*, 160–161
    measles, 162–163
    papovaviruses, 163–164
  epidemiology, 145–146
  future developments, 164–165
  leukemia, 452, 456
  meningitis, 148–154
    antibiotic therapy, 151
    bacterial, 152
    clinical approach, 153–154
    *Cryptococcus neoformans*, 148–150
    *Listeria monocytogenes*, 150
    *Strongyloides stercoralis*, 153
  pathophysiology, 146–148
Insulinoma:
  encephalopathy, 406–407
  peripheral neuropathy, 407
  seizures, 407
Interferons:
  intrathecal, 274–277
  systemic, 277–280

Interleukin-2, 281–283
Interleukin-2/lymphokine activated killer cells, 280–281
Intestinal adenocarcinoma (*see* Small bowel tumors or Colorectal carcinoma)
Intravascular lymphoma (*see* Angioendotheliomatosis)

Jaw pain, with vincristine, 92

Ketoconazole, encephalopathy, 379

Lambert-Eaton (myasthenic) syndrome (*see* Neuromuscular junction disorders)
Leptomeningeal metastases:
  bladder cancer, 391
  breast cancer, 50, 312, 314–315
  carcinoid, 405
  clinical presentation:
    cranial neuropathy, 51–52
    diagnosis, 51, 53
    encephalopathy, 51–52
    focal deficits, 51–52
    headache, 51–52
    spinal deficits, 52–53
  colorectal cancer, 410
  diagnostic tests:
    angiography, 55
    CSF chemistries, 53–54
    CSF cytology, 54
    CSF tumor markers, 54–55
    computed tomography, 55
    MRI, 55
    myelography, 55

# Index

[Leptomeningeal metastases]
  differential diagnosis, 55–59
  epidemiology, 50–51
  Ewing's sarcoma, 443
  gastric carcinoma, 49, 402
  gastrointestinal cancer, 397
  head and neck cancer, 359–360
  infarction, brain, 138
  leukemia, 49, 450–454
    clinical features, 451
    diagnosis, 451–454
    prognosis, 451
    prophylaxis in acute lymphoblastic leukemia, 451, 454
    risk of developing, 451
  lung cancer, 50, 302
  lymphoma, 466, 467–471
    clinical features, 468
    diagnosis, 468–469
    epidemiology, 467
    management, 469–471
  malignant melanoma, 343–344
  management:
    algorithm, 61
    antibodies, 62–63
    arabinosylcytosine, 60, 64
    chemotherapy, 59–61
    complications, 63–64
    methotrexate, 60–62, 64
    Ommaya reservoir, 60, 63–64
    radiotherapy, 59
    thio-TEPA, 60, 64
  multiple myeloma, 494–495
  pathogenesis, 48–50
  pathology, 46–48
  pediatric cancer, 512–513
  polyneuropathy, 83
  rhabdomyosarcoma, 425–430
  uterine carcinoma, cervical, 384–385
Letterer-Siwe disease (*see* Histiocytoses)
Leukoencephalopathy:
  cyclosporine, 270, 272–273
  interferon, intrathecal, 275, 277
  interleukin-2, 282, 283
  methotrexate, 244, 324–325, 367, 437–438

Leukemias:
  brain abscess, 452, 456
  chloroma, 452, 457
  encephalopathy, hyperammonemic, 453, 458–459
  epidemiology, 449–450
  Guillain-Barré syndrome, 453, 460
  hemorrhage, cerebral, 452, 454–455
  $HTLV_1$-associated myelopathy, 453, 460
  leptomeningeal metastases, 450–454
  mental neuropathy, 453, 459
  myasthenia gravis, 453, 461
  mycotic aneurysm, 452, 456–457
  myopathy, 453, 461
  optic neuropathy, 453, 459
  progressive multifocal leukoencephalopathy (PML), 453, 457–458
  sinus thrombosis, cerebral, 452, 455
  subdural hematoma, 452, 455–456
  Wernicke's encephalopathy, 453, 458
Levamisole, 267–269
LHermitte's sign:
  cisplatin, 247, 367
  radiotherapy, 228–229, 363
*Listeria monocytogenes* meningitis, 150
  leukemia, 452, 456
  lymphoma, 466, 475
Lumbosacral plexopathy:
  breast cancer, 322–323
  chemoembolization, complication, 378–379
  cisplatin, 248
  gastrointestinal cancer, 397
  radiotherapy for genitourinary cancer, 377 (*see also* Radiotherapy)
  testicular carcinoma, 391
  uterine carcinoma, cervical, 384
Lumbar radiculopathy with leukemia, 453, 457
Lumbosacral metastases with colorectal carcinoma, 410
Lung cancer:
  brachial plexopathy, 303–305
  brain metastases, 298–300
  encephalopathy, 305

[Lung cancer]
  epidemiology, 295–298
  leptomeningeal metastases, 302
  paraneoplastic syndromes, 302–303
  spinal metastases, epidural, 300–302
Lymphoma:
  brain metastases, 466, 471
  cerebrovascular disorders, 476
  chemotherapy complications, 476–477
  epidemiology, 465–467
  infections, nervous system, 466, 475–476
  intravascular (angioendotheliomatosis), 466, 472–473
  leptomeningeal metastases, 466, 467–471
  paraneoplastic syndromes, 466, 477–478
  primary, CNS:
    AIDS, 478, 479, 480
    clinical features, 478–479
    epidemiology, 478
    management, 479–480
    pathogenesis, 479
    pathology, 479
  peripheral neuropathy, 466, 473
  prophylaxis, CNS, 473–474
  small bowel, 408–409
Lymphocytic leukemia, acute:
  hemorrhage, cerebral, 452, 454–455
  mental neuropathy, 453, 459
  prophylaxis, CNS, 451, 454
  subdural hematoma, 452, 455–456
Lymphocytic leukemia, chronic:
  optic neuropathy, 453, 459
  progressive multifocal leukoencephalopathy (PML), 453, 457–458

Malignant glioma (*see* Brain tumors)
Malignant melanoma (*see* Melanoma)
Mastectomy pain (*see* Pain syndrome, postmastectomy)
Measles encephalitis, 162–163

Medulloblastoma (*see* Brain tumors)
Melanoma:
  brain metastases, 336–343
    anticonvulsant therapy, 340–341
    chemotherapy, 343
    radiotherapy, 341–342
    surgery, 342
  clinical presentation, 335–336
  L-DOPA therapy, 344–345
  epidemiology, 334
  metastases, noncutaneous, 345–346
  ocular, 346
  peripheral neuropathy, 344
  primary CNS, 345–346
  spinal metastases, epidural, 343
  survival, 344
Meningitis (*see* Infections, meningitis)
Meningitis, aseptic:
  lymphoma, 466, 475
  methotrexate, 242–243
  OKT3 therapy, 284–286
Meningoencephalitic syndrome with histiocytosis, 523
Meningioma with genitourinary cancer, 379
Mental neuropathy:
  breast cancer, 323–324
  leukemia, 453, 459
  multiple myeloma, 498
Meralgia paresthetica (*see* Mononeuropathy, lateral femoral cutaneous)
Metastases:
  brain (*see* Brain metastases)
  meningeal (*see* Leptomeningeal metastases)
  peripheral nerve (*see* Nerve metastases)
  spine (*see* Spinal metastases)
Methotrexate:
  leptomeningeal metastases, treatment, 60–62, 64
  leukoencephalopathy, 244, 324–325, 437–438
  lymphoma, 466, 476
  meningitis, aseptic, 242–243, 324
  MRI findings, 438

# Index

[Methotrexate]
  myelopathy, transverse, 243
  stroke-like syndromes, 243, 437–438
Methylprednisolone (*see also* Glucocorticoids)
  animal data in epidural spinal cord compression, 207
  epidural spinal cord compression, actions in, 207
  toxicity, 210–213
Monoclonal antibody therapy, neurotoxicity, 284–286
Monoclonal gammopathy of unknown significance (MGUS): polyneuropathy, 492–494, 497
Mononeuropathy:
  cisplatin, 248
  cranial nerves, other, 84, 87
  facial (Bell's palsy), 84, 86–87
  femoral, 88
  *Herpes zoster*, 83
  lateral femoral cutaneous (meralgia paresthetica), 85, 88–89
  median (carpal tunnel syndrome), 85, 87–88
  metastatic (*see* Nerve metastases)
  multiplex, 92–93, 186–187
  peroneal, 85, 88
  radiotherapy-related, 92
  sciatic, 89
  trigeminal, 84, 87
  ulnar, 85, 88
  vincristine, 84, 92
Mood disturbances with levamisole, 268
Motor neuron disease:
  multiple myeloma, 495, 498
  paraneoplastic, 183, 184
  paraproteinemia, 81
Mucin emboli with breast cancer, 329
Mucormycosis, 155–156
Multiple myeloma (*see* Plasma cell dyscrasias)
Mycotic aneurysm with leukemia, 452, 456–457
Myelogenous leukemia (*see* Leukemias)
Myelopathy:
  arabinosylcytosine, 251–252

[Myelopathy]
  cyclosporine, 273
  $HTLV_1$-associated, 453, 460
  methotrexate, 243
  paraneoplastic, 179–182
  pediatric cancer, 510–512
  radiation, 228–229, 363
  thio-TEPA, 255
Myalgia:
  levamisole, 268
  vincristine, 251
Myasthenia gravis (*see* Neuromuscular junction disorders)
Myopathy (including polymyositis and dermatomyositis):
  acute necrotizing, 192
  carcinoid, 406
  Didemnin B, 96
  disuse atrophy, 97
  glucocorticoid, 96, 209–211
  iatrogenic, 96
  immunotoxins, 287
  inflammatory, 97, 191–192
  leukemia, 453, 461
  multiple myeloma, 498
  neuromyopathy, 192
  ovarian carcinoma, 387
  paraneoplastic, 94, 97, 191–192
  vincristine, 251

Nasal carcinoma, 355
Nasopharyngeal carcinoma, 355
Nerve metastases:
  brachial plexus, 84, 90
  clinical features, 89–90
  cranial nerves, 84, 91–92
  lumbosacral plexus, 84, 90–91
  other (distal branches), 91
Neuroblastoma, 519–520
  opsoclonus-myoclonus, 177, 513–514
Neurogenic bladder, after colorectal surgery, 409
Neurolymphomatosis, 466, 473

Neuromuscular junction disorders:
  clinical features, 93–94
  iatrogenic (drug), 96
  Lambert-Eaton (myasthenic)
    syndrome, 94–95, 189–191
    multiple myeloma, 498
    small cell lung cancer, 302–303
  myasthenia gravis, 94, 95–96
    leukemia, 453, 461
    lymphoma, 478
    thymoma, 95–96
Neuromyotonia, paraneoplastic, 79–80, 189
Neuropathies (*see* Polyneuropathy or Mononeuropathy)
Niacin deficiency with carcinoid, 406
Nitrosoureas, neurotoxicity, 253–254
  myelopathy, 512
*Nocardia asteroides* brain abscess, 155
Nonbacterial thrombotic endocarditis (NBTE), 131–132
  breast cancer, 329
  lymphoma, 476
Numb chin (*see* Mental neuropathy)

Ocular melanoma, 346
Ocular toxicity:
  arabinosylcytosine, 252
  cisplatin, 247
Ocular metastases with breast cancer, 312, 317
Olfield syndrome, 411
Oligodendroglioma (*see* Brain tumors)
Ommaya reservoir, complications, 477
  lymphoma, 466
Ophthalmoplegia with multiple myeloma, 498–499
Opsoclonus-myoclonus (*see also* Neuroblastoma and Paraneoplastic syndromes), 176–179
  breast cancer, 336
  pediatric neural crest tumors, 513–514
Optic neuropathy:
  BCNU-related, 254

[Optic neuropathy]
  leukemia, 453, 459
Oral (oropharyngeal) cancer cancers, 355
Orbital rhabdomyosarcoma, 431
Osteosarcoma:
  brain metastases, 434–435
  epidemiology, 433–434
  intracerebral, primary, 435
  methotrexate toxicity, 437–438
Ototoxicity with cisplatin, 247, 367, 378
Ovarian cancer:
  brain metastases, 385–386
  cerebellar degeneration, 386–387
  leptomeningeal metastases, 386
  paraneoplastic syndromes, 382–387

Pain:
  gastrinoma, 408
  gastrointestinal cancer, 375
  mastectomy, 327–328
  pancreatic cancer, 402–403
  pediatric cancer, 507–509
Pancoast's syndrome, 303–305
Pancreatic cancer:
  neurological complications, 402–403
  pain, 402–403
Paranasal sinus cancer, 355
Paraneoplastic syndromes:
  autonomic neuropathy, 188–189
  cerebellar syndromes, 169–174
    anti-Yo, 170–172
    diagnostic approach, 173–174
    Hodgkin's disease, 172
    Lambert-Eaton myasthenic syndrome, 172–173
  classification, 168–169
  encephalomyelitis, 174–176
    anti-HU, 174–175
    autonomic dysfunction, 176
    brainstem encephalopathy, 176
    cerebellar degeneration, 175
    diagnostic tests, 176
    limbic encephalitis, 175
    motor neuron dysfunction, 175

# Index

[Paraneoplastic syndromes]
   neuropathology, 176
   sensory neuropathy, 175
  epidemiology, 167–169
  gastrointestinal cancer, 398
  lung cancer, 302–303
  management, 192–194
   antineoplastic therapy, 193
   immunosuppression, 193–194
  motor neuron disease, 183–184
  multiple myeloma, 498
  muscle disorders:
   acute necrotizing, 192
   dermatomyositis, 191–192
   neuromyopathy, 192
   polymyositis, 191–192
  myelopathy, 179–182
  natural history, 192–193
  neuromuscular junction, 189–191
  neuromyotonia, 189
  neuropathy:
   chronic, sensorimotor, 187–188
   Guillain-Barré, 186
   sensorimotor, subacute, 186–188
   vasculitic, 186–187
  opsoclonus-myoclonus, 176–179
   with anti-Ri, 177–178
   with neuroblastoma, 177, 513–514
   without anti-Ri, 178–179
  pediatric cancer, 513–514
  peripheral nervous system syndromes, 77, 183–189
  polyneuropathy, 77
  prostate carcinoma, 383
  retinopathy, 179
Paraproteinemias (*see* Plasma cell dyscrasias)
Paresthesias with suramin, 255
Parkinsonism:
  arabinosylcytosine, 252
  bone marrow transplantation, 504
Perineural spread:
  basal cell carcinoma, 346–457
  head and neck cancer, 359
Perioral numbness with taxol, 255
Pernicious anemia with gastric carcinoma, 400–401

Pituitary metastases:
  breast cancer, 312, 317–318
  carcinoid, 405
Pituitary tumors:
  MEA-I, 408
  gastrinoma, 408
Plasmacytoma (*see also* Plasma cell dyscrasias):
  brain, 500
  spinal, epidural, 499
Plasma cell dyscrasias:
  brain plasmacytoma, 500
  cranial neuropathy, 498
  epidemiology, 490
  hyperviscosity syndrome, 494
  leptomeningeal metastases, 494–495
  motor neuron disease, 81, 495–498
  paraneoplastic syndromes, 498
  peripheral neuropathy, 80–82, 490–494
  spinal metastases, epidural, 499
Polymyositis (*see* Myopathy, inflammatory)
Pneumococcal meningitis with lymphoma, 466, 475
POEMS syndrome, 491–492
Polyneuropathy:
  acute inflammatory (Landry-Guillain-Barré syndrome), 82, 186
  amyloid with plasma cell dyscrasias, 490–491, 496
  arabinosylcytosine, 252
  chemotherapy-related, 75–77
  cisplatin, 75, 246–247, 378
  clinical features, 74
  diagnostic tests, 74–75
  etoposide (VP-16), 254
  hepatoma, 411
  immunotoxins, 287–288
  insulinoma, 407
  interferon, 279–280
  interleukin-2, 283
  leptomeningeal metastases, 83
  lymphoma, 466, 473
  malignant melanoma, 344
  metastatic infiltration, 82–83
  monoclonal gammopathy of unknown significance (MGUS), 492–497

[Polyneuropathy]
  multiple myeloma, 491–492, 496, 498
  osteosclerotic multiple myeloma, 491–492, 496
  paraneoplastic, 77–80, 183–189
    chronic progressive sensorimotor, 79, 187–188
    neuromyopathy, 79–80, 189
    subacute sensory, 77–79, 184–185
  paraproteinemia-related, 80–82, 490–494, 497
  procarbazine, 253
  taxol, 254–255, 378
  vasculitic, 186–187
  vincristine, 75, 76, 249–250, 433
  Waldenstrom's macroglobulinemia, 492, 497
Prednisolone (*see* Glucocorticoids)
Prednisone (*see* Glucocorticoids)
Primary CNS lymphoma (*see* Lymphoma, primary CNS)
Procarbazine neurotoxicity, 253
Progressive multifocal leukoencephalopathy (PML), 163–164, 453, 457–458
Prostate cancer:
  brain metastases, 383
  paraneoplastic syndromes, 383
  pathogenesis of neurological complications, 380
  skull metastases, 382
  spinal metastases, epidural, 380–382
  subdural hematoma, 382–383
Purkinje cell degeneration (*see* Paraneoplastic syndromes, cerebellar; Cerebellar degeneration)

Radionecrosis, brain (*see* Radiotherapy, neurological complications)
Radiotherapy, neurological complications:
  breast cancer, 326, 327
  cranial nerves, 229–230, 363
  external beam, 222–225

[Radiotherapy, neurological complications]
  acute effects, 222
  cerebrovascular disorders, 225
  cranial nerves, 229–230
  hyperfractionation, 225
  intellectual sequelae, 222–225
  neuroendocrine dysfunction, 230–231
  peripheral nerve, 229–230, 363–364
  radionecrosis, 225, 363
  subacute/chronic effects, 222
  heavy particle beam, 227
  intracavitary, 227–228
  interstitial, 226
  lymphoma, 466, 477
  mechanisms of neurotoxicity, 228
  second malignancies, after, 231–232
  spinal cord, 228–229, 363
  stereotactic radiosurgery, 226–227
    cranial nerves, 230
    neuroendocrine dysfunction, 231
Radiotherapy, treatment methods:
  external beam, 220
  interstitial, 220–221
  stereotactic, 221
Renal carcinoma, 387–388
  brain metastases, 387–388
  with cerebellar hemangioblastoma, 379
  spinal metastases, epidural, 388
Renal embryonal tumors with embryonal CNS tumors, 380
Retinoblastoma:
  epidemiology, 520
  extraocular, 520
  intraocular, 520
  management, 521
  second malignancies, 521
Retinopathy, 179
  with tamoxifen, 325
Rhabdomyosarcoma:
  brain metastases, 432–433
  chemotherapy complications, 433
  clinical features, 424–425
  cranial neuropathy, 431
  epidemiology, 424
  leptomeningeal metastases, 425–430
  orbital involvement, 431
  spinal metastases, epidural, 431–432

# Index

Sarcomas:
  brain metastases, 418–422
  epidemiology, 417–418
  spinal metastases, epidural, 422–424
Seizures:
  brain metastases, 5
  chemotherapy, 505, 506
  cyclophosphamide, 269–272
  immunotoxins, 288
  malignant melanoma, 340–341
  osteosarcoma, brain metastases, 435
  pediatric cancer, 504–506
  vincristine, 251
SIADH (*see* Syndrome of inappropriate antidiuretic hormone secretion)
Sinus thrombosis, cerebral, 134–135
  asparaginase, 252–253
  breast cancer, 329
  leukemia, 452, 455
  neuroblastoma, 506, 520
Skull metastases:
  breast cancer, 311–313
  carcinoid, 404–405
  Ewing's sarcoma, 441–443
  neuroblastoma, 520
  prostate cancer, 382
Small bowel tumors:
  adenocarcinoma, 408
  lymphoma, 408–409
Spinal epidural fistula with esophageal cancer, 399
Spinal metastases, epidural:
  breast cancer, 318–319
  carcinoid, 404
  clinical presentation:
    pain, 27–28
    sensory loss, 28–29
    sphincter dysfunction, 29
    unusual presentations, 29
    weakness, 28
  diagnostic tests:
    approach, 32–34
    computed tomography, 31–32
    imaging studies, 30–32
    lumbar puncture, 30
    MRI, 32
    myelography, 31–32

[Spinal metastases, epidural]
  epidemiology, 23–24
  Ewing's sarcoma, 440–441
  head and neck cancer, 360
  hepatoma, 411
  Hodgkin's disease, 466, 471
  leukemia, 457
  location, 25–26
  lung cancer, 300–302
  lymphoma, 466, 471
  malignant melanoma, 343
  management:
    chemotherapy, 34–35
    glucocorticoids, 35, 206–209
    radiotherapy, 35
    surgery, 35–36
  multiple myeloma, 499
  neuroblastoma, 519
  osteosarcoma, 435–437
  pathogenesis, 24–25
  pathology, 26
  pathophysiology, 26–27
  pediatric cancer, 510–512
  plasmacytoma, solitary, 499
  primary tumors, 27
  prostate carcinoma, 380–382
  renal carcinoma, 388
  rhabdomyosarcoma, 431
  sarcomas, 422–424
  testicular cancer, 390
Spinal metastases, intramedullary, 36–41
  breast cancer, 319
  clinical presentation, 37–38
  diagnostic tests, 38
  differential diagnosis, 38–40
  epidemiology, 36
  location, 36
  management, 40–41
  pathogenesis, 36–37
Stomach cancer (*see* Gastric carcinoma)
Stroke (*see* Cerebrovascular disorders)
*Strongyloides stercoralis* meningitis, 153
Subacute combined degeneration with gastric carcinoma, 400–401
Subacute sensory neuronopathy, 77–79, 184–185 (*see also* Paraneoplastic syndromes)

Subdural hematoma:
  breast cancer, 328
  leukemia, 452, 455–456
  leptomeningeal metastases, 126
  prostate cancer, 382–383
Superior sagittal sinus thrombosis (*see* Sinus thrombosis)
Suramin neurotoxicity, 255
Syncope with head and neck cancer, 359

Taxol neurotoxicity, 254–255, 378
T-cell leukemia and $HTLV_1$-associated myelopathy, 453, 460
Testicular cancer:
  brain metastases, 390
  lumbosacral plexopathy, 391
  spinal metastases, epidural, 390
Thalamic gliomas in children, 517
Thio-TEPA:
  leptomeningeal metastases, 60, 64
  neurotoxicity, 255
Thrombocytopenia, brain hemorrhage, 128–130
Thrombophlebitis (*see* Brain tumors, management)
Tic doloreux (*see* Mononeuropathy, trigeminal)
*Toxoplasma gondii*, brain abscess, 156–157
Transient focal deficits (TIA-like):
  interleukin-2, 282, 283
  methotrexate, 243, 437–438
Transverse myelopathy (*see* Myelopathy)
Tremor with cyclosporine, 269–270
Tryptophan deficiency with carcinoid, 406
Tumor embolism, 137–138
  breast cancer, 329
Turcot syndrome, 411

Uterine cervical carcinoma:
  brain metastases, 384
  encephalopathy, 385
  leptomeningeal metastases, 384–385
  lumbosacral plexopathy, 384
Uterine endometrial cancer, 385

Varicella-zoster encephalitis, 160–161 (see *Herpes zoster*)
Venous thrombosis, cerebral, 134–135
  asparaginase, 252–253
  breast cancer, 329
Vincristine:
  autonomic dysfunction, 250
  coma, 251
  cortical blindness, 251
  cranial neuropathies, 250
  hyponatremia, 250
  intrathecal, 250–251
  myopathy, 251
  peripheral neuropathy, 75, 76, 249–250
  rhabdomyosarcoma, 433
  seizures, 251
VP-16 (*see* Etoposide)

Waldenstrom's macroglobulinemia:
  hyperviscosity syndrome, 494
  peripheral neuropathy, 492
Wernicke's encephalopathy, 397–398, 453, 458
Wilm's tumor, 521

*Zygomycoses*, 155–156

# About the Editor

RONALD G. WILEY is Professor of Neurology and Pharmacology at Vanderbilt University Medical School, Nashville, and a Neurologist and Chief, Laboratory of Experimental Neurology, at the V. A. Medical Center, Nashville, Tennessee. The author or coauthor of over 80 professional papers, book chapters, and books, and a referee for numerous scientific journals, Dr. Wiley is a fellow of the American Academy of Neurology and a member of the Society for Neuroscience, the Society for Neuroimmunology, and the American Neurological Association, among others. He received the B.S. degree (1972) in the honors program in medical education and the Ph.D. degree (1975) in pharmacology from Northwestern University, Evanston, Illinois, and the M.D. degree with distinction (1975) from Northwestern University Medical School, Evanston, Illinois. Board certified in internal medicine and neurology, Dr. Wiley trained in internal medicine (1975–1977) at the Peter Bent Brigham Hospital, Boston, Massachusetts, and in neurology (1977–1980) at New York Hospital, New York, New York.